Pediatric Surgical Oncology

Pediatric Surgical Oncology

Richard J. Andrassy, M.D.

A.G. McNeese Professor and Chairman
Department of Surgery
University of Texas Medical School at Houston
Chief, Pediatric Surgical Oncology
M.D. Anderson Cancer Center
Houston, Texas

W.B. SAUNDERS COMPANY
A Division of Harcourt Brace & Company
Philadelphia   London   Toronto   Montreal   Sydney   Tokyo

W.B. SAUNDERS COMPANY
A Division of Harcourt Brace & Company

The Curtis Center
Independence Square West
Philadelphia, Pennsylvania 19106

Library of Congress Cataloging-in-Publication Data

Pediatric surgical oncology / [edited by] Richard J. Andrassy.

p.   cm.

ISBN 0–7216–6378–8

1. Cancer—Surgery.   2. Tumors in children—Surgery.   3. Tumors in
  children—Treatment.   I. Andrassy, Richard.   [DNLM: 1. Neoplasms—in
  infancy & childhood.   2. Neoplasms—therapy.   QZ 275P3715 1998]

RD651.P43   1998   616.99′4059′083—dc21

DNLM/DLC   96-53983

PEDIATRIC SURGICAL ONCOLOGY   ISBN 0–7216–6378–8

Printed in the United States of America.

Last digit is the print number: 9   8   7   6   5   4   3   2   1

Contributors

Richard J. Andrassy, M.D., F.A.C.S., F.A.A.P.

A.G. McNeese Professor and Chairman, Department of Surgery, University of Texas Medical School at Houston; Chief, Pediatric Surgery, University of Texas M.D. Anderson Cancer Center, Houston, Texas

General Principles • Melanomas and Other Rare Tumors • Abdominal Complications

Richard G. Azizkhan, M.D.

Professor of Surgery and Pediatrics and Chief of Division of Pediatric Surgery, State University of New York at Buffalo School of Medicine and Biomedical Sciences; Surgeon-in-Chief, Children's Hospital of Buffalo, Buffalo, New York

Neonatal Tumors

Deborah Belchis, M.D.

Assistant Professor of Pathology and Pediatrics, Pennsylvania State University College of Medicine; Children's Hospital, Penn State–Milton S. Hershey Medical Center, Hershey, Pennsylvania

Nonrhabdomyosarcoma Soft-Tissue Sarcomas in Children

C. Thomas Black, M.D.

Associate Professor of Surgery and Pediatrics, University of Texas Medical School at Houston and University of Texas M.D. Anderson Cancer Center, Houston, Texas

Neuroblastoma • Primary Bronchopulmonary Tumors

John C. Bleacher, M.D.

Attending Pediatric Surgeon, Scottish Rite Children's Medical Center, Atlanta, Georgia

Hepatoblastoma

Henry W. Cheu, M.D.

Deceased

Endocrine Tumors

Walter Jakob Chwals, M.D.

Associate Professor, Department of Pediatric Surgery, University of Chicago School of Medicine, Chicago, Illinois

Nutritional Support

Barry R. Cofer, M.D.

Pediatric Surgeon, Surgical Director, Extracorporeal Life Support Program, Wilford Hall U.S.A.F. Medical Center; Critical Care Air Transport Team Physician, Lackland AFB, Texas; Assistant Professor of Surgery, Edward F. Hebert School of Medicine, Bethesda, Maryland

Rhabdomyosarcoma

Cynthia A. Corpron, M.D.

Fellow in Surgical Oncology (Pediatrics), University of Texas Medical School at Houston and University of Texas M.D. Anderson Cancer Center, Houston, Texas

Melanomas and Other Rare Tumors • Abdominal Complications

Peter W. Dillon, M.D.

Associate Professor of Surgery and Pediatrics, The Pennsylvania State University College of Medicine; Chief, Division of Pediatric Surgery, Children's Hospital, Penn State–Milton S. Hershey Medical Center, Hershey, Pennsylvania

Nonrhabdomyosarcoma Soft-Tissue Sarcomas in Children • Neonatal Tumors

John J. Doski, M.D.

Clinical Assistant of Surgery, Department of Surgery, Uniformed Services University of the Health Sciences, F. Edward Hebert School of Medicine, Bethesda, Maryland; Staff Surgeon, Pediatric and Adult Trauma and Pediatric and General Surgery, Wilford Hall Medical Center, Lackland AFB; Brooke Army Medical Center, Ft. Sam Houston, Texas

Endocrine Tumors

Patricia J. Eifel, M.D.

Professor of Radiation Oncology, University of Texas Medical School at Houston; Director, Radiation Oncology Residency Training Program, University of Texas M.D. Anderson Cancer Center, Houston, Texas

Principles of Radiotherapy

Edward G. Ford, M.D.

Surgical Specialists, Fort Collins, Colorado

Gastrointestinal Tumors

v

Daniel M. Hays, M.D.
Professor of Surgery and Pediatrics, University of
Southern California School of Medicine, Los
Angeles, California
Pediatric Surgical Oncology: The Background

George W. Holcomb, III, M.D.
Associate Professor, Department of Pediatric Surgery,
Vanderbilt University School of Medicine, Nashville,
Tennessee
Minimally Invasive Surgery

Jeffrey R. Horwitz, M.D.
Instructor in Surgery, University of Texas Medical
School at Houston, Houston, Texas
Vascular Access

John F. Kuttesch, Jr., Ph.D., M.D.
Assistant Professor of Pediatrics, University of Texas
Medical School at Houston; Assistant Professor of
Pediatrics and Assistant Pediatrician, University of
Texas M.D. Anderson Cancer Center, Houston, Texas
Principles of Chemotherapy for Solid Tumors

Kevin P. Lally, M.D., F.A.A.P., F.A.C.S.
Professor and Chief of Pediatric Surgery, University
of Texas Medical School at Houston; Chief of
Surgery, Hermann Hospital, Houston, Texas
Vascular Access

Scott Lankford, M.D.
Chief Resident, Radiation Oncology, University of
Texas M.D. Anderson Cancer Center, Houston, Texas
Principles of Radiotherapy

Michael P. LaQuaglia, M.D.
Associate Professor of Surgery, Cornell University
Medical College; Associate Attending Surgeon, Chief,
Pediatric Surgical Service, Memorial Sloan-Kettering
Cancer Center, New York, New York
Metastases from Solid Tumors

Judy B. Massengill, M.D.
Assistant Professor, Department of Anesthesiology
Critical Care, University of Texas Medical School at
Houston; Assistant Anesthesiologist, University of
Texas M.D. Anderson Cancer Center, Houston, Texas
Anesthesia, Sedation, and Pain Management

Kimberly Kenfield Nesbitt, M.D.
Assistant Professor, Department of Anesthesiology,
University of Texas Medical School at Houston;
Assistant Anesthesiologist, University of Texas M.D.
Anderson Cancer Center, Houston, Texas
Anesthesia, Sedation, and Pain Management

Kurt D. Newman, M.D.
Professor of Surgery and Pediatrics, George
Washington University School of Medicine and
Health Sciences; Vice Chairman, Pediatric Surgery,
Children's National Medical Center, Washington,
D.C.
Hepatoblastoma • Thyroid Malignancy

Vivian H. Porche, M.D.
Assistant Professor, Department of Anesthesiology
Critical Care, University of Texas Medical School at
Houston; Assistant Anesthesiologist, University of
Texas M.D. Anderson Cancer Center, Houston, Texas
Anesthesia, Sedation, and Pain Management

David M. Powell, M.D.
Assistant Professor of Surgery and Pediatrics, George
Washington University School of Medicine; Attending
Surgeon, Children's National Medical Center,
Washington, D.C.
Thyroid Malignancy

R. Beverly Raney, M.D.
Professor of Pediatrics, University of Texas Medical
School at Houston; Professor, Department of
Pediatrics, University of Texas M.D. Anderson
Cancer Center, Houston, Texas
Principles of Chemotherapy for Solid Tumors

Frederick J. Rescorla, M.D.
Associate Professor of Surgery, Section of Pediatric
Surgery and Department of General Surgery, Indiana
University School of Medicine; Staff Surgeon, James
Whitcomb Riley Hospital for Children, Indianapolis,
Indiana
Pediatric Germ-Cell Tumors

Michael L. Ritchey, M.D.
Associate Professor, Department of Surgery and
Pediatrics, University of Texas at Houston Medical
School; Chief of Pediatric Urology, Hermann
Hospital, Houston, Texas
Wilms' Tumor

Frank M. Robertson, M.D.
Assistant Professor of Surgery, Department of
Surgery, Uniformed Services University of the Health
Sciences, F. Edward Hebert School of Medicine,
Bethesda, Maryland; Chief, Pediatric Surgery,
Wilford Hall Medical Center, Lackland AFB, Texas
Endocrine Tumors

Nicholas C. Saenz, M.D.

Assistant Professor of Surgery, Cornell University Medical College; Assistant Attending Surgeon, Memorial Sloan-Kettering Cancer Center, New York, New York

Metastases from Solid Tumors

Robert S. Sawin, M.D.

Associate Professor of Surgery, University of Washington School of Medicine; Chief, Division of General and Thoracic Surgery, Children's Hospital and Medical Center, Seattle, Washington

Molecular Biology and Tumor Markers

Thomas Whalen, M.D.

Associate Professor of Surgery and Pediatrics, University of Medicine and Dentistry of New Jersey—Robert Wood Johnson Medical School; Head of the Division of Pediatric Surgery, Children's

Regional Hospital at Cooper Medical Center, Camden, New Jersey

Hodgkin's and Non-Hodgkin's Lymphoma

Eugene S. Wiener, M.D.

Professor of Surgery (Pediatric), Training Director, Pediatric Surgical Residency, University of Pittsburgh School of Medicine; Surgeon in Chief, Chief of General Pediatric Surgery, and Benjamin R. Fisher Professor of Pediatric Surgery, Children's Hospital of Pittsburgh, Pittsburgh, Pennsylvania

Rhabdomyosarcoma

Alan W. Yasko, M.D.

Associate Professor of Surgery, University of Texas Medical School at Houston; Chief, Section of Orthopedic Surgery, Department of Surgical Oncology, University of Texas M.D. Anderson Cancer Center, Houston, Texas

Osteosarcoma and Other Bone Tumors

To Lt. Colonel Henry W. Cheu (1959–1996)

and Sally Cheu (1990–1996)

They will be dearly missed

by all of us who had the privilege

and pleasure to know them.

Preface

It has been twelve years since Dr. Daniel Hays edited a text entitled *Pediatric Surgical Oncology*.* Many advances in treatment and improvement in survival have been made since that time. Because pediatric surgical oncology and treatment protocols continue to evolve at a rapid rate, this new text is not intended to be an all-inclusive summary of present treatment modalities. It does provide a single source for current practice trends, written by acknowledged experts who are active clinically.

The introductory chapter of this text, by Dr. Daniel Hays, provides an excellent overview of the historical development of the specialties related to the care of children with cancer. Dr. Hays has been actively involved in the worldwide development of pediatric surgical oncology, and no one is better qualified to provide a first-hand review of many of the key players. He has also stimulated many of the contributors in this book, including this author and editor, toward a career interest in surgical oncology. It is therefore very appropriate that he has provided the lead chapter, and I can hardly add to his narrative.

The majority of the contributors to *Pediatric Surgical Oncology* are active members of the surgical committee of the Children's Cancer Group. In many cases, they are the surgical representatives on the committee for the study of the specific tumor that they have written about in this book. Most of these tumors are rare and, therefore, are seen only sporadically in the practice of most family practitioners, pediatricians, and surgeons. Over the past few years, many surgical and pediatric residents have asked for a single reference source to review the general principles for pediatric solid tumor evaluation, diagnosis, and modern treatment techniques. Because of the rarity of these tumors, it remains extremely important that support for cooperative groups, such as the Children's Cancer Group, Pediatric Oncology Group, and Intergroup Rhabdomyosarcoma Study, just to mention a few, continues in order to improve patient survival and decrease treatment-related complications.

It is hoped that this text will provide a ready reference source for family practitioners, pediatricians, general surgeons, pediatric surgeons (particularly those in training), and physicians involved in the multidisciplinary care of children with cancer.

Richard J. Andrassy, M.D.

---

*Hays DM: *Pediatric Surgical Oncology*. Orlando: Grune and Stratton, 1986.

Acknowledgments

I wish to thank the authors of the individual chapters for sharing their time and expertise and Richard Lampert and Jeff Gunning of the W.B. Saunders Company for their invaluable help in keeping this project on course. Special thanks also to Flora Roeder, Editor in the Department of Surgery, without whose help I would never have completed this project.

Contents

Chapter

1

Pediatric Surgical Oncology:
The Background

• *Daniel M. Hays*

BEFORE CHEMOTHERAPY AND RADIOTHERAPY: THE SURGEONS AND PATHOLOGISTS ALONE

As we well know, the earliest specialists in the field of pediatric surgical oncology were the surgeons of nineteenth-century European university clinics who operated regularly upon children with cancer, predominant among them, Billroth[1] (1860), Jessup[2] (1877), Kocher[3] (1878), Israel[4] (1894), and Wilms[5] (1899) (Fig. 1–1). Jessup (Leeds) may have performed the first successful nephrectomy for nephroblastoma and Kocher the first transperitoneal nephrectomy. Illustrative of the reluctance of surgeons to make large abdominal incisions in this era, Walker[6] (1905), in the United States, suggested transperitoneal ligation of renal vessels followed by a second flank incision for nephrectomy.[6] Relative to the results of surgery in Europe and North America in the pre-radiotherapy era, a collected series of 145 children operated upon for Wilms' tumor had only four known 3-year survivors.[7] The most common operative procedure performed in this series was biopsy.

The reports of these surgeons followed studies of pediatric tumors by contemporary pathologists and physicians, including classic clinical descriptions of childhood cancer such as botryoid rhabdomyosarcoma by Wilks and Moxon (1875)[8] and nephroblastoma by Osler (1879).[9] Pioneering general surgeons (the only type of surgeons known at that time) and tumor pathologists were active in this field on both sides of the Atlantic

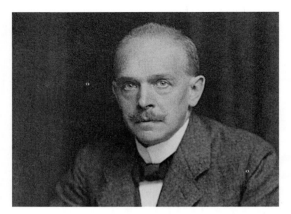

Figure 1–1 • Max Wilms (1867–1918), trained in pathology and surgery, was the chief of the Department of Surgery in the Universities of Basel and then Heidelberg. He described seven children who had what undoubtedly were nephroblastomas, as a part of a monograph on "mixed tumors" published in 1899. At no time did he imply that this was an original clinical observation. The emphasis was on the embryonic mesodermal origin of this tumor. He died at the age of 51, apparently from an infection contracted during an operation on a French prisoner of war during World War I. (Courtesy of the Library of the College of Physicians of Philadelphia.)

(and possibly on the very steps of Japan)[10, 11] for decades before there were specialists in pediatrics, let alone pediatric surgeons or oncologists! In general, physicians in disciplines that we now label internal medicine or pediatrics had little interest in childhood (or adult) cancer. Imaginative practitioners, some well-meaning, some scoundrels, did dispense forms of cancer therapy that in the twentieth century would be labeled highly "unconventional."

THE ROENTGENOLOGISTS

Early surgeons and pathologists with an interest in childhood cancer were joined by a second group of therapists following the discoveries by Roentgen (1895)[12] and the introduction of brachytherapy after the identification of radium by the Curies (1898).[13] Radiotherapy was administered by clinicians with very diverse backgrounds, and even by surgeons, until the 1940s. During the decades between 1930 and 1950, several radiologists in teaching centers became specifically concerned with the treatment of children's tumors. Some of them, as well as some

surgeons, became enthusiasts for this new modality. They advocated, for example, radiotherapy as the sole therapy for Wilms' tumor (Friedlander,[14] 1916) or routine preoperative irradiation for *all* children with Wilms' tumor (Geraghty,[15] 1916). Others were already conscious of the vulnerability of children to the adverse effects of radiotherapy.[16] It is difficult for surgeons today to imagine working in an environment in which there were no cancer chemotherapists or pediatricians with any interest in solid tumors (Wollstein,[17] 1927; Mixter,[18] 1932), relatively few individuals trained in even general radiotherapy, no units designed for the care of children with cancer, and neither a National Cancer Institute nor an American Cancer Society to provide financial or even moral support.

LEADERS EMERGE WORLDWIDE

Most of the founders of the developing specialty of pediatric surgery, including Ladd in Boston, Higgins in London, Harrenstein in Amsterdam, and White in Glasgow, among many, had major concerns about the care of children with cancer. W. E. Ladd (Fig. 1–2) viewed this as an area in which general or urologic surgeons, who operated upon children infrequently, might make major errors in management. He is reported to have entered a local general hospital and personally carried a child out of that institution and into, of course, the Boston Children's Hospital. He strongly advocated the abdominal as opposed to the flank approach for nephroblastomas, although the flank approach was more commonly used at that time.[19, 20] He opposed routine preoperative (but not postoperative) irradiation. At one time, Ladd's recommendation for children with nephroblastomas included postoperative radiotherapy to both the local site and pulmonary areas.[21] Surgery for nephroblastoma without delay and with minimal abdominal palpation was the dictum on his service and likewise on that of his successor in Boston, Robert E. Gross.[22, 23] This urgency was carried to the extreme of performing elective surgery at midnight!

Ladd was among the few early surgeons who made a serious attempt by modern standards to excise large abdominal tumors, including for example, transection and excision of the vena cava inferior to the renal veins. In his advocacy of aggressive surgery, Ladd stressed the experience

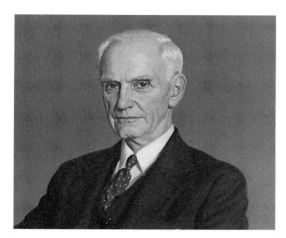

Figure 1–2 • William E. Ladd (1885–1979), chief of the Surgical Service at the Boston Children's Hospital (1934–1944), introduced major new concepts regarding the management of nephroblastoma and neuroblastoma. He vigorously endorsed the transabdominal approach to Wilms' tumor and discouraged routine preoperative radiotherapy. He was a superb surgical technician and was among the first to seriously attempt complete excision of the massive abdominal tumors of childhood. The short-term operative results he obtained were excellent, but his patients usually succumbed to the results of later dissemination.

with solid tumors at the Boston Children's Hospital (Ladd,[21, 20, 23] 1938, 1941). By 1941 this hospital could point to 14 long-term survivors treated for Wilms' tumor (there were only 16 reported such "survivors" in the entire English literature prior to that time) and seven survivors with neuroblastoma. In addition, six patients treated for ovarian tumors (possibly malignant), two treated for teratoma, and two treated for fibrosarcoma were still living. Ladd also recognized the menace of cancer associated with congenital colonic polyposis and performed prophylactic colectomies.

In the early 1940s, when the concept of "pediatric surgical oncology" first interested me, the concerns of medical specialists had changed little since Billroth's day. The Tumor Clinic at Boston Children's Hospital was attended by surgeons, a radiologist, and pathologists. Leukemia was the province of the hematologist, but children with solid tumors, including Hodgkin's disease and brain tumors,[24] were referred to surgeons for management. Preoperative and postoperative care were entirely in the hands of surgeons, with surveillance for recurrence carried out by surgeons, pathologists, and radiotherapists, in this center and other institutions. Most patients at some point in their course received orthovoltage (250 V) radiotherapy, and adverse effects of this on the growth of bone and soft tissue structures had been recognized.[16]

The overall survival rate among children with solid tumors in the era in which surgery and radiotherapy were the only modes of therapy, was probably less than 10% *generally* in Europe and the United States,[7, 17, 19] and close to 20% in the most advanced centers. The clinic for the surveillance of children with solid tumors at Boston Children's Hospital, one of the few such clinics existent in the United States during the years 1944 to 1946, maintained contact with (1) more than a dozen patients who had undergone surgery for Wilms' tumor and (2) a similar group of patients with neuroblastoma, probably half of whom suffered from what we would identify as Stage 4s (formerly Stage IV-s) disease. This entity was readily recognized by the staff of that clinic, although it was still to be labeled. Other long-term survivors in this clinic included one or two each with diagnoses of fibrosarcoma, osteosarcoma (then called osteogenic sarcoma), malignant lymphoma (then called lymphocytic sarcoma and reticulum-cell sarcoma), and Hodgkin's disease. There seemed to be few, if indeed any, survivors of Ewing's tumor, rhabdomyosarcoma, synovial or other sarcomas.

Surgeons and surgeons-in-training examined all patients coming to this Tumor Clinic in Boston, but the most active participant was a young pathologist, Sydney Farber, who a decade later began clinical trials with chemotherapeutic agents at the same institution.[25] During his years on the surgical service of the Boston Children's Hospital, after Ladd's retirement in 1945, Orvar Swenson was perhaps the most consistent participant in the clinic among the attending surgeons. Swenson has proposed Farber as the initial advocate of the "team approach" to cancer therapy,[26] which subsequently spread to pediatric institutions and then to all institutions, nationally. Pediatric hospitals are clearly where this concept began!

In discussing his early years at the Children's Hospital of Philadelphia (CHP), C. Everett Koop (Fig. 1–3) recalls that his intense interest in childhood tumors was shared by hardly anyone—surgeon or physician—in Philadelphia.[27] In trav-

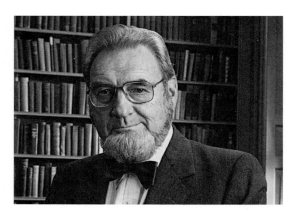

Figure 1–3 • C. Everett Koop (1916–), professor of pediatric surgery, University of Pennsylvania School of Medicine (1959–1985), and surgeon-in-chief, Children's Hospital of Philadelphia (1948–1981), recognized the wide spectrum of clinical presentations exhibited by children with neuroblastoma, evaluated aggressive surgical approaches, noted the effects of irradiation, and studied the problems in developing a classification system for this unique tumor, which had defied the conventional staging systems.

eling nationally, rarely did he meet a physician or surgeon who approached this field with any enthusiasm. A notable exception was Harold W. K. Dargeon, who operated a four-bed ward in the Memorial Cancer Hospital on Central Park West, New York City. Dargeon was almost unique among pediatricians in his single-minded concern for this group of patients.[28] Koop surveyed the records of the CHP when he arrived there in 1946 and found that with few exceptions the only survivors were children with localized and resectable (or Stage 4s) neuroblastoma. His initial studies were directed toward determining the effects of aggressive surgery with "debulking" of unresectable neuroblastomas, emphasizing accurate staging, and assessing the therapeutic and other effects of radiotherapy.[29, 30]

A decade later H. William Clatworthy in Columbus, Ohio (Fig. 1–4) undertook the task of convincing surgeons that radical surgery was not always required for cure, or even the preferred approach, for some pediatric cancer patients who were treated with even the chemotherapeutic agents available in the 1960s and 1970s.[31] Recognizing that a large proportion of pediatric cancer surgery was performed by general, thoracic, and urologic surgeons, his publications were directed toward a wide audience of surgeons and pediatricians.

Clatworthy, Harold Nixon (London), Antonio Gentil-Martins (Lisbon), and later Judson Randolph (Washington, DC) developed series of successful hepatic resections for primary malignant liver tumors during the 1960s. Randolph subsequently became the first surgeon associated with a pediatric cancer cooperative group (1968).

In Europe during this period, Monerreo (Madrid), Gentil-Martins (Lisbon), Carcassone (Marseilles), and Dennison (Glasgow) made contributions in this field and were instrumental in founding the International Society of Pediatric Oncology (SIOP), while Zachary (Sheffield) was a principal in the development of the first pediatric cooperative group in the United Kingdom. In Japan, a surgical cooperative group study of 403 pediatric patients with malignant tumors treated from 1963 to 1972 was reported by M. Ishida (Tokyo). Concurrently, M. Kasai (Sendai) and K. Ikeda (Fukuoka) developed techniques for the excision of hepatic and biliary tract tumors. Ultrasound was used extensively in delineating intra-abdominal masses by Hirai (Tokyo) in the

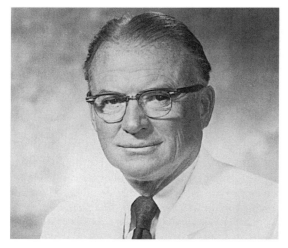

Figure 1–4 • H. William Clatworthy, Jr. (1917–) professor and head of the Division of Pediatric Surgery, Ohio State University, and head of the Department of Surgery, The Children's Hospital, Columbus, OH (1962–1990), advanced the concept that in some situations the addition of effective chemotherapy to the management scheme for childhood tumors (rhabdomyosarcoma, notably) made the survival rates following the more radical surgical procedures no higher than those that followed more conservative surgical approaches. Further, he noted that the latter permitted more opportunities for organ and limb preservation.

early 1960s. The Japanese Pediatric Surgical Society, led by T. Ueda, appointed a committee on cancer in 1970, preceding the formation of the Cancer Committee of the American Pediatric Surgical Association by four years. A national study of neuroblastoma initially led by S. Sawaguchi, Y. Tsuchida, I. Okabe, and I. Watanabe was started the same year.

The next generation of pediatric surgeons in the United States, Thomas Boles, Alfred De Lorimier, Robert Filler, Jay Grosfeld, Daniel Hays, Robert Izant, Dale Johnson, Thomas Santulli, E. I. Smith, James Talbert, and Jessie Ternberg, made contributions in both institutional studies and the development of cooperative group trials for the management of neuroblastomas, nephroblastomas, hepatic tumors, and rhabdomyosarcoma.

Major contributions to our understanding of the nature of neoplasia and the principles of therapy have been made during the last half century, propelled by farsighted investigators, including many pediatric oncologists. Surgeons played little part in this evolution, although clinical research in oncology has been a major interest of a sizable group of pediatric surgeons in the United States, Europe, and Japan. Basic research in the United States by surgeons in this area has been limited in scope. Discoveries in the field of angiogenesis factors by Judah Folkman of Boston constitute a notable exception.

The concept of a pediatrician with an interest confined to oncology (or hematology/oncology) was still developing in the 1950s. The practice of pathologist-clinicians, such as Sydney Farber, directing the surveillance of pediatric cancer patients, and subsequently playing a major role in their therapy, was common in the United States during this era (1950–1960). Farber sought the assistance of pediatric specialists early in the development of his clinic in Boston. Many of the new breed of pediatric hematology-oncologists were trained by pathologist-clinicians.

The Pediatric Oncologists

When they arrived in force in the 1960s, pediatric oncologists rapidly assumed a leadership role in generating clinical trials of competing therapy regimens. Initially, these were primarily focused on leukemia and secondarily on lymphomas. Slowly, and in some instances quite reluctantly,

pediatric oncologists accepted responsibility for the management of children with unresectable or recurrent solid tumors and included them in chemotherapy therapeutic programs and clinical trials. Pediatric surgeons in some areas administered chemotherapy, because they believed the needs of these patients were not being met. This practice was condemned by some hematologist-oncologists and highly encouraged by others. "Prophylactic" chemotherapy, administered to children with apparently completely excised (and frequently irradiated) solid tumors, became standard practice only after the beginning of the intergroup studies, that is, the National Wilms' Tumor Study (NWTS) and subsequently the Intergroup Rhabdomyosarcoma Study (IRS) in the late 1960s and early 1970s.

Cooperative Groups; Intergroup, National, and International Studies

Acute Leukemia Chemotherapy Cooperative Study Group A (ALCCSGA), later Children's Cancer Study Group A (CCSGA) still later, CCSG, and finally CCG, was one of the three original cooperative groups established by the National Institutes of Health (NIH) in 1955, and the only one devoted entirely to childhood tumors.[32] It began with ten participating hospitals. Two additional cooperative groups, the Southwest Cancer Chemotherapy Study Group and Acute Leukemia Group B, both of which were primarily concerned with adult forms of cancer, organized large pediatric sections.

From their origin, these cancer cooperative groups supported by the NIH included studies of childhood leukemia and, from 1960, studies of patients with disseminated pediatric solid tumors. Surgeons were not included in these study committees. From 1961 through 1969 pediatric members of the cooperative groups became increasingly interested in localized and surgically resectable tumors and more convinced of the possibility that adjuvant chemotherapy might increase survival among these patients. Surgical "consultants," including Judson Randolph and Alexander Bill, were invited to attend CCSG meetings in the late 1960s preparatory to the opening of the first study (NWTS, 1968) of adjunctive therapy in a localized solid tumor. CCSG representatives, led by James A. Wolff, met with the members of the Surgical Section of the American Academy of Pediatrics in 1967 and 1968 to solicit comment and encourage surgical participation in the developing NWTS.

In 1969 the CCSG appointed a Surgical Committee, the members of which rapidly increased their scope within the group, including membership on the Executive Committee and participation in the activities of all solid-tumor study committees. The composition of this Surgical Committee demonstrates the interest in oncology among the nationally recognized leaders of pediatric surgery in the United States in that era (Fig. 1–5). The Surgical Committee of CCSG applied for and received separate federal funding (independent of the CCSG grant) from 1978 to 1984.

Pediatric surgeons were included in the surgical committees of both the Southwest Cancer Chemotherapy Study Group, later the Southwest Oncology Group (SWOG), headed by Jessie Ternberg and E. Ide Smith, and the Cancer and Acute Leukemia Group B (CALGB), headed by Alex Haller and John White, although both groups were primarily interested in therapy trials for adult malignant disease. When the pediatric sections of SWOG and CALGB dissolved their affiliations with these original groups in 1979–1980 and merged as the separate Pediatric Oncology Group (POG), the pediatric surgeons from SWOG and CALGB united, wrote a constitution and bylaws, and secured the same general prerogatives that had been obtained by the pediatric surgeons in CCSG. Biemann Othersen, Dennis Shermeta, James Talbert, as well as Ternberg and Smith, were among the leaders in the new organization.

Patients treated in member institutions of the cooperative groups were enrolled in randomized trials, which in the case of solid-tumor studies ordinarily continued from 4 to 6 years. Membership in a group required that all cancer patients treated in participating institutions be registered with a common statistical center. Exemptions were required if eligible patients were not entered in appropriate trials. Group protocols were developed by pediatric oncologists with cooperating pediatric surgeons, pathologists, radiotherapists and statisticians. They were essentially com-

2125 – 13TH STREET, N. W.
WASHINGTON, D. C. 20009

WALLACE WERBLE
PRESIDENT
ROBERT H. PARROTT, M. D.
DIRECTOR

WILLIAM A. HOWARD, M. D.
CHAIRMAN OF MEDICAL STAFF
DONALD F. SMITH
ADMINISTRATOR

MEMORANDUM

TO: Surgical Committee, Children's Cancer Study Group A

Dr. Alexander Bill	Dr. H. William Clatworthy
Dr. Dale Johnson	Dr. William Kiesewetter
Dr. C. Everett Koop	Dr. Tague Chisholm
Dr. Thomas Santulli	Dr. Orvar Swenson

FROM: Dr. Judson Randolph and Dr. Daniel Hays

DATE : September 28, 1970

Figure 1–5 • The composition of the Surgical Committee of CCSGA in 1970 reflects the major interest in pediatric oncology of the leadership of surgical divisions associated with medical schools and the heads of the surgical services of children's hospitals nationally. Each member of the committee could be included in one or both categories. Their affiliations were the University of Washington (Bill), University of Pennsylvania (Koop), Columbia University College of Medicine (Santulli), Ohio State University (Clatworthy), University of Pittsburgh (Kiesewetter), University of Minnesota (Chisholm), and the Northwestern University (Swenson).

parisons of the survival resulting from the use of each of two (or more) competing chemotherapy or chemotherapy-radiotherapy regimens, with surgery continuing to be as nonvariable a factor as it was possible to make it!

Groups of children with acute lymphocytic leukemia or disseminated neuroblastoma were ideally suited to the cooperative-group approach, as the volume of patients available was large and the durations of survival relatively short, thus significant improvement in outcome was readily recognized. In contrast, it was realized that an individual pediatric cooperative group did not ordinarily have the patient resources to conduct studies of either (1) tumors of low incidence or (2) tumors in which the survival rates were relatively high, that is, in which all regimens were relatively effective. Small differences in effectiveness in treating such tumors were difficult to recognize in patient groups of the size found in CCSG or later in POG, and these difficulties led to the "national" or "intergroup" studies.

The first of these was the National Wilms' Tumor Study (1969), which combined the resources of the American Academy of Pediatrics, the existing pediatric group (CCSG), the pediatric sections of the two adult cooperative groups, and also "independent" institutions treating childhood cancer, thus becoming a truly "national" study. The NWTS has become a model of effective interdisciplinary activity, as well as providing guidelines for studies of all tumors with relatively high survival rates. The NWTS Committee, led by Giulio D'Angio, has completed four studies (NWTS 1–4, 1969–1994), and a fifth (NWTS 5), led by Daniel Green, is under way. The Intergroup Rhabdomyosarcoma Study (IRS), headed by Harold M. Maurer, was organized in 1970 by representatives of the existing three pediatric groups (CCSG, SWOG, and CALGB) and opened for patient entry in 1972. Since 1980 the IRS has been continued by representatives of CCSG and POG. Three studies (IRS I, II, and III) have been completed, and a fourth (IRS IV) is in progress.

Of major interest in regard to both the NWTS and IRS is the prominent role that pathologists have assumed in directing therapy. It should probably have been apparent that when a perceptive pathologist was presented with literally thousands of examples of a "rare" pediatric tumor, he or she would find significant differences between different segments of such a sample, and that new and possibly therapy-directing concepts should result. Such has been the case, as during the course of the NWTS and the IRS major recommendations regarding therapy have been made on the basis of histologic distinctions rather than on the basis of clinical stage alone—as they were in the original NWTS and IRS studies. Separate and distinct tumors have been isolated from what were previously considered single entities. The renal clear-cell and rhabdoid sarcomas are now recognized to be unique tumors, not Wilms' tumor variants. Soft-tissue Ewing's tumors and the peripheral neuroectodermal tumors are recognized as being distinct from rhabdomyosarcoma.

Leaders in this movement toward more precise identification of tumor types within large categories have been J. Bruce Beckwith, and William A. Newton, Jr. Both the NWTS and the IRS pathologists are regarded as having achieved major insights into the descriptive histopathology of the tumors within their scope, as well as factors influencing the outcome and the most effective management of patients with these tumors. Contributions of the Intergroup Hodgkin's Disease in Childhood Study (1975–1981), were less impressive; data on the adverse long-range effects of therapy may be the most significant accomplishment of that study. The Intergroup Ewing's Sarcoma Study (1972–1981) made contributions related to the effectiveness of doxorubicin and recognition of the poor prognosis associated with specific tumor sites and histologic variants. Less formal collaboration between the pediatric cooperative groups (CCG and POG) has been achieved by adopting a common protocol for the same tumor and stage. This collaboration has been effective in hepatoma and medulloblastoma trials, and a similar study of malignant germ-cell tumors is in progress.

The first multi-institutional pediatric cancer studies in the United Kingdom were authorized by the Medical Research Council of Great Britain (MRCGB) in 1970. Primarily concerned with nephroblastoma, these studies confirmed the effectiveness of vincristine in Wilms' tumor therapy, as described by Wataru Sutow in the United States.[33] The MRCGB has been succeeded by the United Kingdom Children's Cancer Study Group, which contributed cases to IRS-III but has declined to participate in IRS-IV because a hyperfractionated radiotherapy substudy was included. In Europe, the International Society of Pediatric Oncology (SIOP), which primarily includes institutions throughout Europe and the Near East, was founded in 1968 and has conducted clinical trials since 1971, with Monerreo (Spain) and Pellerin and Bourreau (France) founding surgical members. Accurate data acquisition was a problem in some SIOP studies during the initial trials, but this has been largely overcome. Pediatric surgeons in SIOP with other nonaffiliated surgeons interested in pediatric oncology formed the International Society of Pediatric Surgical Oncology (IPSO) in 1992 with Jack Plaschkes (Switzerland) and this contributor, Daniel M. Hays (United States), its initial presidents.

In the United States the NCI-supported cancer cooperative groups have played a more prominent role in pediatric oncology than have similar groups in adult oncology. At present, more than 94% of patients less than 15 years of age in the United States with solid tumors are treated according to a group research protocol, either as direct (and usually partially funded) participants or otherwise.[34] Among adults with cancer, it is probable that not more than 20% are enrolled in such studies. The significance of the pediatric cooperative group studies appears in subsequent sections. Their contribution to the *general* field of oncology has been impressive, and they are regarded as models for certain types of therapy trials for cancer patients of all ages.

Surgeons in the Pediatric Cooperative Groups

The role of pediatric surgeons, as well as that of surgeons in surgical specialties, associated with the pediatric cooperative groups in the United States has evolved gradually during two decades. As the basic function of these groups was the testing of chemotherapeutic agents and regimens, and to a lesser extent assessment of the contribution of radiotherapy, the activities of the surgeon in the groups were adapted to this goal. Although there was considerable "testing" of surgical approaches or procedures carried out in the course of group studies, no randomized trial that attempted to answer a strictly surgical question was deemed feasible.

As noted, surgical approaches of several types have been employed during group trials, and because of the large number of patients involved, a reasonable evaluation of these innovations has at times been possible. Some of these procedures were "revivals" of operations originating in adult oncology where they were no longer in general use. The original "second look" procedure of Owen Wangensteen[35] was an operation at a selected interval in the postoperative course carried out in a high-risk patient group, the purpose of which was to identify recurrent abdominal cancer before it became apparent clinically. The patient was apparently tumor free, asymptomatic, and, of course, not on chemotherapy, while the involved clinicians were without the benefit of even basic scans to identify recurrences.

Modern pediatric oncologic versions of the second look may be quite different. In some, the procedure is performed in patients who are known to have gross tumor at the end of the initial surgical procedure, with the second look, designed to remove what may be residual tumor following chemotherapy or chemotherapy/radiotherapy regimens, or to determine that no recognizable tumor exists. Although such procedures have fallen into disuse in the management of most cancers in adults, variations have been used with increasing frequency in children. This has been encouraged by the inclusion of these procedures in the protocols of group trials such as the IRS. Another example of an abandoned "adult" cancer operation now used in pediatrics is partial cystectomy. This procedure, once performed by urologists in adults with vesical neoplasms, has been successfully employed in the management of bladder rhabdomyosarcomas in children.

THE PAST DECADE

The initial volume with this title, *Pediatric Surgical Oncology*, published about 10 years ago, was the first textbook devoted exclusively to this subject. The present volume is more comprehensive, and Richard J. Andrassy has assembled a group of contributors reflecting a much wider and deeper range of expertise.

Changes that have occurred in this field since the first publication are legion, and only a few are summarized here, more as a reminder of how rapidly changes occur in this field than as an attempt to be inclusive. Many other changes in the field are described in the chapters on specific tumor types. As a beginning, venous access became a major part of the workload of most pediatric surgeons concerned with oncology during this interval, and laparoscopy was recognized as a factor of significance in pediatric oncology almost entirely during this period. Tubes for decompression are now placed in the stomach or distally far less frequently than a decade ago. Organ transplant for the cancer patient was regarded as almost always associated with a failure in tumor control a decade ago. Its problems are far from solved today, but there have been successful kidney, liver, heart, and even intestinal transplants in patients with cancer or with the sequelae of cancer therapy. Laparotomy, widely used for staging children with Stage I-II Hodgkin's disease a decade ago, is now reserved for the few with very specific indications, for example, ovarian transposition. A policy of scheduled or at least anticipated secondary surgery for children with pediatric tumors has been expanded, encompassing tumor types not previously considered and a wider application among those tumors than was standard ten years ago.

Concepts regarding hepatoblastoma are exemplary. The prevalent dictum a decade ago was that survival among children with all malignant hepatic tumors was dependent upon initial tumor extirpation. In respect to hepatoblastoma, at present the smallest or most readily excised tumors are treated by primary resection, but a larger group of patients are undergoing delayed procedures following chemotherapy.

In respect to neuroblastoma, the most significant advances in the past decade have not been in therapy per se, but rather have issued from a recognition of the basic processes that indicate the intrinsic malignancy of the tumor and thus direct a modulation of therapy for each specific patient group. Ten years ago the controversy over the relative efficacy of the Evans-Randolph-D'Angio staging classification (CCG) versus the St. Jude system, as modified by POG, was active and unresolved. The principal means of making a specific preoperative diagnosis was the determination of the levels of serum or urinary catecholamines, usually restricted to VMA or HVA. Since then, an International Neuroblastoma Staging System that includes elements of both the CCG and POG systems has evolved. Multiple new tumor "markers," or prognostic indicators, are established or under study worldwide. Serum

neuron-specific enolase was briefly regarded as the definitive prognostic indicator in the United States, whereas LDH levels were and still are preferred in Germany. Later it became apparent that N-*myc* copy number or expression was a remarkably accurate indicator of outcome for children with all stages of neuroblastoma.

Although a policy of resection of residual primary neuroblastomas (Stage III) after a response to chemotherapy had been employed for over 15 years, the results relative to ultimate survival have improved somewhat during the past decade.

Early in this decade, the National Wilms' Tumor Study (NWTS) Committee redefined its study population, eliminating the usually lethal rhabdoid tumors and providing intensive chemotherapy regimens for the bone-metastasizing clear-cell tumors. As redefined, nephroblastoma became the only common pediatric tumor in which the results of therapy have been so successful that it is difficult to develop practical clinical trials. Studies have been reduced to those that test the efficacy of different methods of administration of standard agents, lower the cost of care, or follow in detail the long-range adverse effects of therapy. NWTS 5 includes the study of molecular markers (1p or 16q deletions) as indicators of treatment resistance.

Of interest to surgeons is a subset of nephroblastoma patients in which the primary tumor is small and there is no invasion of the vasculature, the capsule, or the renal sinus. A group of such children has been treated with surgery alone with high survival rates. At the other extreme, there is an increasing number of patients now treated by gross "tumorectomy," or partial nephrectomy, a policy influenced by recognition of the fact that many patients with bilateral nephroblastoma who have neither undergone complete tumor excision nor received renal irradiation have nevertheless survived—some on intensive and some on relatively nonintensive chemotherapy regimens! Most patients with nephroblastoma continue to be treated with excision of the primary tumor by nephrectomy, but little effort is made, as it was in some clinics a decade ago, to excise all adjacent node groups or potential extensions. Partial nephrectomy, initially or following chemotherapy, remains controversial except for bilateral disease.

In respect to rhabdomyosarcoma, the patients with peripheral neuroectodermal tumors

(PNET) and Ewing's sarcoma of soft tissue, formerly treated by the IRS protocols, were excluded from those studies during this decade. A classification of rhabdomyosarcoma was developed by a large international group of pathologists during 1993–1994 that is based on established outcome. This classification recognizes for the first time a category of spindle-cell rhabdomyosarcomas, with a particularly favorable prognosis occurring most frequently in patients with tumors in paratesticular or orbital sites. Rhabdomyosarcoma remains a tumor without a specific *clinical* marker, but an extremely sensitive indicator of prognosis in the form of ploidy studies has been developed. During this decade, there has been a clear movement toward less radical surgery for rhabdomyosarcoma in some sites, particularly those primary in the genito-urinary tract and the head and neck areas. This approach has been less well established and is probably less successful in the management of trunk and extremity tumors. Secondary surgery, either immediate—as following early recognized incomplete excision—or delayed—as following a chemotherapy or chemotherapy/radiotherapy response—has become standard.

At the onset of this decade, germ-cell tumors were treated by radical (or less than radical) surgery, irradiation, and variations on vincristine, actinomycin D and cyclophosphamide (VAC) therapy, without noticeable recognition of the major contributions of such people as Einhorn and Golbey in the chemotherapy of the closely related tumors of adults. At the end of the decade, it was apparent that the introduction of platinum-based compounds and bleomycin into the regimens for germ-cell tumors in children was highly effective, in some situations limiting the indications for radical surgery or for local irradiation.

Early in this decade excisions of multiple pulmonary metastasis had a period of widespread use or study, which has been somewhat contracted to procedures for metastatic osteosarcoma and nephroblastoma, but rarely other tumors in pediatric patients.

In summary, during the past decade, surgeons have attempted an adaptation to the current trend of incremental (but far from consistent) increases in the effectiveness of chemotherapy/radiotherapy regimens as determined through group trials without ignoring the individual patient's right to the benefits of early, at times radical, surgery. This trend presents a fine line for the surgeon to walk! Moreover, changes in the practice of the pediatric surgeon, oncology oriented or not, have been influenced during the past decade by what would previously have been regarded as entirely extraneous economic factors. These have assumed an importance not seen before in this century. It is a tribute to surgeons, and their pediatric associates, that progress in scientific areas nonetheless continues. Surprisingly, in the area of pediatric surgical oncology, very significant progress has been made.

References

1. Billroth T: *Untersuchungen uber den feineren Bau and die Entwicklung der Brustdusen-qeschwulste. Verchows Arch Pathol Anat* 18:51–81, 1860.
2. Jessup J: Annotations: Extirpation of the kidney. *Lancet* 1:889, 1877.
3. Kocher T, Longhaus T: *Eine Nephrotomie wegen Nierensarcom, Zugleich ein Beitrag zur Histologie des Nierenkrebses. Dtsch Z Chir* 9:312, 1878.
4. Israel J: *Erfahrungen uber Nierenchirurgie. Arch Klin Chir* 47:302, 1894.
5. Wilms M: *Die Misschengeschulste der Niere.* Leipzig: Arthur Georgi, 1899.
6. Walker G: Transperitoneal ligation of the renal vessels. *JAMA* 45:1647, 1905.
7. Walker G: Sarcoma of the kidney in children: A critical review of the pathology, symptomatology, prognosis and operative treatment as seen in 145 cases. *Ann Surg* 26:529–602, 1897.
8. Wilks S, Moxon W: *Lectures on Pathological Anatomy*, 2nd ed. London: Longman, Brown, Green, Longman, Roberts & Co., 1875.
9. Osler W: Two cases of striated myo-sarcoma of the kidney. *J Anat Physiol* 14:229–233, 1879.
10. Schottlander F: *Erevin von Baelz 1849–1913, Leben & Wirkere eines Deutchen Aertges in Japan Ausland & Heimat.* Stuttgart: Verlags-Aktiengesellschaft, 1925.
11. Sansom GB: *The Western World & Japan.* London: Cresset Press, 1950.
12. Roentgen WC: On a new kind of ray (preliminary communication). Translation of a paper read before the Physikalische-Medicineschem Gesellsehaft of Wurzberg on December 28, 1985. *Br J Radiol* 4:32, 1931.
13. Curie P, Curie Mme P, Bemout G: *Sur une nouvelle substance fortement radioactice contenue dans la pechblende. Comp Rend Acad Sci* (Paris) 127:1215–1217, 1898.
14. Friedlander A: Sarcoma of the kidney treated by the roentgen ray. *Am J Dis Child* 12:328–330, 1916.

15. Geraghty JT, Vesical tumors. *NY Med J* 104:838–840, 1916.
16. Neuhauser EBD: Wittenborg MH, Berman CZ, et al: Irradiation effects of roentgen therapy on the growing spine. *Radiology* 59:637–650, 1952.
17. Wollstein M: Renal neoplasms in young children. *Arch Path* 3:1–13, 1927.
18. Mixter CG: Malignant tumors of the kidney in infancy and childhood. *Ann Surg* 96:1017–1027, 1932.
19. Wharton LR: Transperitoneal nephrectomy for malignant tumors of the kidney. *Surg Gynecol Obstet* 60:689–694, 1935.
20. Ladd WE, White RR: Embryoma of the kidney (Wilms' tumor). *JAMA* 117:1858–1863, 1941.
21. Ladd WE: Embryoma of the kidney (Wilms' tumor). *Ann Surg* 108:885–902, 1938.
22. Gross RE, Newhauser, EBD: Treatment of mixed tumors of the kidney in childhood. *Pediatrics* 6:843–852, 1950.
23. Ladd WE, Gross RE: *Abdominal Surgery of Infancy & Childhood.* Philadelphia: W.B. Saunders Co, 1941.
24. Cushing H: Surgery of the head. In Keen WW (ed): *Surgery: Its Principles and Practice,* vol. 3. Philadelphia/London: W.B. Saunders Co., 1908.
25. Farber S, Toch R, Sears EM, et al: Advances in chemotherapy of cancer in man. In Greenstein, JP, and Haddow, A. (eds): *Advances in Cancer Research,* vol. 4. New York: Academic Press, 1956, pp. 1–71.
26. Swenson O: Personal communication.
27. Koop CE: Personal communication.
28. Dargeon HWK: Cancer in childhood and a discussion of certain benign tumors. St. Louis: C.V. Mosby Co., 1940.
29. Koop CE, Kiesewetter WB, Horn RC: Neuroblastoma in childhood: Survival after surgical insult to tumor. *Surgery* 38:272–278, 1955.
30. Koop CE: Neuroblastoma: Two years' survival and treatment correlations. *J Pediatr Surg* 3:178, 1968.
31. Kilman JW, Clatworthy HW Jr, Newton WA Jr, et al: Reasonable surgery for rhabdomyosarcoma: A study of 67 cases. *Ann Surg* 178:346–351, 1973.
32. Zubrad CG, Schepart S, Teiter J, et al: The Chemotherapy Program of the National Cancer Institute: History, analysis and plans. *Cancer Chemotherapy Reports* 50:349–381, 1966.
33. Sutow WW: Chemotherapy in childhood cancer (except leukemia): An appraisal. *Cancer* 18:1585–1589, 1965.
34. Ross JA, Severson RK, Pollock BH, et al: Childhood cancer in the United States. *Cancer* 77:201–207, 1996.
35. Wangensteen O, Tongen LA: Second look in cancer surgery. *Lancet* 71:303–307, 1951.

General Principles

• *Richard J. Andrassy, M.D.*

This chapter provides an overview of the general principles of pediatric surgical oncology. Details are provided in the individual chapters of this book, authored by acknowledged experts in their fields. Areas of controversy, newer developments, and some commentary on the chapters are included in this overview.

Survival rates for children with solid tumors have improved dramatically during the last two decades. Much of this improvement can be attributed to the multimodal approach to therapy. Refinements in chemotherapy and radiation therapy have allowed for less radical, or less mutilating, operative intervention in many patients. The recognition that preoperative chemotherapy can not only be cytoreductive but can also improve resectability and decrease blood loss and postoperative complications has changed the overall approach to many tumors. Advances in surgical technique and intraoperative monitoring have also contributed to better survival rates. Improved techniques for liver resection, chest-wall reconstruction, and insertion of prosthetic devices, and the use of minimally invasive techniques, have greatly enhanced patient outcome.

Less need for radical resection does not, however, correlate with less need for surgical input. Initial staging, biopsy, enteral and parenteral access, and later resection at second or third look still play invaluable roles. In fact, very few patients with tumors are "cured" without some form of surgical intervention. Because of the multimodal approach to these tumors and the importance of the timing of various therapies, the surgeon has truly become an integral member of the team, beginning with initial protocol design.

The surgeon should also be aware of the relatively high incidence of second malignancies in children cured of an initial tumor.[1] These second malignancies have included early occurrence of breast[2] and colon tumors and melanomas[3] and a variety of other malignancies.[4]

BRIEF OVERVIEW OF METABOLIC CONSIDERATIONS IN PEDIATRIC CANCER

Patients with cancer frequently have associated cachexia with significant weight loss and malnutrition. The reasons for this association are obviously multifactorial and may be related directly to the tumor, such as increased metabolic rate, circulating peptides leading to anorexia, and decreased intake resulting from poor appetite or gut involvement. Other reasons appear to be involved, including increased whole-body protein breakdown, increased lipolysis, and increased gluconeogenesis. Many hormonal, metabolic, and cytokine abnormalities occur in the malnourished cancer patient as well. Release of certain cytokines, such as tumor necrosis factor, interleukin-1, interleukin-6, and others may increase the cancer cachexia. Malnutrition in cancer patients leads to intolerance of chemotherapy and radiation therapy as well to as increased local and systemic infections. Survival as related to treatment may therefore be affected.

For many years, oncologists hesitated to provide nutritional support to cancer patients for fear that the tumor would grow disproportionately to the repletion of the host. It was subsequently demonstrated that the tumor will continue to take from the host until the host is severely malnourished and that starvation should play no role in cancer therapy. Rather, adjunctive nutritional support, either parenterally or enterally, supports the host during therapy with surgery, chemotherapy, or radiation. Numerous studies have demonstrated that the nutritionally repleted patient will tolerate therapy better with fewer complications.

Studies have also shown that enteral nutrition protects the gut and is safer and more effective than intravenous nutrition. Nutrients such as glutamine and arginine may play a role in protecting the gut and enhancing immune response. Overnutrition, however, may be harmful, because there are changes in the metabolism of certain nutrients that may lead to undesirable immunologic effects. The extensive and up-to-date overview on nutrition for pediatric oncology patients is provided by Dr. Walter Chwals (Chapter 24).

VASCULAR ACCESS

Probably the single most frequent operation that the pediatric surgeon performs in caring for the child with a malignancy is that for vascular access. Centrally placed, long-term venous catheters have gained widespread use for chemotherapy, antibiotic, administration, and blood drawing. These catheters have made the care of the child easier, both for the child and the care giver.

Achieving vascular access safely and maintaining long-term patency are critical to the management of the patient. The development of new external and subcutaneous implantable devices improves the quality of life. Attention to detail in placement of the catheters and in long-term maintenance is critical for the safety of these techniques. An extensive discussion of techniques for placement as well as prevention and management of complications is provided by Drs. Lally and Horowitz in Chapter 8.

ENTERAL ACCESS

The use of the patient's gastrointestinal tract to maintain nutritional status during chemotherapy or radiation therapy or following operative intervention has the advantages of being physiologic, safe, effective, and relatively inexpensive. Nutritional support via the gut is no longer limited by the patient's ability or willingness to eat or drink as a variety of techniques are available for administering defined-formula diets that complement total parenteral nutrition. Mauer and coworkers,[5] in reviewing the literature in this area, concluded that enteral nutrition can be successful in maintaining nutritional status in children with low-nutritional-risk cancers (such as acute lymphocytic leukemia), in well-nourished children with less advanced disease, and in children with advanced disease who are in remission and receiving maintenance treatment. Rickard and coworkers[8, 9] reported that an enteral nutrition program was successful in maintaining appropriate weight for height in children with Wilms' tumor[6, 7] or neuroblastoma.[8, 9] In very-high-risk patients with severe malnutrition, there should be a transition from parenteral nutrition to enteral feedings as tolerated.[10]

It is difficult to document that nutritional support improves the patient's prognosis, but nutritional status does correlate with freedom from relapse in children with solid tumors.[11] Nutritional status also correlates with an improved sense of well-being, less lethargy, decreased irritability, increased normal daily activities, fewer delays in providing antineoplastic treatment, and lower complication rates.[7, 8, 11]

Patients who require nonvolitional enteral feeding should be evaluated before the site and route of feeding are decided upon. Confirming the route of access to the gut, ordering the diet, and administering the diet properly are all important aspects of safe and effective enteral nutrition. Selection of the route of access depends upon the portion of the child's gastrointestinal tract to be accessed and used for feeding and the anticipated duration of feeding and whether or not the patient is an operative candidate.

Access may be achieved nonoperatively or operatively. Either the stomach or small bowel may be accessed nonoperatively or operatively, and the clinician must sometimes choose between the two. Delivering the formula into the stomach ensures its exposure to the maximal amount of small bowel absorptive surface available—an important consideration in a patient with a limited amount of small bowel. In addition, the stomach's physiologic mandate of serving as a reservoir where the diet is mixed and its toxicity adjusted before it is metered into the small bowel permits greater latitude in selecting the diet and the technique for administration than would be the case if the small bowel were accessed directly. This greater ease and flexibility with which intragastric feeding is performed is purchased at the expense of increased risk of reflux, vomiting, and aspiration.

Instillation of the defined formula into the small bowel virtually eliminates the problems of gastric overload, reflux, vomiting, and aspiration that are associated with intragastric feeding. This advantage is particularly important in the anorexic or vomiting child receiving chemotherapy. In addition, intrajejunal feeding is not affected by the many mechanical and inflammatory processes in the upper abdomen that may limit gastric emptying. Intrajejunal feeding may be done concurrently with nasogastric decompression as

an early postoperative feeding.[12] The patient may take whatever oral intake is physiologically possible without significant interference with the intrajejunal feeding.

Many techniques for intrajejunal access have been described[13] that offer ready access to the gastrointestinal tract for short- or long-term feeding. Tolerance of enteral feeding may be affected by a number of clinical conditions, including whether the patient is receiving antibiotics or suffers bowel-wall edema secondary to low oncotic pressure, peritonitis, or obstruction.[14, 15]

Gastrostomy tubes, generally of the temporary (Stamm) variety, are frequently employed for intragastric feeding and decompression. These gastrostomy openings close spontaneously after removal of the tube. Gastrostomy feedings have all the advantages and disadvantages described for gastric tubes but obviate the need for a nasogastric tube. Gastrostomy tubes may be placed operatively or endoscopically without need for operative intervention.[16]

Numerous small-caliber nasoenteral catheters are available for nonoperative access of the gastrointestinal tract. The smaller size allows for more comfortable intubation and maintenance. Newer, less viscous formulas allow for administration through smaller-caliber tubes. The smaller catheters also decrease the effect on the gastroesophageal junction and decrease the incidence of reflux and aspiration. These smaller catheters have been utilized for both short-term inpatient and long-term outpatient feedings with success.

Considerable evidence exists that enteral feeding may play a role in gut mucosal protection, decreased bacterial translocation, and decreased local and systemic sepsis.[17] Thus, it is important that the physician caring for the child with cancer be familiar with the different routes of access and the products available for enteral nutrition.

BIOPSIES

Surgeons play a key role in the initial diagnosis of pediatric malignancies. The correct choice of biopsy technique requires knowledge of the natural history of the disease, the resources of the institution, and the patient's further needs for surgical intervention. Consultation with other members of the multimodal team is very important in determining the optimal biopsy technique based on suspected histology and neoplasm site.

One approach to rapid histologic diagnosis involves fine needle aspiration (FNA) and core needle biopsy. The biopsy may be done in the operating room, clinic, or radiologic suite. Improvements in technology and increased training in cytopathologic techniques have led to widespread applications in adults with tumors. Because several pediatric tumors have the histologic picture of "small-, round-, blue-cell tumors," immunohistochemical techniques may be required for final diagnosis.

Several series have shown the usefulness of FNA biopsy in children. In 156 patients who underwent FNA biopsy at M.D. Anderson Cancer Center, diagnosis was obtained in 90% of the patients with solid tumors, but in only 47% with lymphomas.[18] These data suggest that although FNA is an excellent tool for diagnosing solid malignancies in the pediatric population, it may be less helpful in diagnosing lymphomas. A negative study finding or insufficient material should be considered nondiagnostic and should be followed by open biopsy when clinical suspicion of malignancy is high.

FNA has the advantage of requiring only local anesthetic for many patients. CT- or ultrasound-guided FNA may allow for biopsy of deeply located lesions that would require laparotomy or thoracotomy for open biopsy. The biopsy may be performed by surgeons, radiologists, or pathologists. As with other techniques, the experience of the clinician performing the procedure is important to the adequacy of the biopsy specimen. The presence of an experienced cytopathologist nearby when the biopsy is being performed is also important. A well-trained cytopathologist can direct the FNA biopsy procedure and may be able to increase the yield. Core needle biopsies may be performed in many of the same situations as FNA biopsies and may provide tissue with intact architecture that is helpful to the pathologist.

Biopsy of any lesion may involve the need for reoperation and wide excision. Longitudinal incisions are frequently better than horizontal incisions on areas such as an extremity (Fig. 2–1). A biopsy to confirm malignancy requires that the biopsy tract be excised at the time of reoperation; if the biopsy site is inappropriately placed, this excision may require much larger incisions or

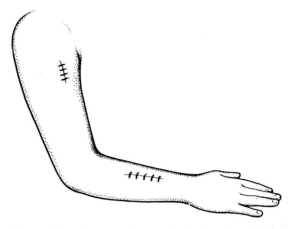

Figure 2–1 • Biopsy of extremity lesions should take into consideration the need for reoperation and wide excision. Longitudinal incisions for biopsy are therefore preferable.

resections than would otherwise be necessary (Fig. 2–2).

Solid-tumor biopsies are traditionally divided into excisional biopsies, in which the entire tumor is included in the specimen, and incisional biopsies, in which only a portion of the tumor is included. In an excisional biopsy, margins should be carefully marked to allow re-resection should the biopsy reveal a positive margin on review. Ideally, excisional biopsies are planned to allow resections that will leave behind only negative margins. If such an excisional biopsy results in too large a resection, then incisional biopsy is more appropriate.

If biopsy margins are not carefully marked on both the specimen and the operative field (usually by sutures or clips), the ability of the surgeon to subsequently obtain negative margins is severely compromised. For example, an inappropriate approach to biopsy may lead to further difficulties in the case of testicular masses. Any testicular mass should be approached through an inguinal rather than a scrotal incision so that proximal control of the cord can be obtained and a wide local excision performed without seeding the scrotum with tumor. The proximal spermatic cord should be examined for free margins. Higher excision may be necessary if tumor is still present. Biopsy of the tumor through the scrotum may lead to further need of scrotal resection and increased risk of local recurrence.

Nephroblastomas have traditionally been ex-

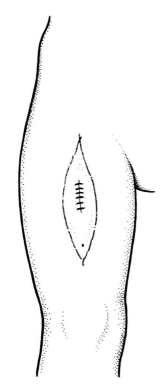

Figure 2–2 • Wide local excision after confirmation of histologic presence of tumor. Re-excision should be considered to ensure negative margins wherever possible.

cised without biopsy, because it was believed that any breach of the tumor capsule would promote intraperitoneal spread. Effective chemotherapy has probably obviated this rationale, but the policy continues because the risk of performing an unnecessary nephrectomy under these circumstances is practically nil. FNA, core biopsy, or incisional biopsy is useful to confirm diagnosis in patients with bilateral Wilms' tumors who will receive preoperative chemotherapy to allow for minimal resection, leaving enough kidney tissue to provide adequate renal function. This approach may also be necessary for larger, unresectable Wilms' tumors that will require preoperative chemotherapy before resection is safe.

The diagnosis of neuroblastoma is frequently made by other studies before the primary tumor is exposed, but in some patients the neuroblastomas are not disseminated and markers are not definite. These cases mandate differentiation between neuroblastomas and other tumors of the abdomen or mediastinum. Obviously, knowledge of the tumor histology will direct the aggressiveness of the local resection.

The diagnosis of rhabdomyosarcoma is usually made by a direct open biopsy, because no helpful markers or specific imaging studies exist for this disease. The pathologist is expected to identify the histologic subgroups of rhabdomyosarcoma to allow adequate staging and direct therapy. For this purpose, several grams of tissue for study are needed. Biopsies of genitourinary rhabdomyosarcomas are frequently done through the endoscope. Although these are predominately embryonal subtypes, larger biopsies are helpful to the pathologist.

The needle biopsies that are performed to establish the diagnosis of prostatic rhabdomyosarcomas are difficult to interpret and must include several cores. Trunk and extremity rhabdomyosarcomas should be approached through excisional or incisional biopsy techniques, with the incision placed so that it will not interfere with the incision required for a subsequent wide local excision. This excision is usually a vertical one in extremities. Wide local excision with clear margins is preferable for definitive surgery whenever possible.

Limb-sparing is an important goal. Fewer than 5% of extremity tumors now require amputation. When biopsy is performed without knowledge of the diagnosis or when the margins are positive, re-excision of the primary site to achieve tumor-free margins improves survival[19]. Regional nodes should be sampled so that appropriate local irradiation can be directed to positive nodes. Surgical removal of the primary site offers the best outcome. After wide local excision, the margins should be checked for tumor.

In patients with ovarian solid tumors, the diagnosis is frequently suggested or indicated by a biochemical marker. The patients may undergo a biopsy or an oophorectomy for biopsy purposes if the tumor involves most of the ovary. If a malignant or teratoid tumor is identified by this procedure, the other ovary is inspected and biopsied or incised longitudinally for inspection of its interior. Biopsy of apparently abnormal areas is then done. Potential abdominal tumor implants or omental nodules should be biopsied for neoplasia. If a solid testicular tumor is identified by biopsy, the previously occluded cord vessels are divided, and the testicle and cord structures up to the internal inguinal ring are removed for examination (Fig. 2–3).

Teratomas and other germ-cell tumors pose major risks in that sampling error may lead to failure in identifying malignant elements. If feasible, excisional biopsies are recommended to allow the pathologist to examine multiple sites within the tumor.

Isolated, deep intrahepatic masses present special biopsy problems. Although needle biopsy cores may not enable a precise diagnosis, if they clearly indicate the presence of a malignant neoplasm confined to a resectable portion of the liver, formal lobectomy is ordinarily performed at the same time. At some institutions, if it is thought that the tumor is a hepatoblastoma, the resectability of which may be increased by initial chemotherapy, resection is delayed. This approach is used quite often at M.D. Anderson Cancer Center.[20, 21]

INTRAOPERATIVE TECHNIQUES

A variety of special techniques may be considered for operating on small children with large tumors. Certain obvious considerations to mini-

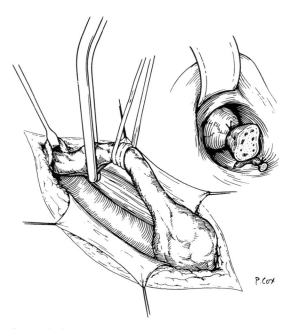

Figure 2–3 • A paratesticular mass should be resected by inguinal orchidectomy, with complete resection of the spermatic cord structures to the level of the internal ring.

mize intraoperative blood loss and the need for massive transfusion in small children with relatively limited blood volume may be helpful. Acute euvolumic hemodilution was first used in patients undergoing cardiopulmonary bypass and is currently used for many types of surgical procedures when significant blood loss is anticipated.[22] This technique involves autologous blood transfusion. After the decision is made that the tumor can be resected, the patient's blood is withdrawn into citrate phosphate dextrose bags at room temperature. A predetermined amount of blood is withdrawn to reduce the hematocrit to 20%. As each cubic centimeter of blood is withdrawn, it is replaced with 3 cc of lactated Ringer's solution containing 2 mEg/L of magnesium. As further intraoperative blood loss occurs, the blood is replaced with equal volumes of lactated Ringer's solution. Blood volume is maintained in this way until the hematocrit falls below 14%. At this point, the patient is transfused with donor blood. After blood loss is controlled, the patient is transfused with his or her own blood and furosemide is given to promote a rapid excretion of the administered crystalloid solution.

When hemodilution techniques are employed, the blood loss has fewer red blood cells; therefore, the actual blood volume lost is decreased. Diluted blood also has decreased viscosity and may enhance tissue profusion. Hemodilution is often combined with two other techniques that complement the hemodilution by decreasing the myocardial work. Deliberate induction of a hypotensive state with deep halothane anesthesia, nitroprusside or nitroglycerin combined with propranolol or labetalol, to prevent reflex tachycardia may keep coronary profusion and cerebral blood flow stable even if systolic and diastolic pressures are reduced by up to 40% of the normal pressures for age. Myocardial workload is thus decreased. The myocardial workload and tissue oxygen demands may be decreased by induced hypothermia to 32°C. The need for oxygen decreases at a rate of 5% to 9% for each 1°C decrease. Combinations of these techniques have been reported on by Schaller and colleagues[22] in their series of surgical resections of pediatric liver tumors. Bank blood transfusion was necessary for only three of the eight patients, and transfusion requirements were markedly decreased. No apparent effect on liver function, blood coagulation, or liver regeneration was noted.

Another method of reducing operative blood loss is radiologic tumor embolization. Preoperative tumor embolization may allow resection with less blood loss, although the technologic limitations of embolization in a pediatric patient may limit its usefulness. Intraoperative arterial embolization to facilitate resection has been described.[23]

Another technique frequently used at M.D. Anderson Cancer Center to minimize blood loss in patients undergoing liver resection is total hepatic vascular occlusion. After dissection of the portahepatis and inferior and superior vena cava, large volumes of lactated Ringer's solution are given to maximize intravascular volume. All clamps are then applied, and during total vascular occlusion, the liver resection is performed. This procedure allows for extensive resection with minimal blood loss. Normothermic hepatic vascular occlusion has been performed for 45–60 minutes without adverse hepatic effects. The relatively avascular field allows for simple dissection. This technique is similar to that in pediatric liver transplantation.

Other techniques for minimizing blood loss—including ultrasonic aspirator, argon laser beam, cryotherapy, and high-speed water jet resection—are beyond the scope of this chapter.

MINIMALLY INVASIVE SURGERY

Minimally invasive surgery for routine laparoscopic procedures such as appendectomy, herniorrhaphy, fundoplication, and cholecystectomy has become quite common. Laparoscopic and thoracoscopic biopsy and staging of malignancies have been done on a more limited basis but have proved valuable.[24] Determining the extent of disease, the resectability of tumor, and the possibility of recurrent or residual tumor is a good indication for laparoscopic intervention. Video-assisted thorascopic surgery has been employed for determining the extent of disease and for performing biopsies on tumors as well as for diagnosing metastatic disease.

In the Children's Cancer Group experience, 25 children with cancer underwent laparoscopic operation.[25] In the 16 cases in which biopsy was performed, diagnostic tissue was obtained in every case. No mortality or morbidity was associated with the laparoscopic operation. The procedure was deemed successful in all cases.

Thoracoscopic diagnosis and management of lesions in children have been common for many years.[26] In children, the most frequent indication for thoracoscopy has been for biopsy or resection of mediastinal and hilar masses. Other indications in children include biopsy of diffuse and localized pulmonary infiltrates, irrigation for empyema with debridement, and other benign conditions. In the Children's Cancer Group experience, the most common indications for thoracoscopy were evaluation of metastatic disease, suspected malignancy in a new mass, and lung biopsy in cancer patients with respiratory failure or pulmonary infiltrates.[25]

Thoracoscopic surgery in children has proved a relatively simple and successful way to obtain adequate tissue. Thus, minimally invasive surgery in the pediatric oncology patient should be at least considered as part of the diagnostic staging and therapeutic evaluation. Dr. George W. Holcomb,[25] a pioneer in minimally invasive surgery for children and the lead investigator of the Children's Cancer Group experience, provides an excellent overview in Chapter 7.

PREOPERATIVE EVALUATION

The evaluation of the pediatric oncology patient before major surgery varies somewhat from that of adults or even nononcologic pediatric patients. As many children with cancer require multiple operations or invasive diagnostic procedures, early consultation with the pediatric anesthesiologist is important. Routine preoperative evaluation is necessary to exclude congenital or familial problems such as a bleeding disorder or malignant hyperthermia. Anemias and coagulation defects are frequent in this population.

Because many children with cancer are immunosuppressed from the disease or the therapy, associated infections or wound-healing problems should be investigated. Many patients may have had treatment with chemotherapy or irradiation prior to surgery and thus may have resulting cardiopulmonary abnormalities. Possible exposure to cardiotoxic drugs may require cardiology consultation and echocardiogram.

Pulmonary function tests may be necessary in patients who have received previous radiation or drugs affecting pulmonary status. Children undergoing pulmonary resection for recurrent metastatic disease may require pulmonary function tests and evaluation of pulmonary status prior to further surgery. Patients with minimal pulmonary reserve may require more vigorous postoperative pulmonary toilet, including incentive spirometry, bronchodilator, and perhaps early antibiotic therapy.

A number of chemotherapeutic agents may adversely affect coagulation status, or platelets. Perhaps the most accurate indicator of adequate coagulation is a normal bleeding time. Generally, a platelet count above 30,000–50,000 is preferable, although platelet transfusion at the time of surgical intervention is often necessary to have adequate levels. Many patients requiring operative placement of indwelling lines or ports may undergo placement with platelet counts even below 5000.

Patients with markedly elevated white blood cell counts secondary to acute leukemia may require leukophoresis or exchange transfusion prior to anesthesia and surgical procedures. Close attention to liver and renal function is important, because many agents adversely affect function of these organs. Routine electrolyte, phosphate, and calcium levels should be evaluated also.

Individual considerations are necessary when dealing with large tumors in certain locations. For example, patients with large anterior mediastinal masses are at risk for respiratory collapse on induction of anesthesia. Many patients with lymphomas, teratomas, or neuroblastomas may present with large anterior mediastinal masses or superior vena cava syndrome. Biopsy using sedation or CT guidance may allow treatment and reduction of tumor mass before the patient undergoes general anesthesia.

Shamberger and coworkers[27] described a prospective evaluation of 31 pediatric patients with anterior mediastinal masses. Patients were evaluated for tracheal cross-sectional area and peak expiratory flow rate. Those patients who had either a tracheal area or peak expiratory flow rate less than 50% of predicted for their age and size underwent only local anesthesia. Under these guidelines, all children underwent uneventful anesthesia. Cross-sectional tracheal area evaluation by CT scan and pulmonary function testing should be performed in all children with large mediastinal masses before a general anesthetic is administered. Patients are classified by the Standard American Society of Anesthesiologists' Physical Status Classification.

ANESTHESIA FOR CANCER SURGERY

The anesthesiologist preparing a child for cancer surgery must consider the cardiorespiratory effects of the tumor itself and the possibility of massive blood or fluid losses as well as specific endocrine effects of the tumor. The location, type, and size of the primary tumor may affect the initiation of anesthesia. Large intra-abdominal masses may affect gastric emptying or may lead to partial small bowel obstruction, requiring changes in the method of anesthesia induction. Intra-operative monitoring has been shown to improve the care of patients during general anesthesia. Such monitoring involves pericardial or esophageal stethoscopes, continuous electrocardiography and pulse oximetry, measurement of end-tidal carbon dioxide, and automated monitoring of blood pressure and body temperature.

Large abdominal tumors and hepatic tumors may require cross-clamping of major vessels to impede venous return to the heart. Resection of these large tumors requires large central venous access for monitoring and infusion. Catheters should be placed in the upper extremities, neck, or superior vena cava. Arterial catheterization for continuous blood pressure monitoring and measurement of blood gases is mandatory. Bladder catheter drainage is important in intra-abdominal surgery for decompressing the bladder as well as monitoring adequate urine output. Adequate profusion is frequently reflected by maintenance of good urinary output. Dr. Kimberly Nesbitt and her colleagues provide an up-to-date review of anesthesia techniques in Chapter 3.

MOLECULAR BIOLOGY AND TUMOR MARKERS

The development of clinically applicable molecular biology and the identification of specific tumor markers will undoubtedly influence cancer therapy experimentally in the coming years. Currently, surgeons are asked to supply additional tissue for histologic evaluation including diagnostic and prognostic factors. High-risk patients may be considered for prophylactic resections. A number of ethical decisions will be part of the decision-making process as regards high-risk patients. New therapies and intensity of treatment may be directed by specific markers or genetic findings. Perhaps genetic manipulation may be a form of therapy in some instances.

Dramatic advances in cellular biology and recombinant DNA technology have focused attention on cancer as a genetic disorder. Pediatric malignancies such as retinoblastoma and Wilms' tumor, which were among the first malignancies to be recognized as occurring in familial clusters, provided important early evidence of a heritable, genetic component of cancer etiology.[28, 29] Development of advanced techniques for the visualization and characterization of chromosomes led to the identification of disease-associated, nonrandom genetic rearrangements in a wide variety of tumors. Gene mapping has made it possible to identify both the precise location and the structural alteration of genes involved in tumor-specific chromosomal rearrangements.[30] An increasing number of malignancies have been recognized as associated with specific genetic alterations. The importance of genetic rearrangements for the diagnosis and classification of patients with cancer is likely to increase.

Cytogenetic studies of leukemias and lymphomas have proceeded much more rapidly than similar studies of solid tumors. Advances in cytogenetic studies for pediatric solid tumors have been the focus for a number of cooperative research efforts. Developments in recombinant DNA technology and molecular biology are having a direct impact on clinical oncology. Types of DNA hybridization analysis in the evaluation of human tumor specimens are discussed in detail by Dr. Robert S. Sawin in Chapter 6.

Genes that are altered in the development of cancer fall into three broad categories: (1) oncogenes, the presence of which may cause cellular transformation; (2) tumor-suppressor genes, the absence of which may cause cellular transformation; and (3) mutator genes.

Proto-oncogenes are genes present in normal cells that, when activated to become *oncogenes*, may lead to the transformation of the cell. The alterations that convert the normal cellular gene to its oncogenic counterpart include gene amplifications, translocations, and point mutations. *Amplifications* result from an increase in the copy number of the gene. *Translocations* refer to the exchange of DNA segments between two chromosomes. *Point mutations* are single nucleotide changes or deletions that can result in an alteration of the gene product.[31] When activated, oncogenes such as *ras*, *neu/erb* B2, and *myc* acquire or gain function and begin to act in a more dominant fashion. Mutations in a single allele may, therefore, contribute to cancer development. About 70 oncogenes have been identified since the first oncogene (*src*) was discovered in 1975.

In contrast with the proto-oncogenes and oncogenes, researchers have also identified about 12 *tumor-suppressor genes*. Tumor-suppressor genes are different from oncogenes in that it is their loss of function, rather than gain of function, that may contribute to cancer development. Although the first known tumor-suppressor gene (Rb) was not cloned until 1986, these genes are now known to be common defects in many cancers. For example, the tumor-suppressor gene p53 is mutated in as many as 50% of human cancers.

The *mutator gene* is responsible for enhancing the fidelity of the DNA replication process. When mutator gene products fail to function, the mutation rate in the cell increases and an inherent predisposition to cancer is observed.

Practical application of some of this knowledge is demonstrated by the extensively studied pediatric tumor, neuroblastoma. Neuroblastoma is the most common extracranial solid malignancy of childhood. The clinical course of neuroblastoma can be unpredictable, with intrastage variability in response to similar treatments common in advanced stages. N-*myc*, a proto-oncogene encoding a gene-regulatory protein, has been demonstrated to be amplified within neuroblastoma cells. The number of copies of the N-*myc* gene in tissue present at different sites is similar to the number present in primary versus metastatic lesions. The copy number is related to the clinical aggressiveness of the tumor and is a prognostic indicator independent of stage and age. N-*myc* amplification associated with any clinical stage or age places the patient at high risk for recurrence. Patients with Stage 3 or 4 disease and high amplification of N-*myc* may benefit from complete versus subtotal resection, whereas aggressive resection of all tumors may not affect survival intervals for those with low amplification of N-*myc*. Patients with Stage 1, 2, or 4 disease with high amplification of N-*myc* should be selected to undergo more aggressive therapy.

Further developments will undoubtedly affect approaches to surgical management of pediatric tumors in the future as well as possible preventive interventions in high-risk patients.

CHEMOTHERAPY

Since the introduction of drug therapy for childhood leukemia almost 40 years ago,[32] the overall prognosis for children with cancer has improved dramatically. The striking increase in survival is directly related to anticancer drugs along with surgical intervention and radiotherapy.[33] The significantly higher response rates achieved by combining active agents into multidrug regimens were initially demonstrated in children with acute lymphoblastic leukemia. Such combination chemotherapy improved both the remission rate and the duration of remission compared with single-agent therapy.[34] The treatment of children with Wilms' tumor serves as a model both for the multidisciplinary, or multimodal, approach and for an adjuvant chemotherapy in patients who are without clinical evidence of residual disease following local therapy with surgery or radiation, but who are at risk for recurrence.

Most of the common pediatric solid tumors, such as rhabdomyosarcoma, lymphoma, Ewing's sarcoma, and osteosarcoma, are now managed with a multimodal approach combining surgery or radiotherapy for the primary tumor and early intensive adjuvant chemotherapy for control of micrometastases.[35] The value of neoadjuvant (preoperative) chemotherapy has been demonstrated in the treatment of several pediatric neoplasms, including osteosarcoma, hepatoblastoma, and rhabdomyosarcoma. The doses and schedules of drug administration are critical in achieving a maximum benefit from chemotherapy.

In patients with no evidence of residual disease following local therapy with surgery or radiation, "prophylactic," or adjuvant, chemotherapy is administered when the risk of recurrent disease at distant sites is high. The efficacy of adjuvant chemotherapy has been established for most of the common pediatric cancers, including Wilms' tumor, Ewing's sarcoma, lymphoma, rhabdomyosarcoma, astrocytoma, retinoblastoma, and osteosarcoma. Specific drugs and treatment protocols are reviewed in Chapter 4 and in the tumor-specific chapters.

RADIOTHERAPY

The surgeon and radiotherapist work collaboratively to control local disease. The rationale for preoperative or postoperative irradiation has been based on the failure patterns of the two modalities of surgery and irradiation. Recurrence after local or radical surgical excision implies residual microscopic disease at the operative margins; recurrence after radiation therapy in general is related to large tumor volume, with an excess of clonogenic tumor cells beyond the number that can be destroyed by locally tolerated doses of radiation.[36] With combined therapy, the goals are to remove all macroscopic disease by surgery, reducing the cell mass, and to eradicate peripheral extensions of disease beyond the operative margins by radiation therapy. The principles of radiotherapy are discussed in Chapter 5.

WILMS' TUMOR (NEPHROBLASTOMA)

The management of Wilms' tumor has been the model by which the multimodal approach to cancer therapy for all tumors has been judged. Surgical excision remains the cornerstone of the management of Wilms' tumor; however, a dramatic improvement in overall survival rate has resulted from the coordinated use of surgery, multiple-drug chemotherapy, and radiation therapy.

Nephroblastoma is the most common solid abdominal tumor in childhood and usually appears as a painless abdominal mass in an otherwise well child. Radical nephrectomy is the primary treatment for unilateral Wilms' tumor. The presence of secondary deposits, caval tumor, bilateral disease, or tumor in a solitary kidney is indication for Tru-Cut or FNA biopsy, chemotherapy, and delayed partial or total nephrectomy.

In a patient with unilateral nephroblastoma, the tumor is almost always excised without biopsy before the institution of chemotherapeutic regimens, even in the presence of dissemination. Some centers recommend needle biopsy and preoperative chemotherapy prior to delayed nephrectomy.

A generous transverse upper abdominal incision is required to facilitate complete exposure of both kidneys. The abdominal contents are examined for liver or peritoneal spread. The contralateral kidney is fully mobilized and examined on both anterior and posterior surfaces in order to detect previously unsuspected bilateral disease. Biopsy of tissue only from the main tumor and contralateral lesion is performed under these circumstances. If the disease is found to be unilateral, the colon and mesentery are dissected from the anterior surface of the tumor and reflected medially. Patients with bilateral tumors are managed with biopsy followed by chemotherapy without attempts at primary resection. Specific surgical management is detailed by Dr. Michael Ritchey in Chapter 9.

NEUROBLASTOMA

Neuroblastoma is the most common extracranial solid tumor of childhood. Surgical therapy may be diagnostic, therapeutic, and palliative. Preoperative surgical evaluation is critically important to aid the surgeon in operative decisions, such as the approach and the extent of resection.

The patient should be adequately monitored at the time of operation by Doppler's pulse-recording and arterial line for blood gas values and blood pressure determinations. When the patient presents with metastatic disease, the most accessible tissues are chosen for diagnosis. FNA or large bore biopsy are being done with increasing frequency. Adequate tissue, usually in the range of 1–5 g, for biologic studies has become more important in selecting the appropriate therapy for neuroblastoma. The tissue should be preserved and frozen rather than placed in a fixative.

Operative procedures include complete gross excision, partial excision, or biopsy. Staging is employed to provide prognostic information, to determine objective criteria for making therapeutic decisions, and to permit comparative evaluation of clinical trials. Staging can be clinical (preoperative), operative (surgical), or postoperative. Several staging systems, including the Evans, the POG, and the International Neuroblastoma Staging System, have been described.

For Stage 1 and resectable 2 and 3 disease, initial resection is routine. In the Children's Cancer Group, patients with Stages 2, 3, and 4 (Evans) with unfavorable histology and N-*myc* greater than three copies are usually managed in identical fashion by delayed excision. Excision at any point during the course of therapy confers an overall survival advantage.

With Stage 4 disease, initial excision of the primary tumor does not appear to increase survival duration. After clinical complete response has been achieved by chemotherapy, delayed excision of the primary is performed if feasible.

In Stage 4s disease, excision of the primary tumor, either initial or delayed, has not been demonstrated to affect survival. If tumor mass remains after metastatic foci have been eliminated, excision of the primary tumor is usually carried out.

Abdominal tumors are usually approached through a generous transverse incision, depending upon the level of the tumor. Adrenal tumors are generally easier to remove than central tumors that surround or are attached to the celiac axis or mesenteric vessels. Usually the tumor can be separated from the kidney unless the renal vessels are involved. Although preoperative evaluation with CT or ultrasound may suggest invasion into the inferior surface of the liver, such has generally not been found in the experience at M.D. Anderson Cancer Center. A plane can be developed with an adequate capsule allowing for resection of the tumor without the need for hepatic resection. As the tumor does not generally invade the vessels, but rather compresses the vessels, an adventitial plane can be developed to separate the tumor from surrounding structures.

Because large tumors may frequently change the course of the vena cava, aorta, or related vessels, care must be taken not to injure the superior mesenteric artery or other vital structures. Numerous large vessels engaged by tumor can lead to intraoperative bleeding but can usually be controlled with packing or electrocautery. Packing, pressure, and paying attention to dissecting the tumor and ligating the major supplying vessels may result in less operative time and blood loss than trying to control each of these tumor-engaged vessels. Experience with dissecting large adrenal tumors or midline masses and familiarity with the anatomy decreases operative time and operative complications. Some surgeons may consider many of these larger lesions unresectable, but at M.D. Anderson Cancer Center, the majority of such tumors could be resected safely by properly entering the capsular plane surrounding the tumor.

Thoracic neuroblastomas are generally removed through a posterior lateral thoracotomy. Extension of the neuroblastoma into the foramina can be done through posterior laminectomy prior to thoracotomy. Frequently the tumor remains extradural and can be freed from the extradural space. Most patients will not need chest-wall resection, but large recurrences or extensions through the intercostal spaces can be managed with a resection of the ribs and an aggressive approach. Free margins can be obtained in this way, frequently in conjunction with partial pulmonary resection. This aggressive approach has proved helpful in treating a number of children with recurrent disease. The policy at M.D. Anderson Cancer Center is to reconstruct the chest with a Gore-Tex patch and muscle flaps. Extensive rib resections are rarely needed in children with neuroblastoma.

Formal lymph node dissection is not performed. Lymph node biopsies are routinely done as part of the excision. The overall complication rate is low. The most common complications include bleeding, diaphragmatic tear during intraoperative dissection, and postoperative atelectasis or late bowel obstruction. For further details on neuroblastoma, see Chapter 10.

RHABDOMYOSARCOMA

Rhabdomyosarcoma is the most common soft-tissue sarcoma in infants and children.[37] Staging for rhabdomyosarcoma is performed in order to classify the extent of the disease for different treatment regimens as well as to compare outcomes. The clinical grouping system developed by the Intergroup Rhabdomyosarcoma Study (IRS) is based upon pretreatment and operative outcome. Its basic premise is that total tumor extirpation at the original operation is the best hope for cure and stratifies cases according to tumor resectability. This premise has led to aggressive and often mutilating procedures in an effort to accomplish complete surgical removal of the primary tumor. The IRS system does not take into account the biologic nature or natural history of the tumor, nor the experience and aggressiveness of the operating surgeon. Attempts have been made to supplant the IRS system with one that takes into account the site and histologic peculiarities of the tumor.

The treatment strategy for rhabdomyosarcoma requires a multidisciplinary approach involving surgeons, oncologists, radiation-oncologists, and pathologists. As with most uncommon tumors, entry into a treatment protocol, such as the IRS-IV, correlates with better outcomes than treatment outside such studies.

Surgical treatment of rhabdomyosarcoma is site-specific. Two general principles are that (1) complete wide excision of the primary tumor and surrounding uninvolved tissues should be performed while preserving cosmesis and function where possible and (2) incomplete excision or tumor debunking is not beneficial and should not be performed, nor should severely mutilating or debilitating excisions. Secondary excision after initial biopsy and neoadjuvant therapy has a better outcome than partial or incomplete resection and should be planned in cases in which primary excision is not possible. What was originally a massive soft-tissue tumor will often show a dramatic reduction in size after chemotherapy or radiation therapy, thereby allowing successful, delayed resection.

When initial excision is not possible, incisional biopsy only is employed, along with biopsy of clinically suspicious-looking lymph nodes as indicated. Pathologic evaluation of clinically uninvolved nodes is site specific, as in cases of extremity lesions and incompletely resected paratesticular tumors. Needle biopsy or FNA may be safer in certain situations but may not provide adequate tissue for special histologic, cytologic, and biochemical studies.

In some patients with extremity or trunk rhabdomyosarcomas, initial tumor resection may appear to be complete, but then positive margins are discovered on histopathologic review, corresponding to Clinical Group IIA—Microscopic Residual Disease. In many of these cases, a *primary re-excision* (PRE) is possible, achieving wider and, it is hoped, negative surgical margins. The report by Hays and coworkers[19] demonstrates the benefit of PRE in this group. In IRS-I and IRS-II, 154 patients with extremity or trunk rhabdomyosarcoma were initially placed in Clinical Group IIA; 41 underwent successful PRE and were converted to Clinical Group I prior to the onset of adjuvant therapy. These patients were compared with 113 patients with microscopic residual disease who did not undergo PRE and 73 patients who were free of disease after the initial resection (Clinical Group I). For the 41 PRE patients, the 3-year Kaplan-Meier survival estimate was 91%, compared with 74% for Group IIA patients who did not undergo PRE and 74% for Clinical Group I patients.

This PRE approach may be applicable to tumors of other locations as well. PRE should be considered even if the margins are apparently negative when the initial resection was not a "cancer" operation or when malignancy was not suspected preoperatively.

Second-look operations (SLO) have been used for several pediatric tumors to evaluate therapeutic response and to remove any residual tumor after completing initial therapy. The utility of SLO was evaluated in IRS-III and shown to be beneficial in Clinical Group III rhabdomyosarcoma patients. Wiener and coworkers[38] evaluated separately 257 patients from IRS-III in Clinical Group II (excluding special pelvic sites). SLO was performed in 21% of patients with complete response (CR), 66% of patients with partial response (PR), and 52% of patients with clinical nonresponse (NR). The performance of SLO changed the response status in a significant number of patients; 12% of presumed CR patients were found to harbor residual tumor, whereas 74% of both PR and NR patients were recategorized as CR after operation. The survival rates for these recategorized PR and NR patients were similar to those for patients confirmed to be CR at re-exploration; clinically NR patients who were reassigned to CR after SLO enjoyed a 73% survival rate compared with an 80% survival rate for all CR patients. Of equal importance, those patients who were recategorized as CR avoided more toxic second-line treatment regimens.

Biopsy of possible metastatic sites, such as the lungs, may also be warranted. The lungs are the most common site for distant metastasis. Pretreatment Stage 4 or Clinical Group IV patients have a significantly worse survival rate. Most patients with lung metastases have not had histologic confirmation. In the experience at M.D. Anderson Cancer Center, single-lung metastases are rare, and biopsy frequently demonstrates an infectious process. It is likely that at least some patients treated as Group IV, because of a single metastasis, may not have had metastatic disease, but rather a benign process. Histologic confirmation of questionable lung metastases, and particularly single-lung lesions, is recommended. This confirmation can be obtained in many cases by thoracoscopic biopsy. Little if any documenta-

tion exists that resection of all metastases improves survival, although such resections have been done at M.D. Anderson Cancer Center for resistant lung disease when the primary tumor has been controlled.

The specific principles of surgical management vary with anatomical location, but, in general, the principle of wide local excision without destroying function is appropriate. The likelihood of growth from microscopic residual neoplasm when simple resection of an undiagnosed soft-tissue tumor has been performed is so high that reoperation is recommended as the initial definitive approach to management.

Head and neck orbital rhabdomyosarcomas are the most common types. Although wide excision is appropriate if it can be performed without significant cosmetic defects, conservative biopsy and chemotherapy are frequently employed. Incidence of cervical node involvement is low; therefore, biopsy is performed only for clinically positive nodes.

The approach to bladder prostate primaries is also more conservative today than was previously the case. Bladder salvage has increased.[39, 40] Anterior pelvic exenteration is no longer considered as initial therapy for pelvic rhabdomyosarcomas.[41]

A paratesticular mass should be resected by inguinal orchiectomy. Complete resection of the spermatic cord structures is done to the level of the internal ring. Initial *retroperitoneal lymph node dissection* (RLND) for paratesticular rhabdomyosarcoma was based upon the management of non-rhabdomyosarcoma testicular malignancies and the high incidence of retroperitoneal lymph node involvement. RLND was performed mainly for staging, and positive nodes were treated with radiation. The role of RLND in paratesticular rhabdomyosarcoma is controversial.[42, 43] It is clear, however, that even with advances in imaging, there is a significant false-negative rate of CT — 14% for IRS-III patients. If positive nodes are not properly treated, recurrence of disease may increase. Perhaps experience with laparoscopic evaluation of the retroperitoneal lymph nodes may allow for better delineation of nodal status without the complications of RLND. These issues are discussed in detail in Chapter 12.

Vaginal rhabdomyosarcoma is accompanied by vaginal discharge or prolapse. The diagnosis is made by vaginoscopy and biopsy of the lesion. Treatment at one time consisted of extensive anterior pelvic exenteration, but when this tumor was found to be very chemosensitive, definitive surgery was delayed until after an initial course of therapy.

Delayed tumor resection may consist of partial vaginectomy. Bladder salvage is possible in most patients. Vaginal tumors originate mainly from the anterior vaginal wall; they may invade the vesicovaginal septum, or bladder wall, because of its proximity. Cystoscopy is warranted during initial evaluation and at intervals during follow-up. Evidence exists that repeated biopsy and chemotherapy without resection may be adequate for many patients.[44] We are now caring for a number of patients in this manner without evidence of recurrence.

Extremity rhabdomyosarcomas represented 19% of all patients in IRS-III.[45] Prognostic factors, including local tissue invasiveness, tumor size, nodal and distal metastases, and site, were previously described.[46] Limb-sparing, wide local excision is the treatment of choice. Amputation is rarely necessary, except perhaps in very distal lesions that can be made Group I by amputation.

Careful determination of margin status is extremely important, and re-resection at initial or subsequent operation is warranted. It has been the policy at M.D. Anderson Cancer Center to recommend re-excision for all patients referred after previous resection, no matter what was previously reported. Patients reported to have had total resection have been found to have residual or even gross disease. Patients reported to have had positive margins have, on occasion, had gross disease present. Thus, re-excision in all cases, particularly when the diagnosis was uncertain at the original operation, may significantly enhance survival.

Lymph node involvement in patients with extremity rhabdomyosarcomas was reported to be between 12% and 17% in IRS-I and IRS-II.[47, 48] LaQuaglia and coworkers[49] reported a 40% incidence of regional node involvement. Few patients in IRS-I and IRS-II underwent lymph node evaluation, whereas the majority did in LaQuaglia's study. In IRS-III, 36 patients had formal lymph node dissections; 17 of these patients had nodal metastasis and 19 did not. Of the 56 patients who underwent only lymph node biopsy, 19 had positive results, and 37 had nega-

tive results. The remaining 97 patients had no histologic confirmation of lymph node status. Thus, 39% of patients had positive results on biopsy.[45] This incidence correlates with that found by LaQuaglia and coworkers[49] and suggests that more frequent evaluation of nodes may be indicated.

Survival rates were significantly better for patients with histologically negative nodes in the study by LaQuaglia and coworkers.[49] Formal lymph node dissection did not improve survival, but all patients with positive nodes underwent irradiation. Histologic evaluation of regional nodes is strongly recommended at M.D. Anderson Cancer Center. Such evaluation enables proper staging and prognostic evaluations. Moreover, positive results warrant nodal irradiation, which may prevent regional recurrence and enhance survival.

Consideration of sentinel node mapping[50, 51] with blue dye or lymphoscintigraphy may prove helpful in determining which nodes to biopsy. Such mapping has proved valuable in treating patients with melanomas and breast cancers and is being evaluated for treating patients with rhabdomyosarcomas. Limited experience at M.D. Anderson Cancer Center with this technique for extremity rhabdomyosarcomas has been encouraging.

In conclusion, the basic surgical principles for treating patients with rhabdomyosarcomas depend upon the site of the primary tumor. Initial surgery should be conservative, with re-excision when possible and second-look surgery used frequently. The advisability of lymph node biopsy varies with site. Treatment of positive node may help decrease the risk of local regional recurrence.

SOFT-TISSUE SARCOMAS OF CHILDHOOD

The most common soft-tissue sarcoma in children is rhabdomyosarcoma; however, 47% of all soft-tissue sarcomas in children have a histology other than rhabdomyosarcoma.[52] These other tumors make up 3% of all tumors in children. Soft-tissue sarcomas in adolescents behave the same as those in adults, but soft-tissue sarcomas in children and infants are associated with a better prognosis.

The most common sites of presentation are

the extremities and trunk, with retroperitoneal occurrence often present. The usual approach to treatment for adults or adolescents is wide local excision, generally with local radiation therapy. Although chemotherapy for soft-tissue sarcomas is controversial, it has often been added in some trials. Treatment for children is site-specific and generally more conservative because the clinical course tends to be more benign than in adolescents. Different biologic behaviors accompany sarcomas of similar histologies in adults as compared with children. For an extensive review of nonrhabdomyosarcoma soft tissue sarcomas, see Chapter 18.

Long-term follow-up and aggressive screening for second malignancies in children previously treated for malignancy are important. At M.D. Anderson Cancer Center,[50] patients presented with malignant fibrous histiocytoma as a second malignant neoplasm.[53] Average time between tumors was 10 years (range .2–36 years). Whereas 50% of the malignant fibrous histiocytomas developed in irradiated fields, the other 50% developed outside irradiated fields, suggesting a genetic predisposition for tumor development.

Second malignant neoplasms are aggressive, associated with only a 33% survival rate at 2 years and a 13% survival rate at 5 years. At M.D. Anderson Cancer Center, 20 patients had second malignant neoplasms after treatment for primary childhood soft-tissue sarcomas.[4] Most primary tumors were rhabdomyosarcomas (13 of 20 patients); half occurred in an extremity (10 of 20 patients). In 90% of patients (18 of 20), there was a complete response to treatment of the primary cancer. Combined chemotherapy and radiation therapy were administered to 11 of the 20 patients. The most common second malignancy was a bone sarcoma (6 of 20). Four of the bone sarcomas developed in the field of radiation treatment. Survival after a second malignancy was only 30%. Two patients developed a third malignant neoplasm.

HEPATOBLASTOMA

Hepatoblastomas are the most frequent malignant liver tumors in children. Hepatocellular carcinomas tend to occur in older children but occasionally occur in younger children in the first few years of life. The most common symptoms of primary liver malignancies are an upper abdominal mass or a generalized abdominal enlargement. The diagnostic evaluation should delineate the following: (1) extent of intrahepatic disease, (2) potential for hepatic resectability, and (3) presence or absence of extrahepatic disease. Minimal evaluation should include the patient history and physical examination plus routine laboratory tests, including liver function studies, clotting studies, CT of the abdomen and chest, alpha-fetoprotein (AFP) measurement, and chest roentgenograms. Hepatic angiography is rarely employed.

Surgical resection continues to be the mainstay of therapy. Past reports indicated a high mortality, significant blood loss, and morbidity associated with resection. Better techniques, such as total hepatic isolation, have reduced blood loss and complications. For many years, preoperative chemotherapy has been advocated at M.D. Anderson Cancer Center to shrink the size of the tumor, making surgical resection simpler and reducing blood loss.[54, 55] Re-resection is employed for locally recurrent hepatic tumors or for inadequate margins obtained at the first procedure. Hepatic tumors metastasize most frequently to the lungs, and an aggressive approach is taken in excision of pulmonary metastases for these tumors.[56]

AFP is a valuable marker for monitoring the residual, recurrent, or metastatic disease following resection of the primary tumor or for monitoring the response of an unresectable primary tumor to therapy. Overall, newer intraoperative techniques and preoperative chemotherapy combined with extensive resection have improved local control, enhanced survival, and reduced postoperative complications (see Chapter 11).

LYMPHOMAS

The surgical role in treating most patients with lymphomas is frequently limited to biopsy, vascular access, or staging. Occasionally patients will present with obstructing non-Hodgkin's lymphoma of the gastrointestinal tract that necessitates biopsy or resection. Surgical staging for Hodgkin's disease is still sometimes used in certain institutions. Surgical staging involves laparotomy with splenectomy; multiple liver biopsies; and sampling of multiple lymph nodes from the splenic hilum, celiac axis, porta hepatis, right and left, high and low periaortic areas, right and left, common and external iliac areas, and a mesenteric lymph node. This procedure should be performed in a concise manner, separating each sample for the pathologist to examine.

Although partial splenectomy and selective splenectomy have been advocated by some investigators, these procedures have a significant risk of false-negative assessment (12%–15%) of the extent of disease. Periaortic lymph nodes should coincide with the large lymph nodes seen on CT scan or lymphangiography. In girls, a bilateral oophoropexy should be performed by mobilizing and tacking the ovaries in the midline behind the uterus to protect them from possible radiation therapy delivered in an inverted-Y port. Bone marrow biopsy should be obtained at the conclusion of the staging laparotomy using the same anesthetic.

Despite the benefits of staging laparotomy, complications related to the procedure are fairly frequent, and the possibility of post-splenectomy sepsis should be considered. All patients are treated with polyvalent pneumococcal vaccine and perioperative and prophylactic antibiotics. Children undergoing staging laparotomy experience a high incidence of subsequent adhesive bowel obstruction. The Children's Cancer Group has reported that 3 of 49 patients who underwent staging laparotomy were rehospitialized for adhesive bowel obstruction.[57] In another series, small bowel obstruction occurred in 10% of the patients, two thirds of them requiring reoperation for correction of the obstruction.[58]

The most common mediastinal malignant neoplasm in children is lymphoma. Roentgenographic evidence of intrathoracic disease appears in 67% of children with Hodgkin's disease and 43% of those patients with non-Hodgkin's lymphoma.[59] Residual mediastinal changes following treatment for Hodgkin's disease are common and do not by themselves suggest a higher rate of disease recurrence.[60] Hyperplasia of the thymus is a normal physiologic response in infants and children during recovery from life-threatening illness. New, recurrent, or residual mediastinal masses in children treated for malignant disease present a diagnostic dilemma. At M.D. Anderson Cancer Center, children with new or recurrent mediastinal masses during or after chemotherapeutic treatment for malignant disease (most had lymphoma) were studied.[61] Those treated with steroids showed resolution of the mediastinal masses in 48 hours to 7 days without recurrences. Those undergoing open biopsy showed only thymic hyperplasias or lymph nodes. Patients with mediastinal masses occurring during or shortly following chemotherapeutic treatments of malignant disease should first be given oral prednisone (60 mg/m²d × 7–10 days). If the patients show a complete or partial resolution, follow-up should include frequent chest roentgenograms or CT and/or a second course of steroids. If the mass fails to respond to steroids, or enlarges, open biopsy through a minithoracotomy or video-assisted thorascopic biopsy will clarify the diagnosis.

GERM-CELL TUMORS

Germ-cell tumors may be gonadal or extragonadal but are most commonly gonadal. As a group, these tumors account for about 3% of malignant disease in children. Sacrococcygeal teratomas (Fig. 2–4) are the most common germ-cell tumors. Biochemical markers, including AFP, β-HCG, and serum lactic dehydrogenase, may be elevated with some of the tumors and are discussed elsewhere.

Gonadal lesions of the testes or ovary as a

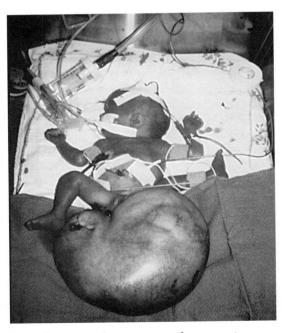

Figure 2–4 • Large sacrococcygeal teratoma in a newborn.

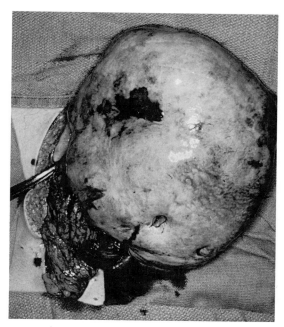

Figure 2–5 • Dysgerminoma of right ovary in a 15-year-old girl. Biopsy of left ovary was negative.

group are seen more frequently in the older child and adolescent. Dysgerminomas of the ovary can become quite large (Fig. 2–5) and are bilateral in 10% to 15% of patients.

Testicular tumors account for 1% of childhood cancers and are the seventh most common pediatric neoplasm. Peak incidence of childhood testicular tumors occurs at 2 years of age.[62] Even large children's centers or cancer centers have a relatively small number of patients. The experience at M.D. Anderson Cancer Center during a 50-year period is shown in Table 2–1.

Table 2–1 • Testicular Tumors at M.D. Anderson Cancer Center (1944–1994) (Age ≤16 Years)

Rhabdomyosarcoma	21
Yolk-sac tumor	33
Teratoma	54
Mixed germ-cell tumor	22
Choriocarcinoma	7
Seminoma	3
Endodermal sinus tumor	12
Unclassified sarcoma	2
Non-Hodgkin's lymphoma	2
Total	156

Benign testicular neoplasms are more common than malignant ones. Teratoma is the most common benign testicular tumor. The most common malignancy is a germ-cell tumor.[63] Testis tumors are rare in African-American and Asian children. The etiology of testicular cancer is unknown. A link exists between cryptochidism and germ-cell tumors of the testes,[64] but tumors in such patients are rare before puberty.[63]

Dr. Frederick J. Rescorla provides an extensive review of germ-cell tumors and their treatment in Chapter 13.

ENDOCRINE TUMORS

Drs. Doski, Robertson, and Cheu provide an extensive review of endocrine tumors of children in Chapter 21, and Drs. Powell and Newman review thyroid malignancy in Chapter 15.

Endocrine malignancies are relatively rare in children, and diagnosis can be delayed. Although carcinoid tumors of the appendix are rare in children and adolescents, they are nevertheless the most common gastrointestinal tumors in this age group. Treatment is discussed in Chapter 20 and in Chapter 16 by Dr. Edward G. Ford on gastrointestinal tumors.

Over a 50-year period at M.D. Anderson Cancer Center, only 22 patients with appendiceal carcinoid tumor were under age 20.[65] (Most patients present with appendicitis or gynecological problems and are usually treated at community hospitals.) The mean age at presentation was 14.6 years. No tumor was more than 2.0 cm in size. Only two patients underwent resection beyond appendectomy. No patient had recurrent or metastatic carcinoid tumor, and all but one patient (who died of ovarian choriocarcinoma) were alive without evidence of carcinoid tumors 1.5 to 30 years after diagnosis.

Thyroid cancer in children is relatively rare. These pediatric tumors differ biologically from adult tumors. A thyroid mass in a child is more than twice as likely to be malignant[66] and is more often larger and multicentric. Children are likely to have a higher rate of lymphatic and pulmonary metastases.[60] Thyroid cancer is more likely to recur in children than in adults.[67] Although controversial, I continue to prefer total or near total thyroidectomy in these patients. As near total or total thyroidectomy prevents recurrence in a multicentric diseased gland and makes further therapy simpler, I believe that in experienced hands, this surgical approach is warranted. With an experienced surgeon, the incidence of recurrent nerve injury should be almost nonexistent and transient or permanent hypoparathyroidism low to absent. This approach remains controversial because improvement in long-term survival has not been demonstrated.

LUNG TUMORS

Primary lung tumors in children are very rare. Metastatic disease to the lungs is common in osteosarcoma, rhabdomyosarcoma, and some other pediatric malignancies and represents the most frequent indication for surgery at M.D. Anderson Cancer Center.

Bronchial carcinoids are the most numerous of the bronchial adenomas, which include adenoid cystic carcinomas and mucoepidermoid adenomas. Cough, hemoptysis, and pneumonia are the usual presenting findings.[69] CT and bronchoscopic evaluation followed by prompt lobectomy offers an excellent long-term prognosis.

Primary squamous cell carcinoma of the lung in children is extremely rare,[70] and delayed diagnosis results in a rapid and usually fatal course. Dr. C. Thomas Black provides a review of other lung tumors in Chapter 17.

MELANOMAS AND OTHER RARE TUMORS

Several of the relatively rare tumors of childhood, including melanoma, colon cancer, and breast cancer, are being seen with increasing frequency in adolescents or young adults as a second malignant neoplasm after initial successful treatment of a primary pediatric neoplasm.[1, 3]

A 40-year review from M.D. Anderson Cancer Center demonstrated 148 patients less than 20 years of age with melanoma[71]; 19%[28] of these were 12 years of age or younger. Stage was not associated with recurrence or survival rates in the younger patients and deserves further evaluation.

Most lesions of the breast in children and adolescents are benign, but early diagnosis is desirable to relieve anxiety.[72] A 40-year review of at M.D. Anderson Cancer Center of patients under age 20 years revealed 16 patients.[73] Four patients were found to have cytosarcoma phyllodes and two, metastatic disease and were excluded. Ten patients had various forms of adenocarcinomas of the breast, including invasive intraductal, invasive lobular, signet ring, and secretory adenocarcinomas. Four had a family history of breast cancer. Delay in diagnosis was frequent. For a further review, see Chapter 20.

MANAGEMENT OF METASTATIC DISEASE

Drs. Nicholas C. Saenz and Michael LaQuaglia provide an excellent overview of the surgical management of metastatic disease in Chapter 22. At M.D. Anderson Cancer Center, an aggressive approach is taken to lung metastases in patients with osteosarcomas, hepatoblastomas, rhabdomyosarcomas, and Wilms' tumors.[56] Occasionally patients are staged and treated as having metastatic disease when only a solitary mass is seen in the lungs. Solitary metastases in patients with rhabdomyosarcomas, for example, are extremely rare and warrant tissue diagnosis. Within the multidisciplinary approach to pediatric solid tumors, aggressive treatment, including surgical excision of metastatic disease, appears to improve prognosis.

NEONATAL TUMORS

Most tumors in the neonatal period are benign. Solid malignant disease in this age group is extremely rare. Problems associated with treatment in the growing, hypermetabolic neonate are challenging. Tolerance of standard chemotherapy or radiation is poor, and response to therapy as well as the biologic nature of the tumors appears to be different in neonates than in older children. Drs. Dillon and Peter W. Azizkhan present an excellent review in Chapter 19.

During 40 years at M.D. Anderson Cancer Center, 45 patients had neonatal malignancies.[74] Of these 45 patients, 32 had solid tumors (Table 2–2). Surgical resection of the primary tumor was performed in 31 infants; 13 of those infants received no additional chemotherapy or radiation therapy, whereas 18 received some combination of surgery and perioperative chemotherapy or radiation therapy or both. Overall survival rate was 78% (25 of 32) with an average follow-up of 8 years.

Table 2–2 • Neonatal Solid Tumors at M.D. Anderson Cancer Center

Soft-tissue sarcoma	13
Brain tumor	5
Neuroblastoma	6
Retinoblastoma	3
Malignant melanoma	2
Hemangiopericytoma	2
Nephroblastoma	1
Total	32

OSTEOSARCOMA AND OTHER BONE TUMORS

The diagnosis of osteosarcoma may be suspected from its appearance on plain radiographs and scans, but definite diagnosis requires pathologic confirmation from a biopsy. The biopsy should be performed by a surgeon familiar with the management of malignant bone tumors, and preferably by the surgeon who will ultimately perform the definitive surgery. Some institutions, including our own, utilize FNA as well as open biopsy for diagnosis.[18]

The presence of metastases at diagnosis is an extremely important prognostic variable and has a major impact on management. The lung is the first site of metastasis in 90% of children with osteosarcomas, and routine posteroanterior and lateral radiographs of the chest reveal metastases in the majority of patients. A CT scan of the chest is more sensitive in revealing pulmonary metastases. As many as 10% to 20% of patients have metastatic nodules found on chest CT that are undetectable on conventional chest radiographs.[75] If there is any doubt that a lesion on CT scan represents metastatic disease, histologic confirmation should be considered. Metastases to other bones may be seen in 10% of patients; therefore, a radionuclide bone scan should be performed to screen for metastatic disease.

Approximately 80% of patients with extremity primaries present without evidence of metastatic diseases. It appears that virtually all these patients have subclinical micrometastatic diseases, even in the absence of clinically detectable metastases.[76] Thus, treatment requires surgical ablation of the primary tumor (amputation or limb-sparing resection). Treatment of micrometastatic disease is with chemotherapy. Selection of amputation versus limb salvage involves consideration of several interrelated factors, including tumor location; size, or extramedullary extent; presence or absence of distant metastatic disease; and patient factors such as age, skeletal development, and life-style preference.

The majority of patients are suitable candidates for management of the primary tumor by limb-sparing surgery, and virtually all these patients can undergo presurgical chemotherapy. After chemotherapy, reassessment of the primary tumor is followed by surgical resection. Reconstruction of the bone and soft-tissue defect to restore the structural integrity of the involved extremity depends upon the extremity involved, the size of the segment requiring reconstruction, and the preferences of the surgeon. Reconstructions utilize allografts, customized endoprosthetic devices, modular endoprosthetic devices, or combination allografts/endoprostheses. For a more extensive review, see Chapter 23 by Dr. Alan Yasko.

From 15% to 20% of patients with osteosarcomas present with clinically detectable metastases. The prognoses for such patients are significantly worse than those for patients presenting with localized diseases.

In general, a curative therapeutic approach entails surgical removal of all visible disease at the primary and metastatic sites in addition to eradication of subclinical sites of disease with chemotherapy. With an aggressive approach, 20% to 40% of patients with extremity primaries presenting with clinically detectable metastases may be cured.

ABDOMINAL EMERGENCIES

Numerous conditions can produce abdominal signs and symptoms in the immunosuppressed or neutropenic child on antineoplastic therapy. Small intestinal intussusception, primarily ileo-ileal, has been seen, with an unusually high incidence following abdominal surgical procedures, particularly when retroperitoneal dissection was performed. Operative intervention and manual reduction are necessary in many cases. Intussusception in children with small bowel lymphomas may be the presenting finding in some patients.

Intestinal-wall tumor lysis with necrosis, perforation, or hemorrhage occasionally occurs, particularly in patients with non-Hodgkin's lymphoma of the small bowel. Typhlitis, enterocolitis, or leukemic cecal infiltration or perforation presents a diagnostic and therapeutic challenge. Mortality is extremely high in these patients, who generally have acute leukemia and respond poorly to operation.

Infections such as fungal abscesses of the spleen or liver may also be present with acute abdominal findings. See Chapter 25 for a more extensive review of acute surgical problems in the pediatric oncology patient.

CONCLUSION

The surgeon must play an active role in the multidisciplinary approach to treating pediatric cancers. The surgeon's involvement in protocol design, diagnosis, timing of surgical intervention, reoperation and therapy, as well as evaluation of complications is essential. As the surgery for these tumors becomes less radical, the surgeon actually plays a greater role in assuring local tumor control, vascular access, and effective long-term follow-up care.

References

1. Smith MB, Xue H, Strong L, et al: Forty-year experience with second malignancies after treatment of childhood cancer: Analysis of outcome following the development of the second malignancy. *J Pediatr Surg* 28:1342–1349, 1993.
2. Bhatia S, Robison LL, Oberlin O, et al: Breast cancer and other second neoplasms after childhood Hodgkin's disease. *N Engl J Med* 334:745–751, 1996.
3. Corpron CA, Black CT, Ross MI, et al: Melanoma as a second malignant neoplasm after childhood cancer. *Am J Surg* 172:459–462, 1996.
4. Rich DC, Corpron CA, Smith MB, et al: Second malignant neoplasms in children after treatment of soft tissue sarcoma. *J Pediatr Surg* 32:369–372, 1997.
5. Mauer AM, Burgess JB, Donaldson SS, et al: Special nutritional needs of children with malignancies: A review. *JPEN* 14:315–324, 1990.
6. Rickard KA, Kirksey A, Baehner RL, et al: Effectiveness of enteral and parenteral nutrition in the nutritional management of children with Wilms' tumors. *Am J Clin Nutr* 33:2622–2629, 1980.
7. Rickard KA, Godshall BJ, Loghmani ES, et al: Integration of nutritional support into oncologic treatment protocols for high- and low-nutritional-risk children with Wilms' tumor: A prospective randomized study. *Cancer* 64:491–509, 1989.
8. Rickard KA, Loghamni ES, Grosfeld JL, et al: Short- and long-term effectiveness of enteral and parenteral nutrition in reversing or preventing protein-energy malnutrition in advanced neuroblastoma: A prospective randomized study. *Cancer* 56: 2881–2297, 1985.
9. Rickard KA, Detamore CM, Coates TD, et al: Effect of nutrition staging on treatment delays and outcome in stage IV neuroblastoma. *Cancer* 52:587–598, 1983.
10. Rickard KA, Foland BB, Detamore CM, et al: Effectiveness of central parenteral nutrition versus peripheral nutrition plus enteral nutrition in reversing protein-energy malnutrition in children with advanced neuroblastoma and Wilms' tumor: A prospective randomized study. *Am J Clin Nutr* 38:445–456, 1983.
11. Rickard KA, Coates TD, Grosfeld JL, et al: The value of nutritional support in children with cancer. *Cancer* 58:1904–1910, 1986.
12. Andrassy RJ, Mahour GH, Harrison MH, et al: The role and safety of early postoperative feeding in the pediatric surgical patient. *J Pediatr Surg* 14:381–385, 1979.
13. Andrassy RJ: Surgical techniques for nutritional support of the pediatric oncology patient. In Hays DM (ed.): *Pediatric Surgical Oncology.* New York: Grune and Stratton, 1986.
14. Ford EG, Jennings LM, Andrassy RJ: Serum albumin (oncotic pressure) correlates with enteral feeding tolerance in the pediatric surgical patient. *J Pediatr Surg* 22:597–599, 1987.
15. Andrassy RJ, Lally KP: Use of albumin in surgical enteral nutrition. *Postgrad Gen Surg* 5:30–33, 1993.
16. Gauderer MWL, Ponsky JL: A simplified technique for constructing a tube feeding gastrostomy. *Surg Gynecol Obstet* 152:83–85, 1981.
17. Andrassy RJ: Role of nutrition in infections. In Fonkalsrud EW and Krummel T (eds.): *Infections and Immunologic Disorders in Pediatric Surgery.* Philadelphia: WB Saunders, 1993, pp. 31–42.
18. Smith MB, Katz R, Black CT, et al: A rational approach to the use of fine-needle aspiration biopsy in the evaluation of primary and recurrent neoplasms in children. *J Pediatr Surq* 28:1245–1247, 1993.
19. Hays DM, Lawrence WJ, Wharam M, et al: Primary re-excision for patients with "microscopic residual" tumor following initial excision of sarcomas of trunk and extremity sites. *J Pediatr Surg* 24:5–10, 1989.
20. Andrassy RJ, Brennan LP, Siegel MM, et al: Preoperative chemotherapy for hepatoblastoma in children: Report of six cases. *J Pediatr Surg* 15:517–522, 1980.
21. Black CT, Cangir A, Choroszy M, Andrassy RJ: Marked response to preoperative high-dose *cis*-platinum in children with unresectable hepatoblastoma. *J Pediatr Surg* 26:1070–1073, 1991.
22. Schaller RT, Schaller J, Furman EB: The

advantages of hemodilution anesthesia for major liver resection in children. *J Pediatr Surg* 19:705–710, 1984.

23. Kitahara S, Makuuchi M, Ishizone S, et al: Successful left trisegmentectomy for ruptured hepatoblastoma using intraoperative transarterial embolization. *J Pediatr Surg* 20:1709–1712, 1995.

24. Green FL: Laparoscopic surgery in cancer treatment. In DeVita VT Jr, Hellman S, Rosenberg SA (eds.): *Important Advances in Oncology.* Philadelphia: JB Lippincott, 1993, pp 157–166.

25. Holcomb GW, Tomita SS, Haase GM, et al: Minimally invasive surgery in children with cancer. *Cancer* 76:121–128, 1995.

26. Rodgers BM, Ryckman FC, Moazam F, et al: Thoracoscopy for intrathoracic tumors. *Ann Thorac Surg* 31:414–420, 1981.

27. Shamberger RC, Holzman RS, Griscom MT, et al: CT quantitation of tracheal cross-sectional area as a guide to the surgical and anesthetic management of children with anterior mediastinal masses. *J Pediatr Surg* 26:1381–1392, 1991.

28. Yunis JJ, Ramsay N: Retinoblastoma and subband deletion of chromosome 13. *Am J Dis Child* 132:161–163, 1978.

29. Riccardi VM, Hittner HM, Francke U, et al: The aniridia-Wilms' tumor association: The critical role of chromosome band 11p13. *Cancer Genet Cytogenet* 2:131–137, 1980.

30. Croce CM: Chromosome translocations and human cancer. *Cancer Res* 46:6019–6023, 1986.

31. Croce CM: Role of chromosome translocations in human neoplasia. *Cell* 49:155–156, 1987.

32. Farber S, Diamond LK, Mercer RD, et al: Temporary remissions in acute leukemia in children produced by folic acid antagonist 4-aminopteroyl/glutamic acid (aminopterin). *N Engl J Med* 238:787–793, 1948.

33. Hammond GD: Keynote address: The cure of childhood cancers. *Cancer* 48(Suppl.):407–413, 1986.

34. Henderson EH, Samaha RJ: Evidence that drugs in multiple combinations have materially advanced the treatment of human malignancies. *Cancer Res* 29:2272–2280, 1969.

35. Hammond GD, Bleyer WA, Hartmann JR, et al: The team approach to the management of pediatric cancer. *Cancer* 41:29–35, 1978.

36. Fletcher GH. Combination of irradiation and surgery. *Int Adv Surg Oncol* 2:55–98, 1979.

37. Mauer HM, Beltangady M, Gehan EA, et al: The Intergroup Rhabdomyosarcoma Study I: A final report. *Cancer* 61:209–220, 1988.

38. Wiener ES, Lawrence W Jr, Hays DM, et al: Survival is improved in clinical group III children with complete response established by second-look operations in the Intergroup Rhabdomyosarcoma Study (IRS-III). *Med Pediatr Oncol* 19:399(abstract), 1991.

39. Hays DM: Bladder/prostate rhabdomyosarcoma:

Results of the multi-institutional trials of the Intergroup Rhabdomyosarcoma Study. *Semin Surg Oncol* 9:520–523, 1993.

40. Hays DM, Lawrence W, Crist W, et al: Partial cystectomy in the management of rhabdomyosarcoma of the bladder. A report from the Intergroup Rhabdomyosarcoma Study (IRS). *J Pediatr Surg* 25:719–723, 1990.

41. Raney RB, Heyn D, Hays DM, et al: Sequelae of treatment in 109 patients followed for five to fifteen years after diagnosis of sarcoma of the bladder and prostate. *Cancer* 71:2387–2394, 1993.

42. Wiener ES, Lawrence W, Hays DM, et al: Retroperitoneal node biopsy in childhood rhabdomyosarcoma. *J Pediatr Surg* 29:171–178, 1994.

43. Olive D, Flamant F, Zucker JM, et al: Para-aortic lymphadenectomy is not necessary in the treatment of localized rhabdomyosarcoma. *Cancer* 54:1283–1287, 1984.

44. Andrassy RJ, Hays DM, Raney RB, et al: Conservative surgical management of vaginal and vulvar pediatric rhabdomyosarcoma: A report from the Intergroup Rhabdomyosarcoma Study III. *J Pediatr Surg* 31:1034–1037, 1995.

45. Andrassy RJ, Corpron CA, Hays DM, et al: Extremity sarcomas: An analysis of prognostic factors from the Intergroup Rhabdomyosarcoma Study III. *J Pediatr Surg* 31:191–196, ,1997.

46. Lawrence W Jr, Gehan EA, Hays DM, et al: Prognostic significance of staging factors of the UICC staging system in childhood rhabdomyosarcoma: A report from the Intergroup Rhabdomyosarcoma Study (IRS-II). *J Clin Oncol* 5:46–54, 1987.

47. Lawrence W Jr, Hays DM, Heyn R, et al: Surgical lessons from the Intergroup Rhabdomyosarcoma Study (IRS) pertaining to extremity tumors. *World J Surg* 12:676–684, 1988.

48. Lawrence W Jr, Hays DM, Heyn R: Lymphatic metastasis with childhood rhabdomyosarcoma. *Cancer* 39:556–559, 1977.

49. LaQuaglia MP, Ghavimi F, Peneberg D, et al: Factors predictive of mortality in pediatric extremity rhabdomyosarcoma. *J Pediatr Surg* 25:238–244, 1990.

50. Wharton DC, Wen DR, Wang JH, et al: Technical details of intraoperative lymphatic mapping for early stage melanoma. *Arch Surg* 127:392–399, 1992.

51. Guiliano AE, Leirgan DM, Guenther JM, et al: Lymphatic mapping and sentinel lymphadenectomy for breast cancer. *Ann Surg* 220:391–401, 1994.

52. Young JL, Miller RW: Incidence of malignant tumors in U.S. children. *J Pediatr Surg* 36:245–258, 1975.

53. Corpron CA, Raney RB, Feig BW, et al: Malignant fibrous histiocytoma as a second malignant neoplasm. *J Pediatr Surg* 31:1080–1083, 1996.

54. Andrassy RJ, Brennan LP, Siegel MM, et al: Preoperative chemotherapy for hepatoblastoma in children: Report of six cases. *J Pediatr Surg* 15:517–522, 1980.

55. Black CT, Cangir A, Choroszy M, Andrassy RJ: Marked response to preoperative high-dose *cis*-platinum in children with unresectable hepatoblastoma. *J Pediatr Surg* 26:1070–1073, 1991.

56. Black CT, Luck SR, Musemeche CA, Andrassy RJ: Aggressive excision of pulmonary metastases is warranted in the management of childhood hepatic tumors. *J Pediatr Surg* 26:1082–1086, 1991.

57. Hays DM, Fryer CJ, Pringle VC, et al: An evaluation of abdominal staging procedures performed in pediatric patients with advanced Hodgkin's disease: A report from the Childrens Cancer Group. *J Pediatr Surg* 27:1175–1180, 1992.

58. Jackovich M, Mendenhall NP, Sombeck MD, et al: Long-term complications of laparotomy in Hodgkin's disease. *Ann Surg* 29:615–624, 1994.

59. Filly R, Blank N, Castellino RA: Radiographic distribution of intrathoracic disease in previously untreated patients with Hodgkin's disease and non-Hodgkin's lymphoma. *Radiology* 120:277–281, 1976.

60. Jochelson MM, Mauch P, Palikian J, et al: The significance of the residual mass in treated Hodgkin's disease. *J Clin Oncol* 3:637–640, 1985.

61. Ford EG, Lockhart SK, Sullivan MP, Andrassy RJ: Mediastinal mass following chemotherapeutic treatment of Hodgkin's disease: Recurrent tumor or thymic hyperplasia? *J Pediatr Surg* 22:1155–1159, 1987.

62. Li FP, Fraumeni JF Jr: Testicular cancers in children: Epidemiologic characteristics. *J Natl Cancer Inst* 48:1575–1581, 1972.

63. Kay R: Prepubertal testicular tumor registry. *J Urol* 150:671–674, 1993.

64. Campbell HE: The incidence of malignant growth in the undescended testicle: A reply and re-evaluation. *J Urol* 81:663–668, 1959.

65. Corpron CA, Black CT, Herzog CE, Sellin RV, Lally KP, Andrassy RJ: A half century of experience with carcinoid tumors in children. *Am J Surg* 170:606–608, 1995.

66. Belfiore A, Giuffrida D, La Rosa GL, et al: High frequency of cancer in cold thyroid nodules occurring at young age. *Acta Endocrinol* 121:197–202, 1989.

67. Winship T, Rosvoll R: Childhood thyroid carcinoma. *Cancer* 14:734–743, 1961.

68. Samaan NA, Schultz PN, Hickey RC, et al: The result of various modalities of treatment of well-differentiated thyroid carcinoma: A retrospective review of 1599 patients. *J Clin Endocrinol Metasis* 75:714–720, 1992.

69. Andrassy RJ, Feldtman RW, Stanford W: Bronchial carcinoid tumors in children and adolescents. *J Pediatr Surg* 12:513–517, 1977.

70. La Salle AJ, Andrassy RJ, Stanford W: Bronchogenic squamous cell carcinoma in childhood: A case report. *J Pediatr Surg* 12:519–521, 1977.

71. Corpron CA, Smith MB, Black CT, Ross MI, Andrassy RJ: Pediatric melanoma: The effect of age on prognosis (in press).

72. Andrassy RJ: Benign breast lesions in children and adolescents. *Cancer Bull* 40:33–35, 1988.

73. Corpron CA, Black CT, Singletary SE, Andrassy RJ: Breast cancer in adolescent females. *J Pediatr Surg* 30:322–324, 1995.

74. Xue H, Horwitz JR, Smith MB, Lally KP, Black CT, Cangir A, Takahashi H, Andrassy RJ: Malignant solid tumors in neonates: A 40-year review. *J Pediatr Surg* 30:543–545, 1995.

75. Neifeld J, Michaelis L, Doppman J: Suspected pulmonary metastases: Correlation of chest x-ray, whole-lung tomograms, and operative findings. *Cancer* 39:383–387, 1977.

76. Link MD, Gookin AM, Horowitz M, et al: Adjuvant chemotherapy of high-grade osteosarcoma of the extremity: Updated results of the multi-institutional osteosarcoma study. *Clin Orthop* 270:8–14, 1991.

Anesthesia, Sedation, and Pain Management

- *Kimberly Kenfield Nesbitt, M.D.* • *Judy B. Massengill, M.D.*
- *Vivian H. Porche, M.D.*

Children with cancer will have far more anesthetic interventions in their lifetimes than any other patient population, including adults with cancer.[1] These interventions pose special problems for the multidisciplinary team of pediatric oncologists, radiologists, surgeons, and anesthesiologists who will treat such children. This chapter focuses on anesthesia-related concerns in the care of children with cancer, beginning with a review of the principles of preoperative evaluation and continuing through intraoperative practices, sedation principles, and postoperative concerns, including methods of pain control. Although it is the anesthesiologist who has the ultimate responsibility for appropriately assessing the condition of the pediatric cancer patient and making known to the parents—and when appropriate, the patient—the risks inherent in particular anesthetic procedures, this chapter is directed toward all members of the treatment team. An improved understanding by all members should lead to more appropriate anesthesia planning and better patient care.

PREOPERATIVE EVALUATION

Purpose

The objective of the preoperative visit is to obtain clinically pertinent information that will help determine the perioperative care of the child undergoing the surgical procedure. The details of prior surgery and radiotherapy or chemotherapy may indicate the need for special attention; some conditions (e.g., thrombocytopenia, neutropenia, organ dysfunction) may lead to technical difficulties and perioperative complications. Anesthesiologists can be requested to provide a variety of services, including airway management, sedation for diagnostic tests and minor procedures, central venous catheter placement, intraoperative care, and general anesthesia. In each case, an appropriate preoperative evaluation must be completed. The overall medical condition of the patient must be assessed, often quickly in emergency cases. This evaluation is also ideally used to establish rapport with the parent and child, provide them with information, and answer their questions while allaying their anxiety. Preparing the patient physically and psychologically for the surgical procedure enhances anesthetic safety. The information obtained by the anesthesiologist allows appropriate perioperative techniques and procedures to be identified and an appropriate anesthetic plan implemented.

A physical-status classification adopted by the American Society of Anesthesiologists (ASA) to summarize the general condition of the patient helps in assessing the relative risk of anesthesia (Table 3–1).[2–4] The usefulness of this classification system is limited, however, because it does not consider the type of the surgical procedure,

nor does it profile potential complications. It primarily serves as a means of communicating overall physical condition. Because these classifications are not age-dependent, they are routinely employed in the anesthetic assessment of the pediatric cancer patient.

Outpatient cancer surgery is common for the otherwise healthy pediatric patient not undergoing a major operation. Such outpatient surgery has proved more cost effective when the patient's physical condition requires no specialized postoperative care.[5] Thus, outpatient surgery is suggested for low-risk patients (i.e., those classified as ASA I and II patients). Other advantages exist for outpatient surgery as well: First, the risk for nosocomial infections in immunocompromised pediatric (e.g., cancer or transplant) patients is lowered by outpatient surgery.[6] Second, long-lasting emotional distress can often be avoided by outpatient surgery because it allows children to immediately return home for a full recovery.[7] Third, hospital interventions can be minimized by outpatient surgery for terminally ill children undergoing palliative procedures (i.e., central line placements, gastrostomy tube insertions), although each case must be considered individually.

Pediatric Anesthesia Considerations

Pediatric cancer patients have special needs and circumstances that require careful consideration in regard to anesthesia. These patients vary

Table 3–1 · Preoperative Classification and Perioperative Mortality Rates of Patients According to the American Society of Anesthesiologists

Class	Definition	Mortality Risk
I	A patient who is normal and healthy except for surgical pathology and who is without systemic disease	1:9,160
II	A patient who has mild systemic disease but no functional limitations	1:10,609
III	A patient who has moderate to severe systemic disturbances as a result of medical or surgical disease and some functional limitation but not to the point of incapacitation	1:347
IV	A patient who has severe systemic disturbance that poses a constant threat to life and is incapacitating	1:134
V	A patient who is moribund and not expected to survive 24 hours with or without surgery	1:64
E	A patient representing an emergency case; the physical status is followed by the letter "E" (e.g., "IIE")	

From Marx GF, Mateo CV, Otkin LR: Computer analysis of postanesthesia deaths. *Anesthesiology* 39:54, 1973; Morgan GE, Mikhail MS: The practice of anesthesiology. In Morgan GE, Mikhail MS (eds): *Clinical Anesthesiology.* Norwalk, CT: Appleton & Lange, 1992, pp. 6–7; and Ross AF, Tinker JH: Anesthesia risk. In Miller RD (ed): *Anesthesia,* 4th ed. New York: Churchill Livingstone, 1994, p. 819.

widely in height, weight, and maturity (both physical and psychological). Thus, a range of equipment sizes is required to administer anesthesia. The type of airway equipment utilized depends on the patient's weight and the breathing characteristics desired during anesthesia.

The increased ratio of *body surface area* (BSA) to weight in infants and children makes them more susceptible to dehydration and temperature instability than adolescents or adults. Fluid requirements and fluid delivery systems vary with patient weight and BSA. Age is also a consideration in determining the patient's ability to tolerate NPO status, bowel preparations, and the like; therefore, intravenous placement may be required preoperatively to prevent dehydration.

Good access to veins and arteries, especially in patients who have received chemotherapy, is still another common preoperative concern. If significant operative blood losses are anticipated, it is important to plan for adequate venous access, including central line placement, along with blood banking, for infants and children who have small intravascular volumes.

Regional anesthesia (either single-shot blocks or continuous infusions of local anesthetics) is usually not used alone but is instead combined intraoperatively with general anesthetics and continued postoperatively for pain management. Ideally, plans for intraoperative and postoperative pain management are discussed with parents and older children at the time of preoperative screening. Regional anesthesia requires preoperative consent. A complete discussion of anesthesia procedures, risks, and benefits should precede the informed consent.

Psychological Preparation

Children are emotionally stressed by any hospital experience involving a surgical procedure. Not only are there long-term psychological implications,[8, 9] but there are also physiologic ones—changes precipitated by stress that may ultimately alter physical well-being.[10] According to Vistainer and Wolfer,[11] children experience five fears related to hospitalization: fear of parental separation, fear of physical harm (pain), fear of the unknown, fear of behavioral expectations (a wish to avoid punishment), and fear of losing control. How these fears are manifest is generally age-related.[14]

As for the parents, they vary greatly, depending upon their own coping skills, in their ability to reduce their child's stress and anxiety. Parents may therefore need advice on how to discuss hospitalization and surgical procedures with their child. Two important principles should be emphasized to parents. First, their child's trust should be maintained at all times, and under no circumstances should he or she be deceived.[12–15] Second, their child's age should dictate what information is shared, and potentially disturbing minor details need not be discussed with younger children. In fact, the age of the child is the most important factor in determining appropriate methods for psychological preparation. Parents may need guidance in deciding what information is reasonable and age-appropriate to share. Preschool-age children should be told of the hospitalization no sooner than 24 hours before it occurs. Conversely, older children and adolescents should participate from the beginning in plans involving their hospitalization.[16]

Preoperative Assessment

The patient's overall condition at preoperative assessment may contrast with the documented medical history. Changes in the patient's mental state, hydration state, nutritional condition, and skin appearance (e.g., bruising and petechiae) might indicate the need for specific laboratory evaluation. Current medications, allergies, and family anesthesia history should be carefully documented.

Prematurity

The pediatric patient born premature (i.e., before 37 weeks gestation or at a birth weight less than 2.5 g) may suffer sequelae of prematurity that leave him or her medically compromised. Therefore, anesthetic risks related to prematurity extend well into childhood and sometimes beyond. Organ dysfunction related to bronchopulmonary dysplasia and congenital heart disease are of particular concern to the anesthesiologist. The patient's condition should be carefully evaluated in regard to such dysfunction and optimized preoperatively. Any neurologic deficits should be documented carefully to provide a baseline against which to contrast postoperative changes. Perioperative respiratory complications (e.g., apnea, laryngospasm, bronchospasm) are significantly more common in premature infants.[17] The susceptibility to apnea in premature infants has been well documented. The incidence is inversely related to age.[18] Studies indicate that outpatient anesthesia is inappropriate for infants less than 50 weeks post conception as they may suffer apnea up to 12 hours after surgery.[19-23] Monitoring for 24 hours after surgery provides a reasonable margin of safety.

Respiratory Assessment

Preoperative respiratory assessment is dictated by a prior history of pulmonary problems or current respiratory insufficiency. A history of prior intubations, dyspneic episodes, and airway tumors should be obtained. Anatomic abnormalities that may affect intubation and ventilation should be carefully assessed. Specifically, tracheobronchial distortion from mediastinal tumor masses may result in the development of voluntary adaptive patterns of ventilation. Radiologic evaluations may be helpful in this regard. A history of alterations in respiratory function with position change allows the anesthesiologist to predict difficulties that may occur during the induction and delivery of anesthesia.

Children must also be evaluated for loose teeth and recent upper respiratory infections. In children with coryza and cough, a careful history must be obtained regarding related symptoms, temperature, and behavior changes (e.g., eating habits, play). Although coryza may be chronic, intraoperative and postoperative airway complications may lead to bronchospasm, mucous plugging, and unexpected hospital admission.[24] The incidence of airway problems in infants and in patients intubated endotracheally is higher in those manifesting symptoms of airway problems before surgery. Conservative management that delays elective surgery 2–4 weeks following an acute upper respiratory tract infection should be discussed with parents and surgeon. The risk of complications appears to decrease after this time.[25] Bronchospastic conditions such as asthma and bronchiectasis should be optimally treated prior to surgery. Children who present with clinical wheezing and significant bronchospasm should not be approved for elective surgery. Surgery should be deferred for 4 weeks after an

acute asthma attack to avoid exacerbating the symptoms.[26]

Routine preoperative chest radiographs are generally not indicated for asymptomatic patients. Cancer patients, however, may require them for a variety of reasons, including fever, coughing, wheezing, and suspected intrathoracic mass. Infection is the most common cause of acute respiratory failure, often in conjunction with neutropenia and immunosuppression in pediatric cancer patients.[27] Diffuse pulmonary infiltrates that produce symptoms resembling those of pneumonia may be seen in leukemia patients. Cardiotoxicity from chemotherapeutic agents (i.e., Adriamycin [doxorubicin]) and underlying myocardial disease, such as congenital heart disease, may result in cardiogenic pulmonary edema.[28] Pleural effusions may result from a variety of conditions in cancer patients. Thoracentesis may be necessary to relieve respiratory symptoms in these patients before anesthesia is conducted.

Leukocytosis is associated with pulmonary thrombosis, which may mimic pulmonary infection. Preoperative thrombolytic therapy is indicated in these cases.[29] Toxic pulmonary effects from radiotherapy and chemotherapy are well described.[30, 31] Patients with a history of bleomycin therapy may present with dyspnea, tachypnea, dry cough, or pleural friction rub.[32] Further evaluation and specific pulmonary consultation is indicated for them. The degree of pulmonary dysfunction can be evaluated by pulmonary function tests (PFTs) and carbon monoxide diffusing capacity. A restrictive pattern on spirometry and a decreased diffusing capacity are the indicators of pathologic changes related to chemotherapy.[33] Unfortunately pulmonary function studies are often difficult to perform in children. Other measures and observations, such as exercise tolerance and activity limitations, are utilized.[30]

There is an increased risk of pulmonary toxicity in patients receiving concomitant chest radiotherapy and cyclophosphamide therapy.[34] Bleomycin toxicity can occur 3–10 days after general anesthesia, with pulmonary infiltration progressing to *adult respiratory distress syndrome* (ARDS).[35, 36] In 1978 Goldiner and coworkers[37] showed that limiting perioperative FIO_2 and minimizing fluid replacement led to a significant reduction in morbidity and mortality related to bleomycin therapy.

Busulfan, BCNU (bis-chloroethyl-nitrosourea), and ifosfamide also place patients at risk for pulmonary dysfunction.[27] Other chemotherapeutic agents, such as doxorubicin and actinomycin, may potentiate the toxicity of chest radiation therapy. In such circumstances, ventilatory support beyond the operative period may allow the acute effects associated with surgery to resolve. Parents and older children should be warned that postoperative mechanical ventilation may be required. When patient history or examination suggests the possibility of pulmonary compromise, the surgeon should carefully appraise the patient by consulting with the anesthesiologist and the pediatric pulmonologist.

Cardiac Assessment

Careful review of a child's history may indicate ongoing cardiac compromise or risk factors for cardiotoxicity related to chemotherapeutic agents. Thus, as part of the physical assessment, blood pressure and heart rate should be documented and the heart auscultated. Even though murmurs may be undetected and clinically insignificant, serious heart defects may be present.[38] New murmurs may occur in cancer patients as a result of severe anemia related to chemotherapy and bone marrow suppression. Innocent murmurs are systolic and tend to be soft and variable, whereas murmurs suggesting structural heart defects tend to be loud, continuous, and transmitted. All diastolic murmurs should be considered pathologic. It is unlikely that an asymptomatic murmur will be related to a defect that will significantly complicate the anesthetic course; nevertheless, antibiotic prophylaxis may be indicated.[39] Certainly, antibiotic prophylaxis is recommended for all patients with proven or suspected cardiac defects (Table 3–2).[40] It is also required for all patients who have undergone surgery to correct a congenital heart defect, with the exception of suture ligation for patent ductus arteriosus or secundum atrial septal defect. A routine preoperative electrocardiogram (ECG) is not a sensitive screening tool in children. When any doubt exists about the presence of cardiovascular disease, a cardiology consultation should be obtained. Echocardiography (ECHO) can usually determine pathology and help estimate cardiac function and myocardial reserve.

Cancer patients have additional potential causes

Table 3–2 • Recommendations for Prophylactic Antibiotic Therapy in Children with Heart Lesions

For Dental/Oral/Upper Respiratory Tract Procedures (Including High-Risk Children)

If able to take oral medication
   Amoxicillin 50 mg/kg 1 hour before procedure
   Amoxicillin 25 mg/kg 6 hours later
If allergic to penicillin
   Erythromycin 20 mg/kg 2 hours before procedure
   Erythromycin 10 mg/kg 6 hours later
If unable to take oral medication
   Ampicillin 50 mg/kg IM or IV 30 minutes before procedure, plus gentamicin 2 mg/kg IM or IV 30 minutes before procedure
   If allergic to penicillin
   Vancomycin 20 mg/kg IV infused slowly over 1 hour, commencing 1 hour before procedure

For Gastrointestinal and Genitourinary Procedures

Ampicillin 50 mg/kg IM or IV 30 minutes before procedure, plus gentamicin 2 mg/kg IM or IV 30 minutes before procedure
If allergic to penicillin
   Vancomycin 20 mg/kg infused slowly over 1 hour commencing 1 hour before procedure, plus gentamicin 2 mg/kg 30 minutes before procedure
If able to take oral medication (for low-risk patients only)
   Ampicillin 50 mg/kg 1 hour before procedure
   Ampicillin 50 mg/kg 6 hours later

From Steward DJ: Preoperative evaluation and preparation for surgery. In Gregory GA (ed): *Pediatric Anesthesia*, 3rd ed. New York: Churchill Livingstone, 1994, p. 187, used with permission.

of myocardial dysfunction that may require careful evaluation and optimization prior to elective surgery. Anthracycline-induced cardiotoxicity is characterized by ECG changes, cardiomyopathies, and dysrhythmias. Cardiomyopathy leading to congestive heart failure is the hallmark of chronic toxicity (occurring in 2% to 10% of patients).[34] Consequently, patients previously exposed to anthracyclines must undergo a full cardiac evaluation prior to surgery. Support for this recommendation comes from several sources. Larsen and coworkers[41] reported an increased frequency of potentially life-threatening dysrhythmias, including supraventricular and ventricular tachycardia, in children treated with doxorubicin. According to VonHoff and coworkers,[42] children younger than 15 years of age treated with daunorubicin and doxorubicin therapy are more likely to develop cardiac failure than adults. Most pediatric studies indicate an increased incidence after the cumulative doxorubicin dose reaches 400–500 mg/m$_2$.[43] Yet, abnormal ECHOs have been reported in 65% of children receiving doses of 228 mg/m$_2$ or more.[44] In the same study, Lipshultz and coworkers[44] demonstrated an even greater risk for cardiotoxicity in leukemia patients under 4 years of age. Most centers routinely and periodically assess these patients for cardiotoxicity because congestive heart failure can develop years after therapy. When Steinherz and colleagues[45] reviewed cases 20 years after childhood treatment, they found a 23% overall incidence of abnormal cardiac function.

Echocardiographic evaluation of left ventricular systolic function, by ejection fraction and fractional shortening, is the most widely used method of assessing cardiotoxicity.[46] Because the myocardium can compensate for early damage, exercise testing can improve the sensitivity of systolic echocardiography.[47] Other contributing factors to toxicity include underlying cardiac disease, mediastinal radiation, and additional cytotoxic drug therapy (cyclophosphamide and bleomycin).[48]

Cardiogenic shock may be the most severe sign of cardiovascular compromise. Prior to surgery patients exhibiting cardiogenic shock may require preoperative optimization with diuretic therapy and inotropic support. The type of intraoperative monitoring and the combination of anesthetic drugs selected will depend upon the degree of cardiac compromise.

Other cardiovascular complications related to malignancy, chemotherapy, and radiation that may develop in the pediatric cancer patient and alter anesthetic management include pericardial effusion and cardiac tamponade. Constrictive pericarditis related to radiation therapy may occur months after treatment.[43]

Renal, Metabolic, and Electrolyte Assessment

In the preoperative care of the routine pediatric patient, urinalysis and electrolyte evaluations are unnecessary. In pediatric cancer patients, however, risk factors for renal dysfunction should be sought. Primary renal tumors (i.e., Wilms' tumors) rarely impair kidney function in children, whereas infiltrative leukemia or lymphoma may cause azotemia and oliguria. Renal insufficiency and electrolyte abnormalities in the pediatric cancer patient are generally related to prescribed therapies, including chemotherapy agents (cyclophosphamide, cisplatin, ifosfamide, and methotrexate), radiation treatments, and antibiotics (aminoglycosides and amphotericin B).[43] A careful drug history and a review of physical findings will help determine the need for further laboratory evaluation. Acute radiation nephritis may appear 6–13 months following exposure to radiation, whereas chronic nephritis may not appear for years.[49] Obstructive nephropathies resulting from external tumor compression and other prerenal etiologies (e.g., hypovolemia, sepsis, renal vascular compression) may cause oliguria or anuria in patients with no history of renal dysfunction. Hypertension related to increased renin secretion may be present in conjunction with Wilms' tumor.

Laboratory studies of patients at risk for renal insufficiency should include urinalysis, BUN, creatinine, and serum electrolytes. Creatinine clearance may be required to demonstrate nephrotoxicity. A urologic consultation may be necessary when the etiology of the renal insufficiency is unclear.

Fluid management in the pediatric cancer patient takes into account the presence of underlying renal, metabolic, and electrolyte abnormalities. Electrolyte abnormalities are commonly seen in the cancer patient (Table 3–3).[50] Preexisting renal dysfunctions can exacerbate these derangements. Acute renal failure may result from metabolic nephropathies. Purine metabolism following tumor-cell breakdown may result in significant uric acid elevations and is particularly common in children with high tumor loads (e.g., those with leukemia or lymphoma). Hyperuricemic nephropathy and fluid overload may result in respiratory failure and cerebral edema. Tumor lysis syndrome, which has been well described, consists of hyperuricemia, hyperkalemia, hypocalcemia, hyperphosphatemia, and renal failure.[51] Its therapy consists primarily of urine alkalinization, aggressive diuresis, and allopurinol administration although calcium supplementation should be considered as well if needed. The preoperative potassium level should be checked in these patients and aggressive treatment for

Table 3–3 • Electrolyte Abnormalities Associated with Treatment of Pediatric Malignancy

Diagnosis	Etiology
Hypokalemia	Amphotericin B
Hyperkalemia	Tumor-cell lysis
	Blood transfusion
Hypocalcemia	Hyperphosphatemia (tumor-cell lysis)
	Citrate binding (blood transfusion)
Hypercalcemia	Bone tumors
	Neuroblastoma
Hyponatremia	Inappropriate antidiuretic hormone secretion (including that caused by vincristine, cyclophosphamide)
	Hydration with hypotonic fluid

From McDowell RH: Anesthesia for children with cancer. *Probl Anesth* 7(4):425–446, 1993, used with permission.

hyperkalemia initiated if indicated. Should hemodialysis be required for any reason, it is best performed within 24 hours of surgery to ensure euvolemia and normal electrolyte levels.[52]

The most common endocrine disorder in childhood is diabetes mellitus. Juvenile diabetics require insulin and are at risk for developing *diabetic ketoacidosis* (DKA) when dosing or metabolic requirements are altered. This catabolic state is often precipitated by infection, trauma, vomiting, or psychological stress. The stress of surgery may also cause changes in glucose and insulin requirements. Leukocytosis and abdominal pain occur in patients with DKA and may be mistakenly attributed to tumor symptoms if the patient is a child with cancer. Proper laboratory evaluation, however, will reveal the hyperglycemia, metabolic acidosis, and ketosis of DKA.

Aggressive hydration is mandatory in children with DKA as renal insufficiency or failure may be the sequela of severe osmotic diuresis and dehydration. Hypoglycemia caused by insulin administration is a risk in presurgical patients who receive insulin and remain NPO. Early consultation with the anesthesiologist will allow proper evaluation of the insulin requirements so that recommendations can be made for preoperative insulin therapy. The minimum preoperative laboratory evaluation for the diabetic pediatric cancer patient includes serum glucose, electrolytes, creatinine, and BUN. Urinalysis is also recommended.

Some tumors are noted for their association with metabolic and electrolyte abnormalities. Brain tumors, specifically craniopharyngiomas, may cause hypopituitarism resulting in hypothyroidism, adrenal insufficiency, and diabetes insipidus.[53] Thyroxine and cortisol replacement therapy should be initiated preoperatively. A euthyroid state must be confirmed clinically. Laboratory assessment may be required if any question about metabolic or electrolyte status remains after a careful history has been obtained and physical examination performed. When the posterior pituitary is involved, an excess of antidiuretic hormone (i.e., SIADH) may result in hyponatremia, low serum osmolality, and decreased urine output. Behavioral changes, headache, nausea, and vomiting may be symptoms related to hyponatremia and/or increased intracranial pressure. Appropriate studies must confirm the etiology prior to surgical intervention.

Patients with neuroblastoma may present with dehydration and significant electrolyte abnormalities caused by vasoactive peptide release resulting in vomiting and diarrhea. Fluid and electrolyte replacement therapy should be initiated preoperatively in these patients.

A preoperative hypertension history may indicate tumor secretion of catecholamines. Pheochromocytoma is classically characterized by catecholamine secretion, primarily norepinephrine.[54] Intravascular volume is decreased by chronic hypertension, and electrolyte abnormalities may result from vomiting and diaphoresis. Owing to chronic catecholamine exposure, cardiomyopathy may develop in these children. If cardiomyopathy is suspected, ECG should be performed as part of the preoperative assessment.

Alpha-adrenergic blockade, which blocks the vasoconstriction that contributes to a contracted volume, is generally started several days prior to surgery. As the fluid deficit lessens, a reduction in hematocrit may indicate a return to normal blood volume. Secretion of catecholamines rarely produces in children the tachycardia and arrhythmias seen in adults.[55] When they do occur, however, as documented by ECG preoperatively, beta-blocker therapy may also be required. In this event, appropriate alpha-blocker therapy (e.g., phenoxybenzamine) must precede the initiation of beta-blocker therapy; otherwise, increased cardiac work resulting from significant afterload pressure may lead to cardiac failure.

Hematologic/Vascular Assessment

For most pediatric patients, a preoperative hemoglobin evaluation is not necessary unless age, medical history, results of physical examination, or considerations of associated therapy dictate otherwise.[56] In the pediatric cancer patient, however, a complete blood count is always necessary and is standard practice for preoperative assessment, despite the possibility that venous access may be limited by scars from previous venous punctures and by chemotherapy-related vascular changes. Abnormalities are frequently revealed in patients with a malignancy related to chemotherapy, radiation, bone marrow infiltration, sepsis, or bleeding disorder. The practice of perioperative transfusion therapy is directed at optimizing oxygen-carrying capacity and thus maintaining the oxygen supply required for the patient's demands. The consideration of acute versus chronic anemia and the adequacy of physiologic compensatory mechanisms supersedes that of maintaining a strict minimum preoperative hemoglobin level.

Other hematologic disorders that may alter intraoperative management include hemorrhage, thrombosis, and blast crisis. Hemorrhage is the second leading cause of death for pediatric leukemia patients; infection remains the leading cause.[57] Because thrombocytopenia, coagulopathy, or a combination of the two may lead to frank hemorrhage in the pediatric cancer patient undergoing surgery, coagulation status and cell counts are also carefully considered when selecting the technique for endotracheal intubation and central line placement.

Patients with thrombocytopenia related to bone marrow infiltration, tumor therapy, or platelet destruction may require transfusion therapy prior to surgery if the platelet count is below 50,000/μL. Some procedures (e.g., craniotomy) may necessitate that platelet counts be maintained at about 75,000–100,000/μL.[58] Borderline platelet numbers should be confirmed manually since machine counting may be unreliable in the presence of platelet aggregates and cellular debris.[51] One unit of platelets generally increases the platelet count by 7000–11,000/mm$_3$ for each square meter of BSA.[58] This guideline for trans-

Table 3–4 • Coagulopathy in Children with Cancer

Etiology	Associated Condition
Thrombocytopenia	Marrow aplasia
	Marrow infiltration
	Consumptive coagulopathy
	Hemodilution
Thrombocytopathy	Antibiotic
	Nonsteroidal anti-inflammatory drugs
Consumptive coagulopathy	Septicemia
	Acute promyelocytic leukemia
Antineoplastic drugs	L-asparaginase
	Actinomycin D
	Anthracyclines
Hepatic insufficiency	Liver tumor
	Viral hepatitis
	Vincristine
	Radiation-induced veno-occlusive disease
Vitamin K deficiency	Actinomycin D
	Antibiotics
	Malnutrition
Acquired von Willebrand's deficiency	Wilms' tumor

From McDowell RH: Anesthesia for children with cancer. *Probl Anesth* 7(4):427, 1993, used with permission.

fusion therapy is, however, of no value in patients with ongoing consumption or alloimmunization. Although thrombocytopenia is the most common hemostatic disorder in pediatric cancer patients, coagulopathies related to other conditions may also occur (Table 3–4).[59] Thus, preoperative laboratory evaluation should include a platelet count and coagulation profile in patients at risk.

Patients with acute leukemia presenting with leukocytosis are known to be at risk for pulmonary and cerebrovascular events related to vascular sludging and hemorrhage. Therefore, the white blood cell count should be reduced preoperatively to below 100,000/μl by leukapheresis or, in the infant, partial-exchange transfusion.[60, 61]

The surgical team should confirm that appropriate blood products are readily available and that the current hematologic status of the patient is reasonable for the procedure required. If irradiated or CMV-seronegative blood products are required, the blood bank will need adequate notification for planning and preparation.

Bone Marrow Transplants

Bone marrow transplants (BMTs) are indicated in *acute myelogenous leukemia* (AML), *acute lymphocytic leukemia* (ALL), lymphoma, and neuroblastoma.[62] Unfortunately, children who undergo BMT are at risk for the complications associated with chemotherapy and radiotherapy as well as several problems specifically associated with BMT. Preparative BMT therapy results in marrow aplasia with profound pancytopenia, and toxic effects of therapy can include severe mucositis, radiation-induced enteritis, cyclophosphamide-induced cardiomyopathy, and hepatic veno-occlusive disease.[63] Common causes of post-transplant morbidity and mortality include opportunistic infections, *graft-versus-host disease* (GVHD), and pulmonary dysfunction related to infectious and noninfectious pneumonitides. Among patients who receive allogeneic BMT, 20% to 35% die as a result of complications and 20% to 50%, suffer acute GVHD despite prophylactic therapy with cyclosporine, alone or in combination with methotrexate and steroids.[64]

Clinical manifestations of GVHD include an erythematous rash on the palms and soles, diarrhea with abdominal pain, and liver dysfunction. Long-term cyclosporine therapy may result in the development of hirsutism, tremors, hypertension, and renal insufficiency.[65] An episode of acute GVHD and increasing age are two factors closely associated with the development of chronic GVHD, which occurs in 20% to 40% of patients who survive transplantation more than 6 months. Findings in the chronic form of this disease are part of a pathologically distinct entity, specifically sclerosis. Sclerosis can manifest as scleroderma, xerostomia, joint contractures, biliary cirrhosis, obliterative bronchiolitis, and immunologic deficiency.[66, 67] Preoperative evaluation and planning of anesthetic management require the careful consideration of pathophysiologic changes that may result from this disease process. The reverse isolation (i.e., to protect patient from infection) necessary in the agranulocytic patient must be maintained throughout the perioperative period and often beyond, when donor-derived immune competence is delayed. The blood bank needs to be notified when blood transfusion therapy may be necessary to ensure that the blood to be transfused is irradiated and CMV-negative.

NPO GUIDELINES

A frequent controversy that arises in preoperative planning for pediatric cancer patients concerns the appropriate duration of fasting. The traditional 8-hour fast recommended for adults is not always appropriate for the pediatric patient. This is due to wide variations in feeding intervals and BSA-to-weight ratios, both of which affect fluid, electrolyte, and metabolic stability. Regardless of duration, the preoperative fast is often uncomfortable for pediatric patients and unpleasant for their caregivers.

In 1946 Mendelson[68] described the pathophysiology of the acid aspiration syndrome now known as Mendelson's syndrome. The early studies indicated that a significant number of anesthetic deaths could be directly attributed to pulmonary aspiration of gastric contents.[69, 70] Several studies also found that both gastric volume and gastric pH contribute to the overall morbidity and mortality risk of acid aspiration.[71–74] Specifically, aspiration of >0.4 ml/kg gastric fluid (versus 25 ml/kg in adult) with a pH <2.5 increases the risk. Particulate matter, if also aspirated, presents a number of other complicating factors, including bronchial obstruction.[75] Many conditions predispose patients to gastric aspiration. These include a full stomach (owing to recent ingestion or acute trauma), delayed gastric emptying (owing to narcotic use, diabetes, uremia, obesity, or abdominal masses), gastrointestinal obstruction, dysphagia, and altered mental status.

Fasting time may be critical in patients without intravenous access, particularly infants and toddlers. Maintaining hemodynamic stability and avoiding dehydration may require preoperative intravenous fluid therapy in patients unable to tolerate oral intake. A number of pediatric studies have reevaluated the standard adult requirements for preoperative fasting by providing clear liquids to children up to 2 hours prior to surgery.[76–78] In 1989, Splinter and coworkers[79] showed that children given 5 ounces of apple juice 2–3 hours before the induction of anesthesia had less gastric volume, thirst, and hunger than those given no fluids preoperatively. Moreover, no demonstrable difference in gastric pH was evident between the two groups. Based upon these findings, revisions in the accepted age-adjusted NPO recommendations have been made (Table 3–5).[80] Questions may arise regarding infants maintained on breast milk. Although it remains controversial, most pediatric anesthesiologists follow the rule of a feeding interval:

Table 3–5 · NPO Guidelines

Age	Formula/Milk/Solids	Clear Liquids	Breast Milk
0–5 months	4 hr	2 hr	Feeding
6–35 months	6 hr	2 hr	Interval
Older than 36 months	8 hr	2 hr	

Adapted from Steward DJ: Preoperative evaluation and preparation for surgery. In Gregory GA (ed): *Pediatric Anesthesia*, 3rd ed. New York: Churchill Livingstone, 1994, pp. 179–195, used with permission.

simply stated, infants feeding at 4-hour intervals should be nursed 4 hours prior to surgery.[80]

INTRAOPERATIVE MANAGEMENT

Premedication

Hospital admission, anesthesia, and surgery are stressful for children. Because premedication significantly reduces their preoperative anxiety and the incidence of postoperative behavioral disturbances,[81–84] clinicians must maintain expertise with a range of available premedicants. Ideally, these premedications allay anxiety, facilitate induction of anesthesia, and cause amnesia. Appropriate premedication can ease the traumatic separation of child from parents, resulting in a more cooperative child and less anxious parents.

The advisability and selection of a premedicant is age- and child-specific. Children less than 6 months old do not typically exhibit "stranger anxiety" and so generally separate readily from their parents without pharmacologic intervention. Conversely, children of 6 months to 6 years old generally benefit from premedication.

Approaches to premedication have undergone a major transformation over the last decade. The traditional method of intramuscular injection has virtually been replaced by other methods of administration, most frequently oral. The oral form of midazolam is one of the most popular premedicants.[85, 86] It must, however, be mixed with juice or flavored syrup to make it palatable. Midazolam has strong anxiolytic, amnestic, and sedative effects that are typically evident within 15 minutes of administration.

Alternatively, premedication can be administered transmucosally to take advantage of the oral or nasal mucosa's rich vascular supply and to avoid first-pass (hepatic) elimination. *Oral transmucosal fentanyl citrate* (OTFC) is a fentanyl-impregnated lozenge mounted on a handle. It is

well tolerated by patients and provides sedation and anxiolysis when administered 30 minutes before outpatient surgery.[82] Although somewhat irritating, sufentanil and midazolam have both been administered nasally for premedication with acceptably rapid onset and good effect.[87] Nasally administered midazolam produces its effects faster than does the orally administered form, and less drug is required to achieve the desired effects.[83]

Rectal administration of premedicants remains a controversial option used primarily in children under the age of 6 years.[84] Midazolam, ketamine, diazepam, and barbiturates have all been administered rectally with effective results.

Children, especially those with cancer, may come to the operating room with established venous access, in which case midazolam, ketamine, barbiturates, or opioids can be administered intravenously and titrated to effect. All children receiving preoperative medication for sedation must be monitored for possible side effects, including respiratory depression, nausea, and vomiting.

Induction

Mask Versus Intravenous Induction

The most common technique for inducing general anesthesia in children is the inhalation of anesthetic vapor. After physiologic monitoring is established, the patient breathes a mixture of nitrous oxide and oxygen (generally 70%/30%). Low concentrations of an anesthetic are then introduced and gradually increased. Halothane has historically been preferred for induction but sevoflurane is increasing in popularity and may soon replace halothane completely.

As children have an aversion to needles, induction is usually done by mask unless there is existing intravenous access or a specific reason for intravenous induction (e.g., a full stomach requiring cricoid pressure). Some anatomic alterations (e.g., mediastinal masses and tracheal compression) may indicate the need for maintenance of spontaneous ventilation and therefore a mask induction. Intravenous induction is rapid and, therefore, reduces the risk of excitement and possible laryngospasm.

Parental Presence

The value of parental presence during the induction of anesthesia is debated, but most pediatric anesthesiologists feel that parental presence comforts and reassures the child. Most parents report that, given the choice, they would participate in their child's induction[88] in order to allay the child's anxiety and satisfy their own sense of duty.[89] More hospitals are therefore employing flexible policies that permit parents to be present if they desire. Special induction rooms can be established for this purpose.

Monitors

Although continuous monitoring is essential to identifying potential problems during anesthesia, it is no substitute for close observation and evaluation by the anesthesiologist. ASA standards mandate that oxygenation, ventilation, circulation, and temperature be continuously monitored during all anesthetic procedures.[90] When large fluid shifts or blood losses are expected, arterial pressure should be continuously measured with an intra-arterial cannula. The radial artery is usually selected for placement of peripheral arterial lines, but alternative sites include the dorsalis pedis and posterior tibial artery. Larger vessels (femoral and brachial) are utilized less often because they pose a greater risk of embolization.[91]

A central venous catheter facilitates the rapid infusion of drugs and large volumes of fluid, provides access for venous blood sampling, and allows measurement of central venous pressure. The veins used most often for central access are the internal jugular, femoral, and subclavian veins.

A pulmonary artery (PA) catheter is indicated in a variety of situations in which oxygenation and hemodynamic stability may be compromised (e.g., large fluid shifts, tumor manipulation, significant blood loss, instrumentation effecting ve-

nous return, critical medical condition). Small, flexible PA catheters are available for pediatric patients. Permanent wedging, a complication of PA catheterization, is more likely to occur in small children because the catheter occupies a greater proportion of the main pulmonary artery. Thus, appropriate size selection is necessary to avoid complications during placement and monitoring.

Endotracheal Tubes

Selecting an endotracheal tube (ETT) for the pediatric patient involves several issues. The ETT must be large enough to permit ventilation but small enough to minimize damage to the trachea while maintaining a seal to prevent aspiration. Tracheal damage occurs when pressure from the ETT against the wall of the trachea exceeds the capillary pressure of the tracheal mucosa, which is believed to be 25–35 mmHg.[92]

The age and medical condition of the child will dictate the size and type (cuffed, uncuffed, reinforced, single- or double-lumen) of the ETT and the leak required to prevent postextubation airway edema (Table 3–6).[217]

Laryngeal Mask

The *laryngeal mask airway* (LMA) is a novel device that helps fill the gap in airway management between tracheal intubation and face mask.[94] The LMA is inserted blindly into the pharynx to form a low-pressure seal around the

Table 3–6 • Recommendations for Size (Internal Diameter) and Type of Endotracheal Tubes

Age	Size	Type
Premature neonate	2.5–3.0	Uncuffed
Full-term neonate	3.0–3.5	Uncuffed
3 months to 1 year	4.0	Cuffed or uncuffed
2 years	4.5	Cuffed or uncuffed
4 years	5.0	Cuffed or uncuffed
6 years	5.5	Cuffed
8 years	6.0	Cuffed
10 years	6.5	Cuffed
12 years	7.0	Cuffed

From Fisher DM: Anesthesia equipment for pediatrics. In Gregory GA (ed): *Pediatric Anesthesia*, 3rd ed. New York: Churchill Livingstone, 1994, p. 216, used with permission.

laryngeal inlet, thus permitting ventilation by gentle positive pressure and inhalation of anesthetics through a minimally stimulated airway.[95] The LMA is relatively simple to insert and is a good choice for the difficult-to-manage airway. Unfortunately, the LMA does not lower the incidence of postoperative sore throat as compared with the noncuffed endotracheal tube[96] and provides no protection against aspiration in patients at risk.

Thermoregulation

Virtually all pediatric surgical patients become hypothermic unless their temperature is actively maintained. Hypothermia results predominantly from anesthetic-mediated interference with thermoregulation, although environmental losses (cold operating rooms, cold preparation solutions, prolonged exposure) also contribute.[93] The newborn is particularly predisposed to hypothermia because of (1) their relatively large BSA, (2) their diminished subcutaneous fat, and (3) their inability to increase heat production through shivering.

Serious potential complications can result from perioperative hypothermia. Platelet function can be decreased,[97] leading to coagulopathy. Severe decreases in core temperature can result in dysrhythmia and myocardial dysfunction. Mild hypothermia can decrease metabolism and increase the duration of action of some muscle relaxants as well as other anesthetic agents, which may lead to delayed awakening.[98] Postanesthetic shivering occurs only in hypothermic patients and can increase oxygen consumption by 200% to 600%.[99] A number of aids are available to help maintain normothermia during the perioperative period, including humidified circuits, warming blankets, heat lamps, fluid warmers, and decreased patient exposure.

Fluid Therapy

Precise intraoperative fluid management is imperative. Calculation of the patient's fluid deficit in routine elective cases is accomplished simply by multiplying the maintenance requirements by the hours spent fasting. This calculation is made more complex in hospitalized and medically compromised patients owing to more variable acute and chronic deficits. Causes of acute fluid losses include bleeding and osmotic diuresis due to

Table 3–7 • 4-2-1 Rule for Maintenance Fluids

Weight	IV Fluid Rate
10 kg	4 ml/kg/hour
11–20 kg	40 ml + 2 ml/kg/hour for every 1 kg weight over 10 kg
>20 kg	60 ml + 1 ml/kg/hour for every 1 kg weight over 20 kg

From Rasch SK, Carter B: *Clinical Manual of Pediatric Anesthesia*. New York: McGraw-Hill, 1994, p. 148, used with permission.

contrast material and other drugs. Causes of chronic losses include drainage from nasogastric tubes and drains, vomiting, diarrhea, and perspiration, especially in febrile patients.

One of the most well-accepted and straightforward methods for calculating standard maintenance fluid requirements is the rule of 4-2-1. By this rule, the fluid rate is calculated from 4 to 2 to 1 ml/kg based on body weight range (Table 3–7).[100] A glucose-containing balanced salt solution is used (D5.2NS in infants less than 6 months and D5.45NS in other patients).

Surgical losses include insensible ones from exposed tissue and third-space accumulation of fluid into adjacent tissues. The amount of fluid loss depends on the extent and location of the surgical procedure. Blood loss also contributes to intraoperative fluid requirements. These losses are replaced with non-glucose containing, balanced crystalloid solutions (e.g., lactated Ringer's, normal saline) or colloids.

TRANSFUSION THERAPY
Red Blood Cell Transfusion

The hematocrit level at which transfusion is warranted depends upon several factors. Concerns over the blood-borne transmission of viruses has prompted surgeons and anesthesiologists to accept lower hematocrit levels than in the past, especially in the presence of stable hemodynamics and normal acid-base balance. Other factors involved in the decision to transfuse include the estimation of oxygen requirements, age-adjusted normal hematocrit, presence of heart disease, and additional anticipated losses. A minimum acceptable hematocrit is used to calculate *estimated allowable blood loss* (EABL):[100]

Table 3–8 • Estimated Blood Volume

Age	Blood Volume (ml/kg)
Preterm infant	90–100
Full-term infant	80–85
Older than 1 year	75

Adapted from Rasch SK, Carter B: *Clinical Manual of Pediatric Anesthesia*. New York: McGraw-Hill, 1994, p. 148, used with permission.

$$^*EABL = \frac{(Hct_i - Hct_{LA}) \times EBL}{Hct_a}$$

Patients with chronic anemia may tolerate a lower acceptable hematocrit if well-developed compensatory mechanisms are established. Prior to transfusion therapy, blood volume loss is replaced with crystalloid solutions at a 3:1 ratio or with colloid solutions at a 1:1 ratio. Age-appropriate estimated blood volumes are shown in Table 3–8.[100]

Indications for Component Therapy

In the absence of laboratory-confirmed abnormalities in the coagulation profile, transfusion of blood components other than packed red blood cells is rarely indicated intraoperatively unless microvascular bleeding ensues or massive surgical losses herald a dilutional coagulopathy. The recommended doses and predicted effects of various blood components are summarized in Table 3–9.[100]

For surgical procedures in which significant blood loss is anticipated, three techniques can be employed to decrease the transfusion requirements. The first, *isovolemic hemodilution*, decreases circulating erythrocyte cell volume in order to conserve red blood cell mass. The second technique, *controlled hypotension*, clearly reduces surgical blood loss.[101] Since physiologic compensation in response to the alterations produced by each of these techniques is different, the two should never be done simultaneously. Older children and adolescents may be eligible for a third technique, *autologous blood donation*, in anticipation of procedures in which transfusion therapy is expected. A small percentage of pediatric cancer patients may qualify for these techniques because of anemia, physiologic debilitation, or multiorgan dysfunction secondary to disease processes or related anticancer therapies.

Central Neural Blockade

Regional anesthetic techniques for children have enjoyed a justified resurgence in popularity. Intraoperative blockade of the neuraxis, whether by the spinal or epidural route, provides excellent analgesia with minimal physiologic alteration. When administered in combination with general anesthesia, epidural or spinal anesthesia reduces and may even abolish the stress response to surgery. It also permits a reduction in the amount of anesthetic agent required. The result is hastened awakening, early ambulation, and shortened recovery-room stay.[102] Regional anesthesia is also useful when general anesthesia is technically difficult or is associated with an increased risk of morbidity and mortality.

Regional anesthesia may offer an alternative to general anesthesia for children with neuromuscular disorders, metabolic derangements, cardiac dysfunctions, pulmonary compromises, or malignant hyperthermias.[103] Emergency situations, when patients are at increased risk of pulmonary aspiration of stomach contents, are another indication.

Absolute contraindications to central neural blockade include (1) patient or parental refusal, (2) coagulopathy, (3) ongoing degenerative axonal

Table 3–9 • Expected Effect of Blood Components

Component	Dose	Effect (Increase)
RBC	3 ml/kg	3% hematocrit
FFP	10 ml/kg	Hemostatic dose (30% coagulation factors)
Platelets	1 unit/10 kg	50,000/μL platelet count
Cryoprecipitate	1 unit/7 kg	50 mg/dL fibrinogen

From Rasch SK, Carter B: *Clinical Manual of Pediatric Anesthesia*. New York: McGraw-Hill, 1994, p. 280, used with permission.

$^*Hct_i$ = initial hematocrit; Hct_{LA} = lowest allowable hematocrit; EBL = estimated blood volume; Hct_a = average of initial and lowest allowable hematocrit.

disease,[104] and (4) infection at the injection site. Relative contraindications include (1) septicemia, (2) abnormal sacral neuroanatomy, such as a myelomeningocele, and (3) preexisting neurologic disease.

The most common regional block performed in North American pediatric centers is the *caudal epidural block*.[105] Its popularity is due to its technical simplicity, its applicability to many pediatric surgical procedures, and its long duration of analgesia achieved with a single injection. Caudal epidural anesthesia is often given to supplement general anesthesia and to provide postoperative analgesia. *Lumbar* or *thoracic epidural anesthesia* is preferred for more rostral pain. The caudal block is relatively simple to perform in children and is less invasive than a spinal (subarachnoid) block. The success rate in one series of 750 consecutive children having caudal block was 96%.[106] Adding a caudal block to the anesthetic regimen reduces postoperative opioid requirements[107] and results in suppression of the endocrine response to surgery.[108] A catheter is usually placed in children who will undergo longer surgical procedures and in those who will require hospital treatment of pain for several days postoperatively.

Spinal (subarachnoid) block can be administered as the sole anesthetic in lower-abdominal and lower-extremity procedures in patients with underlying cardiac and pulmonary dysfunction that precludes a general anesthetic.

SPECIFIC DISEASE STATES

Leukemia

Patients with leukemia are at risk for anemia, coagulopathy, and other consequences of immunosuppression and chemotherapy that may affect their anesthetic care. Mucositis or infiltration of the oropharynx may result in difficult intubation, pharyngeal hemorrhage, or both. Hyperleukocytosis and early cytotoxic treatment are relative contraindications to general anesthesia.[109] Hyperleukocytosis may be triggered by surgery; therefore, the white blood cell count should be reduced prior to general anesthesia. Hyperleukocytosis can mimic hypoxemia leukemic cells in blood drawn for routine blood gas analysis.[109] To avoid leukostasis, transfusion of packed red blood cells should not be done in pediatric leukemic patients. Moreover, only HLA and CMV-compatible blood components should be administered to them.

Central Nervous System Tumors

Surgery is part of the initial management of virtually all pediatric brain and central nervous system tumors. It is a means of both rapidly confirming diagnosis and relieving symptoms caused by space-occupying intracranial masses and associated hydrocephalus.

There are four fundamental approaches to reducing intracranial pressure (ICP): (1) posture (i.e., head elevated >30°), (2) hyperventilation, (3) cerebral spinal fluid drainage, and (4) drug therapy. Hyperosmolar drugs, such as mannitol and urea, are effective in reducing intraoperative ICP. Other diuretics, particularly furosemide and ethacrynic acid, have been given to reduce ICP, especially when pulmonary edema and increased intravascular fluid volume coexist. Corticosteroids, such as dexamethasone and methylprednisolone, also are effective, in this case by lowering peritumoral edema.

Anesthesia in pediatric patients with brain or CNS tumors is induced with agents that produce rapid and reliable anesthesia while minimizing effects on cerebral blood flow and optimizing cerebral oxygen consumption. The trachea is intubated once an adequate depth of anesthesia is achieved and complete skeletal muscle paralysis is confirmed in order to prevent an increase in ICP from higher venous pressure. Following intubation, ventilatory rate and tidal volume are regulated to maintain $PaCO_2$ levels between 25 mmHg and 30 mmHg. Positive end-expiratory pressure that may impair cerebral venous drainage and increase ICP should be avoided.

Anesthesia is usually maintained with a combination of opioids, inhalation anesthetics, and muscle relaxants. The use of nitrous oxide is controversial. Some discourage its administration if the patient is sitting because of the presumed risks of venous air embolism and pneumocephalus. Administration of inappropriate fluid compositions (e.g., D5W, D5.45) and excessive infusion volumes may increase cerebral edema and compromise cerebral perfusion.

Continuous intra-arterial monitoring is utilized for rapidly detecting blood pressure changes that correspond to alterations in cerebral perfusion pressure. Capnography provides a breath-by-breath guide to the adequacy of hyperventilation and serves as a monitor for venous air embolism. A urinary catheter is essential for prolonged surgery and monitoring diuresis resulting from drug administration. A central venous catheter is useful in managing fluid therapy and in aspirating air in the case of venous embolism. A peripheral nerve stimulator is helpful in monitoring and ensuring the persistence of skeletal muscle paralysis.

Venous air embolism is a potential hazard whenever the patient's positioning is such that the operative site is above the level of the heart, creating reductions in venous pressure. Patients undergoing neurosurgery are especially at risk because the venous attachments to bone and dura that prevent collapse may be compromised. During posterior fossa surgery, the incidence of venous air embolism is reportedly as high as 30% to 50%.[110, 111]

Early detection of a venous air embolism is essential to successful treatment. The most sensitive methods for detecting this embolism are transesophageal echocardiography[112] and venous Doppler technique. The latter is technically less difficult and thus more widely utilized. Other detection methods, in order of decreasing sensitivity, are increased end-tidal nitrogen concentration,[113] increased pulmonary artery pressure, decreased end-tidal carbon dioxide concentration, increased central venous pressure, decreased cardiac output, decreased blood pressure, and detection of a mill wheel–like sound through the esophageal stethoscope.

Venous air embolism can be managed several ways, including limiting air entrainment (by flooding of the surgical field or aspirating through the central venous catheter), increasing central venous pressure (with head-down position), delivering positive end-expiratory pressure, maximizing oxygenation (by discontinuing use of nitrous oxide and air), and supporting hemodynamic function.

Abdominal Tumors

Most abdominal tumors are retroperitoneal. Wilms' tumor (nephroblastoma) and neuroblastoma are the most common solid tumors, accounting for 15% of all abdominal malignancies. Pheochromocytoma, although rare in children (less than 5% of reported cases),[114] has serious anesthetic implications.

Any intra-abdominal mass may delay gastric emptying and hence necessitates a rapid-sequence induction with cricoid pressure and endotracheal tube placement. Placement of large-bore peripheral catheters is required as patients can be at increased risk for hemorrhage, depending on the size and location of the mass. Neuroblastoma and other retroperitoneal masses, such as Wilms' tumor, can interfere with renal vascular flow and have been associated with elevated levels of renin and cortisol.[115] Control of hypertension associated with such lesions may be facilitated by an angiotensin-converting enzyme inhibitor such as enalapril.

Because they are associated with the adrenal medulla, pheochromocytomas produce, store, and secrete catecholamines. Anesthetic drugs can exacerbate the life-threatening cardiovascular effects of the catecholamines. Preoperative treatment with alpha blockers and re-expansion of the intravascular fluid compartment reduces the frequency of many of the hemodynamic alterations, including blood pressure fluctuations, myocardial dysrhythmia and dysfunction, congestive heart failure, and cerebral hemorrhage. No clear advantage exists for one anesthetic drug over another, but drugs that are known to liberate histamines and catecholamines should be avoided.[116] Manipulation of the tumor may produce marked elevations in blood pressure, which are controlled with nitroprusside and phentolamine. Tachydysrhythmias are treated with intravenous beta blockers. The reduction in blood pressure that may occur following ligation of the tumor's venous supply should be anticipated and met with intravascular volume expansion.

Upper Airway Tumors

Neoplastic lesions originating in the upper airway are rare in children. Cervical adenopathy is the most common clinical presentation of Hodgkin's disease and, less frequently, non-Hodgkin's lymphoma.[117] It can occasionally displace or obstruct the trachea. Superior vena cava syndrome from the same disease may cause obstruction by venous engorgement of laryngopharyngeal structures.

A variety of options exist for establishing control of the airway in a patient with an airway tumor. The choice depends upon the location and extent of tumor involvement. The safest method involves controlling the airway in an awake, spontaneously breathing patient. The challenge to the anesthesiologist in the case of the younger child involves providing necessary sedation without compromising respiratory function. Utilizing the fiberoptic bronchoscope, intubation can be performed under direct vision while airway pathology is evaluated. A standard pediatric bronchoscope (outer diameter 3.6 mm) will advance through an endotracheal tube (ETT) 4.5 mm or larger. Smaller bronchoscopes are available (outer diameter 2.2 mm) that will pass through an ETT of 2.5 mm or larger. Another option is to perform an "awake look" laryngoscopy in an awake, spontaneously breathing child who is topically anesthetized. This procedure is done to visualize the vocal cords and assure successful intubation of the trachea. Inhalation anesthetic can provide suitable conditions for intubating a spontaneously breathing child who is unable to tolerate the procedure with sedation alone. Surgical tracheostomy is also an option for emergency airway management.

Thoracic Tumors

As most pulmonary neoplastic lesions in children have metastasized from extrapulmonary sites, wedge resection is performed more frequently than lobectomy or pneumonectomy. Thoracic procedures present a number of special considerations. Supraventricular tachyarrhythmias occurring intraoperatively may be caused by cardiac manipulation. Arrhythmias during one-lung ventilation may be a sign of inadequate ventilation or poor oxygenation. Peripheral arterial cannulation has become essential to the management of patients undergoing major thoracic surgical procedures for both monitoring and blood sampling. Monitoring of central venous pressure can also be beneficial in selected patients.

In adults, ventilation for thoracic procedures is commonly accomplished with one-lung anesthesia. The smallest endobronchial tube available is 28 French (Mallinckrodt), which corresponds to an outer diameter of 9.3 mm, limiting the use of double-lumen tubes in infants and young children.

Selective ventilation in the infant and small child can be achieved by two methods. The first involves intubation of the dependent mainstem bronchus. Placement can be ensured by fiberoptic bronchoscopy with the patient in lateral decubitus position. The second method employs a Fogarty embolectomy catheter as a bronchial blocker. If selective ventilation is not accomplished by either method, the procedure can be performed with both lungs ventilated and surgical packing of the operative lung.

Anterior Mediastinal Mass

Most anterior mediastinal masses are lymphomatous in origin. Others can originate from cervical masses that extend deep into the mediastinum. In either case, severe respiratory and cardiovascular complications have been described in pediatric patients with such masses. The resulting airway obstruction is multifactorial. Trapping of air and obstructing of expiration following onset of positive-pressure ventilation are common,[118] likely resulting from a ball-valve effect. Cardiovascular changes resembling venous obstruction or tamponade may occur very rapidly, as the hyperdistended lung places further pressure on the tumor and great vessels, thus inhibiting venous return to the heart or obstructing pulmonary artery blood flow.[119, 120] The safe delivery of an anesthetic may be necessary to provide conditions for obtaining a tissue specimen for pathology evaluation, prior to the initiation of anticancer therapy. The response of lymphomatous tumors to radiation or chemotherapy is normally dramatic. Indeed, following radiation or chemotherapy, the appearance of the tumor must be reevaluated and a dynamic study of pulmonary function performed with flow-volume loops in a variety of positions.

The position for induction of anesthesia must be one that produces the least cardiopulmonary compromise—usually the semi-Fowler's position. A rigid bronchoscope should be immediately available, and the surgical team should be present at the time of induction. Numerous case reports document life-threatening airway crisis and even death following the onset of positive-pressure ventilation in children with mediastinal tumors.[121, 122] Induction of anesthesia is generally performed while maintaining spontaneous ventilation in the absence of muscle relaxants. Although some intrathoracic masses can be excised in spontaneously breathing patients,[123] positive-pressure ventilation normally becomes necessary once the chest is opened. If ventilation suddenly becomes difficult or impossible, a rapid change in patient position (usually from supine to prone or lateral) may relieve pressure on the airway. Occasionally, cardiopulmonary bypass equipment is required.

Extremity Tumors

Phantom Limb Pain with Amputation

As with adults, both phantom sensations and pain are common in children and adolescents following limb amputation.[124] The phenomenon in children and adolescents, however, often tends to decrease more in frequency and intensity over time.[125] At least one study suggests a correlation between the presence of preoperative pain in the diseased extremity and the later occurrence of phantom pain in children and adolescents, implying that as in adults, preoperative regional anesthesia may help prevent phantom pain.[126]

Infectious Disease Considerations

All children with cancer are at risk for immunosuppression. Neutropenia caused by marrow infiltration or treatment-related aplasia is associated with increased risk of serious bacterial, fungal, and opportunistic infections. Other factors associated with immunocompromise include the nature of the malignancy (e.g., lymphoma, leukemia), and whether the patient has received a bone marrow transplant, particularly if graft-versus-host disease is present. Hospitalization in and of itself predisposes the patient to infection owing to the disruption of physical barriers by indwelling catheters, invasive procedures, and exposures to multiple antibiotics and drug-resistant microorganisms. Consequently, it is especially important that sterile techniques be employed during all invasive procedures. Frequent handwashing and avoidance of unnecessary stopcocks are recommended.[127] Neutropenic patients should be identified, and their caretakers should routinely wear gown, mask, and gloves.

PEDIATRIC PAIN MANAGEMENT

Public awareness and multiple research studies have brought effective pain management to the forefront of patient care. Multiple etiologies of pain are associated with malignancies. In addition, the cancer patient frequently experiences pain related to procedures and surgical interventions. The psychological and physiologic side effects of inadequate pain management are well documented in the scientific and clinical literature.[128, 129] These undesirable effects include stimulation of the endocrine and metabolic pathways and elevation of stress hormones, which translate into increased cardiac work, increased ICP, decreased transcutaneous oxygenation, increased serum glucose with decreased utilization, diminished gastrointestinal function, fluid retention, alteration in coagulation, catabolic breakdown of tissue, and poor healing.[130] Impairment of the immune response has also been demonstrated,[131] which may be particularly problematic for the cancer patient.

The research supporting these adverse findings was done primarily in adult patients. A few well-cited studies by Anand and coworkers[132, 133] clearly demonstrated similar phenomena in the pediatric population. In addition, sensitization of peripheral pain receptors has been demonstrated.[134] Such sensitization can lead to a heightened experience of acute pain and development of chronic pain syndrome.[135] Historically, pain in the pediatric population has been vastly undertreated.[136, 137] Societal perceptions, physician's attitudes, and lack of scientific data have perpetuated myths about the pain experience of infants and children. For example, it was once commonly held that owing to their immature nervous systems, neonates and infants do not experience or remember pain as adults do. Even now, unfounded concerns about narcotic addiction continue to prevent physicians from giving children adequate analgesia. Fortunately, research has encouraged a heightened sensitivity in clinical practice to pain problems in children and adults alike. Cost-containment concerns in health care have prompted studies demonstrating that adequate pain therapy is associated with decreased complication rates, shorter ICU stays, and lower mortality rates.[138, 139]

Pain Assessment

In 1990 the World Health Organization published its Consensus Conference report on the Management of Pain in Childhood Cancer. In regard to the assessment of pain, two principles were accepted as patient-care standards:[140]

1. Systematic assessment of pain is necessary in the management of cancer as most children with cancer experience significant pain at some time in the disease course. The etiology of this pain may be related to the disease process and associated therapy as well as to invasive procedures for diagnosis and monitoring.

2. Ongoing assessment of pain throughout the course of the illness is necessary as factors that alter the pain experience change with time and must be continuously evaluated.

A variety of specific obstacles prevent adequate pain management in the pediatric population at large. For example, one must consider a large spectrum of ages and age-related development. Parental involvement and coping responses must also be carefully considered when caring for the child who is experiencing or anticipating pain.

A number of age-specific tools have been suggested. These assessment tools take into account physical and behavioral responses, including self-reporting in verbal patients with appropriate cognitive development. Clinicians have become more acutely aware of the physiologic changes and behavioral responses related to pain in the care of neonates and infants. Pain-assessment tools are not universally utilized, and foolproof scales have yet to be developed. Nevertheless, a number of clinically validated methods exist for assessing postoperative pain in children.[141] Comprehensive therapy takes into account the multifactorial experience of pain and the related issues that contribute to its severity. Some of these factors include cultural and familial expectations (e.g., parental response and attitude), environmental factors (e.g., past experiences, sounds, smells), and situational cues (the child's expectations and sense of control, responses of medical personnel).[142]

Infant Pain Scales

Results of studies evaluating pain in infants have varied significantly. This variation has often been attributed to developmental and age discrepancies as well as to different medical procedures. In addition, a number of common distress responses may depend upon the behavioral state of the same infant at any given time. No single behavior or physiologic response is unequivocally reliable in measuring an infant's pain. Therefore, it is inappropriate to interpret an absent or a variable response to a noxious stimulus as lack of pain. Recommendations are to monitor behavior trends and to provide analgesia consistent with the extent of tissue damage and the region of involvement in infants. Additional research is necessary to assess the ability of infants to express a varied response to stress, distress, and pain.

CHEOPS (Children's Hospital of Eastern Ontario Pain Scale)

The Children's Hospital of Eastern Ontario Pain Scale (CHEOPS) developed by McGrath[143] uses sequential observations of six behaviors (crying, facial expression, verbal expression, torso position, touch behavior, and leg position) to assess pain. Physiologic changes (including vital signs) are not part of the overall evaluation. As in the assessment of infant pain, one must carefully avoid implying pain severity based solely on the child's behavioral response to an acute pain experience.

Faces Scales

Scales that employ cartoon faces to help assess pain have proved effective. The Oucher scale was designed for pain assessment in young children (3–7 years of age).[144] Beyer and Aradine[145] showed that many children as young as 3 years of age were able to comprehend the rank order of faces showing increments of discomfort. The six pictures of a child's face demonstrate levels of severity ranging from "no pain" to "most pain." Once the tool is understood by the child, it is no longer language-dependent. Whaley and Wong[146] (1987) also employed cartoon faces with varied expressions to stratify pain severity. A follow-up study by Wong and Baker[147] demonstrated efficacy for this tool in pain assessment.

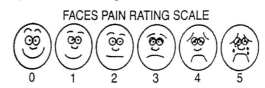

FACES PAIN RATING SCALE

0 1 2 3 4 5

Face 0: no hurt; Face 1: hurts little bit; Face 2: hurts little more; Face 3: hurts even more; Face 4: hurts whole lot; Face 5: hurts worst. From Whaley L, Wong D: Nursing Care of Infants and Children, 3rd ed. St. Louis: C.V. Mosby Co., 1987, p. 1070, used with permission.

Visual Analog Scale

A number of self-reporting tools for pain assessment are based on a number or color-intensity line. One number scale that ranges from 1 (no pain) to 10 (worst imaginable pain) has been comfortably, reliably, and validly used with children as young as 5 years of age.[148] The clinician must remember, however, that the intervals along the scale may be interpreted differently by different children.

Pain Journals

Older children and adolescents can keep a journal to accurately record their pain experience. These journals can be especially helpful in managing chronic pain. Patterns of pain can indicate the need for dosing and scheduling changes in medication.

Pain Management

The special pain concerns of the pediatric cancer patient include acute pain and onset of a new pain symptomatology that can persist as chronic pain. Tumor invasion involving bony infiltration, visceral extension with capsular distension, and neural compression are significant causes of pain. Leukemias, lymphomas, and solid abdominal tumors produce significant pain related to visceral infiltration and distension. Bone, soft tissues, nerve roots, and plexuses can be involved in sarcomas (osteosarcoma, Ewing's sarcoma, and rhabdomyosarcoma). Neuroectodermal tumors are associated with extremely severe pain related to tumor invasion that may include the epidural space.

Headaches are a common complaint of patients with primary or metastatic involvement of the brain, especially when involving the posterior fossa. Therapy for this malignancy may involve surgical intervention and other painful procedures including bone biopsy and lumbar puncture.

Complications of cancer therapy can include peripheral neuropathies related to vincristine or cisplatin treatment.[149] Phantom limb deafferentation pain may follow amputation and limb-salvage procedures.[150] Patients treated with chemotherapy (i.e., Adriamycin [doxorubicin], methotrexate, fluorouracil) or radiation to the head and neck may develop mucositis, a particularly uncomfortable condition.[151]

Non-Narcotic Analgesia

Non-narcotic analgesic drugs include salicylate, acetominophen, and nonsteroidal anti-inflammatory drugs. In general, these analgesics are ideal for managing mild to moderate pain. Acetaminophen remains the most popular analgesic in the pediatric population, although, its dose-response curve for analgesia in this population is unknown. Two studies suggest that common oral dosing of 10 mg/kg is probably too conservative. Berde[148] reports that 15–20 mg/kg can be safely administered every 4 hours. Moreover, this dose may need to be increased for rectal administration, as Rusby and coworkers[152] showed that plasma levels remained low 40 minutes after a rectal dose of 35 mg/kg. The analgesia at this dose was, however, reportedly equivalent to that produced by intravenous ketorolac (1 mg/kg).[152] No children involved in Rusby's study had any significant hepatic dysfunction.

Aspirin remains an effective therapy, especially when the pain has an inflammatory component. Even so, problems associated with aspirin (Reye's syndrome, gastrointestinal upset, and platelet dysfunction) have contributed to a decline in its prescription.[153, 154] The larger group of nonsteroidal anti-inflammatory drugs (NSAIDs) includes indomethacin, which has been shown to have opioid-sparing properties in children postoperatively.[155] Orthopedic-related pain is especially appropriate for NSAID therapy alone or in conjunction with narcotics.

Vetter and Heiner[156] compared ketorolac with a placebo in patients receiving opioids following orthopedic operations. In the ketorolac group, pain scores and drug side effects were lower. Morphine use fell 38%.[156] Other advantages of ketorolac alone or in combination with narcotics include decreased respiratory depression, sedation, and nausea. Yet, ketorolac therapy is still controversial in light of its reported side effects. Rusby and coworkers[152] reported greater blood loss in conjunction with ketorolac and the need for additional intervention to achieve homeostasis. No clinical bleeding episodes were identified, but one institution reported significant post-tonsillectomy bleeding believed to be related to ketorolac.[157] Thus, it is prudent to refrain from administering ketorolac to patients with coagulopathy, nephropathy, gastropathy, or hypovolemia. Furthermore, studies in adult patients indicate that a 1 mg/kg loading dose of ketorolac is unnecessary.[154] Instead, giving the minimum dose for the shortest period possible (0.2–0.5 mg/kg every 6 hours for 48 hours) is probably the best guideline for safe and effective administration.

In patients with bone marrow suppression or platelet dysfunction, NSAIDs and salicylates are best avoided. It is also advisable to provide alternative pain therapy for at least 5 to 7 days before surgical intervention in patients receiving aspirin or other NSAIDs. This delay allows time for platelet recovery.

Narcotic Analgesia

Children may vary as much as adults in terms of individual experience with pain and response to pharmacologic agents. The pain experience will vary according to location and extent of tissue involved, neurologic and cardiovascular status, pain chronicity, and amount and type of prior pain experience. Parents and caregivers' fear of addiction in children—based more on myth than on fact—has often created a reluctance to administer sufficient narcotics. Tolerance often occurs in the patient with longstanding or chronic pain, but addiction is rare and, in general, not a relevant subject for consideration in the treatment of the severe pain common in cancer.[158, 159]

The severity of pain and the underlying medical condition should dictate the agent and dose required for therapy. Narcotics can be administered in a number of routes: oral, intramuscular (IM), intravenous (IV), and neuraxial are the most common. Following non-narcotic therapy, codeine and oxycodone are reasonable progressive agents. Agonist-antagonist agents (i.e., nalbuphine) are generally not recommended for long-term use or for use in patients already receiving narcotic therapy—they may precipitate a withdrawal response. Oral morphine is regarded by many as the drug of choice in children with cancer who have significant pain.[160] Methadone, another alternative, provides excellent analgesia with longer duration. The elixir form may be better for pediatric patients unable to swallow pills or tablets.

In light of so many painless methods for delivering narcotics, intramusclar injections are completely unnecessary and offer no advantage. Some children in pain will even deny their discomfort in order to avoid a shot. Intravenous

Table 3–10 • Opioid Analgesics for Pediatric Pain

Drug	Equipotent IV Dose (mg/kg)	Comments
Morphine	0.1	Histamine release, vasodilation Use caution with asthmatics or patients with hemodynamic compromise
Meperidine	1.0	Metabolite produces seizures—not recommended for chronic use Catastrophic interaction with MAO inhibitors
Methadone	0.1	Very effective by the IV, IM, or PO route
Fentanyl	0.001	Chest wall rigidity Decreases heart rate but causes minimal hemodynamic changes
Codeine	1.2	Oral use only
Hydromorphone (Dilaudid)	0.015–0.02	Associated with less itching and nausea than morphine May be used by either IV or epidural route
Oxycodone	0.15	Better oral bioavailability than morphine Often used when weaning from IV to oral pain medications

From Houck CS, Berde CB, Anand KJS: Pediatric pain management. In Gregory GA (ed): *Pediatric Anesthesiology*, 3rd ed. New York: Churchill Livingstone, 1994, p. 751, used with permission.

Table 3–11 • Narcotics for Analgesia in Children

Name	Relative Potency	Dosage	Comments
Morphine (MS)	1 1	IV 0.02–0.05 mg/kg IM 0.1–0.2 mg/kg/dose q 2–4 hours PO 0.3–0.5 mg/kg/dose q 4 hours	Duration: child, 2–3 hours; neonate, 14 hours Enterohepatic circulation is important for elimination
Sustained-release MS (MS Contin)	1	PO 0.3–0.6 mg/kg/dose q 12 hours	BID useful in outpatient care
Hydromorphone (Dilaudid)	6	PO 0.05–0.1 mg/kg/dose q 6 hours (maximum: 5 mg/dose)	Possibly less dysphoria and nausea, vomiting
Meperidine (Demerol)	0.1	PO, IM 1.0–1.5 mg/kg/dose q 4 hours IV 0.1–0.25 mg/kg/dose	Duration: child, 3–4 hours; neonate, 24 hours Risk of CNS toxicity from normeperidine metabolite accumulation Increased euphoria and dysphoria
Fentanyl	80	IV 1.0–1.5 μg/kg/dose q 1–2 hours	Duration: 3–4 hours
Methadone (Dolobid)	1 0.5	IV 0.1 mg/kg/dose q 6–12 hours PO 0.2 mg/kg/dose q 6–12 hours	Duration: 12–24 hours Less sedation, nausea, and dysphoria than morphine
Propoxyphene (oxycodone)	1	PO 0.05–0.15 mg/kg/dose q 4–5 hours	Duration: 4–5 hours Lower dependence liability
Codeine	0.8	PO 0.5–1.0 mg/kg/dose q 4–6 hours (maximum: 5 mg/dose)	Duration: 3–4 hours High incidence of constipation

From Eige SA, Bell C: Pediatric pain management. In Bell C, Hughes CW, Oh TH (eds): *Pediatric Anesthesia Handbook.* St. Louis: Mosby-Year Book, 1991, p. 507; Greene MG (ed): *Harriet Lane Handbook*, 12th ed. St. Louis: Mosby-Year Book, 1991; and Koren G, Maurice L: Pediatric uses of opioids. *Pediatr Clin North Am* 36:1141–1156, 1989.

opioids are often prescribed for children postoperatively and for pain related to other acute and chronic etiologies.

In patients who have been receiving ongoing narcotic therapy, the dosing required may be much greater than expected for the child's size and type of acute pain problem. When narcotics are altered or changed, the prescribing physician must be careful to provide an equivalent dose of opioid therapy (Table 3–10).[161] Pharmacists and service personnel can be helpful in this regard. The safe starting doses of commonly administered intermittent intravenous narcotics are listed in Table 3–11.[162–164] The dosing limit for drug therapy, however, should be primarily determined by patient response. Give as much as is required to make the patient comfortable.[165] Epidural and intrathecal narcotic therapy offer

additional routes of administration for patients suffering postoperative and chronic pain.

Although side effects may commonly develop during narcotic therapy, they can be treated and hence pain management can be continued. All opioids produce a dose-dependent respiratory depression that affects both tidal volume and respiratory rate. The compensatory response to hypoxia and hypercarbia is also affected. Atelectasis can develop quite easily in this setting, but respiratory exercises that encourage coughing and deep breathing may attenuate the occurrence. Other side effects include nausea, pruritus, constipation, urinary retention, and sedation. In the hypovolemic patient, hypotension may occur, especially in association with morphine boluses, which can be attributed to histamine release.

Adjunctive medication therapy should be provided to treat troublesome side effects. Stool softeners are often routinely prescribed for the patient requiring ongoing narcotic therapy. Diphenhydramine and low-dose naloxone (1.0 µg/kg/hour) offer effective treatment for bothersome pruritus. Some patients are uncomfortable with the sedation associated with narcotic therapy. Stimulants such as dextroamphetamine (0.1–0.2 mg/kg PO) not only decrease the respiratory depression, sedation, and nausea seen with narcotics but also increase the analgesic effect.[166]

Patient-Controlled Analgesia

Patient-controlled analgesia (PCA) was first discussed by Sechzer[167] (1969) and was used primarily for adults and adolescents.[167] Considered helpful for all forms of acute pain, including cancer pain, PCA has been widely accepted in North America since the mid-1980s.[168] It has been utilized for severe chronic pain in cancer patients and non-cancer patients at home as well as in the hospital. The principle behind PCA is to give patients control over their own opioid administration. Factors determining opioid requirements include prior opioid use, pain tolerance, tissue involvement extent, and concurrent drug therapy. In addition to intermittent, or "demand" dosing, a basal infusion can provide a low level of continuous analgesia by maintaining a minimum opiate blood level.

With PCA, patients can obtain pain relief when discomfort is initially experienced and need not suffer from delays in nursing response and administration. PCA is the only specialized analgesic technique that has been shown to be cost-effective; it reduces the nursing staff workload.[169] The PCA infusion system is portable, too, allowing the patient to walk with the device. Patients can deliver doses of pain medication to themselves prior to painful procedures and tests even when away from the nursing floor. Overall, the total dose of narcotic required for adequate relief of symptoms is less with PCA than with traditional routes of administration. This lower dose requirement can be explained by the immediate treatment of symptoms around the clock and less opioid blood level variability afforded by PCA.[170]

PCA has been successful in young children as well as adolescents. A randomized prospective comparison of IM morphine and patient-controlled morphine in children conducted by Berde and coworkers[171] demonstrated that pain scores in the PCA group were significantly lower and patient satisfaction higher than in the IM group. The PCA group also demonstrated less somnolence. Somnolence requiring naloxone therapy did, however, occur in 2 of the first 1500 study patients who received concurrent antiemetic and antipruritic therapy.[172] The importance of patient selection, appropriate drug selection and dosing, and adequate monitoring cannot be overemphasized.

Patient Selection for PCA

The factors most important for successful PCA use in children are (1) age, (2) the physical ability to push the button, and (3) the cognitive ability to comprehend the cause-and-effect relationship involved in pushing the button.[173] Any response by a child to the effect that pushing the button "makes the pain go away" demonstrates comprehension. With appropriate instruction, virtually all 7-year-old children can independently operate the device and titrate analgesics to a personal level of tolerable pain.[171] PCA has been used successfully in children as young as 4 years of age, but additional support and encouragement were required of parents and nurses.[174] Children inflicted with mental-status changes and children with mental handicaps must be individually evaluated regardless of age. Parents should not be put in the position of providing 24-hour care for their ill child, but they can assist with reinforcement of teaching. Beware of parents transferring their own personal concerns about opioid use (i.e., drug addiction) to the child. But parents must also be taught not to overmedicate their child by pushing the PCA button for him or her in anticipation of pain. Parental concerns are best solicited and addressed prior to initiation of therapy.

PCA Dosing

The ideal drug for the PCA prescription would have rapid onset, moderately long duration of action, and minimal side effects. Although no such perfect drug exists, a number of drugs, each with unique characteristics and potential side effects, have been given successfully. When choosing a dosing regimen, one must take into account the patient's clinical condition, prior opioid therapy, and adjuvant drug therapy.

In general, the bolus dose should be enough for the patient to perceive some analgesic effect without side effects. If the relief of pain symptoms is inadequate, the bolus dose can be increased by 50%. Patients who require long-term narcotic therapy should have the prescribed doses adjusted to reflect current tolerance. The concentration should be adjusted to provide a bolus dose of at least 0.5 ml.

To avoid the accumulation of opiate by reflux into the maintenance line, a one-way valve should be incorporated into the system.[175] The PCA infusion should be connected as closely as possible to the intravenous catheter to avoid dead-space infusion buildups. The maintenance IV fluid infusion rate should be adequate to allow bolus doses to be received prior to completion of the lockout interval. Analgesics should be titrated prior to initiation of the PCA system.

Opiate-naive patients should be started on a conservative dosing schedule. For postoperative pain, the basal infusion should not exceed a dose that would be considered safe in an opiate-naive patient.[174] One study produced results suggesting that a basal infusion is advantageous, especially in the first 48 hours postoperatively.[176] A safe nighttime basal infusion rate can best be assessed by carefully reviewing the hourly requirements during the day. One half the average hourly daytime requirement is a safe dose for basal infusion. Dosing data for children are simply anecdotal, and most recommendations are extrapolated from adult data.[177]

An initial dose of morphine (0.05–0.1 mg/kg) may be required in the postoperative patient to provide analgesia before PCA therapy. Intraoperative delivery of narcotics should be taken into consideration when prescribing postoperative narcotic therapy. Morphine may be titrated at the bedside (0.03–0.05 mg/kg at 8-minute intervals) to achieve patient comfort. A safe starting dose for demand PCA with morphine is 0.01–0.03 mg/kg, with a lockout interval of 5–8 minutes. When a basal infusion is required, 0.01 mg/kg/hour is a reasonable initial dose.

Morphine fulfills most of the desirable drug criteria and is the drug most commonly prescribed for PCA; however, a variety of other agents have been used successfully. Meperidine is an acceptable alternative for short-term (24-to 48-hour) therapy. Its active metabolite, normeperidine, is primarily excreted in the urine but may accumulate, resulting in neurotoxicity. The dose for meperidine is approximately 10 times that recommended for morphine. Because of its short duration of action, fentanyl is less desirable for demand PCA dosing, unless a background basal infusion is prescribed. Basal infusions of 0.3–2 μg/kg/hour may be utilized, with bolus demand doses of 0.3–1.5 μg/kg.[178] Six-minute lockout intervals are within safe dosing guidelines. Owing to the rapid onset of its effect, fentanyl may be selected for PCA when required for painful procedures and treatments. In this situation a "demand only" prescription can be ordered, with a lockout interval as short as 3 minutes.[174] Hydromorphone and methadone have also been given successfully in PCA. The slow onset of hydromorphone and the long half-life of methadone, however, may present a less than ideal pharmacokinetic profile for PCA, and neither appears to offer an advantage over morphine, meperidine, or fentanyl.

Continuous Narcotic Infusions

Because of age, mental or physical handicaps, and other related issues, some pediatric cancer patients may not be able to use a PCA pump. Continuous IV opioid infusion is an effective analgesic alternative. Morphine is the most common agent for this purpose. Infusions, however, require a bolus loading dose to establish a blood level. This loading dose is often administered in the operating room, with the continuous infusion established later in the postanesthesia care unit.

In the narcotic-naive patient, morphine sulfate 0.05–0.1 mg/kg IV generally provides adequate pain relief. This dose may need to be decreased by one half to one third in patients with limited morphine clearance (e.g., those with hepatic insufficiency or neonates).[161] In pediatric patients over 1 month old, the metabolic pathways actually clear morphine to a greater extent than in adults.[179] Initial infusion rates of 10–30 μg/kg/hour provide adequate analgesia in most patients without producing hypercarbia as a result of respiratory depression. Higher rates of infusion have been given successfully in patients with narcotic tolerance without untoward effects.

Fentanyl may be continuously infused in those patients unable to tolerate the histamine release caused by morphine. Infusion rates of 1–2 μg/kg/hour usually produce adequate analgesia, following an initial bolus of 1–2 μg/kg. As with morphine, infants younger than 3 months old and children with hepatic insufficiency require dose reductions. It is not uncommon for fentanyl requirements to increase daily in order to maintain the same level of analgesia, apparently representing a fairly rapid tolerance to fentanyl.

The potential problem of overmedication in a patient receiving a continuous infusion of narcotic, either alone or in conjunction with a PCA dosing program, presents special considerations for monitoring. Patient somnolence or cessation of demand PCA dosing should alert the caregiver to the need for alterations. Frequent observation and vital-sign monitoring every 4 hours are mandatory. In addition, continuously monitored respiratory assessment (i.e., pulse oximetry) is required.

Preventing and Managing Narcotic Side Effects

Regardless of the route of administration, a variety of side effects may accompany the administration of narcotics. Oversedation and respiratory depression are of greatest concern in ongoing narcotic therapy. All types of narcotic infusions for analgesia require diligent nursing assessment and monitoring. The nursing staff should provide careful observation, with hourly monitoring of the patient's mental alertness and respiratory function. Because narcotic requirements may vary dramatically among patients, clinical vigilance is mandatory. As sedation always precedes respiratory depression, the onset of sedation is an important clinical sign of ensuing overdose. In such a case, appropriate action must be taken immediately: the infusion rate decreased and monitoring by the nursing staff subsequently increased. In patients receiving continuous infusions and those with significant alterations of hepatic function or neurologic status, continuous respiratory monitoring with pulse oximetry and more intensive nursing supervision are recommended.

Nausea has been reported to occur in 33% of patients receiving narcotic therapy.[171, 180] Various antiemetics have been recommended to relieve this side effect, including scopolamine, metoclopramide, Phenergan (promethazine), trimetho-benzamide, ondansetron, and prochlorperazine. The different treatments are directed at the different possible etiologies, including delayed gastric emptying, chemoreceptor trigger zone activity, and vestibular stimulation. Although no agent has been shown to be specific for narcotic-induced nausea, each agent may have its own side effects. Increased sedation and dystonia are of primary concern.

Confusion and dysphoria may occur with high-dose narcotic therapy or with combination therapy that includes NSAIDs, psychotropic drugs, and sedative-hypnotics. In the presence of mental-status changes, hypoxia must be ruled out prior to other potential etiologies. Corrective interventions may include modifying the medication regimen.

Constipation is a common problem related to narcotic analgesia. Prophylactic measures for prevention may include stool softeners; increased fluids, including fruit juices; and ambulation, when possible. Effective treatments include lactulose, suppositories, enemas, and other standard therapies.

Relative Potency

Patients who require ongoing narcotic therapy for chronic or acute pain management will require larger doses of medication than narcotic-naive patients. The narcotic requirements for postsurgical patients will be based upon preoperative narcotic therapy and relative potencies of selected postoperative narcotics. Narcotic tolerance, a decrease in susceptibility to the effects of a drug resulting from continued use, should be considered as well. Tolerance may be seen within the first week of initiating drug therapy. Cross-tolerance between drugs is not predictable.

Preventing Withdrawal Reactions

The risk of significant pain exacerbation and deleterious effects from acute narcotic withdrawal make mandatory a careful drug history specifically eliciting information on any pain medications. Concerns about drug withdrawal and addiction should be considered only when therapy is to be decreased or discontinued. Such concerns should not be addressed when drug therapy is initiated for management of pain. Drug withdrawal, the abstention from drugs to which one is habituated,[181] also known as abstinence syndrome,[182] may produce a variety of symptoms, including restlessness, agitation, low-grade fever, vomiting, anorexia, and increased blood pressure. Habituation can be observed as early as the first week of continuous drug therapy. Following a prolonged course of narcotic or benzodiazepine therapy, a gradual reduction in drug therapy by 10% to 20% per day may prevent acute deleterious withdrawal reactions. The longer a patient has been on drug therapy, the slower the required weaning process. When patients are on IV or epidural narcotics, continuous infusions should be discontinued first, allowing narcotic therapy to be provided by intermittent demand doses.

Pain Consultants

With the advancement of pain management as a specialty, multidisciplinary practitioners have developed both independent and collaborative treatment-based consultation services. Through careful clinical evaluation and assessment, appropriate and effective therapy can be recommended that will effectively treat pain and pain syndromes. Pain specialists may include anesthesiologists, pediatricians, neurologists, oncologists, internists, and neurosurgeons. A comprehensive practice incorporates support staff with individual expertise. Representative disciplines may include nurses, psychologists, physical and occupational therapists, and pharmacists. When standard therapy is not effective, or when the side effects of the therapy are preventing an optimal outcome, a pain-management consultation should be obtained. Management of chronic pain in the outpatient setting may be proposed. Other treatment options for maximizing the results from standard pain therapy may be available for consideration, including central, regional, and local nerve blocks as well as adjuvant pharmacologic interventions.

Caudal and Epidural Catheters

When indicated, caudal and epidural catheters can be placed in the surgical patient while he or she is in the operating room for postoperative pain management. Surgical procedures that may be associated with significant pain include thoracotomy, laparotomy, limb salvage, and amputation. Catheters can also be placed for the sole purpose of acute and chronic pain management outside the operating room environment, provided that sterile technique is not compromised. The indications for an epidural approach, outside the perioperative period, include acute and chronic cancer-related pain,[183, 184] phantom limb pain,[185] ischemia related to vasculitis or arterial lines,[186–188] and sickle-cell vaso-occlusive crisis.[189] Tobias and coworkers[190] have clearly demonstrated the efficacy of this technique in the pediatric cancer patient. Despite variations in patient size, age, diagnosis, and surgical procedure, epidural catheterization has been shown to be clearly beneficial for the respiratory, cardiovascular, and metabolic status. Patients with effective epidural pain control do not demonstrate the typical postsurgical neuroendocrine stress response that can lead to morbidity and mortality.[138]

Although a variety of drugs have been used in the epidural space, current clinical practice generally favors narcotics, local anesthetics, or a combination of the two. Combination therapy improves analgesia while limiting some common adverse effects.[191] Drug-related side effects may include reactions to narcotics, local anesthetics, or both. The local anesthetics provide neural blockade that may pertain to sensory, motor, and sympathetic nerves.

Epidural Side Effects and Complications

Adverse effects may result from placement of the epidural catheter or from drug administration through the catheter. The most common complications are dural puncture, bleeding, and infection. Nerve injury or trauma related to the procedure is rare, provided the practitioner is experienced.

The epidural space contains an extensive venous plexus. Uncontrolled bleeding can result in the formation of an epidural hematoma, which can lead to paralysis resulting from compromise of spinal cord perfusion. Therefore, patients with suspected coagulopathies should be evaluated by PT, PTT, bleeding time, and platelet count. Epidural analgesia is contraindicated in patients with qualitative or quantitative thrombocytopenia (platelet counts <100,000/mm³ or abnormal bleeding time). PT and PTT should be less than 1.5 times that of the control.

The incidence of dural puncture may be higher in the pediatric population (8% to 10%).[192] Frontal headaches can occur that are exacerbated by upright positioning. This problem is usually self-limited, but if the headaches persist, an epidural "blood patch" can be performed.

Infections from epidural catheters in acute (3–5 day) pain management are extremely uncommon[193] even in the immunocompromised cancer patient. DuPen and coworkers[194] studied 350 cancer patients with long-term epidural catheterization for chronic pain management.[194] All 19 patients who developed deep-track or epidural-space infections were successfully treated with catheter removal and antibiotic therapy. Rare case reports do exist of infections requiring surgical decompression and drainage. Maintenance of sterile technique during catheter placement and dressing changes, careful skin/site assessment, and routine temperature monitoring are the standard preventive measures.

Should the catheter ever become dislodged or disconnected, the anesthesiologist or pain consultant must be notified immediately. The contaminated catheter tip must not be reconnected to the infusion system. Berde and coworkers[195] recommend that the catheter be tunneled subcutaneously at the time of initial placement for chronic pain purpose[195]; this technique helps prevent infection and minimizes the risk of catheter dislodgment.[196]

Drug therapy and catheter utilization may cause additional side effects. Children have compensatory mechanisms that maintain cardiac output and blood pressure during epidural blockade.[197] A high sympathetic block (T1–4) can be associated with inhibition of the cardiac accelerators, resulting in bradycardia, but this is generally not a problem associated with blood pressure alterations in pediatric patients. The drastic drop in blood pressure that can occur in adults from a sympathetic blockade is also not common in children unless dehydration is severe.

Motor blockade related to local anesthesia can lead to weakness in the motor groups supplied by the nerve roots affected by infusion distribution. During ambulation, the patient should be assisted to prevent a fall. Providing a dilute local anesthetic solution (i.e., bupivacaine 0.1–0.2%) may decrease the incidence and severity of motor blockade.

Careful catheter placement by skilled practitioners and close monitoring during administration of drug boluses can prevent life-threatening complications that might otherwise result from inadvertent intrathecal or intravascular injection. Respiratory embarrassment and severe hypotension are evidence of accidental intrathecal injection. Respiratory support must be provided until the symptoms abate, approximately 4–6 hours later. Although there is a remote chance that a catheter may migrate, this is primarily a concern only when injecting a bolus immediately after the catheter is placed. Intravascular injection of more than 2.5 mg/kg of bupivacaine can result in cardiovascular and central nervous system toxicity. Symptoms may include dysrhythmia and cardiovascular collapse as well as neurologic symptoms of altered mental status and seizures. A small test bolus with local anesthetic and epinephrine may provide evidence of inadvertent injection. All subsequent bolus doses should be carefully monitored, although a test dose is not required each time.

Narcotic-related respiratory depression may be related to cephalad spread of the drug in the CSF to brainstem respiratory centers, or it may result from systemic absorption into the epidural venous plexus. This form of respiratory depression is immediately reversible with naloxone. The cephalad spread is less likely with fentanyl than morphine. Sedation may be the first symptom of severe and impending respiratory depression.

A number of fairly common side effects are primarily attributed to peridural narcotics and include nausea, pruritus, urinary retention, and sedation. Although less common with fentanyl, these bothersome complications of therapy can be seen with any narcotic regardless of the route of administration. Symptom management can be helpful with specific pharmacologic intervention: antiemetics for treating the nausea and vomiting and antihistamines to relieve the pruritus (both seen in about 8% of pediatric patients).[198] Many children needing epidural pain therapy will also require a urinary catheter for postsurgical monitoring. Careful assessment of urinary output and identification of retention symptoms in patients without Foley catheters can indicate the need for additional interventions. Should one or a combination of these narcotic-related problems not respond to conservative symptom management, a low-dose infusion of naloxone may be required for patient comfort. At the University of Texas M.D. Anderson Cancer Center, doses of naloxone as low as 0.1–1 μg/kg/hour have been very effective in controlling the bothersome adverse effects of peridural narcotic therapy. Local anesthetics alone can be utilized in a continuous epidural infusion if narcotic effects continue to interfere with and diminish the benefits of good pain management.

Safety and Monitoring

Safe and effective delivery of epidural analgesia requires careful education of and instructions to the nursing staff. Routine assessments of the patient's vital signs and mental status as well as ongoing respiratory assessment (i.e., monitored pulse oximetry) are mandatory. Emergency supplies, including airway-management equipment and resuscitative drugs, must be immediately available. Naloxone must be located at the bedside in case respiratory depression becomes severe. When children are receiving continuous epidural infusions, it is important that *no one* other than the pain-service personnel prescribe sedative medications, including benzodiazapine, narcotics, and the like. Otherwise, cumulative and synergistic drug effects could lead to life-threatening respiratory complications.

Regional and Local Nerve Blocks

Children with cancer may present with a variety of pain complaints due to regional or local nerve involvement in the tumor process. Medical, surgical, and radiologic interventions may cause nerve-related injury resulting in pain. When standard pain therapy measures are not effective, consultation with a pediatric anesthesiologist or a multidisciplinary pain team may be helpful. In addition to epidural catheters, a variety of local and regional nerve blocks can be utilized to inhibit the transmission of pain via nerve pathways. Local anesthetics have been given to treat somatic and neuropathic pain. Surgical wounds have been directly infused with local anesthetics administered continuously through small catheters placed into the incision site.[199] Intrapleural analgesia has been performed successfully in children with procedural pain related to medias-

tinal masses.[200] Results have been mixed about insertion of wound and pleural catheters. Questions of their safety and efficacy have prevented their widespread acceptance.

Nerve blocks involving the celiac and brachial plexus have been performed successfully for pain caused by tumor progression. Pain refractory to narcotic therapy may respond to neurolytic blocks. Although these blocks can provide effective long-term pain relief for many patients, the symptoms may worsen again following the intervention.[201] Continuous infusions of local anesthetics via catheters placed within the plexus sheath may be effective; however, the easy dislodgment of the catheter and the risk of local anesthetic toxicity keep such infusions from being generally useful.

Adjuvant Therapies

A number of pharmacologic agents have been found to ease specific chronic pain syndromes. Although not developed for this purpose, this group of unrelated drugs, prescribed in small doses, has gained wide acceptance in the area of pain management.

Tricyclic antidepressants and anticonvulsants have been successfully given in the management of neuropathic pain. Some specific indications include phantom limb pain, painful peripheral neuropathies related to vincristine therapy, radiation plexopathy, and tumor pain related to direct nerve involvement.[202] These agents work directly on the pain-processing area of the central nervous system[203] and also potentiate narcotic therapy.[204] Amitriptyline 0.5–1.0 mg/kg at bedtime is a recommended starting drug and dose.

Corticosteroids are beneficial for pain management in the presence of spinal cord compression, tumor-related increased intracranial pressure, and widespread bony metastases. The recommended starting dose is a bolus of 10–15 mg/m² followed by intermittent doses of 4–10 mg/m² every 6 hours. Steroid therapy should be quickly tapered once the tumor has shrunk in response to anticancer therapy.[202]

PEDIATRIC SEDATION

Over the last several years there has been an increase in the number of diagnostic, radiologic, and minor surgical procedures for pediatric patients performed outside the operating room.[205] Successful performance of these tests and procedures (e.g., lumbar punctures, bone marrow biopsies and aspirations, chest tube placements, wound care, tissue biopsies, radiologic examinations and procedures) requires that the pediatric patient be sedated or anesthetized. Complications have arisen when those prescribing medications for these purposes are not familiar with the pharmacokinetics and pharmacodynamics of the drugs selected. As a consequence of several sedation-related deaths in dental offices in the early 1980s,[206] guidelines for sedation were formulated by the American Academy of Pediatrics in 1985[207] and revised in 1992.[208] The ASA has also developed guidelines for the safe delivery of general anesthesia and *monitored anesthesia care* (MAC) both inside and outside the operating room.[209]

In discussing patient management for sedation, some specific terms must be clearly defined. Conscious sedation, deep sedation, and general anesthesia differ in regard to the personnel, monitoring equipment, and type of drugs required for each. These requirements have been issued by the ASA as guidelines for monitoring and management of pediatric patients.[209]

Conscious sedation implies a level of pharmacologically produced consciousness in which a patient is able to respond to verbal or gentle physical stimuli.[208] Despite a depressed level of consciousness, the patient's protective respiratory reflexes remain intact. Monitoring of the patient must include continuous pulse oximetry (heart rate and oxygen saturation) and assessment of mental status, with intermittent evaluation of blood pressure and respiratory rate. This care can be provided by the physician performing the procedure or by a nonphysician assistant responsible for monitoring the child.[208]

In procedures and tests in which pain can be significant or absolute immobility is required, deep sedation may be indicated. In this state the patient may not respond easily to verbal or tactile stimuli. A heightened level of vigilance by the caregiver is necessary because of the potential loss of protective airway reflexes and the increased risk of airway obstruction. A specially trained physician or nurse must be present whose sole responsibility involves the monitoring and airway management of the child.[210] Monitoring modalities required for deep sedation include all those described for conscious sedation. Although not strictly required, capnography can be indicated for specific patients. Intravenous access is mandatory for all patients undergoing this level of sedation.

When deep sedation is inappropriate or inadequate due to the patient's condition or the required procedure, general anesthesia may be indicated. This state of unconsciousness renders the patient completely unresponsive. An anesthetized patient has total loss of protective respiratory reflexes and is unable to maintain a patent airway without assistance. Placement of an endotracheal tube may be required (e.g., if aspiration is a risk or if there is anatomic airway compromise) but is not always necessary. Anesthesia personnel are the required providers of this care.

In all sedations and anesthetic procedures done outside the operating room, age-appropriate emergency equipment must be immediately available, including suction, airway supplies (oxygen, Ambubag, intubation equipment), and resuscitative drugs. Accepted guidelines for NPO status must be followed in cases requiring deep sedation or general anesthesia and are suggested for any sedation. Recommended drugs and dosages for sedation are included (Table 3–12).[218]

Special Considerations for Radiologic Procedures

Magnetic resonance (MR) imaging is a highly specialized radiologic diagnostic tool. The highly static magnetic field (0.12–2.00 T) generated and the radio frequency energy transmitted during image acquisition can damage standard ventilators and monitoring equipment.[211] MR imaging–compatible equipment containing nonferrous alloys has been specifically designed. When magnetic fields fluctuate, localized currents can occur in wires (e.g., ECG leads), resulting in heat generation and dermal burns.[212] Anesthesia equipment can cause artifacts and interfere with the quality of the image.[213]

Children with radiosensitive tumors may require *external-beam radiation* (XRT) daily for several weeks.[214] Although the treatments are not painful, sedation or general anesthesia may be necessary to ensure the patient's complete immobility. Because of the high radiation doses utilized in such therapy, all personnel must leave the room during treatment.[215, 216] Standard monitor-

Table 3–12 • Common Sedation Drugs, Dosages, and Routes

Drug	Effect	Route/Dosage
Morphine	Sedation and analgesia	PO 0.3 mg/kg
Fentanyl	Sedation and short-term analgesia	IV 0.05–0.15 mg/kg q 3 hours
		IV 0.05–1.0 µg/kg q 5 minutes
		Up to 4.0–5.0 µg/kg
Meperidine	Sedation and analgesia	IV 1.0 mg/kg q 3 hours
Hydromorphone	Analgesia	IV 0.015 mg/kg q 3 hours
Alfentanil	Sedation and short-term analgesia	IV 1.5–3.0 µg/kg q 5 minutes × 3
Midazolam	Sedation and amnesia	IV 0.5 mg/kg q 5 minutes × 2
		PO 0.5–0.75 mg/kg for toddlers
		PO 0.3–0.5 mg/kg for older ages
		IM 0.1–0.2 mg/kg
		PR 0.3–0.7 mg/kg
Diazepam	Sedation and amnesia	IV 0.1 mg/kg
		PO 0.1–0.5 mg/kg
		PR 0.1–0.5 mg/kg
Chloral hydrate	Sedation	PO 25–100 mg/kg
		PR 25–100 (maximum: 2.0 g)
Pentobarbital	Sedation	IV
Ketamine	Sedation, amnesia, and analgesia	IV 0.5–1.0 mg/kg

From Yaster M, Maxwell L: Opioid agonists and antagonists. In Schecter NL, Berde CB, Yaster M (eds): *Pain in Infants, Children and Adolescents.* Baltimore: Williams & Wilkins, 1993, p. 147, used with permission.

ing, previously discussed, must be accomplished via closed-circuit television.

References

1. Wingo PA, Tong T, Bolden S: Cancer statistics, 1995. *CA: Cancer Clin* 45(1):8–30, 1995.
2. Ross AF, Tinker JH: Anesthesia risk. In Miller RD (ed): *Anesthesia,* 4th ed. New York: Churchill Livingstone, 1994, p. 819.
3. Marx GF, Matteo CV, Otkin LR: Computer analysis of postanesthesia deaths. *Anesthesiology* 39:54, 1973.
4. Morgan GE, Mikhail MS: The practice of anesthesiology. In Morgan GE, Mikhail MS (eds): *Clinical Anesthesiology.* Norwalk, CT: Appleton & Lange, 1992, pp. 6–7.
5. Pineault R, Conandriopoulos AP: Randomized clinical trial of one-day surgery: Patients' satisfaction, clinical outcomes, and costs. *Med Care* 23:171, 1985.
6. Otherson AB, Clatworthy HW: Outpatient herniorrhaphy for infants. *Am J Dis Child* 78:116, 1968.
7. Steward DJ: Outpatient pediatric anesthesia. *Anesthesiology* 43:268, 1975.
8. Chapman AH, Leob DG, Gibbons MJ: Psychiatric aspects of hospitalizing children. *Arch Paediatri* 73:77, 1956.
9. Vernon DTA, Schulman JL, Foley JM: Changes in children's behavior after hospitalization. *Am J Dis Child* 111:581, 1966.
10. Schmeling DJ, Coran AG: Hormonal and metabolic response to operative stress in the neonate. *JPEN* 17:215, 1991.
11. Vistainer MA, Wolfer JA: Psychological preparation for surgical pediatric patients: The effect on children's and parents' stress responses and adjustment. *Pediatrics* 56:187, 1975.
12. Steward DJ: Preoperative evaluation and preparation for surgery. In Gregory GA (ed): *Pediatric Anesthesia,* 3rd ed. New York: Churchill Livingstone, 1994, p. 182.
13. Korsch BM: The child and the operating room. *Anesthesiology* 43:251, 1971.
14. Krane EJ, Davis PJ, Smith RM: Preoperative Preparation. In Motoyama E (ed): *Smith's Anesthesia for Infants and Children,* 5th ed. St. Louis: C.V. Mosby, 1990, p. 201.
15. Lockhart CH: Preoperative preparation of the child for hospitalization, anesthesia, and surgery. In *Annual Refresher Course Lectures,* American Society of Anesthesiologists, 1984, p. 125.
16. Krane EJ, Davis PJ, Smith RM: Preoperative preparation. In Motoyama E (ed): *Smith's Anesthesia for Infants and Children,* 5th ed. St. Louis: C.V. Mosby, 1990, pp. 202–204.
17. Steward DJ: Preterm infants are more prone to complications following minor surgery than are term infants. *Anesthesiology* 56:304–306, 1983.
18. Kurth CD, Spitzer AR, Broennle A, et al: Postoperative apnea in preterm infants. *Anesthesiology* 66:483–488, 1987.
19. Liu LM, Cote CJ, Goudsouzian NG, et al: Life-threatening apnea in infants recovering from anesthesia. *Anesthesiology* 59:506–510, 1983.

20. Welborn LG, Rice LJ, Hannallah RS, et al: Postoperative apnea in former preterm infants: Prospective comparison of spinal and general anesthesia. *Anesthesiology* 72:838–842, 1990.

21. Warner LO, Teitelbaum DH, Caniano DA, et al: Inguinal herniorrhaphy in young infants: Perianesthetic complications and associated preanesthetic risk factors. *J Clin Anesth* 4(6):455–461, 1992.

22. Welborn LG, Ramirez N, Oh TH, et al: Postanesthetic apnea and periodic breathing in infants. *Anesthesiology* 65:658–661, 1986.

23. Mestad PH, Glenski JA, Binda JRE: When is output surgery safe in preterm infants? *Anesthesiology* 69:a744, 1988.

24. Liu LM, Ryan JF, Cote CJ, et al: Influence of upper respiratory infections on critical incidents in children during anesthesia. *Abstracts of the World Congress of Anesthesiology,* 1988.

25. Cohen MM, Cameron CB: Should you cancel the operation when a child has an upper respiratory tract infection? *Anesth Analg* 72:282, 1991.

26. Steward DJ: Preoperative evaluation and preparation for surgery. In Gregory GA (ed): *Pediatric Anesthesia,* 3rd ed. New York: Churchill Livingstone, 1994.

27. McDowell RH: Anesthesia for children with cancer. In Kirby FF, Brown DL (eds): *Problems in Anesthesia: Cancer Pain Management.* Philadelphia: J.B. Lippincott, 1993, pp. 425–449.

28. Goorin A, Borow K, Goldman A, et al: Congestive heart failure due to Adriamycin cardiotoxicity: Its natural history in children. *Cancer* 47:2810–2816, 1981.

29. Marraro G, Uderzo C, Marchi P, et al: Acute respiratory failure and pulmonary thrombosis in leukemic children. *Cancer* 67:696, 1991.

30. Kreisman H, Wolkove N: Pulmonary toxicity of antineoplastic therapy. *Semin Oncol* 19:508–520, 1992.

31. Busch DB: Radiation and chemotherapy injury: Pathophysiology, diagnosis, and treatment. *Crit Rev Oncol Hematol* 15:49–89, 1993.

32. Waid-Jones MI, Coursin DB: Perioperative considerations for patients treated with bleomycin. *Chest* 99:997, 1991.

33. Sorenson PG, Rossing N, Rorth M: Carbon monoxide diffusing capacity: A reliable indicator of bleomycin-induced pulmonary toxicity. *Eur J Respir Dis* 66:333, 1985.

34. Desiderio DP: Chemotherapy-anesthetic drug interactions. In Kirby RR, Brown DL (eds): *Problems in Anesthesia: Cancer Pain Management.* Philadelphia: J.B. Lippincott, 1993, pp. 425–446.

35. Donhue JP, Rowland RG: Complications of retroperitoneal lymph node dissection. *J Urol* 125:338–340, 1981.

36. Hulbert JC, Grossman JE, Cummings KB: Risk factors of anesthesia and surgery in bleomycin-treated patients. *J Urol* 130:163–164, 1983.

37. Goldiner PL, Carlon GD, Cvitkovic E, et al: Factors influencing postoperative morbidity and mortality in patients treated with bleomycin. *BMJ* 1:1664–1667, 1978.

38. Rosenthal A: How to distinguish between innocent and pathologic murmurs in childhood. *Pediatr Clin North Am* 31:1229, 1984.

39. Child JS: Infective endocarditis: Risks and prophylaxis. *J Am Coll Cardiol* 18:337, 1991.

40. Steward DJ: Preoperative evaluation and preparation for surgery. In Gregory GA (ed): *Pediatric Anesthesia,* 3rd ed. New York: Churchill Livingstone, 1994, p. 187.

41. Larsen R, Jakacki R, Vetter V, et al: Electrocardiographic changes and arrhythmias after cancer therapy in children and young adults. *Am J Cardiol* 70:73–77, 1992.

42. VonHoff DD, Rocencweig M, Layard M, et al: Daunomycin-induced cardiotoxicity in children and adults: A review of 110 cases. *Am J Cardiol* 62:200–208, 1977.

43. Gordan JB, Yeager AM: Management of the child with malignant disease in the pediatric intensive care unit. In Rogers MC (ed): *Textbook of Pediatric Intensive Care.* Baltimore: Williams & Wilkins, 1992, pp. 1223–1261.

44. Lipshultz S, Colan S, Gelber R, et al: Late cardiac effects of doxorubicin therapy for acute lymphoblastic leukemia in childhood. *N Engl J Med* 324:808–815, 1991.

45. Steinherz L, Steinherz P, Tan C, et al: Cardiac toxicity 4 to 20 years after completing anthracycline therapy. *JAMA* 266:1672–1677, 1991.

46. Hale JP, Lewis IJ: Anthracyclines: Cardiotoxicity and its prevention. *Arch Dis Child* 71:448, 1994.

47. Weesner KM, Bledsoe M, Chauvenet A, et al: Exercise echocardiography in the detection of anthracycline cardiotoxicity. *Cancer* 68:435–438, 1991.

48. Allen A: The cardiotoxicity of chemotherapeutic drugs. *Semin Oncol* 19(5):529–530, 1995.

49. Schilsky RL: Renal and metabolic toxicities of cancer chemotherapy. *Semin Oncol* 9:75, 1982.

50. McDowell RH: Anesthesia for children with cancer. *Probl Anesth* 7(4):425–446, 1993.

51. Stokes DN: Tumor lysis syndrome and the anesthesiologist: Intensive care aspects of pediatric oncology. *Semin Surg Oncol* 6:156, 1990.

52. Everts EA: Anesthesia for organ transplantation. In Cote CJ, Ryan JF, Todres ID, et al (eds): *A Practice of Anesthesia for Infants and Children,* 2nd ed. Philadelphia: W.B. Saunders, 1993, p. 379.

53. Petrozza PH: Craniopharyngioma. In Stehling L (ed): *Common Problems in Pediatric Anesthesia,* 2nd ed. St. Louis: Mosby-Year Book, 1992, pp. 366–367.

54. Wall RT: Endocrine fascinomas: Endocrine abnormalities the anesthesiologist may face that

have important anesthetic implications. *Annual Refresher Course Lectures and Clinical Update Program* 143:1–4, 1994.

55. McGowan FX, Chlebowski SM: Anesthetic management of children with renal and endocrine dysfunction. In Bell C, Hughes CW, Oh TH (eds): *The Pediatric Anesthesia Handbook*, St. Louis: Mosby-Year Book, 1991, pp. 343–344.

56. Cote CJ, Todres ID, Ryan JF: Preoperative evaluation of pediatric patients. In Cote CJ, Goudsouzian NG, Ryan JF, et al (eds): *A Practice of Anesthesia for Infants and Children*, 2nd ed. Philadelphia: W.B. Saunders, 1993, p. 43.

57. Gordan JB, Yeager AM: Management of the child with malignant disease in the pediatric intensive care unit. In Rogers MC, Helfaer MA (eds): *Handbook of Pediatric Intensive Care*, 2nd ed. Baltimore: Williams & Wilkins, 1995, pp. 698–670.

58. Cote CJ: Strategies for blood product management and blood salvage. In Cote CJ, Ryan JF, Todres ID, et al (eds): *A Practice of Anesthesia for Infants and Children*, 2nd ed. Philadelphia: W.B. Saunders, 1993, p. 186.

59. McDowell RH: Anesthesia for children with cancer. *Probl Anesth* 7(4):427, 1993.

60. Myers TJ, Cole SR, Klatsky AU, et al: Respiratory failure due to pulmonary leukostasis following chemotherapy of acute nonlymphocytic leukemia. *Cancer* 51:1808, 1983.

61. Priest JR, Ramsay NK, Latchaw, et al: Thrombotic and hemorrhagic strokes complicating early therapy for childhood acute lymphoblastic leukemia. *Cancer* 46:1548, 1980.

62. O'Reilly RJ, Papadopoulos E: Allogenic bone marrow transplantation. In Holland JF, Frei I, Bast RC, et al (eds): *Cancer Medicine*, 3rd ed. Philadelphia: Lea & Febiger, 1993, pp. 998–1016.

63. Vogelsang GB, Hess AD, Santos GW: Acute graft-versus-host disease: Clinical characteristics in the cyclosporin era. *Medicine* 67:163, 1988.

64. Appelbaum FR: Bone marrow transplantation. In Stein JH, et al (eds): *Internal Medicine*, 2nd ed. Boston: Little, Brown and Company, 1987, pp. 966–969.

65. Sullivan KM, Shulman HM, Storb R, et al: Chronic graft-versus-host disease in 52 patients: Adverse natural course and successful treatment with combination immunosuppression. *Blood* 57:267, 1981.

66. Sanders JE: Bone marrow transplantation for pediatric leukemia. *Pediatr Ann* 20:671–676, 1991.

67. DeSantes KB, Cowan MJ: Pediatric bone marrow transplantation. *Curr Opin Pediatr* 4:92–101, 1992.

68. Mendelson CL: The aspiration of stomach contents into the lungs during obstetric anesthesia. *Am J Obstet Gynecol* 52:191–205, 1946.

69. Morton HJV, Wylie WD: Anaesthetic deaths due to regurgitation or vomiting. *Anaesthesia* 6:190–205, 1981.

70. Edwards G, Morton HJV, Pask EA, et al: Deaths associated with anaesthesia: A report on 1,000 cases. *Anaesthesia* 11:194–220, 1956.

71. Teabeaut JR II: Aspiration of gastric contents: An experimental study. *Am J Pathol* 28:51–62, 1952.

72. Alexander IGS: The ultrastructure of the pulmonary alveolar vessels in Mendelson's syndrome. *Br J Anesth* 40:408–414, 1968.

73. Greenfield LJ, Singleton RP, McCaftree DR, et al: Pulmonary effects of experimental graded aspiration of hydrochloric acid. *Ann Surg* 170:74–86, 1969.

74. Morgan TJ: Pulmonary edema produced by intrathecal injection of milk, feeding mixtures, and sugars. *Am J Dis Child* 86:45–50, 1953.

75. Wynne JW, Modell JH: Respiratory aspiration of stomach contents. *Ann Intern Med* 87:466–474, 1977.

76. Cote CJ, Goudsouzian NG, Liv LMP, et al: Assessment of risk factors related to the acid aspiration syndrome in pediatric patients: Gastric pH and residual volume. *Anesthesiology* 56:70–72, 1982.

77. Sandhar BK, Goresky GV, Maltby JR, et al: Effect of oral liquids and ranitidine on gastric fluid volume and pH in children undergoing outpatient surgery. *Anesthesiology* 71:327–330, 1989.

78. Schreiner MS, Triebwasser A, Keon TP: Ingestion of liquids compared with preoperative fasting in pediatric outpatients. *Anesthesiology* 72:593–597, 1990.

79. Splinter WM, Stewart JA, Muir JG: The effect of preoperative apple juice on gastric contents, thirst, and hunger in children. *Can J Anaesth* 36:55–58, 1989.

80. Steward DJ: Preoperative evaluation and preparation for surgery. In Gregory GA (ed): *Pediatric Anesthesia*, 3rd ed. New York: Churchill Livingstone, 1994, pp. 179–195.

81. McCluskey A, Meakin GH: Oral administration of midazolam as a premedicant for paediatric day-case anaesthesia. *Anaesthesia* 49:782–785, 1994.

82. Gerwels JW, Bezzant JL: Oral transmucosal fentanyl citrate premedication in patients undergoing outpatient dermatologic procedures. *J Dermatol Surg Oncol* 20:823–826, 1994.

83. Malinovsky JM, Populaire V: Premedication with midazolam in children. *Anaesthesia* 50:351–354, 1995.

84. Spear RM, Yaster M: Preinduction of anesthesia in children with rectally administered midazolam. *Anesthesiology* 670–674, 1991.

85. Gregory GA: Pharmacology. In Gregory GA (ed): *Pediatric Anesthesia*, 3rd ed. New York: Churchill Livingstone, 1994, p. 33.

86. McCluskey A, Meakin GH: Oral administration of midazolam as a premedicant for paediatric day-case anaesthesia. *Anaesthesia* 49:782–785, 1994.

87. Karl HW, Keifer AT: Comparison of the safety and efficacy of intranasal midazolam or sufentanil for preinduction of anesthesia in pediatric patients. *Anesthesiology* 76:209–215, 1992.

88. Vessey JA, Bogetz MS: Parental upset associated with participation in induction of anaesthesia in children. *Can J Anaesth* 41(4):276–280, 1994.

89. Braude N, Ridley SA: A prospective study of parental attitudes to their presence at induction. *Ann R Coll Surg Engl* 72:41–44, 1990.

90. Standards for basic intra-operative monitoring. The American Society of Anesthesiologists, Park Ridge, Illinois, 1993.

91. Sellden H, Krister N: Radial arterial catheters in children and neonates: A propsective study. *Crit Care Med* 15:230–232, 1987.

92. Tonneson AS, Vereen L: Endotracheal tube cuff residual volume and lateral wall pressure in a model trachea. *Anesthesiology* 55:680, 1981.

93. Roizen MF, Sohn YJ: Operating room temperature prior to surgical draping: Effect on patient temperature in recovery room. *Anesth Analg* 59:852–855, 1980.

94. Pennant JH, White PF: The laryngeal mask airway. *Anesthesiology* 79:144–163, 1993.

95. Brain AI: The laryngeal mask: A new concept in airway management. *Br J Anaesth* 55:801–804, 1983.

96. Splinter WM, Smallman B: Postoperative sore throat in children and the laryngeal mask airway. *Can J Anaesth* 41(11):1081–1083, 1994.

97. Valeri RC, Cassidy G: Hypothermia-induced reversible platelet dysfunction. *Ann Surg* 205:175, 1987.

98. Heier T, Caldwell JE: Mild intraoperative hypothermia increases duration of action and spontaneous recovery of vecuronium blockade during nitrous oxide-isoflurane anesthesia in humans. *Anesthesiology* 74:815, 1991.

99. Horvath SM, Spurr GB: Metabolic cost of shivering. *Anesthesiology* 68:843, 1988.

100. Rasch SK, Carter B: *Clinical Manual of Pediatric Anesthesia.* New York: McGraw-Hill, 1994, pp. 148–280.

101. Thompson GF, Miller RD: Hypotensive anesthesia for total hip arthroplasty: A study of blood loss and organ function (brain, heart, liver, and kidney). *Anesthesiology* 48:91, 1978.

102. Shandling B, Steward DJ: Regional analgesia for postoperative pain in pediatric outpatient surgery. *J Pediatr Surg* 15:477–480, 1980.

103. Berkowitz A; Rosenberg H: Femoral nerve block with mepivacaine for muscle biopsy in malignant hyperthermia patients. *Anesthesiology* 62:651–652, 1983.

104. Vandam LD, Dripps RE: Exacerbation of pre-existing neurologic disease after spinal anesthesia. *N Engl J Med* 255:843–849, 1956.

105. Pullertis J, Holzman RS: Pediatric neuraxial blockade. *J Clin Anesth* 4:342–354, 1993.

106. Dalens B, Hasnaoui A: Caudal anesthesia in pediatric surgery: Success rate and adverse effect in 750 consecutive patients. *Anesth Analg* 68:83–89, 1989.

107. Blaise G, Roy WL: Postoperative pain relief after hypospadias repair in pediatric patients: Regional anesthesia versus systemic analgesics. *Anesthesiology* 65:84–86, 1986.

108. Nakamura T, Takasaki M: Metabolic and endocrine responses to surgery during caudal anesthesia in children. *Can J Anaesth* 38:969–973, 1991.

109. Groeben H, Heyll A, Peters J: Pathophysiologic and anesthesiologic characteristics of patients with leukemia. *Anaesthesist* 41(8):438–447, 1992.

110. Michenfelder JD, Miller RH, Gronert GA: Evaluation of an ultrasonic device (Doppler) for the diagnosis of venous air embolism. *Anesthesiology* 36:164, 1972.

111. Buckland RW, Manners IM: Venous air embolism during neurosurgery: A comparison of various methods of detection in man. *Anesthesia* 31:633, 1976.

112. English JB, Westenshown D, Hodges MR, et al: Comparison of venous air embolism monitoring methods in supine dogs. *Anesthesiology* 48:425–429, 1978.

113. Matjasko J, Petrozza P, Mackenzie CF: Sensitivity of end-tidal nitrogen in venous air embolism in dogs. *Anesthesiology* 55:343–348, 1981.

114. Motoyama EK, Spear RM, Deshpande JK, et al: Clinical anesthesia. *Anesthesia for Infants and Children*, 5th ed. St. Louis, Missouri: C.V. Mosby Co, 1990, p. 792.

115. Weinblatt ME, Heisel MA, Siegel SE: Hypertension in children with neurogenic tumors. *Pediatrics* 71:947–951, 1983.

116. Roizen MF, Horrigan RW, Koike M, et al: A prospective randomized trial of four anesthetic techniques for resection of pheochromocytoma. *Anesthesiology* 57:A43, 1982.

117. Ternberg JL: Hodgkin's and non-Hodgkin's lymphoma. In Welch KJ, et al (eds): *Pediatric Surgery*, 4th ed. Chicago: Year Book Medical Publishers, 1986, pp. 256–265.

118. Bray RJ, Fernandes FJ: Mediastinal tumor causing airway obstruction in anaesthetized children. *Anaesthesia* 37:571–575, 1982.

119. Wolfe TM, Chalapathi CR: Anesthesia for selected procedures. *Semin Pediatr Surg* 1:74–80, 1992.

120. Mackie AM, Watson CB: Anaesthesia and mediastinal masses: A case report and review of the literature. *Anaesthesia* 39:899–903, 1984.

121. Ferrari LR, Bedford RF: General anesthesia prior to treatment of anterior mediastinal masses in pediatric cancer patients. *Anesthesiology* 72:991–995, 1990.

122. Halpen S, Chatten J, Meadows AT, et al: Anterior mediastinal masses: Anesthesia hazards and other problems. *J Pediatr* 102:407–410, 1983.
123. Sibert KS, Biondi JW, Hirsch NP: Spontaneous respiration during thoracotomy in a patient with a mediastinal mass. *Anesth Analg* 66:904–907, 1987.
124. Krane EJ, Heller LB: The prevalence of phantom sensation and pain in pediatric amputees. *J Pain Symptom Manage* 10(1):21–29, 1995.
125. McGrath PA, Hillier LM: Phantom limb sensations in adolescents: A case study to illustrate the utility of sensation and pain logs in pediatric clinical practice. *J Pain Symptom Manage* 7:46–53, 1992.
126. Bach S, Noreng MF, Tjellden NU: Phantom limb pain in amputees during the first 12 months following limb amputation after preoperative lumbar epidural blockade. *Pain* 33:297–301, 1988.
127. Walrath JB, Stopcock: Bacterial contamination in invasive monitoring systems. *Heart Lung* 9:100, 1979.
128. McGrath PA: Psychological aspects of pain perception. In Schecter NL, Berde CB, Yaster M (eds): *Pain in Infants, Children, and Adolescents.* Boston: Williams & Wilkins, 1993, pp. 39–63.
129. Anand KJS, Hickey PR: Halothane-morphine compared with high-dose sufentanil for anesthesia and postoperative analgesia in neonatal cardiac surgery. *N Engl J Med* 326:1–9, 1992.
130. Anand KJS: The stress response to surgical trauma: From physiological basis to therapeutic implications. *Prog Food Nutr Sci* 10:67–132, 1986.
131. Fitzgerald M, Anand KJS: Developmental neuroanatomy and neurophysiology of pain. In Schecter NL, Berde CB, Yaster M (eds): *Pain in Infants, Children, and Adolescents.* Boston: Williams & Wilkins, 1993, pp. 23–25.
132. Anand KJS, Hickey PR: Pain and its effects in the human neonate and fetus. *N Engl J Med* 317:1321–1329, 1987.
133. Anand J, Sippel WG, Aynsley-Green A: Randomized trial of fentanyl anesthesia in preterm babies undergoing surgery: Effects on the stress response. *Lancet* 1:62–66, 1987.
134. Fitzgerald M, Millard C, McIntosh N: Cutaneous hypersensitivity following peripheral tissue damage in newborn infants and its reversal with topical anesthesia. *Pain* 39:31–36, 1989.
135. Dubner R, Basbaum AI: Spinal dorsal horn plasticity following tissue or nerve injury. In Wall PD, Melzack R (eds): *Textbook of Pain.* 3rd ed. New York: Churchill Livingstone, 1994, pp. 225–241.
136. Beyer JE, DeGood DE, Ashley LC, et al: Patterns of postoperative analgesic use with adults and children following cardiac surgery. *Pain* 17:71–81, 1983.
137. Schecter NL: The undertreatment of pain in children: An overview. *Pediatr Clin North Am* 36:781–794, 1989.
138. Yeager MP, Glass DD, Neff RK, et al: Epidural anesthesia and analgesia in high-risk surgical patients. *Anesthesiology* 66:729–736, 1987.
139. Murrell D, Gibson PR, Cohen RC: Continuous epidural analgesia in newborn infants undergoing major surgery. *J Pediatr Surg* 28:548–552, 1993.
140. McGrath PJ, et al: Report of the Subcommittee on Assessment and Methodologic Issues in the Management of Pain in Childhood Cancer. *Pediatrics* 86:814, 1990.
141. Tyler DC, Ahn T, Douthit J, et al: Toward validation of pain measurement tools for children: A pilot study. *Pain* 52:301–309, 1993.
142. McGrath PA: Evaluating a child's pain. *J Pain Symptom Manage* 4:189–214, 1989.
143. McGrath PA: Advances in pain research and therapy. In Fields HL, Dubner R, Cervero F (eds): *The CHEOPS: A Behavioral Scale to Measure Postoperative Pain in Children.* New York: Raven Press, 1985.
144. Berg J: *The Oucher: A User's Manual and Technical Report.* Evanston, IL: Judson Press, 1984.
145. Beyer JE, Aradine CR: Content validity of an instrument to measure young children's perception of the intensity of their pain. *J Pediatr Nurs* 1:386, 1986.
146. Whaley L, Wong D: *Nursing Care of Infants and Children,* 3rd ed. St. Louis: C.V. Mosby Co., 1987, p. 1070.
147. Wong D, Baker C: Pain in children: Comparison of assessment scales. *J Pediatr Nurs* 14:9–17, 1988.
148. Berde CB: Pediatric analgesic trials. In Max MB, Portenoy RK, Laska EM (eds): *Advances in Pain Research Therapy: The Design of Analgesic Clinical Trials.* New York: Raven Press, 1991, pp. 445–555.
149. Mollman JE, Glover LJ, Hogan WM, et al: Cisplatin neuropathy. *Cancer* 61:2192, 1988.
150. Subhash J: Nerve blocks. In Warfield CA (ed): *Principles and Practice of Pain Management.* New York: McGraw-Hill, 1993, p. 389.
151. Gootenberg JE, Pizzo PA: Optimal management of acute toxicities of therapy. *Pediatr Clin North Am* 38:282, 1991.
152. Rusby LM, Houck CS, Sullivan LJ, et al: A double-blinded evaluation of ketorolac tromethamine versus acetaminophen in pediatric tonsillectomy: Analgesia and bleeding. *Anesth Analg* 80:226–229, 1995.
153. Hurwitz ES, Barret MJ, Bregman D, et al: Public Health Service study on Reye's syndrome and medication: Report of pilot phase. *N Engl J Med* 313:849, 1985.

154. Houck CS, Berde CB, Anand KJS: Pediatric pain management. In Gregory GA (ed): *Pediatric Anesthesia*. 3rd ed. New York: Churchill Livingstone, 1994, p. 749.

155. Maunukesela EL, Ryhanen P, Janhunen L: Efficacy of rectal ibuprofen in controlling postoperative pain in children. *Can J Anaesth* 39:226–230, 1992.

156. Vetter TR, Heiner EJ: Intravenous ketorolac as an adjuvant to pediatric patient-controlled analgesia with morphine. *J Clin Anesth* 6:110–113, 1994.

157. Gunter JB, Varughese AM, Harrington JF, et al: Recovery and complications after tonsillectomy in children: Comparison of ketorolac and morphine. *Anesth Analg* 81:1136–1141, 1995.

158. Porter J, Jick H: Addiction rare in patients treated with narcotics. *N Engl J Med* 302:1231, 1980.

159. Portenoy RK: Chronic opioid therapy in nonmalignant pain. *J Pain Symptom Manage* 5:s46, 1990.

160. Houck CS, Berde CB, Anand KJS: Pediatric pain management. In Gregory GA (ed): *Pediatric Anesthesiology*, 3rd ed. New York: Churchill Livingstone, 1994, pp. 758–760.

161. Houck CS, Berde CB, Anand KJS: Pediatric pain management. In Gregory GA (ed): *Pediatric Anesthesiology*, 3rd ed. New York: Churchill Livingstone, 1994, p. 751.

162. Eige SA, Bell C: Pediatric pain management. In Bell C, Hughes CW, Oh TH (eds): *Pediatric Anesthesia Handbook*. St. Louis: Mosby-Year Book, 1991, p. 507.

163. Greene MG (ed): *Harriet Lane Handbook*, 12th ed. St. Louis: Mosby-Year Book, 1991.

164. Koren G, Maurice L: Pediatric uses of opioids. *Pediatr Clin North Am* 36:1141–1156, 1989.

165. Nahata MC, Miser AW, Miser JS, et al: Variations in morphine pharmacokinetics in children with cancer. *Dev Pharmacol Ther* 8:182–188, 1985.

166. Zelter LK, Anderson CT, et al: Pediatric pain: Current status and new directions. In Lockhart JD (ed): *Current Problems in Pediatrics*. St. Louis: Mosby-Year Book, 1990, p. 462.

167. Sechzer PH: Objective measurement of pain. *Anesthesiology* 29:209–210, 1968.

168. White PF: Use of patient-controlled analgesia for management of acute pain. *JAMA* 259:243–247, 1988.

169. Ready LB: The economics of patient-controlled analgesia. In Ferrante FM, Ostheimer GW, Covino BG (eds): *Patient-Controlled Analgesia*. Oxford: Blackwell Scientific Publications, 1990, p. 191–197.

170. Ferrante FM, Orav EJ, Rocco AG, et al: A statistical model for pain in patient-controlled analgesia and conventional intramuscular opioid regimens. *Anesth Analg* 67:457–461, 1988.

171. Berde CB, Lehn BM, Yee JD, et al: Patient-controlled analgesia in children and adolescents: A randomized, prospective comparison with intramuscular administration of morphine for postoperative analgesia. *J Pediatr* 118:460–466, 1991.

172. Berde CB: Acute postoperative pain management in children. *Annual Refresher Course Lectures*, American Society of Anesthesiologists, 1994, p. 224.

173. Houck CS, Berde CB, Anand KJS: Pediatric pain management. In Gregory GA (ed): *Pediatric Anesthesiology*, 3rd ed. New York: Churchill Livingstone, 1994, pp. 751–752.

174. Gaukroger PB: Patient-controlled analgesia in children. In Schecter NL, Berde CB, Yaster M (eds): *Pain in Infants, Children and Adolescents*. Baltimore: Williams & Wilkins, 1993, p. 204.

175. Patient-controlled analgesic infusion pumps. *Health Devices* 17:137–167, 1988.

176. McKenzie R, Rudy T, Tanisira B: Comparison of PCA alone and PCA with continuous infusion on pain relief and quality of sleep. *Anesthesiology* 73:a787, 1990.

177. Owen H, Plummer JL, Armstrong I, et al: Variables of patient-controlled analgesia: Bolus size. *Anesthesia* 44:7–10, 1989.

178. Omoigui S: *The Anesthesia Drug Handbook*, 2nd ed. St. Louis: Mosby-Year Book, 1995, pp. 127–132.

179. Polaner DM, Berde CB: Postoperative pain management. In Cote CJ, Ryan JF, Todres ID, et al (eds): *A Practice of Anesthesia for Infants and Children*, 2nd ed. Philadelphia: W.B. Saunders Co., 1993, pp. 455–456.

180. Gaukroger PB, Tomkins DP, van der Walt JH: Patient-controlled analgesia in children. *Anesthesia Intensive Care* 17:264–268, 1989.

181. In Miller BF, Keane CB (eds): *Encyclopedia and Dictionary of Medicine, Nursing, and Allied Health*, 5th ed. Philadelphia: W.B. Saunders Co., 1992.

182. Doberczak TM, Kandall SR, Wilets I: Neonatal opiate abstinence syndrome in term and preterm infants. *J Pediatr* 118:933–937, 1991.

183. Pilon RN, Baker AR: Chronic pain control by means of an epidural catheter: Report of a case with description of the method. *Cancer* 37:903–905, 1976.

184. Zenz M, Schappler-Scheele B, Neuhaus R, et al: Long-term peridural morphine analgesia in cancer pain. *Lancet* 1:91, 1981.

185. Bach S, Noreng MF, Tjellden NU: Phantom limb pain in amputees during the first 12 months following limb amputation, after preoperative lumbar epidural blockade. *Pain* 33:297–301, 1988.

186. Anderson CT, Berde CB, Sethna NF, et al: Meningococcal purpura fulminans: Treatment of vascular insufficiency in a 2-year-old child with lumbar epidural sympathetic blockade. *Anesthesiology* 71:463–464, 1989.

187. Tobias JD, Haun SE, Helfaer M, et al: Use of

continuous caudal block to relieve lower extremity ischemia caused by vasculitis in a child with meningococcemia. *J Pediatr* 6:1019–1020, 1989.

188. Sanchez ZV, Seggedin ER, Moser M, et al: Role of lumbar sympathectomy in the pediatric intensive care unit. *Anesth Analg* 67:794–797, 1988.

189. Finer P, Blair J, Rowe P: Epidural analgesia in the management of labor pain and sickle cell crisis: A case report. *Anesthesiology* 68:799–800, 1988.

190. Tobias JD, Oakes L, Rao B: Continuous epidural anesthesia for postoperative analgesia in the pediatric oncology patient. *Am J Pediatr Hematol Oncol* 14:216–221, 1992.

191. Rucce TS, Cardamone M, Migliori P: Fentanyl and bupivacaine mixtures for extradural blockade. *Br J Anaesth* 57:275–284, 1985.

192. Dalens B, Tanguy A, Haberer JP: Lumbar epidural anesthesia for urologic and upper abdominal surgery in infants. *Anesthesiology* 65:87–90, 1986.

193. Baker AS, Ojemann RG, Swartz MN, et al: Spinal epidural abscess. *N Engl J Med* 293:463, 1975.

194. DuPen SL, et al: Infection during chronic epidural catheterization: Diagnosis and treatment. *Anesthesiology* 73:905–909, 1990.

195. Berde CB: Regional analgesia in the management of chronic pain in childhood. *J Pain Symptom Manage* 4:232–237, 1989.

196. Sethna NF, Wilder RT: Regional anesthetic techniques for chronic pain. In Schecter NL, Berde CB, Yaster M (eds): *Pain in Infants, Children and Adolescents.* Baltimore: Williams & Wilkins, 1993, p. 219.

197. Payen D, et al: Pulsed Doppler: Ascending aortic, carotid, brachial, and femoral artery blood flows during caudal anesthesia in infants. *Anesthesiology* 67:681–685, 1987.

198. Ballantyne JC, Loach AB, Carr DB: Itching after epidural and spinal opiates. *Pain* 33:149–160, 1988.

199. Thomas DF, Lambert WG, Williams KL: The direct perfusion of surgical wounds with local anaesthetic solution: An approach to postoperative pain? *Ann R Coll Surg Engl* 65:226–229, 1983.

200. Swinhoe CF, Pereira NH: Intrapleural analgesia in a child with a mediastinal tumor. *Can J Anaesth* 41:427–430, 1994.

201. Cousins MJ, Dwyer B, Gibb D: Management of pain associated with childhood cancer. In Schecter NL, Berde CB, Yaster M (eds): *Pain in Infants, Children, and Adolescents,* 2nd ed. Philadelphia: J.B. Lippincott Co., 1988, pp. 1053–1084.

202. Miser AW: Management of pain associated with childhood cancer. In Schecter NL, Yaster M, Berde CB (eds): *Pain in Infants, Children and Adolescents.* Baltimore: Williams & Wilkins, 1993, p. 421.

203. Feinmann C: Pain relief by antidepressants: Possible modes of action. *Pain* 23:1–8, 1985.

204. Botney M, Fields H: Amitriptyline potentiates morphine analgesia by direct action on the central nervous system. *Ann Neurol* 12:160, 1983.

205. Keeter S, Benator RM, Weinberg SM, et al: Sedation in pediatric CT: National survey of current practice. *Radiology* 175:745–752, 1990.

206. Goodson JM, Moore PA: Life-threatening reactions after pediodontic sedation: An assessment of narcotic, local anesthetic, and antiemetic drug interaction. *J Am Dent Assoc* 107:239–245, 1983.

207. American Academy of Pediatrics (AAP). Committee on Drugs (Section on Anesthesiology): Guidelines for the elective use of conscious sedation, deep sedation, and general anesthesia in pediatric patients. *Pediatrics* 76:317–321, 1985.

208. Guidelines for monitoring and management of pediatric patients during and after sedation for diagnostic and therapeutic procedures. *Pediatrics* 89:1110–1115, 1992.

209. American Society of Anesthesiologists: Position on Monitoring Anesthesia (approved October 1986); Guidelines for Patient Care in Anesthesiology (approved October 1967, amended October 1985); Standards for Basic Intra-Operative Monitoring (approved October 1986, amended October 1990); 1986.

210. Joint Commission on Accreditation of Healthcare Organizations (JCAHO): *Accreditation Manual for Hospitals.* Oakbrook Terrace, IL: JCAHO, 1991.

211. McCullough EC, Baker JHL: Nuclear magnetic resonance imaging. *Radiol Clin North Am* 20:3, 1982.

212. Rejger VS, Cohn BF, Vielvoye GJ, et al: A simple anesthetic and monitoring system for magnetic resonance imaging. *Eur J Anaesthesiol* 6:373–378, 1989.

213. Patterson SK, Chesney JT: Anesthetic management for magnetic resonance imaging: Problems and solutions. *Anesth Analg* 74:123, 1992.

214. Glanber D, Audenaert S: Anesthesia for children undergoing craniospinal radiotherapy. *Anesthesiology* 56:801, 1987.

215. Bashein G, Russell A, Momil S: Anesthesia and remote monitoring for intraoperative radiation therapy. *Anesthesiology* 64:805, 1986.

216. Pandya J, Martin J: Improved remote cardiorespiratory monitoring during radiation therapy. *Anesth Analg* 65:529, 1986.

217. Fisher DM: Anesthesia equipment for pediatrics. In Gregory, GA (ed): *Pediatric Anesthesia,* 3rd ed. New York: Churchill Livingstone, 1994, p. 216.

218. Yaster M, Maxwell L: Opioid agonists and antagonists. In Schecter NL, Berde CB, Yaster M (eds): *Pain in Infants, Children and Adolescents.* Baltimore: Williams and Wilkins, 1993, p. 147.

Principles of Chemotherapy for Solid Tumors

• *John F. Kuttesch, Jr., Ph.D., M.D.* • *R. Beverly Raney, M.D.*

Although cancer is often considered rare in children and adolescents, it is actually one of the leading causes of death in these age groups. The important role of surgery in pediatric solid tumors cannot be disputed. Significant survival advantage exists in patients undergoing total surgical resection. Most pediatric solid tumors, however, have metastatic potential leading to tumor progression.

Significant improvement in the survival among this group is due, in part, to the development of combined modality therapy with the addition of chemotherapy and/or radiotherapy (Table 4–1). The incidences and types of childhood malignancies are different and more diverse than those of adult malignancies. The most common childhood

Table 4–1 • Changes in Survival for Children with Malignant Solid Tumors

	1960–1963	1986–1992
All sites	28	71
Bone and joints (Ewing's sarcoma, osteosarcoma, chondrosarcoma)	20	65
Neuroblastoma	25	63
Soft tissue sarcoma (including rhabdomyosarcoma)	38	72
Wilms' tumor	33	93
Central nervous system tumors	35	61

From Parker SL, Tong T, Bolden S, et al: Cancer statistics, 1997. CA Cancer J Clin 47:5–27, 1997.

malignancies are more chemosensitive than the most common adult malignancies (i.e., carcinomas). A role for chemotherapy in cancer treatment was first suggested by Goodman and colleagues,[1] who reported the effectiveness of mechlorethamine in patients with lymphoma, and by Farber and colleagues,[2] who reported the effectiveness of aminopterin in children with acute lymphocytic leukemia.

In the 1960s, the effectiveness of combined therapy that incorporated chemotherapy was first demonstrated in Wilms' tumor and later in rhabdomyosarcoma and other embryonal solid tumors of childhood.[3] In the past five decades, several classes of drugs have been developed and incorporated into the treatment of childhood malignancies.[3, 4] Our current therapies have been empirically derived. The development of both in vitro and in vivo models within the last two decades has led to a better understanding of the physiology and molecular biology of these diseases and to an identification of the potential molecular targets for the development of new therapies.[5, 6] The goals of this chapter are to describe the underlying pharmacologic principles of cancer chemotherapy and to then review the different classes of chemotherapy agents and their clinical utility.

PRINCIPLES OF CLINICAL PHARMACOLOGY

The goal for the rational development of therapeutic approaches in the treatment of cancer is the identification of selective agents or modalities.[4, 7–9] Selectivity may be based on several factors: (1) favorable biologic differences between normal tissues and malignant tissues, (2) favorable differences in distribution of the therapeutic target, and (3) favorable differences in distribution of the therapeutic agent. A major limitation in successful treatment is the lack of selective antitumor agents. The clinical use of these drugs is affected by several issues: (1) tumor cell heterogeneity; (2) patient population heterogeneity; (3) patient clinical performance status; and (4) pharmacologic interaction between combinations of drugs.

The development of "resistance" must also be addressed. Clinical resistance to an antitumor agent can be defined as a lack of selectivity, whether intrinsic or acquired. The result is an equal or a greater effect of the drug on normal rather than on tumor tissue, thus limiting its usefulness. All these issues must be considered in the future development of therapeutic approaches in cancer therapy.

CLINICAL PHARMACOLOGY

Many of the current chemotherapeutic agents act at specific phases of the cell cycle.[10] These agents are more effective against mitotically active cells. Agents that specifically act on processes such as DNA synthesis, DNA transcription, or mitosis are classified as cell-cycle specific. This category includes the antimetabolites, topoisomerase I and II inhibitors, and antitubulin agents. Cell-cycle nonspecific agents act nonselectively at many stages of the cell cycle. Alkylating agents are the best examples.

The investigations of Skipper and colleagues[11, 12] established several key principles that have guided the development of cancer therapeutics through our current era.[11, 12] These can be summarized as follows:

1. A single clonogenic cell can give rise to a lethal tumor. Complete eradication (total cell kill) of this clonal population is necessary for cure.
2. The host's immune system plays a negligible role in cure except when the tumor cell burden is minimal.
3. The cell killing by chemotherapeutic agents follows first-order kinetics (i.e., a constant proportion of the tumor burden will be killed).

These principles were the initial basis for the development of multiple agents (combination therapy). As we have gained a greater understanding of cell biology, these principles may need to be readdressed based on the following observations. Biologic agents that affect immune modulation enhance the cytotoxicity of conventional chemotherapeutic agents when given in combination.[13] Roberts and coworkers[14] suggest that residual leukemic clones may exist in pediatric patients who are clinically cured of disease. Virtually all current chemotherapeutic agents cause cell damage–induced apoptosis, also known as programmed cell death. In experimental systems, relative drug resistance of tumor cell populations has been associated with alterations in biologic mechanisms associated with regulation of apoptosis.[15-18] Future targets for development of new therapies will include the signal transduction elements associated with tumor suppressor genes and apoptosis.

Clinical pharmacology is a field that encompasses the study of drugs from the elucidation of their mechanism of action to their clinical evaluation and usage (Table 4–2).[8, 9] In the context of the clinical use of an agent, the pharmacologist attempts to understand its pharmacodynamics and pharmacokinetics. Pharmacodynamics refers to the interactions between the drug and the organism (dose-effect relationship). Pharmacokinetics is the drug's disposition in the body, including its absorption, bioavailability, distribution, metabolism, and excretion.

Pharmacodynamic studies define the therapeutic action of cancer drugs.[19, 20] In in vitro systems, pharmacodynamic models show the relationships between dose exposure and effects, usually cell kill in the case of antitumor agents. Dose exposure can be measured as the concentration multiplied by the exposure time. Pharmacodynamic models become very complex in in vivo systems in which pharmacokinetic, biochemical, and cell kinetic parameters must be considered simultaneously in both normal tissue and tumor tissue.

Pharmacokinetics is a discipline that also deals with the characterization and quantitation of a drug's disposition.[21] Sensitive analytic methods have been developed for the measurement and quantitation of many anticancer agents. The ultimate goal of pharmacokinetic monitoring of the classic chemotherapeutic agents is to define the optimal drug delivery needed to achieve the therapeutic goal of maximal tumor cell kill with acceptable toxicity. The major limitation of most classic antitumor agents is their small therapeutic index. With plasma pharmacokinetics as surrogate measures of systemic drug exposure, investigators can adjust the administered drug dose individually. Thus, pharmacokinetic monitoring may benefit the patient.[22-24] The classic example in cancer chemotherapy is the pharmacokinetic monitoring of methotrexate followed by administration of leucovorin as an antidote.[22, 25] In several cases (carboplatin, etoposide, cytosine arabinoside), this pharmacokinetic approach has led to decreased intrapatient variability. Theoretically, it should also decrease the incidence of toxicity.

Current studies suggest that the dose intensity of chemotherapeutic regimens can influence the clinical response of patients with malignancies. The outcome of therapy, however, can be influenced by many factors. Broad variability is found from patient to patient in the pharmacokinetics of drugs. The cancer chemotherapeutic agents have a low therapeutic index. Their toxicities are life-threatening. Inadequate therapy leads to poor outcome. With pharmacokinetic monitoring, several investigators have addressed and are continuing to study the concept of systemic dose exposure both to optimize and to standardize the use of selected agents.[19, 23]

Table 4–2 • Terminology in Clinical Pharmacology

Plasma Sample

C_{max}	Maximum observed concentration
T_{max}	Time at which C_{max} occurs
AUC	Area under the concentration-time curve over the dosing interval
C_{ave}	Average serum concentration at steady state, computed as the ratio of AUC divided by 24
C_{min}	Minimum serum concentration over 24 hours
K_e	Elimination rate constant computed as the magnitude of the slope from the log-linear regression of concentration versus time during the elimination phase
$T_{1/2}$	Terminal half-life

Urine Sample

Cl_{renal}	Renal clearance computed as the amount of drug or metabolites excreted in urine over an interval divided by the area under the curve over the same interval

CHEMOTHERAPEUTIC AGENTS

There are several classes of chemotherapeutic agents (Table 4–3). Representatives of each class interfere with the growth of certain normal and malignant cells. Each has certain side effects that tend to be similar among drugs within each class. These are described by class, together with their spectrum of activity. Characteristic early and late toxicities are detailed.

Table 4–3 • Drugs Commonly Used for Treatment of Pediatric Solid Tumors

Drug	Route*	Mechanism of Action	Toxicities†	Antitumor Spectrum
Alkylating Agents				
Mechlorethamine (Mustargen, HN₂, nitrogen mustard)	IV	Alkylation; crosslinking	M, N and V, A, phlebitis; vesicant, mucositis; NT (HD)	Hodgkin's, brain tumors
Cyclophosphamide (Cytoxan, CTX)	IV PO	(Prodrug) alkylation; crosslinking	M, N and V, A, cystitis, water retention; cardiac (HD)	Sarcomas, neuroblastoma, lymphomas
Ifosfamide (IFOS)	IV	(Prodrug) alkylation; crosslinking	M, N and V, A, cystitis, NT, renal	Sarcomas, germ cell tumors
Melphalan (Alkeran, L-PAM)	IV PO	Alkylation; crosslinking	M, N and V, mucositis and diarrhea (HD)	Rhabdomyosarcoma; sarcomas, neuroblastoma
Lomustine (CeeNU, CCNU)	PO	Alkylation; crosslinking	M, N and V, renal and pulmonary	Brain tumors
Carmustine (BiCNU, BCNU)	IV	Alkylation; crosslinking	M, N and V, renal and pulmonary	Brain tumors
Cisplatin (Platinol, CDDP)	IV	Platination; crosslinking	M (mild), N and V, A, renal, NT, ototoxicity, allergic	Hepatoblastoma, germ cell, osteosarcoma, brain tumors, neuroblastoma
Carboplatin (CBDCA)	IV	Platination; crosslinking	M (Plt), N and V, A, hepatic (mild)	Brain tumors, germ cell, neuroblastoma
Dacarbazine (DTIC)	IV	(Prodrug) alkylation	M (mild), N and V, flu-like syndrome, hepatic	Neuroblastoma, sarcomas, Hodgkin's
Procarbazine (Matulan, PCX)	PO	(Prodrug) alkylation; free-radical formation	M, N and V, NT, rash, mucositis	Hodgkin's, brain tumors
Antimetabolites				
Methotrexate (MTX)	PO, IM, IV	Interferes with folate metabolism	M (mild), mucositis, rash; hepatic, renal, NT (HD)	Osteosarcoma, lymphoma, leukemia (ALL)
5-Fluorouracil (5-FU)	IV	(Prodrug) inhibits thymidine synthesis; incorporated into RNA, DNA	M (bolus), mucositis, N and V, diarrhea, skin, NT, ocular	Hepatic neoplasms
Antibiotics				
Adriamycin (doxorubicin, ADR)	IV	Topoisomerase II inhibitor	M, mucositis, N and V, A, vesicant, cardiac (acute and chronic)	Most solid tumors
Bleomycin (Blenoxane, BLEO)	IV, IM, SC	DNA strand breaks	Lung, skin, hypersensitivity, Raynaud's disease	Germ cell tumors, lymphoma
Dactinomycin (actinomycin D, ACT-D)	IV	Intercalation; DNA strand breaks	M, N and V, A, mucositis, vesicant, hepatic	Wilms' tumor, sarcomas

Table 4–3 • Drugs Commonly Used for Pediatric Solid Tumors *(Continued)*

Drug	Route*	Mechanism of Action	Toxicities†	Antitumor Spectrum
Plant Alkaloids				
Vincristine (Oncovin, VCR)	IV	Mitotic inhibitor; binds tubulin	NT, A, SIADH, hypotension, vesicant	Leukemia (ALL), lymphomas, most solid tumors
Vinblastine (Velban, VLB)	IV	Mitotic inhibitor; binds tubulin	M, A, mucositis, mild NT, vesicant	Histiocytosis, Hodgkin's, testicular tumors
Etoposide (VePesid, VP-16)	IV	Topoisomerase II inhibitor	M, A, N and V, mucositis, mild NT, hypotension, allergic	Leukemia (ALL, ANL), lymphomas, testicular, neuroblastoma, sarcomas, brain tumors
Teniposide (VM-26)	IV	DNA strand breaks	Same as etoposide	Same as etoposide
Miscellaneous				
Topotecan	IV	Topoisomerase I inhibitor	M, GI	Sarcoma, neuroblastoma
Prednisone	PO	Receptor-mediated lympholysis	Metabolic	Lymphoma, leukemia
L-Asparaginase (L-ASP)	IM	Decreased protein synthesis	Hypersensitivity, coagulopathy, pancreatitis	Lymphoma, leukemia

*IV, intravenous; PO, oral; IM, intramuscular; SC, subcutaneous

†M, myelosuppression; N and V, nausea and vomiting; A, alopecia; NT, neurotoxicity; GI, gastrointestinal toxicity; HD, high dose; SIADH, syndrome of inappropriate secretion of antidiuretic hormone

Alkylating Agents

Mode of Action

Alkylating agents are highly reactive chemical compounds that covalently bind alkyl groups in the place of hydrogen atoms in DNA, RNA, and protein. They have broad utility because they inhibit cell reproduction whether the cell is synthesizing DNA, undergoing mitosis, or resting. Their primary cytotoxic effects are damage to the DNA template and inhibition of DNA synthesis. Cells are most sensitive to damage in the G1, S, or M phase of the cell cycle.[26] Several groups of drugs are considered as alkylating agents: (1) mustards, (2) nitrosoureas, and (3) nonclassic alkylating agents.

Mustards

Nitrogen mustard, or mechlorethamine, is the parent compound in its group; related agents are cyclophosphamide, ifosfamide, and melphalan.[27] Mechlorethamine, a bifunctional alkylating agent, spontaneously forms a reactive intermediate that alkylates a wide spectrum of molecules. It has a propensity to alkylate the N–7 position on guanine residues. The pharmacokinetics of this agent are not well understood because of its rapid degradation. The major toxicities produce myelosuppression, nausea, and vomiting. The drug has an anticholinergic effect and is a potent vesicant.

Cyclophosphamide and ifosfamide are prodrugs that require activation by the hepatic microsomal oxidative enzymes. Cyclophosphamide is administered widely in the treatment of pediatric malignancies, in bone marrow transplant regimens, and in immunosuppression. Ifosfamide has a spectrum of antitumor activity similar to that of cyclophosphamide.[28] The pharmacokinetics of cyclophosphamide do not appear to be dose dependent. A dose-dependent saturable metabolism of ifosfamide may exist. Noncumulative my-elosuppression is the major dose-limiting toxicity of these two agents. Both agents have significant oral bioavailability. Hemorrhagic cystitis is another common toxicity of the oxazaphosphorines, especially ifosfamide. Acrolein and other reactive metabolites are the causal agents. With the current practice of hydration and mesna (2-mercaptoethane sulfonate) use, hemorrhagic cystitis is rather unusual.[29]

Both agents may be nephrotoxic. Cyclophosphamide can be associated with a syndrome of inappropriate antidiuretic hormone (SIADH)–like syndrome.[30] Ifosfamide can cause proximal renal tubular dysfunction similar to that in Fanconi's syndrome.[14, 31] Ifosfamide can also cause reversible CNS toxicity with somnolence, lethargy, and/or disorientation and occasionally seizures, attributed to accumulation of chloroacetaldehyde, another by-product of metabolism. Acute cardiotoxicity has been associated with cyclophosphamide when given in doses in excess of 100 mg/kg.

Melphalan (L-phenylalanine mustard) has limited use in pediatric malignancies.[32] It has a role at doses that are myeloablative in autologous bone marrow–rescue regimens and has an activity in rhabdomyosarcoma at less myelotoxic doses.[32–34] Myelosuppression and cumulative bone marrow damage are the primary effects of toxicity. Gastrointestinal toxicity may also occur. All these agents may cause infertility. A potential risk exists for the development of second malignancies.

Nitrosoureas

Nitrosoureas are a group of lipid-soluble alkylating agents. DNA alkylation and crosslinking are the primary mechanisms of antitumor activity.[35, 36] In addition, a secondary product, an isocyanate moiety, may contribute to the antitumor activity and toxicity through inhibition of DNA repair. The most active compounds of this class used clinically are a series of 2-chloroethyl derivatives that include bis-chloroethyl-nitrosourea (BCNU), chloroethyl-cyclohexyl-nitrosourea (CCNU), and methyl-CCNU. BCNU is given by intravenous administration; CCNU and methyl-CCNU are given orally.

These agents widely distribute and easily penetrate into the CNS, which has led to their broad use in neuro-oncology. The side effects are defined temporally into three categories: (1) vomiting acutely; (2) myelosuppression beginning at 3 to 4 weeks after administration and often lasting for 2 weeks; and (3) pulmonary fibrosis, usually after several months of treatment. Bone marrow hypoplasia can develop after long-term dosing. Renal and liver damage can also occur.

Dacarbazine, dimethyl triazeno imidazole carboxamide (DTIC), requires demethylation via hepatic microsomal activation to form the reactive alkylating metabolite, aminoimidazole-4-carboxamide (AIC).[37, 38] It is provided as a secondary agent in treatment of solid tumors and of Hodgkin's disease. DTIC can undergo photodegradation to form reactive derivatives. DTIC is given parenterally and has highly variable oral bioavailability. Temozolomide, an analog, has been developed and has excellent oral bioavailability. The primary dose-limiting toxicity involves the gastrointestinal tract. In rare cases, DTIC has been associated with liver failure and death (secondary to veno-occlusive disease).

Procarbazine, a methylhydrazine analog, requires metabolic activation to form alkylating and reactive metabolites via the cytochrome P-450 enzyme complex.[39] This agent has good oral bioavailability. Its metabolism is modulated by long-term administration and by barbiturates, phenytoin, and sedative hypnotics. Since this agent is an effective monoamine oxidase inhibitor, foods containing tyramine are contraindicated. The primary effects of its toxicities include nausea, vomiting, and myelosuppression. High doses or long-term therapy can result in neurotoxicity. Procarbazine is used primarily in patients with Hodgkin's disease.

Platinum Compounds

Cisplatin (CDDP) and carboplatin are heavy-metal coordination complexes exerting their antitumor effects by platination of DNA.[40, 41] These analogs are spontaneously activated in aqueous solution. CDDP is more reactive than carboplatin. Normal saline (0.9% NaCl) is necessary to stabilize CDDP. Both CDDP and carboplatin share a similar spectrum of antitumor activity; however, the spectrum of dose-limiting toxicities is different. CDDP produces significant and potentially nonreversible nephrotoxicity (decreased glomerular filtration rate and renal blood flow and tubular dysfunction with loss of ions, especially magnesium and calcium) and ototoxicity.[42–44] Brisk diuresis with mannitol and careful attention to fluid balance are essential to minimize renal toxicity. Carboplatin produces significant thrombocytopenia and myelosuppression.[41, 45] These agents are active primarily against malignant germ-cell tumors, hepatoblastomas, osteosarcomas, and neuroblastomas.

ANTIMETABOLITES

Antimetabolites are chemical analogs of endogenous substrates of DNA, RNA, and protein synthesis. The most important are analogs of purines (6-thioguanine, 6-mercaptopurine, 2-chloroadenosine), pyrimidines (arabinosyl cytosine, 5-fluorouracil), and folates (methotrexate, trimetrexate). These agents are cell-cycle and S-phase specific, with the maximal cytotoxic effect occurring in cells undergoing DNA synthesis. In clinical use, therefore, these agents are highly schedule dependent.

Methotrexate

Methotrexate (MTX) is used widely in the treatment of pediatric malignancies. It can be administered orally and parenterally.[46] Methotrexate is the first antitumor agent for which pharmacologic dose targeting was utilized in order to standardize dose exposure and monitoring.[42, 47] Leucovorin (5-formyl tetrahydrofolate) is given as a "rescue" agent to bypass the metabolic block produced by methotrexate.

Methotrexate is a folic acid analog that is a tightly binding inhibitor of dehydrofolate reductase, an enzyme that converts folate to tetrahydrofolate. Depletion of tetrahydrofolate results in decreased pools of DNA precursors, especially thymidine, and inhibits DNA synthesis. Intracellular polyglutamation of methotrexate enhances its cytotoxicity. The primary liver metabolite is 7-hydroxymethotrexate. This agent has a volume of distribution equivalent to that of body water and is primarily eliminated by the kidneys, through both glomerular filtration and tubular excretion. Elimination is delayed in patients with ascites and pleural effusions, which act as reservoirs. This delayed elimination can result in excess toxicity.

The primary effects from the toxicities of methotrexate are myelosuppression and gastrointestinal mucositis. These may be prevented by leucovorin. Nephrotoxicity may be prevented by fluid hydration and alkalization. Renal dysfunction during methotrexate infusion is a medical emergency requiring close monitoring and aggressive leucovorin dosing. Hepatic toxicity is usually transient.

Acute, subacute, and chronic neurotoxicity can occur after high-dose therapy. Combined high-dose methotrexate and cranial radiation may lead to devastating neurotoxicity.

Several common drugs may interfere with methotrexate elimination by competing for renal tubular secretion. These include salicylates, sulfisoxazoles, penicillins, and nonsteroidal anti-inflammatory agents.

Methotrexate is poorly diffusible into cerebrospinal fluid, but can be injected via lumbar puncture for prophylaxis or treatment of acute lymphocytic leukemia (ALL), non-Hodgkin's lymphoma, medulloblastoma, or rhabdomyosarcoma arising in cranial parameningeal sites (greatest dose 15 mg). Dilution for lumbar instillation should be accomplished using buffered normal saline.

Side effects of intrathecal administration include meningismus (headache, fever, vomiting, pleocytosis, back pain), and rarely seizures or other neurologic signs. Convulsions are now very unusual since preservative-free methotrexate is available.

Purine Analogs

Two closely related purine analogs are in clinical use: 6-mercaptopurine (6-MP) and 6-thioguanine (6-TG).[48] Both are orally administered compounds used in patients with ALL (6-MP), acute myeloid leukemia (6-TG), and non-Hodgkin's lymphoma and Langerhans' cell histiocytosis (6-MP). Both have very few toxic effects other than myelosuppression. Nausea and vomiting are unusual side effects, as are mouth ulcers and liver damage.

Pyrimidine Analogs

Two primary pyrimidine analogs are in clinical use. Cytosine arabinoside (Ara-C) is an analog of deoxycytidine and has several effects on DNA biosynthesis.[49, 50] Ara-C is useful in patients with acute leukemia and non-Hodgkin's lymphoma. It can be given singly or along with methotrexate (often with hydrocortisone) via lumbar puncture for prophylaxis or treatment of these diseases and parameningeal sarcoma.

Side effects consist predominantly of vomiting and myelosuppression. Sometimes, fevers of 40° to 41°C are noted during and/or after infusion. Acute cerebellar toxicity has been noted after administration of high dosages intravenously.[51, 52] Chemical conjunctivitis has also been observed at doses of 3 g/m.[2] Prevention is by prophylactic instillation of glucocorticoid eyedrops during Ara-C infusion.

The agent 5-fluorouracil (5-FU) is commonly used in adults with gastrointestinal cancer. It has, however, very limited utility in pediatric oncology. The major diseases for which it is given to children are malignant hepatic neoplasm (hepatoblastoma, hepatocellular carcinoma) and colon cancer.[53, 54] 5-FU can be administered orally or intravenously. Similar to Ara-C, its side effects consist primarily of vomiting and myelosuppression.

ANTITUMOR ANTIBIOTICS

Modes of Action

There are three antibiotics produced by various *Streptomyces* organisms that have activity against many pediatric malignant tumors. Of interest is that all three compounds bind to DNA and act to prevent DNA replication and RNA transcription. Combinations of these agents with radiation may result in increased toxicity because of increased normal tissue damage.

Actinomycin D

This yellow-colored compound was the first of the actinomycin family to be introduced. First found to be active in rodent tumors, it was then given to children with metastatic Wilms' tumor in 1956 with striking results.[55] Actinomycin D (AMD) also has demonstrable activity in children with rhabdomyosarcomas, Ewing's sarcomas, and malignant germ cell tumors.[56] Actinomycin D's toxic effects are vomiting, mucositis, and myelosuppression. Often, the platelet count is suppressed more than the neutrophil and red blood cell counts.

Because it is excreted in the liver and can intensify the reaction of tissues to therapeutic radiation, special caution is required when giving AMD to a child with a right-sided flank tumor that is in or next to the liver. A radiation "recall" phenomenon can also occur after the completion of radiotherapy when AMD is readministered.[57] This effect can lead to cutaneous erythema and inflammatory changes or to functional impairment of deeper structures, such as in pulmonary fibrosis or hepatopathy. Similar to nitrogen mustard and BCNU, AMD is a vesicant and can cause serious burns if leakage into subcutaneous tissue occurs during intravenous administration.

Doxorubicin (Adriamycin)

This red-colored antibiotic has a spectrum of oncolytic activity similar to that of AMD but broader. Doxorubicin (Adriamycin, ADR) and its congener, daunomycin, have demonstrated efficacy in children with leukemia, Hodgkin's and non-Hodgkin's lymphomas, Wilms' tumors,[58] rhabdomyosarcomas, Ewing's sarcomas,[59] osteogenic sarcomas,[60] and liver tumors.[61] Doxorubicin is given intravenously and temporarily imparts a reddish-orange hue to the urine afterward. It is similar to actinomycin D in being excreted in the liver, in producing radiation recall, and in causing a severe chemical burn if leakage occurs under the skin. Some children experience a peculiar blushing or reddening of the veins through which the material is flowing, sometimes with itching, but true allergic reactions are rare. The notable acute side effects are mucositis and myelosuppression (chiefly neutropenia), which become most pronounced during the second week after administration. Alopecia is common, but vomiting is rather mild compared with the emetogenic effects of actinomycin D, cisplatin, and nitrogen mustard.

The major long-term toxic effect, however, is cardiac failure, usually following cumulative doses in excess of 450 mg/m[2] of body surface.[62] Some evidence exists that babies are more susceptible to cardiac failure at doses less than 400 mg/m[2] than are older children.[63] Since both ADR and daunomycin (used primarily for treating acute leukemia and lymphoma in children) intensify radiation effects, the dose of either is usually limited to 300 mg/m[2] of body surface in patients who receive radiation to the heart (i.e., incidental to the presence of a pulmonary or mediastinal tumor). Echocardiography or radionuclide angiocardiography is employed to monitor for signs of left ventricular (LV) dysfunction. Reduction of LV ejection fraction to under 50% is an indication to withhold ADR or daunomycin.[64]

Bleomycin

The third antitumor antibiotic, bleomycin, has rather limited usefulness in pediatric oncology. The primary indications are malignant germ-cell tumors and Hodgkin's disease.[65] Bleomycin is usually given intravenously. Occasionally, subcutaneous or intramuscular injections are employed. It is unusual in that myelosuppression after its administration is unexpected, although febrile reactions during prolonged intravenous infusion are rather common. These reactions can usually be controlled, at least in part, by acetaminophen. The skin may become pigmented or develop a rash after prolonged administration.

More serious, however, is long-term pulmonary toxicity, chiefly pulmonary fibrosis, which may be dose related and can be augmented by administration of high concentrations of oxygen (e.g., during anesthesia) or pulmonary radiation therapy.[65] Serial pulmonary function tests should be obtained at the beginning of treatment and after 100 units/m² of body surface and 200 units/m² have been delivered. Fortunately, pulmonary restrictive changes so discovered do not necessarily progress to fibrosis, but it is our practice to discontinue bleomycin if the predicted pulmonary function values are diminished by 25% or more below the baseline. A cumulative maximum total of 400 units (mg) should not be exceeded in adults (200–240 u/m² in children).

MICROTUBULE BINDING AGENTS
Mode of Action

There are two drugs in this category currently in use in pediatric oncology. These agents probably act by binding to the cellular microtubules. This action inhibits mitotic spindle formation, and the cells are thus interrupted in mitosis.

Vinca Alkaloid Group

This group contains two major related agents, vincristine and vinblastine. There are some dif-

ferences between the compounds in terms of oncolytic activity and side effects. Vincristine is most useful for induction of remission in children with ALL and for patients with lymphomas, Wilms' tumors, neuroblastomas, rhabdomyosarcomas, Ewing's sarcomas,[66, 67] and intracranial tumors.[68] Vincristine is myelosuppressive after four or more weekly injections, but affects the red blood cells more than the white blood cells or platelets.

Vinblastine is given primarily to children with malignant germ-cell tumors, Hodgkin's disease, and Langerhans' cell histiocytosis. This agent is also myelosuppressive, but produces granulocytopenia more often than arrest of red blood cells.

Both agents are strong vesicants, but neither causes vomiting. Constipation is expected after two or more weekly doses of either agent. A stool softener should be given routinely unless the child develops diarrhea.

Interference with microtubules may also produce neurotoxicity (chiefly ileus, peripheral neuropathy, cranial nerve paresis with ptosis and hoarseness with or without jaw pain, and weakness).[69, 70] Transient cortical blindness has also been noted after vincristine administration.[71]

OTHER NATURAL PRODUCTS
Semisynthetic Epipodophyllotoxins

This group of agents is derived from the mandrake plant. Etoposide (VP–16) is commercially available, as is its congener teniposide (VM–26). Their spectrum of activity differs: VP–16 is most active in patients with malignant germ-cell tumors, rhabdomyosarcomas, and histiocytic malignancies,[72, 73] whereas VM–26 is active in patients with acute lymphoblastic leukemias, Ewing's sarcomas, intracranial tumors, and neuroblastomas.[74, 75] Vomiting and myelosuppression, chiefly granulocytopenia, are the expected side effects. Both products are given intravenously over 60 minutes or more, in order to avoid hypotension.

Corticosteroids

Glucocorticosteroids are produced in the adrenal cortex and have many physiologic properties. Their precise mechanism of action is still unclear.

The synthetic analogs of glucocorticosteroids, chiefly prednisone and dexamethasone, are widely utilized as lympholytic agents in children with leukemia, lymphoma, and Langerhans' cell histiocytosis.[76] They are also used for the alleviation of acute CNS edema caused by primary or metastatic intracranial or paraspinal neoplasms. Prolonged administration (over 1 to 2 weeks) is associated with increased appetite and weight gain, hypertension, decreased glucose tolerance, and other findings typical of Cushing's syndrome. Statural growth may be adversely affected, as may muscle strength.

Because the adrenal glands are readily suppressed by exogenous glucocorticoids, a period of gradual discontinuation is necessary if either drug is given for more than 3 to 4 weeks at therapeutic dosages. Usually, the dosage is reduced by 50% every 4 days in order to taper the drug safely. A rebound increase in intracranial pressure can occur occasionally, especially when that was the initial indication. Because vomiting can result either from raised intracranial pressure or from insufficient glucocorticoids (adrenal insufficiency), careful clinical judgment and attention to the possibility of blood-pressure alterations and fluid shifts are mandatory in treating patients with glucocorticoids, especially when given over several weeks' time.

Antiglucocorticosteroids

Probably the least frequently used drug in pediatric oncology is the corticoid antagonist o,p'-DDD (mitotane). This drug damages mitochondria of the adrenal cortical cells and thereby reduces secretion of the glucocorticoids.

Mitotane has been given as an adjuvant to surgical management of patients with adrenocortical carcinomas. This disease is rare in children; only seven cases were reported over 20 years at the Children's Hospital of Philadelphia.[77] The drug is given orally and usually causes vomiting and diarrhea. Lethargy, somnolence, and skin eruptions may also occur.

THERAPEUTICS

The ultimate goal of chemotherapy for cancer is cure of the patient with minimal toxicity. The limitations in therapeutics include several issues. The tumor cell population is heterogeneous and may demonstrate a broad range of chemosensi-

tivity. The development of a resistant tumor cell population can lead to tumor progression.

Patients have broad heterogeneity in their sensitivities to the toxic effects of the oncolytic agents. The clinician must balance the oncolytic effect of each agent with its spectrum and expected severity of toxicity.

Drug Resistance

As discussed previously, the occurrence of intrinsic and/or acquired resistance to chemotherapeutic agents is also a limiting factor in the successful treatment of malignant tumors. Several mechanisms, associated with pharmacologic resistance to specific classes of antitumor agents, have been described in in vitro and in vivo laboratory studies (Table 4–4).[78–82] The clinical importance of these mechanisms of drug resistance is unclear because of the lack of consistent clinical correlative data. In consideration of multimodal therapy, the clinical relevance of individual factors in resistance to specific chemotherapeutic agents may be difficult to identify. These mechanisms of resistance may be associated with important physiologic functions in normal tissues. Molecular events that interfere with apoptosis and lead to the development of chemoresistance—independent of the chemotherapeutic agent—have been suggested and must be considered.[18]

Table 4–4 • Mechanisms of Drug Resistance

Alteration in Intracellular Drug Distribution

Impaired transport	Alkylating agents, antimetabolites
Increased efflux	Vinca alkaloids, anthracyclines

Alteration in Cellular Metabolism

Decreased metabolic activation	Antimetabolites
Increased metabolic inactivation	Alkylating agents Antimetabolites
Altered expression of target	Antimetabolites Vinca alkaloids Epipodophyllotoxins
Increased expression of DNA repair mechanisms	Alkylating agents
Altered Apoptotic Mechanisms	All agents

Combination Chemotherapy

From early experience with single chemotherapeutic agents, we empirically determined that combinations of these agents were necessary to cure chemosensitive tumors.[83] Goldie and Coldman[84-86] based a concept for rational design of combination chemotherapy on the hypothesis that each tumor cell population is composed of multiple subpopulations of cells that are less sensitive to a specific agent than to other agents. In the theoretical design of drug combinations, agents should be selected that (1) permit maximal log cell kill within an acceptable range of toxicity, (2) offer a broader range of coverage of resistant clones, and (3) alter the development of resistant clones. Clinically, the major principles for rational design of combination therapy[7] are as follows:

1. The investigator should select only those agents that have activity against the target tumor.
2. The agents selected should have nonoverlapping toxicities, thereby minimizing their severity.
3. These agents must be given at their optimal doses and schedule.
4. The combination itself must be given at constant intervals.

Clinical Investigations

The major objective of clinical trials is to define the effect of an intervention (such as chemotherapeutic agent) in patients with a specific disease. Endpoint measures in such studies may include response measures, survival, disease control, and/or toxicity. In the current era, the clinical trial is the culmination of experimental in vitro and in vivo studies that suggest a clinical role for the agent.

The first two stages of investigational drug testing in humans are Phase I and Phase II clinical trials.[4, 7, 87] Appropriate patients for these studies are those who have tumor progression or recurrence after standard therapy and those who have tumors known to be refractory to conventional therapy. Using the information obtained in the Phase I trial, the goal of the Phase II clinical trial is to determine the effect of the agent in a specific disease (i.e., the cancer diagnosis).

Agents may also be tested by employing a Phase II window model.[32] In this model, an investigational agent that has shown promising activity in the earlier Phase I trial is tested in patients who are chemonaive, prior to receiving a standard treatment regimen. Endpoints of evaluation in Phase II trials include response rate, disease control interval, or survival interval. Drug toxicity is also monitored closely in Phase II trials. Once the agent has been shown to be effective in this setting, it may be incorporated into Phase III studies. Current results of Children's Cancer Group Phase III trials for solid tumors are presented in Table 4–5.

Phase I and II investigational trials in children cannot be done until early phases of adult trials have been completed and after the maximum tolerated dose (MTD) has been defined in adult patients.[87] Generally, pediatric trials are initiated at dose schedules using approximately 80% of the MTD established in the adult trials, because there is a limited number of pediatric patients eligible for these trials and selection of a higher starting dose may potentially be of greater therapeutic benefit in these patients. Retrospective reviews have suggested that pediatric patients generally tolerate higher dose levels (ranging from 0.75- to 2.8-fold) of these agents than adults.

Caution must be taken, however, in future studies of biologic and cytotoxic agents. Current frontline therapy for childhood disease is more dose intense. Patients entering investigational trials will therefore be heavily pretreated and at risk for greater toxicity. The tolerance to biologic agents by children cannot be predicted. In fact, children may only tolerate smaller doses of biologic agents than determined in adults, as noted in some trials of retinoids.[88]

As we have gained a better understanding of tumor cell biology and genetics, novel targets for drug development, such as growth receptor complexes, signal transduction pathways, and gene mutations, are being identified. The design of clinical trials to evaluate agents or modalities directed toward these targets may need modification to define their safety, toxicity, and effectiveness. Issues relevant to their clinical pharmacology, such as methods of administration, mechanism of delivery to target, and disposition, must be addressed.

Table 4–5 • Frontline CCG and Intergroup Studies of Extracranial Malignant Solid Tumors in Children and Adolescents*

Study No.	Disease	Chemotherapeutic Agents	Chemotherapeutic Duration	XRT, Gray	Results	Reference Number
CCG–521	Advanced Hodgkin's	MOPP + ABVD vs. ABVD + EF/XRT	48 weeks 26 weeks	0 21	EFS at 4 yr. = 78% EFS at 4 yr. = 87% (P>0.05)	90
CCG–502	Lymphoblastic lymphoma	LSA2L2 vs. ADCOMP	18 months	15–lymph nodes	EFS at 5 yr. = 84%-localized, 67%-disseminated; LSA2L2 vs. ADCOMP (P>0.05)	91
CCG–5911	Advanced nonlymphoblastic lymphoma	CHOP, HD/MTX, ETP/ARA-C vs. CHOP, HD/MTX, ETP/IFO, DECAL	33 weeks 26 weeks	0 0	EFS at 2 yr. = >90%-standard risk; >60%-high risk patients	92
CCG–3881	Low- and intermediate-risk neuroblastoma	CPM, CPT, DOX, ETP	38 weeks	15	PFS at 3 yr. = 95%-Stage I 83%-Stage II 96%-Stage III 74%-Stage IV 79%-Stage IV-S	93–95
CCG–321 (P2)	High-risk neuroblastoma	CPM, CPT, DOX, ETP, ± BMT for selected Stage II, III, IV patients	1 year	0	PFS at 3 yr. = 45%	96
CCG–461 (IG)	National Wilms' Tumor Study–IV	VCR, AMD VCR, AMD VCR, AMD, DOX±CPM	18–24 weeks, Stage I, FH 18–65 weeks, Stage II, FH 24–65 weeks, Stages III and IV, FH and all CCSK	10.8	RFS at 4 yr. = 87 to 93%-Stage I 82 to 84%-Stage II 74 to 91%-Stages III, IV, CCSK	97
CCG–631 (IG)	Rhabdomyosarcoma, undifferentiated sarcoma, extraosseous Ewing's (IRS–III)	VCR, AMD ± DOX for Group I + II + favorable Group III, FH VCR, AMD, CPM (VAC) + DOX + CPT, for Group I + II, UH; VAC ± DOX + CPT ± ETP for Groups III and IV	1 year 2 years	0, Group I; 41.4, Group II 41.4 to 50.4, Group III, IV	PFS at 5 yr. = 84%-Group I 74%-Group II PFS at 5 yr. = 66%-Group III 28%-Group IV	98

82

Study	Disease	Treatment	Duration		Outcome	Ref
CCG–7881 (IG)	Ewing's sarcoma	VAC, DOX vs. same + IFO, ETP	1 year	45 microresidual; 55.8, gross residual	EFS at 3 yr. = 50% EFS at 3 yr. = 69% (P = 0.0005)	99
2 CCG–limited-institution Pilot Studies	Localized osteosarcoma	IFO, ADR, HD/MTX or same + CPT	42 weeks	0	DFS at 3 yr. = 75% DFS at median of 30 months = 78%	100, 101
CCG–8891 (IG)	(Malignant) germ-cell tumors, low-risk	Observation for immature teratoma and Stage I testis; BLE, ETP, CPT for Stage I + II ovary and Stage II testis	0 / 9 weeks	0	DFS at median of 33 mo. for immature ovarian teratoma = 98%; altogether EFS at 3 yr. = 92%	102
CCG–8882 (IG)	Malignant germ-cell tumors, high-risk	BLE, ETP, CPT vs. BLE, ETP with double-dose CPT, for Stages III, IV gonadal and all stages of extragonadal tumors	9–16 weeks	0	EFS at 3 yr ~ 77%	103
CCG–8881 (IG)	Hepatoblastoma	CPT, VCR, 5-FU vs. CPT, DOX	18–24 weeks	0	EFS = 95%-Stages I, II; 61 to 62%-Stage III; 23 to 33%-Stage IV	104, 105
	Hepatocellular carcinoma	Same as above	18–24 weeks	0	EFS = 100%-Stage I; 12%-Stage III; 8%-Stage IV	

Abbreviations: CCG = Children's Cancer Group; IG = Intergroup Study with the Pediatric Oncology Group; No. = number; XRT = radiation therapy; MOPP = mustargen (HN₂), Oncovin (vincristine, VCR), prednisone (PDN), procarbazine (PCZ); ABVD = Adriamycin (ADR), bleomycin (BLE), vinblastine (VBL), dinethyl triazeno imidazole carboxamide (DTIC); EF = extended field; LS2L2 = VCR, PDN, daunomycin (DNM), arabinosyl cytosine (ARC), 6-thioguanine, L-asparaginase (ASP), cyclophosphamide (CPM), hydroxyurea, methotrexate (MTX), bis-chloroethyl-nitrosourea (BCNU); ADCOMP = ASP, DNM, CPM, VCR, MTX, PDN; CHOP = CPM, hydroxyldaunomycin (DOX), VCR, PDN; HD/MTX = high-dose MTX; ETP = etoposide; IFO = ifosfamide; DECAL = dexamethasone, ETP, cisplatin (CPT), ARC, ASP; BMT = bone marrow transplantation; AMD = actinomycin D; 5-FU = 5-fluorouracil; FH = favorable histology; CCSK = clear cell sarcoma of the kidney; UH = unfavorable histology; EFS = event-free survival; PFS = (tumor) progression-free survival; RFS = (tumor) relapse-free survival; DFS = disease-free survival

References

1. Goodman LS, Wintrobe MM, Dameshek W, et al: Nitrogen mustard therapy. Use of methyl-bis (beta-chloroethyl)amine hydrochloride for Hodgkin's disease, lymphosarcoma, leukemia and certain allied and miscellaneous disorders. *JAMA* 132:126–1321, 1946.
2. Farber S, Diamond LK, Mercer RD, et al: Temporary remission in acute leukemia in children produced by folic acid antagonist, 4-aminopteryl-glutamic acid (aminopterin). *N Engl J Med* 4:1–71, 1956.
3. Crist WM, Kun LE: Common solid tumors of childhood. *N Engl J Med* 324:461–471, 1991.
4. Balis FM, Poplack DG, Holcenberg JS: General principles of chemotherapy. In Pizzo PA, Poplack DG (eds): *Principles and Practice of Pediatric Oncology*, 2nd ed. Philadelphia: J.B. Lippincott, 1993, pp. 197–246.
5. Mulder JH: Basic cancer chemotherapy: Experimental models—strategy. *Cancer Clin Trials* 1:129–134, 1978.
6. Goldin A, Venditti JM: Progress report on the screening program at the Division of Cancer Treatment, National Cancer Institute. *Cancer Treat Rev* 7:167–176, 1980.
7. DeVita VTJ: Principles of cancer management: chemotherapy. In DeVita VTJ, Hellman S, Rosenberg S (eds): *Cancer Principles and Practice of Oncology*, 5th ed. Philadelphia: Lippincott-Raven, 1994, pp. 333–348.
8. Chabner BA, Myers CE, Coleman CN, et al: The clinical pharmacology of antineoplastic agents (part 2). *N Engl J Med* 292:1159–1168, 1975.
9. Chabner BA, Myers CE, Coleman CN, et al: The clinical pharmacology of antineoplastic agents (part 1). *N Engl J Med* 292:1107–1113, 1975.
10. Calabresi P, Chabner BA: Chemotherapy of neoplastic diseases. In Hardman JG, Limbird LE, Molinoff PB, et al (eds): *Goodman and Gilman's The Pharmacological Basis of Therapeutics*, 9th ed. New York: McGraw-Hill, 1995, pp. 1225–1232.
11. Skipper HE, Schabel FM Jr, Wilcox WS: Experimental evaluation of potential anticancer agents. XIV. Further study of certain basic concepts underlying chemotherapy of leukemia. *Cancer Chemother Rep* 45:5, 1965.
12. Skipper HE, Schabel FM Jr, Wilcox WS: Experimental evaluation of potential anticancer agents. XII. On the criteria and kinetics associated with "curability" of experimental leukemia. *Cancer Chemother Rep* 35:1, 1964.
13. Bukowski RM, McLain D, Finke J: Clinical pharmacokinetics of interleukin 1, interleukin 2, interleukin 4, tumor necrosis factor, and macrophage colony-stimulating factor. In Chabner BA, Longo DL (eds): *Cancer Chemotherapy and Biotherapy: Principles and Practice*, 2nd ed. Philadelphia: Lippincott-Raven, 1996, pp. 609–638.
14. Roberts WM, Estrov Z, Ouspenskaia MV, et al: Measurement of residual leukemia during remission in childhood acute lymphoblastic leukemia. *N Engl J Med* 336:317–323, 1997.
15. Reed JC: BCL-2: Prevention of apoptosis as a mechanism of drug resistance. *Hematol Oncol Clin North Am* 9:451–473, 1995.
16. Nooter K, Boersma AW, Oostru RG, et al: Constitutive expression of the *c-H-ras* oncogene inhibits doxorubicin-induced apoptosis and promotes cell survival in a rhabdomyosarcoma cell line. *Br J Can* 71:556–561, 1995.
17. Bloch CA, Castle VP: Bcl-2 inhibits chemotherapy-induced apoptosis in neuroblastoma. *Cancer Res* 54:3253–3259, 1994.
18. Lowe SW, Ruley HE, Jacks T, et al: p53-Dependent apoptosis modulates the cytotoxicity of anticancer agents. *Cell* 74:957–967, 1993.
19. Evans WE: Clinical pharmacodynamics of anticancer drugs: a basis for extending the concept of dose-intensity. *Blutalkohol* 56:241–248, 1988.
20. Ratain MJ, Schlisky RL, Conley BA, et al: Pharmacodynamics in cancer therapy. *J Clin Oncol* 8:1739–1753, 1990.
21. Rosen G, Caparros B, Hubos AG, et al: Preoperative chemotherapy for osteogenic sarcoma: selection of postoperative adjuvant chemotherapy based on the response of the primary tumor to preoperative chemotherapy. *Cancer* 49:1221–1230, 1982.
22. Collins JM: Pharmacokinetics and clinical monitoring. In Chabner BA, Longo DL (eds): *Cancer Chemotherapy and Biotherapy: Principles and Practice*, 2nd ed. Philadelphia: Lippincott-Raven, 1996, pp. 17–29.
23. Clark JW: Targeted therapy. In Chabner BA, Longo DL (eds): *Cancer Chemotherapy and Biotherapy: Principles and Practice*, 2nd ed. Philadelphia: Lippincott-Raven, 1996, pp. 691–708.
24. Collins JM, Grieshaber CK, Chabner BA: Pharmacologically guided phase I clinical trials based upon preclinical drug development. *J Natl Cancer Inst* 82:1321–1326, 1990.
25. Jaffe N, Frei EI, Traggis D, et al: Adjuvant methotrexate and citrovorum-factor treatment of osteogenic sarcoma. *N Engl J Med* 291:994–997, 1974.
26. Baserga R: The cell cycle. *N Engl J Med* 304:453–459, 1981.
27. Colvin OM, Chabner BA: Alkylating agents. In Chabner BA, Collins JM (eds): *Cancer Chemotherapy Principles and Practice*. Philadelphia: J.B. Lippincott, 1990, pp. 276–313.
28. Jurgens H, Treuner J, Winkler K, et al: Ifosfamide in pediatric malignancies. *Semin Oncol* 16:46–50, 1989.
29. Burkert H: Clinical overview of mesna. *Cancer Treat Rev* 10:175–181, 1983.

30. Bode U, Seif SM, Levine AS: Studies on the antidiuretic effect of cyclophosphamide: Vasopressin release and sodium excretion. *Med Pediatr Oncol* 8:295–303, 1980.

31. Newbury-Ecob RA, Noble VW, Barbor PRH: Ifosfamide-induced Fanconi syndrome. *Lancet* 1:1328, 1989.

32. Horowitz ME, Etcubanas E, Christensen ML, et al: Phase II testing of melphalan in children with newly diagnosed rhabdomyosarcoma: A model for anticancer drug development. *J Clin Oncol* 6:308–314, 1988.

33. Graham-Pole J, Lazarus HM, Herzig RH, et al: High dose melphalan for the treatment of children with refractory neuroblastoma and Ewing's sarcoma. *Am J Pediatr Hematol Oncol* 6:17–26, 1984.

34. Lazarus HM, Herzig RH, Graham-Pole J, et al: Intensive melphalan chemotherapy and cryopreserved autologous bone marrow transplantation for the treatment of refractory cancer. *J Clin Oncol* 1:359–367, 1983.

35. Mitchell EP, Schein PS: Contributions of nitrosoureas to cancer treatment. *Cancer Treat Rep* 70:31–41, 1986.

36. Kann HE: Comparison of biochemical and biological effects of four nitrosoureas with differing carbamoylating activities. *Cancer Res* 38:2363–2366, 1978.

37. Aunbuch SD: Nonclassical alkylating agents. In Chabner BA, Collins JM (eds): *Cancer Chemotherapy Principles and Practice*. Philadelphia: J.B. Lippincott, 1990, pp. 314–340.

38. Gottlieb JA, Baker LH, Quagliana JM, et al: Chemotherapy of sarcomas with a combination of Adriamycin and dimethyl triazeno imidazole carboxamide. *Cancer* 30:1632–1638, 1972.

39. Prough RA, Tweedie DJ: Metabolism and action of anti-cancer drugs. In Powis G, Prough RA (eds): *Procarbazine*. London: Taylor & Francis, 1987, pp. 29–47.

40. Zwelling LA: Cisplatin and new platinum analogs. In Pinedo HM, Chabner BA (eds): *Cancer Chemotherapy, Annual*. New York: Elsevier, 1986, pp. 97–116.

41. Wagstaff AJ, Ward A, Benfield P, et al: Carboplatin: A preliminary review of its pharmacodynamic and pharmacokinetic properties and therapeutic efficacy in the treatment of cancer. *Drugs* 37:162–190, 1989.

42. Daugaard G, Abildgaard U: Cisplatin nephrotoxicity. *Cancer Chemother Pharmacol* 25:1–9, 1989.

43. McHaney VA, Thibadoux MA, Hayes FA, et al: Hearing loss in children receiving cisplatin chemotherapy. J Pediatr 102:314–317, 1983.

44. Cersosimo RJ: Cisplatin neurotoxicity. *Cancer Treat Res* 16:195–211, 1989.

45. Van Echo DA, Egorin MJ, Aisner J: The pharmacology of carboplatin. *Semin Oncol* 16:1–6, 1989.

46. Allegra CJ: Antifolates. In Chabner BA, Collins JM (eds): *Cancer Chemotherapy Principles and Practice*. Philadelphia: J.B. Lippincott, 1990, pp. 110–153.

47. Stoller RG, Hande KR, Jacobs SA, et al: Use of plasma pharmacokinetics to predict and prevent methotrexate toxicity. *N Engl J Med* 297:630–634, 1977.

48. McCormack JJ, Johns DG: Purine and purine nucleoside antimetabolites. In Chabner BA, Collins JM (eds): *Cancer Chemotherapy Principles and Practice*. Philadelphia: J.B. Lippincott, 1990, pp. 234–252.

49. Chabner BA: Cytidine analogues. In Chabner BA, Collins JM (eds): *Cancer Chemotherapy Principles and Practice*. Philadelphia: J.B. Lippincott, 1990, pp. 154–179.

50. Stentof J: The toxicity of cytarabine. *Drug Safety* 5:7–27, 1990.

51. Preisler HD, Early AP, Raza A, et al: Therapy of secondary acute nonlymphocytic leukemia with cytarabine. *N Engl J Med* 30:21–23, 1983.

52. Winkleman MD, Hines JD: Cerebellar degeneration caused by high-dose cytosine arabinoside: a clinicopathologic study. *Ann Neurol* 14:520–527, 1983.

53. Myeres CE: The pharmacology of the fluoropyrimidines. *Pharmacol Rev* 33:1–15, 1981.

54. Grem JL: Fluorinated pyrimidines. In Chabner BA, Collins JM (eds): *Cancer Chemotherapy Principles and Practice*. Philadelphia: J.B. Lippincott, 1990, pp. 180–224.

55. Farber S, Roch R, Sears EM, et al: Advances in chemotherapy of cancer in man. *Adv Cancer Res* 4:1–71, 1956.

56. Hustu HO, Holton C, James DJ, et al: Treatment of Ewing's sarcoma with concurrent radiotherapy and chemotherapy. *J Pediatr* 73:249–251, 1968.

57. D'Angio GJ, Garber S, Maddock CL: Potentiation of x-ray effects by actinomycin D. *Radiology* 73:175–177, 1959.

58. D'Angio GJ, Beckwith JB, Breslow NE, et al: Wilms' tumor: An update. *Cancer* 45:1791–1798, 1980.

59. Nesbit MEJ, Perez CA, Tefft M, et al: Multimodal therapy for the management of primary, nonmetastatic Ewing's sarcoma of bone: An Intergroup Study. *Monogr Natl Cancer Inst* 56:255–262, 1981.

60. Cortes EP, Holland JF, Wang JJ, et al: Amputation and Adriamycin in primary osteosarcoma. *N Engl J Med* 29:998–1000, 1974.

61. Evans AE, Land VJ, Newton WA, et al: Combination chemotherapy (vincristine, Adriamycin, cyclophosphamide, and 5-fluorouracil) in the treatment of children with malignant hepatoma. *Cancer* 50:821–826, 1982.

62. Goorin AM, Borow KM, Goldman A, et al: Congestive heart failure due to Adriamycin cardiotoxicity: its natural history in children. *Cancer* 47:2810–2816, 1981.

63. Pratt CB, Ransom JL, Evans WE: Age-related Adriamycin cardiotoxicity in children. *Cancer Treat Rev* 62:1381–1385, 1978.

64. Alexander J, Dainiak N, Berger HJ, et al: Serial assessment of doxorubicin cardiotoxicity with quantitative radionuclide angiocardiography. *N Engl J Med* 300:278–283, 179

65. Cooper KR, Hong WK: Prospective study of the pulmonary toxicity of continuously infused bleomycin. *Cancer Treat Rev* 65:419–425, 1981.

66. James DHJ, George P, Hustu O, et al: Chemotherapy of localized inoperable malignant tumors of children. *JAMA* 189:636–638, 1964.

67. Sutow WW: Vincristine (NSC–67574) therapy for malignant solid tumors in children (except Wilms' tumor). *Cancer Chemother Pharmacol* 52:485–487, 1968.

68. Rosenstock JG, Evans AE, Schut L: Response to vincristine of recurrent brain tumors in children. *J Neurosurg* 45:135–140, 1976.

69. Kaufman IA, Kung FH, Koenig HM, et al: Overdosage with vincristine. *J Pediatr* 89:671–674, 1976.

70. O'Callaghan MJ, Ekert H: Vincristine toxicity unrelated to dose. *Arch Dis Child* 51:289–292, 1976.

71. Byrd RL, Rohrbaugh TM, Raney RBJ, et al: Transient cortical blindness secondary to vincristine therapy in childhood malignancies. *Cancer* 47:37–40, 1981.

72. Chard RLJ, Krivit W, Bleyer WA, et al: Phase II study of VP–16–213 in childhood malignant disease: A Children's Cancer Study Group Report. *Cancer Treat Rev* 63:1755–1759, 1979.

73. Zijlstra JG, DeJong S, DeVries EGE, et al: Topoisomerases, new targets in cancer chemotherapy. *Med Oncol Tumor Pharmacol* 7:11–18, 1990.

74. Rivera G, Avery T, Pratt C: (NSG-122819; VM-26) and 4'-demethylepipodophyllotoxin 9-(4,6-O-ethylidene-β-D-glucopyranoside) (NSC–141540; VP–16–213) in childhood cancer: preliminary observations. *Cancer Chemother Pharmacol* 59:743–749, 1975.

75. Rozencweig M, VonHoff DD, Henney JE, et al: VM 26 and VP 16–213: A comparative analysis. *Cancer* 40:334–342, 1977.

76. Vietti TJ, Sullivan MP, Berry DH, et al: The response of acute childhood leukemia to an initial and a second course of prednisone. *J Pediatr* 66:18–26, 1965.

77. Raney BJ, Meadows AT, D'Angio GJ: Adrenocortical carcinoma in children: Experience at the Children's Hospital of Philadelphia, 1961–1980. *In* Humphrey GB, Grindey GB, Dehner LP (eds): *Adrenal and Endocrine Tumors in Children*. Boston, Martinus Nijhoff Publishers, 1983, pp. 303–305.

78. Beck WT, Danks MK: Mechanisms of resistance to drugs that inhibit DNA topoisomerases. *Semin Cancer Biol* 2:235–244, 1991.

79. Cole SPC, Sparks KE, Fraser K, et al: Pharmacological characterization of multidrug resistant MRP–transfected human tumor cells. *Cancer Res* 54:5902–5910, 1994.

80. Black SM, Wolf CR: The role of glutathione-dependent enzymes in drug resistance. *Pharmacol Ther* 51:139–154, 1991.

81. Bugg BY, Danks MK, Beck WT, et al: Expression of a mutant DNA topoisomerase II in CCRF–CEM human leukemic cells selected for resistance to teniposide. *Proc Natl Acad Sci USA* 88:7654–7658, 1991.

82. Clapper ML, Tew KD: Alkylating agent resistance. *Cancer Treat Rev* 48:125–150, 1989.

83. DeVita VT, Schein PS: The use of drugs in combination for the treatment of cancer: rationale and results. *N Engl J Med* 288:998–1006, 1973.

84. Goldie JH, Coldman AJ, Gudauskas GA: Rationale for the use of alternating non-cross-resistant chemotherapy. *Cancer Treat Rep* 66:439–449, 1982.

85. Goldie JH, Coldman AJ: A mathematical model for relating the drug sensitivity of tumours to their spontaneous mutation rate. *Cancer Treat Rep* 63:1727–1733, 1979.

86. Goldie J, Coldman A: Quantitative model for multiple levels of drug resistance in clinical tumors. *Cancer Treat Rep* 67:923–931, 1983.

87. Pratt CB: The conduct of Phase I–II clinical trials in children with cancer. *Med Pediatr Oncol* 19:304–309, 1991.

88. Smith MA, Adamson PC, Balis FM, et al: Phase I and pharmacokinetic evaluation of ALL-trans-retinoic acid in pediatric patients with cancer. *J Clin Oncol* 10:1666–1673, 1992.

89. Parker SL, Tong T, Bolden S, et al: Cancer Statistics, 1997. *CA Cancer J Clin* 47:5–27, 1997.

90. Hutchinson R, Fryer C, Krailo M, et al: Comparison of MOPP/ABVD with ABVD/XRT for treatment of advanced Hodgkin's disease in children (CCG–521). *Proc Am Soc Clin Oncol* 11:340 (abstract 1166), 1992.

91. Tubergen DG, Krailo MD, Meadows AT, et al: Comparison of treatment regimens for pediatric lymphoblastic non-Hodgkin's lymphoma: A Childrens Cancer Group Study. *J Clin Oncol* 13:1368–1376, 1995.

92. Cairo MS, Krailo M, Morse M, et al: The efficacy of two short but intensive regimens (CCG "Orange" and "French" LMB-89-C) in children with advanced non-lymphoblastic lymphoma. *Proc Am Soc Clin Oncol* 15:431 (abstract 1335), 1996.

93. Matthay K, Seeger R, Haase G, et al: Treatment and outcome of stage III neuroblastoma based on prospective biologic staging. *Med Pediatr Oncol* 23:173 (abstract 0–15), 1994.

94. Matthay KK, Seeger RC, Atkinson J, et al: A prospective Childrens Cancer Group Study of stage II neuroblastoma treated with surgery

alone. *Proc Am Soc Clin Oncol* 12:414 (abstract 1420), 1993.

95. Haase GM, Atkinson JB, Stram DO, et al: Surgical management and outcome in non-metastatic neuroblastoma: comparison of the Childrens Cancer Group and the International Staging Systems. *J Pediatr Surg* 30:289–295, 1995.

96. Haase GM, O'Leary M, Ramsay NKC, et al: Aggressive surgery combined with intensive chemotherapy improves survival in poor risk neuroblastoma. *J Pediatr Surg* 26:1119–1124, 1991.

97. Green D, Breslow N, Beckwith J, et al: A comparison between single dose and divided dose administration of dactinomycin and doxorubicin. A report from the National Wilms Tumor Study Group. *Proc Am Soc Clin Oncol* 15:457 (abstract 1433), 1996.

98. Crist W, Gehan EA, Ragab AH, et al: The Third Intergroup Rhabdomyosarcoma Study. *J Clin Oncol* 13:610–630, 1995.

99. Grier H, Krailo M, Link M, et al: Improved outcome in non-metastatic Ewing's sarcoma and PNET of bone with addition of ifosfamide and etoposide to vincristine, Adriamycin, cyclophosphamide, and actinomycin: A Childrens Cancer Group and Pediatric Oncology Group Report. *Proc Am Soc Clin Oncol* 13:421 (abstract 1443), 1994.

100. Miser J, Arndt C, Smithson W, et al: Treatment of high-grade osteosarcoma with ifosfamide, mesna, Adriamycin, high-dose methotrexate with or without cisplatin. Results of two pilot trials. *Proc Am Soc Clin Oncol* 13:421 (abstract 1442), 1994.

101. Arndt C, Miser J, Pritchard D, et al: Treatment of high-grade osteosarcoma with ifosfamide, mesna, Adriamycin, high-dose methotrexate and cisplatin. *Med Pediatr Oncol* 27:227, 1996.

102. Cushing B, Giller R, Cohen L, et al: Surgery alone is effective treatment of resected ovarian immature teratoma in children: A Pediatric Intergroup Report (POG 9048/CCG 8891). *Proc Am Soc Clin Oncol* 15:461 (abstract 1449), 1996.

103. Hawkins E, Issacs H, Cushing B, et al: Occult malignancy in neonatal sacrococcygeal teratomas. A report from a combined Pediatric Oncology Group and Childrens Cancer Group Study. *Am J Pediatr Hematol Oncol* 15:406–409, 1993.

104. Ortega J, Douglass E, Feusner J, et al: A randomized trial of cisplatin, vincristin, 5-fluorouracil vs. DDP/doxorubicin IV continuous infusion for the treatment of hepatoblastoma: Results from the Pediatric Intergroup Hepatoma Study (CCG–8881/POG–8945). *Proc Am Soc Clin Oncol* 13:416 (abstract 1421), 1994.

105. Douglass E, Ortega J, Feusner J, et al: Hepatocellular carcinoma in children and adolescents: Results from the Pediatric Intergroup Hepatoma Study (CCG 8881/POG–8945). *Proc Am Soc Clin Oncol* 13:420 (abstract 1439), 1994.

Principles of Radiotherapy

• *Scott Lankford, M.D.* • *Patricia J. Eifel, M.D.*

Pediatric oncology has served as a model for the multidisciplinary approach to cancer therapy in general. Systemic chemotherapy has dramatically improved survival rates for children with many solid tumors, but drug therapy alone is often insufficient to control gross disease, particularly in the primary tumor site. Instead, locoregional control often depends upon the careful application of surgery, radiation therapy, and chemotherapy, timed and measured to achieve a high rate of local control with minimized morbidity. Optimization of the ratio between disease control and morbidity requires close cooperation among all members of the management team, including the child's pediatric oncologist, a surgical oncologist, an anesthesiologist, a radiation oncologist who specializes in the treatment of children, pediatric and radiation oncology nurses, dieticians, play therapists, radiotherapists, and other support personnel.

Control of local disease with acceptable morbidity relies on close communication among these disciplines at all levels of treatment planning. Seemingly routine surgical decisions, such as the placement of an operative incision, can have a profound impact on subsequent radiation treatment volumes and morbidity. Carefully placed surgical clips can help the radiation oncologist to localize surgical margins, thus aiding in the design of precise treatment fields. The sequence of drugs, surgery, and irradiation can influence the volume and morbidity of irradiation, the severity of drug-radiation interactions, the likelihood of delays in treatment, and the speed of surgical wound healing. Thus, a basic understanding of radiotherapeutic principles is essential to a good surgical oncology practice.

In this chapter, we review the fundamental physical and biologic principles governing radiotherapy. We also discuss some of the clinical considerations that influence radiotherapeutic decisions, giving particular attention to those that are specific to pediatric radiation oncology practice.

PHYSICAL PRINCIPLES

The last decade of the nineteenth century marked a revolution in physics with the discovery of X rays by Roentgen and the discovery of radioactivity by Becquerel. No one at that time could have imagined the far-reaching ramifications of the collective genius of these two men. Before the turn of the century, while Marie Curie diligently perfected techniques to purify and quantify radioactive elements, the therapeutic qualities of ionizing radiation already were being tested by physicians in Europe and North America. Today sophisticated computerized linear accelerators deliver precisely focused beams of electromagnetic radiation to deep-seated tumors. Despite the increasing complexity of radiotherapy equipment and techniques, however, the guiding principles of radiotherapy have not changed.

Types of Ionizing Radiation Used in Therapy

Ionizing radiations lie on the high-energy portion of the electromagnetic spectrum. They differ from nonionizing electromagnetic radiations such as visible light because of their ability to excite, or ionize, atoms in an absorbing material. These ionizations produce highly reactive *free radicals* that participate in the biochemical reactions responsible for therapy effects.

The nuclear decay of certain radioactive elements (e.g., cobalt 60) produces ionizing radiations of characteristic energies called *gamma rays*. Electromagnetic ionizing radiations can also be produced artificially by bombarding fast-moving electrons onto a target such as tungsten. By varying the energy of the accelerated electrons, therapeutic X rays of different energies can be produced, each having a distinct absorption profile in tissue (Fig. 5–1). Both X rays and gamma rays are composed of discrete quanta of energy called *photons*. They are distinguished only by whether they are produced by extranuclear forces (X rays) or intranuclear forces (gamma rays).

Particulate ionizing radiations are used therapeutically as well. Their absorption characteristics differ markedly from photons. The most commonly used particle is the *electron*, or *beta particle*. Electrons produced by a linear accelerator are made available for treatment simply by removing the tungsten target from their path. Unlike photons, electrons deposit their energy in superficial tissues to a depth that is related to the electron energy and thus deliver little radiation to deeper tissues (see Fig. 5–1). For this reason, electrons are ideally suited for treating tumors close to the skin surface, whereas photons are best for deeper lesions.

Other ionizing particles have been investigated for their therapeutic value. These include neutrons, protons, π mesons, and helium nuclei. Heavy, charged particles such as protons can be especially helpful because they deposit most of their energy at a discrete depth in tissues (see Fig. 5–1).[1] The point at which they deposit their energy is called the *Bragg peak*. This characteristic of proton beams enables the radiotherapist to deliver a very high dose of ionizing radiation to a deeply seated tumor while sparing the surrounding normal tissues. Although the expense of proton-beam irradiation has limited its use, the sharply defined beams produced with this technique have proved particularly useful for some special problems such as ocular melanomas.

Radiation Interactions with Tissue

At the atomic level, ionizing radiation is absorbed by tissues in an energy-dependent manner through three distinct mechanisms: the photoelectric effect, Compton scatter, and pair production. The characteristics of these mechanisms of energy absorption determine whether they are used for diagnostic or therapeutic X rays.

Relatively low-energy photons (<40 keV) interact predominantly by the *photoelectric effect*. At these energies, the incident photon's energy is absorbed by an inner-shell electron of a tissue atom, exciting the electron and ejecting it from the atom. This leaves a hole in the inner orbital shell that is filled when an outer-shell electron

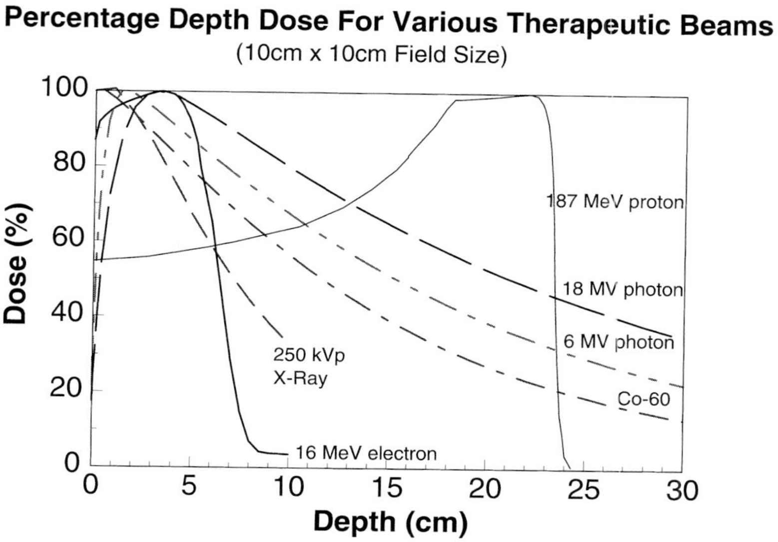

Percentage Depth Dose For Various Therapeutic Beams
(10cm x 10cm Field Size)

Figure 5–1 • The relationship between the doses of radiation deposited at various distances from the surface of an absorbing tissue (percentage depth doses) and the type and energy of the radiation beam. Note that the dose from a 250 kVp X-ray beam is greatest at the skin surface. Megavoltage beams (e.g., cobalt 60, 6 MV, and 18 MV) deliver a lower dose to the skin surface; as the energy of the beam increases, the depth of maximum dose also increases. Particle beams (e.g., electron and proton beams) have markedly different absorption characteristics that can be exploited in special clinical situations.

falls into its place, emitting a photon of characteristic energy that is rapidly absorbed.

Photoelectric absorption is highly dependent on the atomic number (Z) of elements in the absorbing tissues. In fact, the probability of a photoelectric interaction increases by a factor of Z^3. Tissues composed of high-Z elements such as the calcium in bone (Z = 20) absorb many more photons than do soft tissues composed primarily of carbon (Z = 6), hydrogen (Z = 1), and oxygen (Z = 8). This differential absorption produces the sharp contrasts between bone and soft tissues that are characteristic of diagnostic X rays.

The increased absorption by bone is, however, a disadvantage for radiotherapy. Kilovoltage units, which were used extensively for therapy before the mid 1960s, were inferior to today's megavoltage beams not only because they delivered high doses to the skin and relatively low doses to deeper tissues, but because the doses absorbed by bone were as much as two to three times higher than those in soft tissue, contributing to a high morbidity.

Megavoltage beams produced by ^{60}Co units

and modern linear accelerators produce photons of 1 to 20 MV that interact with tissues predominantly by means of the *Compton effect*, or *Compton scatter*. In this process, the incident photon is scattered by a loosely bound outer-shell electron, imparting some of its energy to the electron and ejecting it from the atom. This ionizes, or excites, the atom, making it highly reactive. The scattered photon and the ejected electron then interact with other atoms to cause additional ionizations.

Compton scatter is essentially independent of the atomic number of the absorbing material. Thus, all solid tissues of similar density absorb approximately the same quantity, or dose, of radiation. The difference between the photoelectric effect and the Compton effect is illustrated by the difference between a diagnostic X-ray film and a port film taken on a megavoltage therapy unit (Fig. 5–2).

A third type of radiation interaction, called *pair production*, becomes significant only at energies greater than 20 MV. At these energies, incident photons interact directly with the atomic

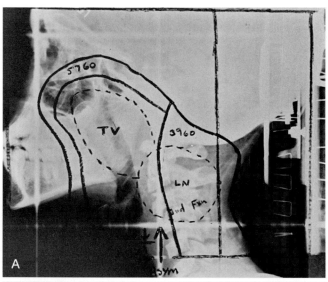

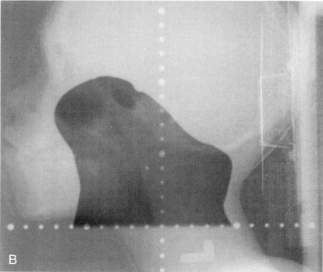

Figure 5–2 • *A*, A simulation film used to plan the treatment of a child with a nasopharyngeal carcinoma. The film is taken with a diagnostic X-ray beam on a treatment simulator. The rectangular delineator marks mimic the position of the accelerator's collimators and define the edges of the beam. The curved lines indicate regions that will be shielded by custom-fabricated blocks. *B*, A port film taken during treatment to confirm proper setup is exposed with a therapeutic (6 MV) X-ray beam. Note that there is very little contrast between bone and soft tissues in the port film (X-ray absorption is mediated primarily by the Compton effect) compared with the simulation film that was exposed with a diagnostic-quality X-ray beam (X-ray absorption is mediated by the photoelectric effect).

nucleus of the absorbing molecule to form an electron and a positron. When these particles recombine, they form characteristic X rays that travel in opposite directions. This type of interaction is of little importance within the range of beam energies used for therapy.

Characteristics of Megavoltage Irradiation

Megavoltage radiotherapy was introduced in the late 1940s with the development of the cobalt unit. Megavoltage beams revolutionized radiotherapy by enabling the delivery of higher doses to deeper-seated tumors, by providing more even dose distributions, and by allowing for significant skin sparing.

One result of Compton-scatter absorption is that the photons penetrating deeper into tissues produce an increasing number of scattered electrons and ionizations that create a "buildup region" just below the surface. For this reason, the dose at the skin surface is significantly less than the maximum dose delivered to deeper tissues. For example, a single appositional 6 MV photon beam delivers its maximum dose (d_{max}) at a depth of approximately 1.5 cm, whereas the skin surface receives only 15% to 25% of that dose (see Fig. 5–1). As a general rule, the d_{max} is reached at a depth that increases with the energy of the incident photon beam. Early kilovoltage beams did not allow for skin sparing, and, as a consequence, the deliverable dose was usually limited by toxic effects to the skin.

Measurement of Radiation Dose

In the early days of radiotherapy, radiation doses from kilovoltage units were determined empirically through observations of clinical effect. One of the most commonly used methods was a scale of skin redness, the *skin erythema dose*. This imprecise method has long been replaced by highly quantitative direct physical measurements of machine output and absorbed doses.

Radiation treatments are prescribed by specifying an absorbed dose to be delivered to some point or volume of tissue and a treatment technique. The absorbed dose is specified in terms of the energy absorbed per unit of absorbing tissue. The current international unit of absorbed dose is the *Gray* (1 Gy = 1 J/kg). About 10 years ago the Gray replaced the *rad* (radiation-absorbed dose) as the unit of absorbed dose: 1 Gy = 100 cGy = 100 rad.

The safe and accurate delivery of therapeutic radiation depends upon the precise calibration of machine output. This is accomplished by placing a sensitive ion chamber in a tissue phantom, usually a tank of water, that simulates the human body. The tissue phantom is then irradiated, and output is measured electronically. Meticulous calibrations must be performed at regular intervals to ensure the continued accuracy of radiation delivery.

Machine output and absorbed doses can also be confirmed by direct measurements with small solid-state thermoluminescent dosimeters. Such dosimeters are very versatile and can be placed directly on a patient to measure the dose of irradiation. In this capacity, they can confirm treatment plans and serve as a secondary form of quality assurance between formal machine calibrations.

BIOLOGIC PRINCIPLES

Shortly after the discovery of ionizing radiation at the turn of the century, investigators recognized that radiation tended to have a differential effect on tumors and normal tissues. This differential effect made ionizing radiation a powerful therapeutic modality. However, it was only after the discovery of DNA and the development of modern mammalian-cell culture techniques that investigators began to learn about the cellular and subcellular responses that lead to clinical radiation effects.

Subcellular Effects

When ionizing radiation interacts with cellular molecules, highly reactive free radicals are formed that participate in biochemical reactions, potentially altering the cell's physiology. If biochemical pathways critical to cell function or to cell replication are disturbed, the cell may die. Normal cells have the capacity to neutralize free radicals before they cause damage and can repair many types of sublethal injury when it occurs. Because malignant cells often lack these abilities, they tend to be more susceptible to damage by free radicals.

Because of the high degree of molecular redundancy within cells, most ionizations produced by a photon beam probably have little impact on cellular function. Interactions with DNA are thought to be responsible for most of the significant cellular effects of radiation. Radiation causes double- and single-strand breaks in DNA, leaving reactive ends that recombine with other broken DNA. The cell dies when the resulting abnormal chromosomes cannot migrate correctly during mitosis. Cells with a rapid mitotic rate, such as those found in many tumors, are more vulnerable to this reproductive cell death than the dormant, postmitotic cells that predominate in surrounding normal tissues.

Although DNA molecules can be ionized directly by incident photons or by secondary scattered electrons, most biologically significant radiation damage is caused by molecular ionizations mediated by *hydroxyl radicals*, resulting from the ionization of water. Hydroxyl radicals have short half-lives, and only those formed in close proximity to DNA are likely to produce effects. The abundance of water in the subcellular environment, however, makes this an important mechanism of radiation damage.

Because oxygen stabilizes free radicals, well-oxygenated tumors are more sensitive to radiation injury than are hypoxic ones. Using in vitro and in vivo models, investigators have demonstrated that this *oxygen effect* can increase the sensitivity of cells to a single dose of irradiation by as much as a factor of 3. The clinical importance of the oxygen effect, however, is still controversial. Fractionated schedules used in clinical radiotherapy may allow reoxygenation of tumor cells between radiation doses, which would reduce the clinical importance of tumor hypoxia. However, a number of investigational treatments (hypoxic cell sensitizers, hyperbaric oxygen) designed to overcome tumor hypoxia have failed to improve local control rates.[2] Nevertheless, because several studies have demonstrated a relationship between severe anemia and decreased local control rates,[3] radiation oncologists usually attempt to maintain patients' hemoglobin levels above 10 g/dl during treatment. Other characteristics of the subcellular environment that can affect cellular radiosensitivity include temperature and pH level.[4]

The physical characteristics of an ionizing radiation beam can also help determine the amount of damage done to irradiated cells. The *linear energy transfer* of a radiation beam quantifies the amount of energy it deposits along its path through tissue. The linear energy transfer of electrons and of most photons used in therapy is the same, meaning that equal doses of electrons and photons produce equivalent effects in tissues. Densely ionizing particles such as neutrons and alpha particles, however, have linear energy transfer values that are many times greater than those of electrons or photons. The *radiobiologic effect (RBE)* of a dose of irradiation is greatly increased with these types of particle irradiation.

Reproductive cell death from DNA damage is not the only means by which radiation kills cells. There is increasing evidence that *apoptosis* ("interphase death") plays an important role in the responses of both tumor and normal tissues. In this process, the cell condenses and forms many small membranous buds that then undergo phagocytosis by neighboring cells. Highly differentiated cells that are either nondividing or slowly dividing, such as nerves and myocytes, are susceptible to this phenomenon. Lethally irradiated lymphocytes appear to undergo apoptotic cell death. Little is known about the biochemistry of apoptosis or the magnitude of its role in radiation therapy; this remains an area of active and exciting research.

Cellular Effects

Irradiated cells undergo a number of morphologic changes that are indistinguishable from those occurring in cells that have been treated with other cytotoxic agents such as nitrogen mustard. Acutely, the cells swell, cytoplasmic vacuoles form, and subcellular organelles become distorted. Critically injured cells can look so deformed that even non-neoplastic cells may appear malignant. This can make it difficult to interpret findings on biopsy specimens taken shortly after treatment.

The radiosensitivities of normal and malignant cell populations vary widely. Figure 5–3 illustrates a typical cell-survival curve after in vitro delivery of a single radiation dose, with the proportion of surviving cells plotted against the dose of radiation. The shape of the initial portion, or *shoulder*, of the cell-survival curve reflects the ability of the cells to accumulate and repair sublethal injury. Many normal-tissue cell populations and some poorly responsive malignant cell populations respond to irradiation with single-dose survival curves that have a broad shoulder. In contrast, most malignant cell populations and some acutely responding normal-tissue cell populations produce survival curves that have relatively narrow shoulders. The narrow shoulder reflects their relatively poor ability to accumulate sublethal injury. *Fractionated irradiation* takes advantage of these differences, allowing cells in normal tissues time to repair sublethal injury between doses (see Fig. 5–3).

Appreciation of the differential fractionation effects on tumors and normal tissues was central to the development of radiation as a useful treatment modality. The fractionation schedule used most frequently today (1.8 to 2.0 Gy per daily fraction) was developed primarily from clinical observations of tumor-control rates and late reactions in normal tissue. Other fractionation schedules that appear to have theoretical advantages are currently the subject of active investigation. In particular, numerous studies have explored the use of *hyperfractionation schedules* that deliver similar doses per day divided into two or three fractions usually separated by at least 6 hours. Laboratory studies have indicated that at least 6 hours are required to complete repair of sublethal injury to normal tissues.

The added tissue sparing of these hyperfrac-

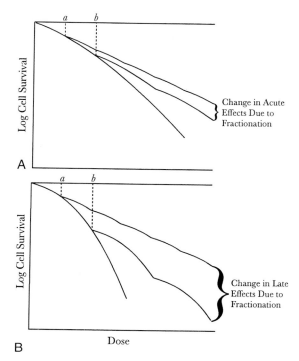

Figure 5–3 • The relationship between radiation dose and the surviving fraction of cells treated with a single dose or a fractionated dose of radiation. *A,* For most tumors and acutely responding normal tissues, the cellular responses to single doses of irradiation are described by curves with relatively narrow initial "shoulders." *B,* Cellular survival curves for late-responding normal tissues have a broader shoulder, suggesting that these cells have a greater capacity to accumulate and repair sublethal radiation injury. When the total dose of radiation is delivered in several smaller fractions, the response to each fraction is similar, and the overall radiation survival curve reflects multiple repetitions of the initial portion of the single-dose survival curve. Note that the total dose required to produce a specific amount of cell killing increases as the dose-per-fraction (*a, b*) decreases. The differential effects of fractionated irradiation on tumor and normal tissues reflect the greater capacity of late-responding tissues to accumulate and repair sublethal radiation injury. (From Karcher KH, Kogelnik HD, Reinartz G (eds): Progress in Radio-Oncology II, pp 287–296, New York, Raven Press, 1982.)

tionated schedules permits delivery of higher total doses of radiation. More standard fraction sizes are used (1.5 to 2.0 Gy), although the overall time is decreased by delivering more than one fraction per day. These schemes have the theoretical advantage of minimizing the opportunity for tumor-cell repopulation, but they tend to be limited by more severe acute reactions.

Hypofractionation schedules use relatively large daily fractions and thus deliver the total dose over a short time. These schedules are rarely used for curative treatment because the large fraction sizes increase late side effects in normal tissue. The reduced number of treatments makes these schedules ideal for palliative irradiation.

The ability to control a solid tumor with radiotherapy depends upon a number of factors. If the tumor-control rate is plotted against the dose of radiation given, a sigmoid curve results (Fig. 5–4). Higher doses of irradiation increase the probability of tumor control, particularly along a narrow dose range where the curve is the steepest. The position of this curve is influenced by tumor size and inherent tumor radiosensitivity. As tumor size and radioresistance increase, the tumor-control probability curve shifts to the right, indicating that higher doses are necessary to cause the same probability of control.

Factors that influence the response of tumors to a dose of radiation include the capacity of cells to repair sublethal injury, the reassortment of cells into sensitive portions of the cell cycle, the repopulation of cells during a fractionated course of irradiation, and the reoxygenation of cells during irradiation. These four factors—repair, reassortment, repopulation, and reoxygenation—have been termed the four "R's" of radiation biology.

With the exception of reoxygenation, these factors also affect the response of normal tissues to irradiation. Variations in the *repair* capacity of tumors influence their response to irradiation. *Reassortment* of cells into the more sensitive M phase of the cell cycle may influence the overall sensitivity of the tumor. *Repopulation* of rapidly dividing tumor cells between treatments can prevent control of even relatively sensitive tumors. Some data suggest that cellular repopulation can be accelerated by various cytotoxic interventions, including chemotherapy, irradiation, and surgery. This factor may influence the efficacy of sequenced treatments. Accelerated radiation fractionation schemes are designed to overcome cellular repopulation but are limited by associated increased acute toxic effects to normal tissues.

The probability of developing a severe late complication in normal tissue is also a function of radiation dose and can be represented by a sigmoid curve similar to the tumor-control probability curve (see Fig. 5–4). Factors influencing

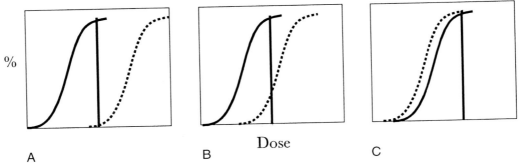

Figure 5–4 • Tumor-control probability curves (solid) and late-complication probability curves (dashed) depicting three clinical situations. A, Ideally, these curves are widely separated and a radiation dose can be selected that will achieve high probability of tumor control with very little risk of complications. B, More commonly a high probability of tumor control is not possible without some risk of late complications in an adjacent normal tissue, but most patients enjoy complication-free tumor control. C, Occasionally the risk of normal tissue injury exceeds the probability of tumor control. In particular, the dose of radiation needed to control tumors in young children is often more than that required to arrest the development of adjacent bone and soft tissues. In such cases, the long-term cosmetic and functional effects of radiation therapy must be weighed against the risk and consequences of local tumor recurrence if radiation therapy is not given.

the shape and position of this curve include (1) the inherent radiosensitivity of various normal tissues and (2) incompletely understood clinical and genetic factors peculiar to each individual.

The therapeutic ratio is represented by the separation between the tumor-control probability curve and the normal-tissue complication curve. When the distance between the curves is great, the therapeutic window is large, and tumor control can readily be achieved with minimal morbidity. When the distance is small, the clinician is often faced with difficult choices between the benefit of tumor control and the severity of effects to normal tissue. Ultimately, all investigational manipulations of radiation treatment (radiation sensitizers, altered fractionation schemes, conformal therapy, and so forth) can be viewed as an effort to increase the distance between these two curves. Because treatments that simply shift both curves equally to the right or left (i.e., have equal effects on tumor control and normal-tissue morbidity) do not improve the patient's outcome, it is important that studies of new interventions consider end results on normal tissue and on tumor control.

Several chemotherapeutic agents are known to sensitize cells to the effects of ionizing radiation. Both doxorubicin and actinomycin D inhibit repair of sublethal radiation injury, reducing the shoulder of the radiation cell-survival curve.[5] These agents increase the effect of irradiation on both tumor and normal-tissue cells. They are often deleted from pediatric chemotherapy regimens during radiotherapy because children who receive these drugs during irradiation may experience severe, acute exacerbations of mucositis and dermatitis within the radiation field 1 to 5 days after administration. Other drugs (e.g., bleomycin, cisplatin, cyclophosphamide) may also influence the response of cells to irradiation, but the character and extent of these damage interactions are less well understood.

When doxorubicin or actinomycin D are delivered after a course of radiation, a "recall" of the radiation reaction may be observed within the previously treated field. Shortly after chemotherapy administration, patients may experience recurrent symptoms of mucositis, dermatitis, or pneumonitis within the radiation field.[6–9] Recall radiation esophagitis may lead to long-term abnormalities in esophageal motility and even severe stricture.[9]

TREATMENT PLANNING AND DOSIMETRY

Therapeutic radiation may be delivered using a radiation source located some distance from the body (*teletherapy*) or using sources that are placed into a body cavity (*intracavitary therapy*), into the tumor itself (*interstitial therapy*), or on the skin surface (*surface molds*). The latter three are all examples of *brachytherapy*. Although brachytherapy has been used for some special problems, most pediatric radiotherapy is delivered using teletherapy external-beam techniques.

The safe and precise delivery of therapeutic radiation requires meticulous planning and accurate dosimetry. The radiation oncologist must have a thorough understanding of clinical oncology, tumor biology, and radiographic anatomy. He or she also must be familiar with the capabilities and the limitations of various treatment machines, treatment-planning methods, radiation beam-shaping devices, and treatment aids.

Treatment Unit Features

Linear accelerators are usually used to deliver external-beam radiotherapy to children. Cobalt

60 beams are rarely utilized to treat children because the beam edge *(penumbra)* is less sharp than that produced by a linear accelerator, making it more difficult to treat small volumes precisely.

The basic characteristics of a therapeutic linear accelerator are illustrated in Figure 5–5. The treatment unit consists of a couch and a treatment head (containing the linear accelerator), each of which has several precisely defined and measured degrees of motion. The treatment head is attached to a rotating gantry that can be positioned at any angle necessary with respect to the patient. Heavy lead or tungsten collimators in the treatment head define a rectangular treatment field to within 1 to 2 mm; the collimators can also be rotated to the desired position. The

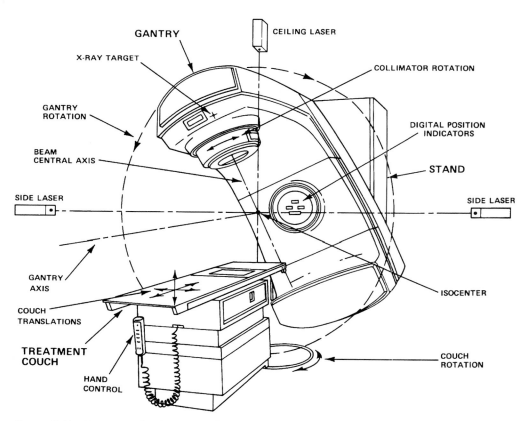

Figure 5–5 • Diagram of a therapeutic linear accelerator. Patients are positioned on the treatment couch with a system of lasers that are aligned precisely with the center of the radiation beam. The size and rotation of the radiation field is defined by collimators in the treatment head, which is mounted on a rotating gantry. The treatment couch can also be rotated about the central axis of the radiation beam. This arrangement gives the radiotherapist flexibility in designing beam angles for a variety of clinical situations. Various beam-modifying devices, such as blocks and wedges, can be attached to a tray beneath the collimator (not shown). (From Karzmark CJ, Nunan CS, Tanabe E: *Medical Electron Accelerators.* New York: McGraw-Hill, Inc, 1993, with permission.)

treatment table can be raised, lowered, and rotated to achieve the desired position of the patient with respect to the treatment head. Specially fabricated beam-modifying devices such as cerrubend blocks (which produce irregularly shaped fields) or lead wedges and compensating filters (which alter the profile of the dose distribution at various depths) can be placed in the accessory tray. The patient is placed on the couch and is aligned with the treatment head using precisely aimed lasers.

Patient-Immobilization Devices

Precise treatment can be delivered only if the patient's position can be accurately reproduced on a daily basis and maintained throughout a 10- to 20-minute treatment. To achieve this, a variety of patient-immobilization devices have been developed. A good immobilization device enables the radiation therapist to quickly, accurately, and reproducibly configure the treatment while maximizing the patient's comfort and minimizing the patient's movements. This is particularly important in pediatric practice, where a well-designed, comfortable immobilization device can make it possible to deliver complex treatments to young children without daily sedation (Fig. 5–6).

Simulation

Once the patient has been evaluated and the overall goal of treatment determined, the first step in treatment planning involves a treatment mockup, or simulation. Critical decisions are made at this time regarding patient positioning and immobilization. Gantry angles and field sizes are determined, beam energies are considered, and, ultimately, the target volume is defined. The target volume is the volume of tissue at risk and includes the tumor volume plus an adequate margin.

The tumor volume can be determined from diagnostic images or from surgical descriptions. These are made more precise by placing surgical clips in defined locations at the time of exploration. In selected cases, radiographic contrast may be used during simulation to localize critical or-

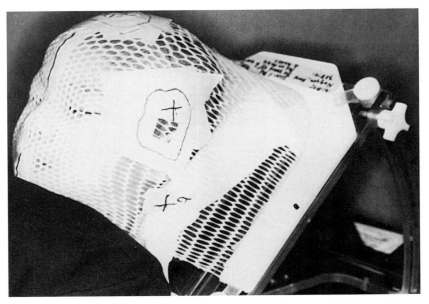

Figure 5–6 • This 5-year-old boy was receiving radiation to his brain for an unresectable astrocytoma. The mask was made of a specially designed plastic (Aquaplast) that becomes pliable in warm water and can be easily shaped. The mask was used to hold his head in a reproducible, stable, and comfortable position. Guides for alignment and positioning of the child were placed on the mask, avoiding the need for marks on his face. After several practice simulations and play therapy with a doll-sized linear accelerator, the child was able to tolerate 6 weeks of daily treatment without sedation.

gans; radiopaque markers may be inserted in tissue, or wires may be placed on the patient's skin to permit radiographic localization of superficial lesions or scars.

The target volume must include areas of possible microscopic tumor infiltration, sites at risk for regional spread, and a margin of tissue to compensate for any uncertainties in the determination of the target volume or any variation in the daily treatment setup. The volume of irradiation and consequent morbidity are affected by the precision of radiographic findings, the accuracy of surgical descriptions of the tumor bed, and the degree of patient immobilization.

Treatment fields are simulated on a machine equipped with a conventional X-ray fluoroscopy unit mounted on a rotating gantry that reproduces the precise movements of a linear accelerator and treatment couch. The radiation oncologist indicates areas to be shielded directly on the simulation film (see Fig. 5–2), which serves as a template from which custom blocks are cut.

Today many departments are equipped with computerized tomography (CT) simulators (combining the features of a CT scanner and a simulator) or with dedicated CT scanners with lasers and flat couches. These produce images of the patient in the treatment position that are used to develop a treatment plan. Doses are calculated using CT numbers to correct for density differences of various tissues, and dose distributions can be superimposed on cross-sectional images of the patient's anatomy.

Beam-Modifying Devices

Custom shielding is done with blocks that are fabricated from a lead alloy (cerrubend) employing the simulation film as a template. These blocks are placed in an accessory tray in the treatment head of the linac (linear accelerator) each day, and they shape the beam as it exits the machine (see Fig. 5–5).

Other beam-modifying devices include wedges, skin bolus, and tissue compensators. Some are placed in the accessory tray of the linac and others are placed directly on the patient. By understanding the various effects these devices have on the therapy beam, the radiation oncologist is able to integrate them into a patient's treatment plan to achieve a favorable distribution of the dose to tumor and normal tissues.

Dosimetric Considerations

Though some target volumes (e.g., the whole brain for leukemia prophylaxis) are most effectively treated with simple appositional arrangements of two treatment fields, the potentially serious late consequences of irradiation in children and the wide variety of tumor sites and distributions often demand complex, multifield treatment arrangements to achieve an optimal therapeutic ratio. In pediatric radiotherapy the advantages of CT-based treatment planning, sophisticated immobilization, treatment-planning optimization, and three-dimensional treatment planning are most apparent. Although it may take several days to generate these complex multifield treatment plans, the added tissue sparing often justifies a short delay.

Once the radiation oncologist has defined a target volume and specified the desired dose to the target volume and critical normal tissues, a final treatment plan is developed through close cooperation with an experienced radiation dosimetrist and a radiation physicist. Most plans are developed through experience and iteration, although the development of computerized optimization programs is currently an active area of research in radiation physics. Three-dimensional reconstructions of the target volume and normal-tissue structures can be used to generate "beam's-eye views" that allow the radiation oncologist to visualize and generate blocks for fields that cross the patient at unusual angles. The quality of the treatment plan is evaluated by the radiation oncologist and dosimetrist utilizing computer-generated isodose plots (Fig. 5–7). Dose-volume histograms that summarize the volume of normal or tumor tissue receiving specific doses may also be helpful.

From these treatment plans the dosimetrist creates a list of treatment beams described in terms of beam energy, beam type, field size, gantry angle, table angle, beam-shaping devices, and so on, and specifies the amount of radiation to be delivered with each beam. Treatment fields are verified on the therapy simulator and carefully checked when they are reproduced on the first day of treatment. Subsequent quality assurance checks with port films verify that the treatment fields are being applied as originally prescribed.

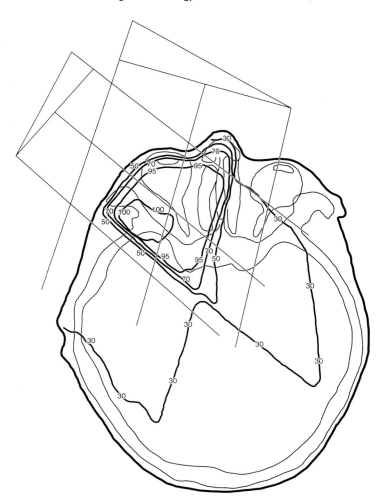

Figure 5–7 • A CT-based plan used to treat a 5-year-old boy with an embryonal rhabdomyosarcoma of the right orbit. The eyes, lenses, bones, and skin surface are outlined using the corresponding CT image. Treatment was delivered using right and left anterior oblique 6 MV photon beams with wedged beam-shaping devices and custom blocks. The numbers on the curvilinear lines (isodose curves) indicate the percentage of the maximum absorbed dose that will be delivered to various tissues. In this case, the treatment dose (50.4 Gy) was specified to the 95% line, meaning that all the tissue within the 95% isodose curve received at least 50.4 Gy.

Special Considerations in Pediatric Radiotherapy Planning

The accurate delivery of radiation requires painstaking attention to detail and necessitates a great deal of patience and cooperation on the part of the patient. Although the actual delivery of a single radiation treatment may take only 1 to 2 minutes, setting up a single treatment field and taking port films for confirmation of the treatment setup may take 10 minutes or longer. Coupling this with the fact that most treatments require multiple radiation fields, it is easy to understand why a patient may be on the treatment table 20 to 30 minutes a day. This requirement can be an enormous challenge for young children.

Children younger than 3 years of age are rarely capable of cooperating with such regimens and usually require sedation with each treatment. Short-acting anesthetic agents now permit children to be anesthetized for short periods without endotracheal intubation, provided there is close monitoring by an experienced pediatric anesthesiologist (see Chapter 3). Such treatments can be delivered only in the context of a close working relationship with a pediatric anesthesiologist and when close-up video cameras are available to monitor the patient from outside the treatment room while the radiation beam is on. Although conscious sedation can sometimes be used for short treatment courses that require no manipulation of the child's head or face (e.g., flank irradiation for Wilms' tumor), a partially sedated child is often more difficult to work with than one who is fully awake.

For older children, anesthesia is replaced by patient, consistent compassion. Extra time must be taken to acclimate children with the staff, the equipment, and the surroundings. Several "pretend" procedures (simulations) may be needed before children will be ready to cooperate, allow themselves to be placed in immobilization devices, and be treated with their parents outside the room. It sometimes helps for a child to bring a familiar toy into the treatment room, listen to a favorite tape of music, or hear a parent's reassurances over the intercom. Certainly, it is important to individualize the treatment routine to the needs of each child.

ROLE OF RADIOTHERAPY IN MULTIDISCIPLINARY CARE

Although the role of radiotherapy in pediatric oncology is still being refined, it has clearly proved itself a highly effective treatment for achieving and maintaining local control of a vari-

ety of neoplasms. Table 5–1 lists some of the pediatric malignancies that are treated with radiation and demonstrates the wide range of indications, treatment volumes, and doses.[10–33]

Two factors add to the challenge of developing an irradiation treatment plan for children that will maximize the chance of cure without causing unacceptable long-term morbidity. First, morbidity is likely to be higher in children because their bones are still developing. Second, the dominant role of chemotherapy in the management of pediatric neoplasms presents unfortunate opportunities for adverse drug-radiation interactions. Furthermore, the techniques used routinely in pediatric radiation oncology must often be more intricate than those used in adult radiation oncology, reflecting both the complex nature of pediatric malignancies as well as the delicate balance between achieving tumor control and preventing severe late complications. Differences of a few

Table 5–1 • Summary of Selected Pediatric Malignancies Treated with Radiotherapy

Disease	Peak Ages (years)	Indications for Radiotherapy	Treatment Volume	Dose Range (Gy)
Acute lymphoblastic leukemia[12, 26]	2–10	CNS prophylaxis CNS involvement	Whole cranium Craniospinal axis	18–24 18–24
Hodgkin's disease[17–19, 28]	15–34, >50	Definitive treatment for early-stage disease	Involved regions plus contiguous lymphatics	30–40
		Combined with CT in young children	Involved regions	15–25
Astrocytoma[31, 32]	Sporadic	Incomplete resection	Tumor bed plus margin	50–55
Craniopharyngioma[22, 30]	0–20, 40–50	Incomplete resection	Tumor plus margin	50–54
Medulloblastoma[24, 25]	5–6	Postoperative regardless of extent of resection	Craniospinal axis (plus boost posterior fossa)	36 (+18–20)
Neuroblastoma[15]	0–2	POG stage C	Tumor bed plus draining lymphatics	25–30
		Palliation	Symptomatic lesions	12–30
Rhabdomyosarcoma[13, 16, 29]	2–5	Postoperative in IRS Group II, III	Tumor bed plus draining lymphatics	40–50
		Lung metastases	Whole lung (plus boost gross residual)	14.4 (+40)
Wilms' tumor[20, 33]	2–3	Favorable histology, Stage III, IV	Tumor bed	10.8
		Unfavorable histology	Tumor bed	12–38°
		Lung metastases	Whole lung (plus boost gross residual)	2 (+7.5)
Ewing's sarcoma[11, 23, 27]	8–25	Definitive treatment of primary site	Prechemotherapy tumor volume plus margin	45–55
Osteosarcoma[21]	10–20	Incomplete surgical resection	Tumor plus margin	50–70
		Palliation	Involved field	30–36
Retinoblastoma[10, 14]	1–2	Sight preservation in a functioning eye	Entire retina, sparing lens if possible	40–45

°Recommended dose increases with age.

CNS = central nervous system; POG = Pediatric Oncology Group; IRS = Intergroup Rhabdomyosarcoma Study.

millimeters in field placement may reduce morbidity by avoiding a developing growth center or may dramatically increase the severity of late deformity if, for example, growth centers are partially treated, causing asymmetric growth. Relatively small differences in radiation dose can also cause dramatically different long-term side effects. Yet these considerations must always be weighed against the risk of a fatal tumor recurrence.

The histopathologic features of a tumor can markedly influence radiotherapeutic treatment strategy. Radiosensitive tumors such as Hodgkin's disease, Wilms' tumor, and ovarian dysgerminoma require lower total doses than do more radioresistant carcinomas and sarcomas. Moreover, the histologic type and grade of a tumor may provide important information regarding biologic behavior, patterns of spread, and radiocurability. For these reasons, an accurate tissue diagnosis is critical to subsequent treatment planning. Rarely, when the risk of biopsy exceeds the risk of inaccurate diagnosis (e.g., in the case of some tumors of the central nervous system), the radiation oncologist must rely upon the specific radiographic features of the disease as well as the judgment of an experienced diagnostic radiologist and neurosurgeon.

The ability to obtain local and regional tumor control is directly related to the primary site and the size of the tumor or degree of local tumor infiltration. These features also affect the risk of treatment-related morbidity. In general, larger tumors require higher doses. Most radiotherapy for solid tumors is given using a *shrinking-field technique*. Treatment is begun with larger fields that encompass the gross disease and surrounding areas likely to contain microscopic disease. The field is then reduced after a dose adequate to control microscopic disease is reached, and the gross disease is boosted to a higher total dose. The higher doses and larger treatment volumes needed to control locally advanced tumors also can lead to more serious morbidity. Accurate staging and judicious use of diagnostic imaging studies enable the best determination of tumor extent and help to ensure optimal radiation delivery.

Most pediatric malignancies are treated with two or three modalities. The sequence of treatments varies according to the disease type and the specific demands of each case. Radiotherapy,

for example, can be given preoperatively or postoperatively and can be delivered concurrently or sequentially with chemotherapy. It is important to define the goals of combined modality treatment early and with input from all the subspecialists. Once a treatment is initiated, it is imperative to maintain continued lines of communication because outcomes and morbidity are a function of all the modalities used.

In pediatric oncology cases, when radiotherapy is combined with surgery, it is usually given postoperatively. Often the irradiation is limited to the surgical bed. In some circumstances, however, undissected areas at risk are treated adjuvantly. Presurgical imaging studies, detailed operative notes, and metallic clips placed intraoperatively to delineate the tumor bed or areas of close or positive margins are all extremely helpful for postoperative radiation treatment planning. Consultation between the surgical and radiation oncologists before surgery and in the operating room often prevent miscommunications that can compromise the overall efficacy of combined-modality treatment.

In selected cases, preoperative irradiation may be preferred over postoperative treatment. Reports of treatment of soft-tissue sarcomas in adults suggest that patients can often be treated effectively with lower doses and smaller treatment volumes when radiation is given before surgery.[34, 35] For children this could mean a significant difference in radiation morbidity. For example, the need to treat the entire surgical bed (including scar and drain sites) of an extremity sarcoma postoperatively can increase the field size dramatically, requiring inclusion of additional joints and long-bone growth centers. The role of preoperative irradiation has not been extensively explored in the treatment of soft-tissue sarcomas in children, but this approach should be considered in selected cases where it might improve the therapeutic ratio of combined treatment.

The interval between surgery and radiation therapy depends upon a number of factors. Preoperative radiotherapy is usually followed by resection within 3 to 6 weeks. The longer times may be necessary if there is significant edema or hyperemia. Protracted delays may increase the risk of surgical dissection, however, because radiation changes may obscure facial planes or cause intra-abdominal adhesions. Postoperative radiotherapy is usually initiated 3 to 4 weeks following surgery, but the time interval may depend upon the extent of the procedure, the rapidity of the wound healing, and the nature of the tumor. For rapidly dividing tumors, treatment may be started before removal of staples and drains. Ideally, there should be some balance between allowing for normal-tissue recovery and reducing the potential for tumor regrowth.

When radiotherapy is combined with chemotherapy, the risk of morbidity such as bone marrow suppression and mucositis is increased, especially when the treatments are given concurrently. Chemotherapy given after irradiation can produce a *radiation recall phenomenon* in which *in-field mucositis* is reactivated. Irradiation of the central nervous system too soon after intrathecal administration of methotrexate can lead to irreversible leukoencephalopathy. Knowledge of potential interactions such as these has improved treatment planning so that treatment tolerance is raised and the risk of severe complications reduced.

Although the primary role of radiation therapy is usually to achieve tumor control at the primary site, irradiation has also been used effectively to treat metastatic disease in selected circumstances. Whole-lung irradiation improves cure rates for patients with metastatic Ewing's sarcoma or rhabdomyosarcoma and has been employed successfully to prevent lung metastases from osteosarcoma. Craniospinal irradiation is an important part of disease management in children with brain tumors (primitive neurectodermal tumors and germ-cell tumors) that have a tendency to spread throughout the neuraxis. Irradiation is also a part of some preparative regimens for bone marrow transplantation.

Unfortunately, there is still a need for effective palliative treatment in pediatric oncology. When locoregional or metastatic disease becomes symptomatic, radiation therapy can often provide very effective and durable symptom relief with little or no morbidity. Because late morbidity in normal tissue is not a concern in this setting, rapid fractionation schedules are often used to minimize inconvenience to the patient. Patients with radiosensitive tumors such as neuroblastoma may experience significant relief within 24 hours of the first fraction of irradiation. Occasionally, radiotherapy is given prophylac-

tically to prevent symptoms such as pathologic fractures in diseased long bones.

Tumor-related symptoms of spinal cord compression, superior vena cava syndrome, airway obstruction, or cranial nerve compression may require emergent intervention with radiation therapy. Under these circumstances, the radiotherapist should be notified immediately and the diagnostic workup should be done quickly so that treatment can begin within 24 hours of symptom onset if possible. Patients should always be started on dexamethasone before irradiation of spinal cord or cranial nerve compression in order to reverse symptoms and to prevent edema that may occur as the tumor reacts to the first few fractions of irradiation.

Normal-Tissue Effects

Some normal tissue is inevitably irradiated when a tumor is treated with radiation. The consequences of this are minimized because ionizing radiation selectively kills tumor cells and spares normal cells that have the capacity to repair radiation damage. The clinical effect of damage to an organ depends both on the repair capacity of parenchymal and stromal cells and on the level of redundancy of that organ. Because radiation dose is limited by the tolerance of normal tissues within the target volume, the anatomic location of a tumor is a major determinant of how safe and how effective treatment is delivered.

Normal-tissue responses to ionizing radiation are of particular concern in pediatric patients because a child's growth and development can be irreversibly altered by treatment. Doses as low as 10 Gy to an epiphyseal growth plate can result in measurable changes, and doses of 30 to 40 Gy can result in nearly total growth arrest. When the location of a tumor demands treatment of an area of developing bone, an experienced pediatric radiotherapist may actually choose to widen the treatment field so as to avoid partial irradiation and consequent asymmetric growth. This is often necessary, for example, when the flank is irradiated following surgery for Wilms' tumor. Although radiation could be directed to only the operative site, it is better to treat the entire width of the adjacent vertebral column because partial irradiation of vertebral growth plates will cause asymmetric growth and result in spinal scoliosis.

Radiation sequelae may be acute or late. Acute effects occur during or shortly after a treatment course and are usually temporary. Late effects, in contrast, may not appear for months or even years after treatment and may cause permanent disability.

Acute Effects of Radiation Therapy

Acute radiation effects vary according to the treatment site and are summarized in Table 5–2. Normal tissues that have a rapid turnover rate and are composed of actively dividing progenitor cells are more susceptible. Acute reactions generally do not occur until the patient has accumulated a dose sufficient to affect a critical proportion of progenitor cells. For example, patients receiving a 5-week course of radiation to the brain usually do not lose their hair until the third or fourth week of treatment. Some reactions, such as nausea, however, can occur after the first treatment. The mechanism for this immediate reaction is not well understood and may involve the release of cytokines into the bloodstream.

Acute reactions are usually temporary because they affect renewable systems that have a high capacity for cellular repair and repopulation. Most such reactions resolve within a few weeks of the completion of radiation treatment. Most symptoms can be managed effectively with medi-

cations such as antiemetics and mild analgesics. However, children who receive more than 30 to 40 Gy to a significant portion of the aerodigestive tract are likely to develop significant nutritional problems. These children should be followed closely, and physicians should be prepared to intervene rapidly with nutritional supplements delivered by nasogastric tube or gastrostomy to prevent weight loss.

The radiation oncologist must be familiar with the expected duration and the potential severity of acute side effects so that symptoms can be anticipated and managed appropriately. Unexpectedly severe symptoms should be evaluated for other causes. For instance, unexpectedly severe or persistent odynophagia may indicate a superimposed infection caused by *Candida*. The child's family must always be carefully informed and reminded about the symptoms that are expected during treatment and convalescence.

Late Effects of Radiation Therapy

Late morbidity from irradiation, like early morbidity, correlates directly with the site of treatment (see Table 5–2).[36, 37] In children, the severity of some late sequelae are inversely correlated with age during treatment. Other factors, including the effects of other treatment modalities and the tissue damage caused by the infiltrating tu-

Table 5–2 · Possible Acute and Late Effects of Radiation Therapy on Normal Tissues

Organ or System	Acute Effects	Late Effects
Skin	Erythema, desquamation, epilation	Telangiectasia, subcutaneous fibrosis, ulceration
Central nervous system	Cerebral edema	Learning or memory deficits, pituitary insufficiency, necrosis, myelitis
Eye	Conjunctivitis	Cataract, keratitis, optic nerve atrophy, dry eye
Upper aerodigestive tract	Mucositis, xerostomia, anosmia, dysgeusia	Xerostomia, dental caries
Lung	Pneumonitis	Pulmonary fibrosis Pericarditis, vascular damage
Gastrointestinal tract	Nausea, diarrhea, edema, ulceration, hepatitis	Stricture, ulceration, perforation, hematochezia
Kidney		Nephropathy, renal insufficiency
Urinary bladder	Dysuria	Hematuria, ulceration, perforation, decreased capacity
Testis or ovary		Atrophy, sterility, ovarian failure
Hematopoietic tissue	Lymphopenia, neutropenia, thrombocytopenia, anemia	Pancytopenia
Bone		Growth arrest, osteonecrosis

mor, may contribute to the child's ultimate disability.

Many of the reports of the long-term sequelae of treatment in children reflect techniques that were in use 20 years or more ago. Severe late sequelae should occur less frequently in patients treated with current techniques and equipment. However, the risk of late effects in developing children should not be underestimated and must be considered by the treating physicians and parents before treatment is begun. Though we know a great deal about the late effects of irradiation, children who are now being cured may expect more than 60 years of cancer survival, and our understanding about extremely long-term effects of the modern combined-modality treatment that they receive is obviously incomplete. This should be explained to the parents in obtaining their informed consent.

Late tissue responses to irradiation cannot be predicted from the severity of acute responses. Late complications in tissues composed of terminally differentiated "nonrenewable" cells (e.g., in the central nervous system) are believed to result from microvasculature damage. Late reactions such as skin thickening and fibrosis may also reflect the inherent radiosensitivity of fibroblasts and other soft-tissue components. In vitro radiosensitivity measurements have shown that fibroblasts obtained from different radiotherapy patients vary greatly in their response to radiation. These measurements tend to correlate with the late morbidity observed in patients who received radiotherapy to the head and neck.[38] They, along with other biologic parameters, are currently being investigated to develop assays to improve our ability to predict an individual's risk for developing late complications.

The late effects of irradiation in children are compounded by the effects of treatment on tissue development. As mentioned, growing bone is particularly sensitive to the effects of radiation.[37, 39, 40] Irradiation of a long-bone epiphyseal growth plate will inhibit subsequent growth of that bone in a manner related to (1) the dose of irradiation, (2) the proportion of that bone's growth that is normally contributed by the irradiated growth center, and (3) the age of the patient. Animal studies suggest that the amount of damage may also be related to radiation fraction size.[41]

The effects of a course of irradiation on bone growth cannot be fully appreciated until the child has completed his or her pubertal growth spurt. Of course, other factors, such as additional damage from tumor or surgical treatment, effects of concurrent chemotherapy, and hormonal deficiencies, can also affect the ultimate severity of growth arrest. Radiation may inhibit development of soft tissues within the radiation field as well.

The late effects of irradiation on cognition are of particular concern in children with brain tumors.[36] Once again, the contribution of radiation to these late deficits may be difficult to distinguish from the effects of tumor damage, increased intracranial pressure, surgical intervention, social disruption, and other factors. Radiation clearly contributes to long-term cognitive deficits, however, in some children. These effects are correlated with the dose, site, and volume of irradiation. They may be particularly severe in children younger than 3 years who have not completed axonal myelination of the nervous system. Symptoms may not be manifest for several years and may range from very subtle learning and memory deficits to frank necrosis and profound disability.

One cannot effectively treat tumors without a risk of late complications. Novel treatment strategies are being developed, however, that may improve the therapeutic ratio. Hyperfractionated radiotherapy may achieve tumor control with reduced fraction sizes and reduced late morbidity. This approach is currently being investigated in children with rhabdomyosarcoma. Unfortunately, the typical twice-daily schedule of hyperfractionated irradiation poses special problems in the pediatric population, particularly for very small children who require anesthesia for adequate immobilization. Advances in radiation therapy, including three-dimensional treatment planning and fractionated stereotactic radiotherapy, may reduce the volume of tissue irradiated and thus be of particular help in pediatric cases.

Second Malignancies

The risk of developing a second malignancy is increased in pediatric cancer survivors. This added risk undoubtedly reflects a combination of treatment-related carcinogenic effects, predisposing genetic defects, and other poorly understood factors such as diet and environment. The role treatment may play in this phenomenon is important to recognize.

Both ionizing irradiation and alkylating agents are capable of inducing malignancies that are histopathologically indistinguishable from those that occur spontaneously. Both hematogenous and solid tumors have been described, although the former are most often attributed to chemotherapy. In general, the risk of developing a treatment-related hematogenous malignancy peaks within several years of treatment and is rare 10 years or more thereafter. The risk of developing a solid tumor, in contrast, is low in the first 5 years but then rises, apparently without reaching a plateau. Prior radiation therapy is usually implicated in the development of solid tumors that occur within the previously irradiated field. The risk of sarcoma development within the radiation field is particularly high for children treated for Ewing's sarcoma or retinoblastoma; these children often have a genetic defect that increases their risk of developing second tumors, particularly within the radiation field. Young children treated with irradiation for Hodgkin's disease have also been found to have an increased risk of second tumors, particularly lung cancer and breast cancer. These risks can be increased if patients are exposed to other known carcinogens such as cigarette smoke.

Fortunately, clinical studies of both pediatric and adult patients have demonstrated that malignancies directly attributable to therapeutic radiation are relatively rare. The Childhood Cancer Research Group reported on second primary malignancies in a large cohort of pediatric cancer survivors.[42] They found the relative risk (observed/expected) of second tumors after radiotherapy alone to be 6; however, the relative risk was 4 after treatment with surgery alone and 9 after combined chemotherapy and radiotherapy. Clearly, this risk must be balanced against the risk of death from the tumor that required treatment in the first place.

SUMMARY

The optimal delivery of therapeutic radiation requires an intimate understanding of clinical oncology and a substantial technical expertise. The role of radiotherapy in pediatric oncology, although firmly established, continues to be refined. There have been dramatic improvements in equipment and techniques as well as advances in our understanding of radiation physics and biology. Ongoing clinical investigations continue to perfect specific aspects of radiotherapy and underscore the importance of close multidisciplinary management of children with cancer. It is imperative that an experienced and qualified radiation oncologist be involved early in the clinical decision-making process of the pediatric cancer patient so that an individualized, optimized treatment plan can be devised.

References

1. Suit H, Urie M: Proton beams in radiation therapy. *J Natl Cancer Inst* 84:155, 1992.
2. Eifel PJ: Does tumor hypoxia influence local control of carcinoma of the cervix? *Gynecol Oncol* 51:139, 1993.
3. Bush R: The significance of anemia in clinical radiation therapy. *Int J Radiat Oncol Biol Phys* 12:2047, 1986.
4. Hall E: *Radiobiology for the Radiologist.* Philadelphia: JB Lippincott Co, 1988.
5. Belli JA: Principles of damage interactions between radiation and chemotherapeutic agents. In Cassady JR (ed): *Radiation Therapy in Pediatric Oncology.* Berlin: Springer-Verlag, 1994, p. 75.
6. Castellino R, Glatstein E, Turbow M, et al: Latent radiation injury of lungs or heart activated by steroid withdrawal. *Ann Int Med* 80:593, 1974.
7. D'Angio G: Delayed consequences of cancer therapy: Proven and potential. *Cancer* 37:979, 1976.
8. Donaldson S, Glick J, Wilbur J: Adriamycin activating a recall phenomenon after radiation therapy. *Ann Int Med* 81:407, 1974.
9. Greco F, Brereton H, Dent H, et al: Adriamycin and enhanced radiation reaction in normal esophagus and skin. *Ann Int Med* 85:294, 1985.
10. Amendola BE, Lamm FR, Markoe AM, et al: Radiotherapy of retinoblastoma. A review of 63 children treated with different irradiation techniques. *Cancer* 66:21, 1990.
11. Ari Y, Kun LE, Brooks MT, et al: Ewing's sarcoma: Local tumor control and patterns of failure following limited-volume radiation therapy. *Int J Radiat Oncol Biol Phys* 31:1501, 1991.
12. Bleyer WA: Acute lymphoblastic leukemia in children. Advances and prospectus. *Cancer* 65 (3 Suppl):1051, 1990.
13. Cassady JR: Contributions of pediatric oncology: Examples derived from advances made in the treatment of rhabdomyosarcoma and neuroblastoma. *Int J Radiat Oncol Biol Phys* 20:1177, 1991.

14. Cassady JR: Retinoblastoma. In Cassady JR (ed): *Radiation Therapy in Pediatric Oncology.* Berlin: Springer-Verlag, 1994, p. 319.

15. Castleberry RP, Kun LE, Shuster JJ, et al: Radiotherapy improves the outlook for patients older than 1 year with Pediatric Oncology Group Stage C neuroblastoma. *J Clin Oncol* 9:789, 1991.

16. Crist W, Gehan EA, Ragab AH, et al: The third Intergroup Rhabdomyosarcoma Study. *J Clin Oncol* 13:610, 1995.

17. Donaldson SS, Link MP: Hodgkin's disease. Treatment of the young child. *Pediatr Clin N Am* 38:457, 1991.

18. Fryer CJ, Hutchinson RJ, Krailo M, et al: Efficacy and toxicity of 12 courses of ABVD chemotherapy followed by low-dose regional radiation in advanced Hodgkin's disease in children: A report from the Childrens Cancer Study Group. *J Clin Oncol* 8:1971, 1990.

19. Gehan EA, Sullivan MP, Fuller LM, et al: The intergroup Hodgkin's disease in children. A study of stages I and II. *Cancer* 65:1429, 1990.

20. Green DM, Beckwith JB, Breslow NE, et al: Treatment of children with stages II to IV anaplastic Wilms' tumor: A report from the National Wilms' Tumor Study Group. *J Clin Oncol* 12:2126, 1994.

21. Harter KW: Osteosarcoma. In Cassady JR (ed): *Radiation Therapy in Pediatric Oncology.* Berlin: Springer-Verlag, 1994, p. 305.

22. Hetelekidis S, Barnes PD, Tao ML, et al: 20-year experience in childhood craniopharyngioma. *Int J Radiat Oncol Biol Phys* 27:189, 1993.

23. Horowitz ME, Neff JR, Kun LR: Ewing's sarcoma. Radiotherapy versus surgery for local control. *Pediatr Clin N Am* 38:365, 1991.

24. Hughes EN, Shillito J, Sallan SE, et al: Medulloblastoma at the Joint Center for Radiation Therapy between 1968 and 1984. *Cancer* 61:1992, 1988.

25. Jenkin D, Goddard K, Armstrong D, et al: Posterior fossa medulloblastoma in childhood: Treatment results and a proposal for a new staging system. *Int J Radiat Oncol Biol Phys* 19:265, 1990.

26. Kun LE, Camitta BM, Mulhern RK, et al: Treatment of meningeal relapse in childhood acute lymphoblastic leukemia. I. Results of craniospinal irradiation. *J Clin Oncol* 2:359, 1984.

27. Nesbit ME, Gehan EA, Burgert O, et al: Multimodal therapy for the management of primary, nonmetastatic Ewing's sarcoma of bone: A long-term follow-up of the First Intergroup Study. *J Clin Oncol* 8:1664, 1990.

28. Oberlin O, Leverger G, Pacquement H, et al: Low-dose radiation therapy and reduced chemotherapy in childhood Hodgkin's disease: The experience of the French Society of Pediatric Oncology. *J Clin Oncol* 10:1602, 1992.

29. Raney RB, Hays DM, Tefft M, et al: Rhabdomyosarcoma and undifferentiated sarcomas. In Pizzo P, Poplack O (eds): *Principles and Practice of Pediatric Oncology.* Philadelphia: JB Lippincott, 1989, p. 635.

30. Regine WF, Mohiuddin M, Kramer S: Long-term results of pediatric and adult craniopharyngiomas treated with combined surgery and radiation. *Radiother Oncol* 27:13, 1993.

31. Swift PS: Brainstem gliomas in children. In Cassady JR (ed): *Radiation Therapy in Pediatric Oncology.* Berlin: Springer-Verlag, 1994, p. 215.

32. Swift PS: Tumors of the supratentorium, ventricular system, and visual pathways, and tumors of the sellar region. In Cassady JR (ed): *Radiation Therapy in Pediatric Oncology.* Berlin: Springer-Verlag, 1994, p. 221.

33. Thomas PRM, Tefft M, Compaan PJ, et al: Results of two radiation therapy randomizations in the third National Wilms' Tumor Study. *Cancer* 68:1703, 1991.

34. Nielsen OS, Cummings B, O'Sullivan B, et al: Preoperative and postoperative irradiation of soft tissue sarcomas: Effect on radiation field size. *Int J Radiat Oncol Biol Phys* 21:1595, 1991.

35. Suit HD, Mankin HJ, Wood WC, et al: Preoperative, intraoperative, and postoperative radiation in the treatment of primary soft tissue sarcoma. *Cancer* 55:2659, 1985.

36. Ang KK, Van Der Kogel AJ, Van Der Schueren E: Effects of therapy on central nervous system functions in children. In Cassady JR (ed): *Radiation Therapy in Pediatric Oncology.* Berlin: Springer-Verlag, 1994, p. 133.

37. Eifel PJ: Acute and chronic normal tissue effects and potential modification in pediatric radiation therapy. In Cassady JR (ed): *Radiation Therapy in Pediatric Oncology.* Berlin: Springer-Verlag, 1994, p. 13.

38. Geara FB, Peters LJ, Ang KK, et al: Prospective comparison of in vitro normal cell radiosensitivity and normal tissue reactions in radiotherapy patients. *Int J Radiat Oncol Biol Phys* 27:173, 1993.

39. Rate W, Butler M, Robertson W, et al: Late orthopedic effects in children with Wilms' tumor treated with abdominal irradiation. *Med Pediatr Oncol* 19:265, 1991.

40. Willman KY, Cox RS, Donaldson RS: Radiation-induced height impairment in pediatric Hodgkin's disease. *Int J Radiat Oncol Biol Phys* 85, 1994.

41. Eifel P, Sampson C, Tucker S: Radiation fractionation sensitivity of epiphyseal cartilage in a weanling rat model. *Int J Radiat Oncol Biol Phys* 19:661, 1990.

42. Hawkins M, Draper G, Kingston J: Incidence of second primary tumours among childhood cancer survivors. *Br J Cancer* 56:339, 1987.

Molecular Biology and Tumor Markers

• *Robert S. Sawin, M.D.*

Fundamentally, cancer is a genetic disease. This does not mean that all cancers are inherited. Rather, it means that alterations in the gene structure or function of either somatic or germ cells result in malignant-cell behavior. Knowledge of molecular biology is no longer the domain of research scientists only, for the intracellular and genetic abnormalities that are being described in increasing detail have great clinical significance. A dramatic example of this clinical relevance is demonstrated by the finding that neuroblastoma tumors displaying amplification of the N-*myc* gene are associated with more malignant behavior than tumors without N-*myc* amplification.[1] Such observations may eventually alter the treatment plans for children with neuroblastoma, including the timing and extent of surgical resection required. In this chapter the basic concepts of molecular biology are reviewed, along with examples of clinically significant abnormalities of cellular biology and genetics. In addition, protein tumor markers used for diagnosis and prognosis are discussed.

CHROMOSOMES AND NUCLEIC ACIDS

All diploid human cells contain 23 pairs of chromosomes, 22 of which are termed *autosomes*. The other pair are sex chromosomes, either XX or XY. Preparations of cells arrested in mitosis by colchicine allow for good visualization of chromosomes, that is, *karyotype analysis*. The use of dyes such as Giemsa stain produces a characteristic pattern of light and dark bands in each chromosome. Each chromosome has a short arm, termed *p*, and a long arm, termed *q*, with a *centromere* dividing the two arms. The size of the chromosome, the location of its centromere, and the banding pattern are unique and thus allow for identification of individual chromosomes. Autosomes are numbered from largest (number 1) to smallest (number 22) by convention. The arms are separated into regions, bands, and subbands, enabling an exact labeling of locations.

Chromosomes are composed of tightly wound double-helical DNA, plus some structural protein and RNA. Each chromosome contains a single molecule of DNA. The DNA is a double-stranded helix of nucleic acids attached to a backbone of deoxyribose and bound together by complementary base pairs. The bases are either *purines*, namely adenine (A) and guanosine (G), or *pyrimidines*, namely thymine (T) or cytosine (C). The purines of one strand are always bound to the pyrimidines of the other strand in a specific fashion: adenine is bound to thymine (A-T) and guanosine is bound to cytosine (G-C). Consequently, the sequence of bases in one strand can be determined by knowing the sequence of the other strand.

DNA can be separated into two strands by heating, which disrupts the weak hydrogen bonds. When cooled, these separate strands will reattach, or *anneal*, in exactly the same position since the base pairs are complementary. This process of separating nucleic acid strands and reannealing is termed *hybridization* and is a valuable characteristic that enables many reliable molecular biology research techniques.

RNA differs from DNA in three basic ways. First, the sugars in the backbone are hydroxylated. Second, the purine uracil (U) is present in RNA instead of thymine. Last, RNA exists as a single-stranded molecule.

Replication. By convention the sequence of base pairs in DNA or RNA is written from the 5′ end toward the 3′ end of the molecule. The DNA sequence that codes for a gene is termed the *sense* strand. The complementary strand is called *antisense*. The complementary structure of DNA allows for exact copies to be made by *replication*, in which the two DNA strands unwind, and then the enzyme DNA polymerase

copies each strand. When completed, replication results in two exact copies of the sense strand and two exact copies of the antisense strand. Next, the sense and antisense strands hybridize, resulting in two double-helical molecules of DNA. If mistakes do occur during the replication process, repair mechanisms are available to the cell. These repair mechanisms are also important in nonreplicating DNA because mutations can occur spontaneously after exposure to toxic substances or after irradiation. Failures of this repair process can result in permanent DNA mutations, some of which lead to uncontrolled cell growth. Patients with xeroderma pigmentosum, for example, have abnormal DNA repair enzymes. They are at risk for developing skin malignancies after exposure to ultraviolet radiation, which causes DNA mutation in skin cells.

Transcription. In the process of *transcription*, RNA is formed in the cell nucleus by the enzyme RNA polymerase, which "reads" the sequence of DNA bases from the antisense strand and forms a complementary strand of RNA, that is, a sense strand. This sense strand is identical to the original DNA base sequence aside from the U replacing the T. The product of transcription is *messenger RNA (mRNA)*, which moves from the nucleus to the cytoplasm. All mRNA molecules are capped on the 5′ end and terminated with a polyadenylated tail (. . . AAAAA) on the 3′ end. This fact can be utilized to help isolate mRNA from cells.

Translation. The mRNA nucleotides (A, U, G, and C) are the "letters" of the genetic code. Each group of three consecutive base pairs encodes for a specific amino acid and is called a *codon*. There are 64 different possible codons that encode for the 20 different amino acids and stop signals. This code is universal and allows molecular genetic analysis of all organisms. The mRNA binds to ribosomes where *ribosomal RNA (rRNA)* begins to synthesize proteins. The *transfer RNA (tRNA)* acts as a decoder in this process. The tRNA molecule has an amino acid attached to one end and a codon recognition site on the other end. The codon recognition site, or *anticodon*, binds to the mRNA, delivering an amino acid for attachment to the growing polypeptide. This process of producing proteins from mRNA is called *translation*.

The DNA in human cells contains approximately 3 billion base pairs, which compose nearly 50,000 genes. The typical gene contains 10,000 base pairs, so that less than one fifth of the total DNA is composed of the genes. The rest of the DNA was once termed "junk DNA" because it had no obvious function. As more is learned about these portions of the DNA that are not part of the genes, it appears that they may have important functions.

Normal cells with 23 pairs of chromosomes are called *diploid*. Cells with abnormal numbers of chromosomes are termed *aneuploid*. Some tumor cells have less than 46 chromosomes (*hypodiploid*), whereas others have more than 46 (*hyperdiploid*). Although the chromosome number can be analyzed by karyotyping cells, the total amount of DNA in tumor cells can be measured more easily using flow cytometry.[2] Flow cytometry correlates well with the number of chromosomes without making it necessary to perform cumbersome cytogenetic analysis, which requires growing the cells in culture, which is not always possible.

Genes can be mapped to fairly specific locations on the chromosome. For example, the location of a gene on the q arm of chromosome 17 could be labeled as 17q21.3, indicating the long arm, region 2, band 1, subband 3.

The ability to identify chromosomes in such detail has led to the observation that some malignant cells have distinctive abnormalities of their chromosomes. The common abnormalities are deletions or insertions of segments of one chromosome into another chromosome. A *translocation* is an exchange of a piece from one chromosome to a different chromosome in a reciprocal fashion. One example of a specific chromosomal anomaly, the translocation of the long arm of chromosomes 11 and 22, is found in most Ewing's sarcoma cells.[3] The finding of this, t(11;22), is so specific that it is often utilized to help verify the diagnosis of Ewing's sarcoma. Similarly, in neuroblastoma patients, the deletion of a portion of the small arm of chromosome 1, designated 1p-, is associated with highly malignant behavior and a poor prognosis.[4] Although precise analysis of these 1p deletions indicates that the break point is often at different locations, almost all of the deletions associated with neuroblastoma are distal to the 1p36.1 locus. This sort of specific chromosomal abnormality suggests that one or more of the genes in that locus are important to modulating cell proliferation.

Another nonrandom chromosomal abnormality seen in malignant cells is termed *loss of heterozygosity (LOH)*. Since each normal human diploid cell has two copies of a gene, one from each parent, the cells are said to be heterozygous for that allele. One allele may be abnormal either because of a somatic mutation or because of a germline mutation from one parent. Occasionally the remaining normal allele is discarded or replaced by a copy of the abnormal allele. Thus, the cell has become homozygous for abnormal allele, or has lost its heterozygosity. Several genetic alterations like LOH have been described for chromosomes 1 and 17 in neuroblastoma[5, 6] and for chromosomes 1 and 16 in Wilms' tumor.[7]

CELL CYCLE

The process of cell proliferation can be viewed schematically as a highly regulated series of steps termed the *cell cycle* (Fig. 6–1).[8] Most nonmalignant cells are in a resting, nonproliferating stage called G0. Cells that are proliferating enter a phase termed *S phase*, during which DNA synthesis occurs. The process of cell proliferation then requires entering the mitosis phase, or *M phase*.

There are checkpoints in the cell cycle prior to S phase (G1) and prior to M phase (G2) that retard progress through the cell cycle. Many genes, and the intracellular proteins for which they encode, act on the cells at these checkpoints. Some of these genes and proteins are stimulating and thus provoke progression from the G1 phase into S phase, whereas many others are inhibitory and prevent this progression, acting as "brakes" to prevent uncontrolled proliferation.

In addition, cells also possess the machinery to actively provoke their own destruction, known as *apoptosis*, or programmed cell death (see Fig. 6–1).[9] Surprisingly, many of the same genes and proteins have both stimulatory and inhibitory activity. Together these same growth-stimulating and growth-controlling signals play a role in developing embryos, in somatic cells of the mature organism, and in neoplastic cells. Thus, the regulation of growth and differentiation is a finely controlled system that can be altered at many

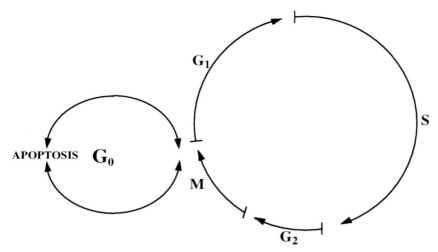

Figure 6–1 • Cell cycle. In this schematic representation of phases through which cells pass when reproducing, resting cells are in G0. Some of the cells in G0 will actively undergo programmed cell death (apoptosis) and others will enter S phase, during which DNA is synthesized. Once DNA is synthesized, the cells can undergo mitosis in M phase. In between these phases are potential stop points, G1 and G2.

different points, resulting in aberrant growth, proliferation, or differentiation. One group of molecules modulating these cellular behaviors is the group called *oncogenes.*

ONCOGENES

In the 1970s viruses were discovered that were capable of inducing malignancies in animals, giving rise to the hypothesis that many human cancers were caused by virus infections. Although this theory has never been substantiated in more than a few examples of tumors (Table 6–1), the molecular genetics of viruses and malignant cells do share some common features.[10] Analysis of genetic material from viruses that could transform normal cells into tumor cells led to the

Table 6–1 • Viruses Associated with Human Cancer

Virus	Cancer
Epstein-Barr (EBV)	Burkitt's lymphoma
	Nasopharyngeal carcinoma
Papilloma virus	Laryngeal papillomatosis
	Cervical carcinoma
HIV	Kaposi's sarcoma
HTLV	T-cell lymphoma

observation that small portions of DNA were the responsible agents. These segments of DNA were called *oncogenes.*[11, 12] One of the early oncogenes identified was the *src* gene isolated from the Rous sarcoma virus. Analysis of this viral oncogene (labeled v-*src*) revealed that it had a great deal of homology with a normal gene from normal chicken cells. This normal *src* gene was later discovered to encode for a protein that helps regulate normal cell growth and physiology.[13] It appears that an ancestor virus of the Rous sarcoma virus had incorporated this normal *src* gene and converted, or mutated, it to a gene capable of transforming cells to tumors.

Because very few human malignancies are caused by viral infections, these viral oncogenes cannot account for the role of genes in the tumorigenesis of the majority of human cancers. An experimental method called *transfection* was used to introduce small fragments of DNA from human cancer cells into normal cells that would ordinarily not produce tumors. In that way, the DNA of these transformed (or transfected) cells could be analyzed and compared with the DNA in normal cells. Any differences in the DNA would presumably account for the development of a malignant phenotype. In one such experiment a gene, transfected from human bladder cancer cells into normal fibroblasts, once isolated and cloned, was found to be nearly identical to a gene in the normal cells, differing only by one base pair. It is hypothesized that this normal gene underwent this mutation, leading to the malignant change in the cells. The normal *src* gene and other genes that are similar to the oncogenes present in normal cells are termed *proto-oncogenes*. Many of these proto-oncogenes encode for proteins involved in the normal control of cell proliferation, and they can undergo amplification or mutation, like the v-*src*, resulting in uncontrolled growth or proliferation. When activated in that manner they are termed *oncogenes*. These oncogenes encode for proteins, sometimes termed *onco-proteins*, that affect their changes in cell growth and proliferation in a number of ways.

The oncogenes and their encoded onco-proteins that exert a positive effect on the growth and proliferation of cells are termed *dominant oncogenes*. Several examples of dominant oncogenes are now known to be important factors in the biology of human malignancies. Table 6–2 shows some of these oncogenes whose expression or overexpression is associated with pediatric tumors. Other oncogenes, termed *tumor suppressor genes*, encode for inhibitory proteins, which can transform cells once mutated. Other alterations inactivate their onco-proteins, leading to a loss of control—analogous to brake failure in a car heading downhill. Table 6–3 shows some of these oncogenes associated with pediatric tumors when both alleles are mutated or inactivated. The mechanisms by which oncogenes affect cell growth or proliferation can be classified into three groups (Fig. 6–2): (1) some oncogenes encode for transmembrane receptors, to which peptide growth factors bind, or for the growth factors themselves, which stimulate activation of secondary messengers, leading to signal trans-

Table 6–2 • Dominant Oncogenes Associated with Pediatric Tumors

Gene	Associated Tumor
N-*myc*	Neuroblastoma
N-*ras*	Neuroblastoma
H/K-*ras*	Neuroblastoma
	Rhabdomyosarcoma
RET	Thyroid carcinoma
	Pheochromocytomas

Table 6–3 • Tumor Suppressor Genes Associated with Pediatric Tumors

Gene	Associated Tumor
RB1	Retinoblastoma
WT1	Wilms' tumor
p53	Neuroblastoma
	Osteosarcoma
NF1	Neurofibromatosis

duction; (2) other oncogenes encode for the secondary messengers or transduction signals themselves, and (3) the remainder encode for intranuclear proteins that regulate transcription.

GROWTH FACTORS AND GROWTH FACTOR RECEPTORS

The peptide growth factors bind to specific receptors on the cell membrane. This interaction between growth factor (or *ligand*) and receptor results in intracellular changes that activate secondary messengers such as G-proteins, cyclic AMP, and protein kinase C.[14] Most cells possess receptors for several different growth factors. Each growth factor usually binds to only one specific membrane receptor, whereas receptors may bind to several ligands. For example, epidermal growth factor (EGF) binds only to the EGF-receptor, but transforming growth factor-α (TGF-α),[15] heparin-binding EGF-like growth factor (HB-EGF),[16] and amphiregulin[17] also serve as ligands for the EGF-receptor.

One cloned proto-oncogene, *RET*, has been determined to encode for a tyrosine kinase membrane receptor that is usually absent or expressed in low levels in normal cells. Malignant cells, particularly those in neuroendocrine malignancies, such as pheochromocytomas, medullary carcinomas of the thyroid, and multiple endocrine neoplasia syndromes, are associated with mutations of the RET proto-oncogene.[18] The ligand that binds to the normal RET receptor protein is unknown. The value of this particular oncogene is that screening for a specific-point mutation of this gene is very sensitive and predictive for the development of multiple endocrine neoplasia.[19]

Neuroblastoma cells demonstrate the important role of growth factors and their recep-

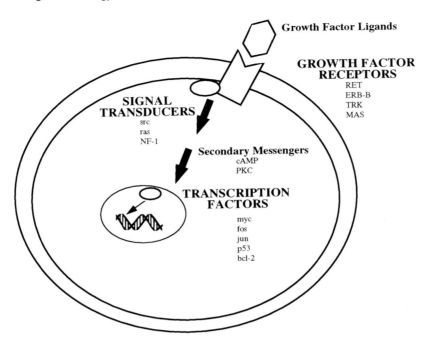

Figure 6–2 • Categories of onco-proteins. Growth factor receptors, signal transducers, and transcription factors are the three major categories of proteins for which oncogenes encode. Examples of each are shown.

tors. Receptors for insulin-like growth factors (IGF-I and IGF-II),[20] nerve growth factor (NGF),[21, 22] and gastrin-releasing peptide (GRP)[23] have all been identified on human neuroblastoma cells. IGF-I and IGF-II stimulation of neuroblastoma cells results in differentiation, with expression of a more mature or benign phenotype.[20] NGF binds to two different membrane receptors, a high-affinity and a low-affinity receptor. The gene that encodes for the high-affinity receptor is termed *Trk-A*. Neuroblastoma tumors lacking TrkA expression have a more malignant behavior.[24] This, along with cell culture findings, suggests that the NGF binding to the receptor promotes differentiation similar to that of IGF-I and IGF-II.[21]

The source of growth factors in different tissues may vary. When the growth factor is secreted by the cells that are to be stimulated, this is termed *autocrine* stimulation.[25] The secretion of the growth factor from surrounding cells is labeled *paracrine* stimulation (Fig. 6–3). *Endocrine* stimulation occurs when remote cells secrete the growth factor into the circulation. Autocrine stimulation is demonstrated in small-cell carcinoma of the lung (SCLC), where GRP is

secreted by the SCLC cells, SCLC tumor growth is stimulated by GRP, and SCLC cells possess thousands of copies of the GRP membrane receptor per cell.[26] Paracrine stimulation is more commonly utilized by other types of cancers and growth factors.

SIGNAL TRANSDUCERS

External signals received by the cell membrane are transmitted to the intracellular biochemical pathways by a group of proteins juxtaposed with the inner surface of the cell membrane. These proteins are termed *signal transducers* and are the protein products of two types of oncogenes. The first, *src* oncogene, was discussed earlier and is the first proto-oncogene identified in the human genome.[13] The *src* gene encodes for a protein called $pp60^{c\text{-}src}$, which is a tyrosine-specific protein kinase.[27] The second type of signal-transducer oncogene is the *ras* family, H-*ras*, K-*ras*, and N-*ras*. The *ras* oncogenes are the most common genes associated with human malignancies, and all of them encode for a protein named $p21^{ras}$, which is related to the G-proteins.[28] These G-proteins either stimulate or inhibit the activity

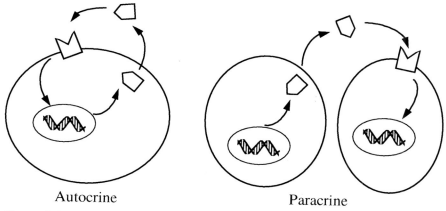

Autocrine Paracrine

Figure 6–3 • Modes of growth factor activity. Autocrine effect is seen in cells that produce the growth factor and its receptor. The growth factor binds to the receptor on the same cell, stimulating intracellular events leading to DNA synthesis, more growth-factor synthesis, and cell proliferation. Paracrine effect is seen when neighboring cells secrete the growth factor, which then binds to its receptor and stimulates DNA synthesis and cell proliferation. When the cells that produce the growth factor are remote from the stimulated cell, the effect is termed endocrine.

of adenylate cyclase, which increases cAMP production. The cAMP acts as a secondary messenger by activating protein kinases. Normal $p21^{ras}$ cycles between an active state and an inactive state, whereas the oncogene-encoded protein is trapped in the active state. Increased expression of the oncogene-encoded $p21^{ras}$ protein has been described in low-stage neuroblastoma tumors and is associated with a good prognosis.[29]

NUCLEAR ONCOGENES

Nuclear oncogenes encode for proteins that regulate the transcription of DNA in the cell nucleus. Many of these proteins bind to the DNA at specific recognition sites and facilitate DNA *dimerization*, which is necessary for transcription. The *myc* family of oncogenes (C-*myc*, L-*myc*, S-*myc*, B-*myc*, and N-*myc*) serves as a good example of this DNA-protein binding.[30] The regulation of this binding and subsequent transcription is finely modulated by other DNA-binding proteins as well. The *myc* onco-protein binds with the *max* protein to form a *myc:max* hybrid.[31] Only this *myc:max* hybrid successfully binds to DNA recognition sites and initiates transcription; thus, an overabundance of *myc* may be offset by a deficiency of *max* protein, reducing the tendency to increase DNA transcription. *Max* can also form *homodimers*, which can suppress

myc:max-mediated transcription. Other nuclear onco-proteins can also compete with the *myc:max* heterodimer for binding sites on the DNA. These include *mad* and *mxi1*.[32]

Other nuclear oncogenes that are important regulators of transcription include *fos* and *jun*.[33] The proteins encoded by these genes hybridize to form a complex termed *AP1*, which binds to a specific sequence of nucleic acids, TGACTCA. The *fos* and *jun* genes are termed *early-response genes*. Their expression is upregulated as a "downstream" event in the cascade initiated by the binding of a growth factor to its receptor.

Not all the oncogene-encoded nuclear transcription factors are promoters of transcription. *WT1*, the proto-oncogene associated with Wilms' tumors, encodes for a protein that suppresses the expression of other genes.[34] Wilms' tumor cells lack the normal *WT1* protein. The retinoblastoma gene *Rb* is another suppressor oncogene, and probably the best understood.[35] Children with familial retinoblastoma inherit one copy of the abnormal gene (allele) from the parent with the disease. That abnormal allele is present in all cells, both germ and somatic. If a mutation of the other allele occurs in the retinal cells, a retinal tumor develops. Patients with nonfamilial or sporadic retinoblastoma develop tumors after retinal cells develop spontaneous mutations of both alleles.

APOPTOSIS

Healthy tissue maintains a balance between cells that are proliferating, cells that are dormant in G_0, and cells that are dying (see Fig. 6–1). In order to keep these different cellular states in balance, fine control mechanisms must be present in the cells. Cells die in two very different ways. *Necrosis* is the pathologic response to an insult such as ischemia or exposure to toxins. It is characterized by cell swelling, lysis of cell membranes, release of lysosomal enzymes, and finally inflammation. In *apoptosis,* cells shrink rather than swell, the cell membranes form blebs, the nuclear chromatin condenses, the nuclear membrane lyses, and the cells finally lyse.[9, 36] Research activity in this area has exploded in the past several years, and it is now apparent that many of the growth factors and onco-proteins participate both in the biochemistry of apoptosis and in cell proliferation.

Negative growth regulators such as tumor suppressers are one such example. The DNA-binding transcription factor *p53,* for instance, is essential to apoptosis to occur. Cells from genetically altered mice with mutant *p53* genes fail to demonstrate radiation-induced apoptosis.[37] Also, *p53* inhibits cell proliferation by halting DNA-damaged cells in phases G_1 and G_2, allowing time for DNA repair mechanisms to work.[8, 38, 39] The importance of this gene is implied by the observation that more than half of human tumors demonstrate mutations or deletions of *p53.*[40–43]

Another example of an oncogene involved in apoptosis is the *bcl-2* gene. The onco-protein encoded by this gene is BCL-2, which prevents apoptosis in normal cells.[44] Genetically altered mice that overexpress the *bcl-2* gene develop a proliferation of lymphocytes, presumably because the cells are incapable of undergoing apoptosis. Eventually, these lymphocytic proliferations become malignant lymphomas.[45] Increased levels of expression of *bcl-2* have also been reported in many other tumor types, including neuroblastoma.[46] These findings suggest the importance of apoptosis in regulating cell number and proliferation.

Experimental studies have also suggested an association between *bcl-2* expression and tumor cell resistance to chemotherapy. It is hypothesized that BCL2 protein prevents the cell from beginning the apoptosis pathway, allowing time for the cell to repair the chemotherapy-induced damage to the genetic material.[46]

MOLECULAR GENETIC TECHNIQUES

As mentioned earlier, the clinician must be familiar with the terms and the techniques of molecular biology in order to comprehend the advances in oncology and the care of cancer patients. For surgeons in particular, clinical decisions may soon be directed by the molecular characteristics of a given tumor. Furthermore, surgeons are essential to obtain the tissue specimens needed to perform these molecular techniques. Following are some of the more common methodologies, most of which take advantage of the hybridization characteristics of nucleic acids.

Southern Blot Analysis. Named after its inventor, E. M. Southern, this technique begins with the isolation of genomic DNA from cells.[47] The DNA is then cut into fragments of different lengths by employing restriction endonucleases, enzymes that cut double-stranded DNA at specific base-pair locations. The DNA fragments are then separated by size with gel electrophoresis. These DNA fragments can be transferred to a membrane (by blotting), and after baking, the DNA is densely adherent to the membrane. Using a radioactively labeled sequence of nucleic acids as a probe, one can search the membrane for the presence of the complementary sequence of DNA to which the probe will hybridize. Nonradioactive, chemiluminescent probes have been developed as well. This technique is used to look for the amplification of N-*myc* in DNA from neuroblastoma cells using a ^{32}P-labeled probe (Fig. 6–4).

Northern Blot Analysis. This technique is similar to the Southern Blot except that cellular RNA is transferred to the membrane rather than DNA. Thus, probing this membrane with a labeled sequence of a gene would result in detectable hybridization only if the gene has been transcribed into RNA. This, then, is a method of analyzing gene expression, in contrast to the Southern Blot, which only assesses the presence of the gene or the number of copies of the gene.

Fluorescent In Situ Hybridization (FISH). This tool allows for identification of specific genes in tumor cells without extracting large

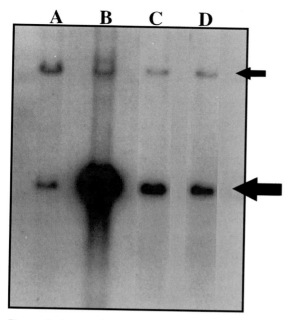

Figure 6–4 • Southern Blot analysis of N-myc oncogene. DNA extracted from neuroblastoma cells is fragmented by restriction endonuclease enzymes, then separated by size using electrophoresis. Radioactive probes for N-*myc* oncogene (*large arrow*) and a standard gene such as the gene encoding for actin (*small arrow*) hybridize to the DNA fragments that contain the appropriate gene sequence. The actin gene signal serves as a control, allowing quantitative comparisons of the amount of N-*myc* DNA relative to the actin DNA. Lane A is a normal patient with a single copy of the actin gene and the N-*myc* gene. Lane B is a positive control with DNA known to contain >100 copies of the N-*myc* gene. Lanes C and D contain DNA from neuroblastoma cells removed from a patient with advanced stage disease. Comparison to lane A and to the actin probe signal allows an estimate of 25 to 30 copies of the N-*myc* oncogene in this patient's tumor cells.

amounts of DNA or RNA. Consequently, the genetic information can be gleaned from small samples those from such as biopsies. The technique utilizes DNA probes labeled with fluorescent molecules. The labeled probe can then be hybridized to the DNA of lysed metaphase cells, which allows for localization of the gene to a specific chromosome. Interphase cells can also be utilized if the goal is merely to assess the number of copies of a gene rather than their location on a specific chromosome (Fig. 6–5).

Polymerase Chain Reaction (PCR). This technique is one of the most powerful tools employed in molecular biology (Fig. 6–6). Like FISH, PCR permits genetic analysis using only small amounts of DNA or RNA. The DNA or RNA to be assessed serves as a template, and, in theory, only a single molecule of DNA is necessary. A primer approximately 20 base pairs long is chosen to anneal to sequences near the gene of interest. The DNA template from the specimen is denatured by heating, then cooled to allow for annealing of the primer to the DNA template. Heat-stable DNA polymerase is added to the reaction, and this begins replication of the DNA template. Thus, at the completion of this reaction, the original DNA template from the specimen of interest has been doubled. Each subsequent repetition of this cycle of heating to denature, cooling to allow annealing of more primer, and DNA replication using the heat-stable DNA polymerase results in a geometric increase in the amount of DNA. In this way more than 8 million copies of the original, single DNA molecule can be generated after only 25 cycles. Reverse transcriptase PCR (RT-PCR) is similar except that the initial template used is RNA. The enzyme, reverse transcriptase, is employed to generate a sense copy of DNA from the RNA template. The regular PCR methodology can then be utilized.

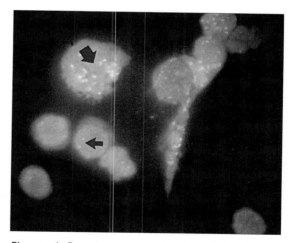

Figure 6–5 • Fluorescent in situ hybridization (FISH). A bone marrow specimen from the same patient as the one in Figure 6–4 contains normal bone marrow cells that have one copy of the N-*myc* gene on each of two chromosomes (*small arrow*), as well as neuroblastoma cells that contain approximately 30 copies of the gene (*large arrow*). The use of FISH permits analysis of N-*myc* amplification on a small number of cells, whereas Southern Blot analysis requires much more tissue.

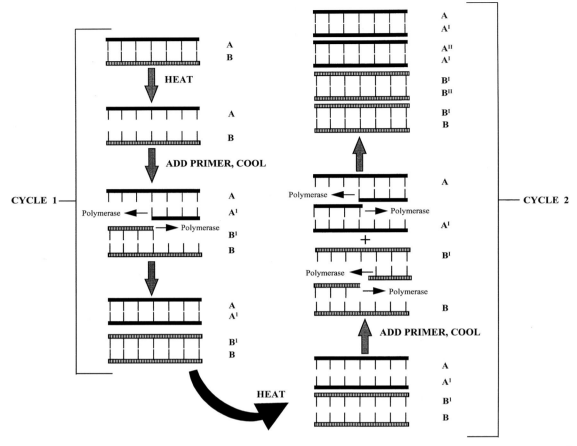

Figure 6–6 • Polymerase chain reaction (PCR). Beginning with only a small amount of DNA and a primer of approximately 20 bases, DNA replication is initiated with a heat-stable DNA polymerase enzyme. Each successive cycle of the PCR reaction doubles the amount of DNA so that large amounts of DNA can be available for analysis.

This method is thus much more sensitive than the Northern Blot in analyzing gene expression.

TUMOR MARKERS

In its broadest sense, the term *tumor marker* represents any measurable or detectable biologic finding associated with malignant cells. Until the identification of the molecular genetic abnormalities in tumor cells, most tumor markers were proteins synthesized by tumor cells. The ideal tumor marker would be (1) easily measured from blood, urine, or tumor sample; (2) elevated (abnormal) only in patients with malignancies (specific); and (3) uniformly elevated (abnormal) early in the course of the disease or recurrence (sensitive). Alternatively, tumor markers may be

reliable predictors of prognosis, enabling aggressive therapy to be individualized for patients with advanced-stage or poor-prognosis tumors. Although such an ideal tumor marker does not exist, several of the following are commonly used in managing pediatric tumors nonetheless.[48, 49]

Alpha-Fetoprotein (AFP). This protein is synthesized by fetal liver, intestine, kidneys, and yolk-sac cells. AFP shares considerable amino acid sequence homology with albumin.[50] During pregnancy, the elevated maternal serum levels and elevated amniotic fluid levels are attributable to fetal production. The newborn serum levels are very high as well. With a serum half-life of five to six days, the AFP levels drop rapidly.[51, 52] Infants with sacrococcygeal teratomas may have persistent elevations of the AFP levels. This elevation raises the suspicion of endodermal sinus tumor foci in the teratoma. Unfortunately, only 60% of children with yolk-sac tumors have elevated AFP levels.[53]

Other tumors are associated with AFP elevations regardless of age, including hepatoblastoma and hepatocellular carcinoma.[54–57] If a patient with a germ-cell tumor, hepatoblastoma, or hepatocellular carcinoma presents with an elevated AFP level, it is an accurate tool for monitoring response to therapy and recurrence in that patient. An injured or regenerating liver following surgical resection will produce AFP, which can be measured in serum. This factor becomes particularly important to consider when one is monitoring AFP levels in a patient who undergoes hepatic resection for hepatoblastoma. Six to 8 weeks must be allowed for hepatic regeneration to be nearly complete before one can attribute elevated AFP levels to recurrent tumor.

β-Human Chorionic Gonadotropin-(β HCG). This glycoprotein is elevated in patients with germ-cell tumors, particularly those derived from trophoblastic tissue.[58] Persistently abnormal HCG levels in such patients treated with chemotherapy indicate residual viable tumor and are predictive of a poor prognosis.[59] Some children with hepatoblastoma also have elevated serum HCG levels.[60, 61]

Lactate Dehydrogenase (LDH). Increased serum LDH levels are seen in patients with malignancies of many types, including germ-cell tumors,[62] neuroblastoma,[63] and lymphoma.[64] Since LDH is a common cytoplasmic enzyme involved in the metabolism of lactic acid, its release into the serum merely reflects cell injury or necrosis. But rapidly proliferating malignant cells also have high rates of cell death. Consequently, LDH may be an indirect measure of the amount of tumor burden. The degree of elevation in serum LDH levels correlates inversely with the prognosis for patients with lymphoma[64] and neuroblastoma.[63, 65] LDH has at least five isozymes, and while the total LDH level may be normal, the pattern of distribution of these isozymes may be altered in malignant cells.[66, 67]

Other Tumor Markers. Neuron-specific enolase was once thought to be a very specific marker of neural crest cell derivative tumors.[68] It has been subsequently established to be rela-

tively nonspecific. The catecholamines homovanillic acid (HVA) and vanillylmandelic acid (VMA) are elevated in patients with neuroblastoma,[69] but they may also be abnormal in patents with the benign variant of ganglioneuroma. The degree of elevation does not correspond to prognosis for neuroblastoma patients. Serum ferritin is a tumor marker used to assess prognosis in neuroblastoma patients,[70] and hyaluronic acid is a tumor marker for pediatric malignancies, notably Wilms' tumor.[71]

Many other putative tumor markers have been identified. Enumeration of all of them is beyond the scope of this chapter. Most await large-scale testing to establish their validity. Some of these proteins are not measurable in serum or urine but may be detected by immunohistochemical staining of tumor cells. These tumor markers can be adjuncts to hematoxylin and eosin staining to aid in accurate diagnosis and typing of biopsy specimens. As additional oncogenes are discovered, the protein products for which they encode can be detected by immunohistochemistry as well. Histochemistry is cheaper, easily automated, and more universally applicable than nucleic acid analysis or cytogenetics. Unfortunately, the data from DNA or RNA analysis do not always correlate with the onco-protein analysis by immunohistochemistry. For example, N-*myc* analysis by Southern Blot and histochemical detection of N-*myc* protein may be disconjugate for a given tumor specimen.[72]

An understanding of the biochemical and molecular principles covered in this chapter is important to the surgeon who cares for children with cancer.[73] Surgeons employ different modes of treatment for these children, including the extent of surgical resection, based on many of these biologic markers. In addition, surgeons are responsible for obtaining tissue and body fluids for measurement of these molecular and biochemical data. Indeed, as genes are identified that are associated with increased risk of developing cancer, surgeons may even make decisions regarding resection of organs before malignancy has actually developed.[19] For all these reasons, knowledge of the basic terminology and concepts of molecular biology is a necessity for all surgeons.

References

1. Seeger RC, Brodeur GM, Sather H, et al: Association of multiple copies of the N-*myc*

oncogene with rapid progression of neuroblastoma. *N Engl J Med* 313:1111–1116, 1985.

2. Williams NN, Day JM: Flow cytometry and prognostic implications in patients with solid tumors. *Surg Gyn Obst* 171:257–266, 1990.

3. Berube D, Passage E, Mattei MG, et al: Fine mapping of the long arm of human chromosome 11 by in situ hybridization using different translocations, including the t(11;22) of Ewing sarcoma. *Cytogenet Cell Genet* 54:142–147, 1990.

4. Mathew CGP, Smith BA, Thorpe K, et al: Deletion of genes on chromosome 1 in endocrine neoplasia. *Nature* 328:524–526, 1987.

5. Fong CT, Dracapoli NC, White PS, et al: Loss of heterozygosity for chromosome 1p in human neuroblastomas: Correlation with N-*myc* amplification. *Proc Natl Acad Sci* 86:3753–3757, 1989.

6. Caron, H: Allelic loss of chromosome 1 and additional chromosome 17 material are both unfavorable prognostic markers in neuroblastoma. *Med Pediatr Oncol* 24:215–221, 1995.

7. Grundy PE, Telzerow PE, Breslow N, et al: Loss of heterozygosity for chromosomes 16q and 1p in Wilms' tumors predicts an adverse outcome. *Cancer Res* 54:2331–2333, 1994.

8. Agarwal ML, Agarwall A, Taylor WR, Stark GR: p53 controls both the G2/M and the G1 cell cycle checkpoints and mediates reversible growth arrest in human fibroblasts. *Proc Natl Acad Sci* 92:8493–8497, 1995.

9. Merlino G: Regulatory imbalances in cell proliferation and cell death during oncogenesis in transgenic mice. *Semin Cancer Biol* 5:13–20, 1994.

10. Morris JDH, Eddleston ALWF, Crook T: Viral infection and cancer. *Lancet* 346:754–758, 1995.

11. Brosman SA, Liu BCS: Oncogenes: Their role in neoplasia. *Urology* 30:1–10, 1987.

12. Bishop JM: Molecular themes in oncogenesis. *Cell* 64:235–248, 1991.

13. Erikson RL, Purchio AF, Erikson E, et al: Molecular events in cells transformed by Rous sarcoma virus. *J Cell Biol* 87:319–325, 1980.

14. Weinberg RA: Molecular mechanisms of carcinogenesis. In Leder P, Clayton DA, Rubinstein E (eds): *Introduction to Molecular Medicine* New York: Scientific American, 1994.

15. Groener LC, Nice EC, Burgess AW: Structure-function relationships for the EGF/TGF-alpha family of mitogens. *Growth Factors* 11:235–237, 1994.

16. Besner GE, Whelton D, Crissman-Combs MA, et al: Interaction of heparin-binding-EGF-like growth factor (HB-EGF) with the epidermal growth factor receptor: Modulation by heparin, heparinase, or synthetic heparin-binding-EGF fragments. *Growth Factors* 7:289–296, 1992.

17. Pathak BG, Gilbert DJ, Harrison CA, et al: Mouse chromosomal location of three EGF receptor ligands: Amphiregulin (Areg), betacelluilin (Btc) and heparin-binding EGF (Hegf1). *Genomics* 28:116–118, 1995.

18. Carlson KM, Dou S, Chi D, Seaverda N, et al: Single missense mutation in the tyrosine kinase catalytic domain of the RET protooncogene is associated with multiple endocrine neoplasia type 2B. *Proc Natl Acad Sci* 91:1579–1583, 1994.

19. Chi DD, Toshima K, Donis-Keller H, Wells SA: Predictive testing for multiple endocrine neoplasia type 2A (MEN 2A) based on the detection of mutations in the RET protooncogene. *Surgery* 116:124–32, 1994.

20. Meghani MA, Martin DM, Singleton JR, Feldman EL: Effects of serum and insulin-like growth factors on human neuroblastoma cell growth. *Regul Pept* 48:217–224, 1993.

21. Suzuki T, Bogenmann E, Shimada H, et al: Lack of high-affinity nerve growth factor receptors in aggressive neuroblastomas. *J Natl Cancer Inst* 85:377–384, 1993.

22. Nakagawara A, Arima-Nakagawara M, Azar CG et al: Clinical significance of expression of neurotrophic factors and their receptors in neuroblastoma. *Prog Clin Biol Res* 385:155–161, 1994.

23. Sawin RS, Brockenbrough J, Ness JC: Gastrin-releasing peptide is an autocrine growth factor for human neuroblastoma. *Surgical Forum*, XLIII:606–608, 1992.

24. Chen J, Chattopadhyay B, Venkatakrishnan G, Ross RA: Nerve growth factor induced differentiation of human neuroblastoma and neuroepithelioma cell lines. *Cell Growth Differ* 1:79–85, 1990.

25. Sporn MB, Todaro GJ: Autocrine secretion and malignant transformation of cells. *N Engl J Med* 303:878–880, 1980.

26. Cuttitta F, Carney DN, Mulshine J, et al: Bombesin-like peptides can function as autocrine growth factors in human small cell lung cancers. *Nature* 316:823–826, 1985.

27. Muthuswamy SK, Muller WJ: Activation of the *src* family of tyrosine kinases in mammary tumorigenesis. *Adv Cancer Res* 64:111–123, 1994.

28. Satoh T, Nakafuku M, Kaziro Y: Function of *ras* as a molecular switch in signal transduction. *J Biol Chem* 267:24149–24152, 1992.

29. Tanaka T, Slamon DJ, Shimoda H, et al: Expression of HA-*ras* oncogene products in human neuroblastomas and the significant correlation with a patient's prognosis. *Cancer Res* 48:1030–1034, 1988.

30. Kato GJ, Dang CV: Function of the C-*myc* oncoprotein. *FASEB J* 6:3065–3072, 1992.

31. Hurlin PJ, Ayer DE, Grandori C, Eisenman RN: The *max* transcription factor network: Involvement of *mad* in differentiation and an approach to identification of target genes. *Cold Spring Harbor Symp Quant Biol* 59:109–116, 1994.

32. Chin L, Schreiber-Agus N, Pellicer I, et al: Contrasting roles for *myc* and *mad* proteins in cellular growth and differentiation. *Proc Natl Acad Sci* 92:8488–8492, 1995.

33. Sassone-Corsi P, Lamph WW, Kamps M, Verma IM: *fos*-associated cellular p39 is related to nuclear transcription factor AP-1. *Cell* 54:553–560, 1988.

34. Call KM, Glaser T, Ito CY, et al: Isolation and characterization of a zinc finger polypeptide gene at the human chromosome 11 Wilms' tumor locus. *Cell* 60:509–513, 1990.

35. Weinberg RA: Positive and negative controls on cell growth. *Biochemistry* 28:8263–8269, 1989.

36. McDonnell TJ, Meyn RE, Robertson LE: Implications of apoptotic cell death regulation in cancer therapy. *Semin Cancer Biol* 6:53–60, 1995.

37. Clarke AR, Purdie CA, Harrison DJ, et al: Thymocyte apoptosis induced by p53-dependent and independent pathways. *Nature* 362:849–852, 1993.

38. Kastan-M-B. Onyekwere-O. Sidransky-D, et al: Participation of p53 protein in the cellular response to DNA damage. *Cancer Res* 51:6304–6311, 1991.

39. Lane DP: Cancer p53, guardian of the genome. *Nature* 362:786–787, 1993.

40. Greenblatt MS, Bennett WP, Hollstein M, Harris CC: Mutations in the p53 tumor suppressor gene: Clues to cancer etiology and molecular pathogenesis. *Cancer Res* 54:4855–4878, 1994.

41. Malkin D, Jolly KW, Barbier N, et al: Germline mutations of the p53 tumor suppressor gene in children and young adults with second malignant neoplasms. *N Engl J Med* 326:1309–1315, 1992.

42. Toguchida J, Yamaguchi T, Dayton SH, et al: Prevalence and spectrum of germline mutations of the p53 gene among patients with sarcoma. *N Engl J Med* 326:1301–1308, 1992.

43. Malkin D, Li FP, Strong LC, et al: Germ-line p53 mutations in a familial syndrome of breast cancer, sarcomas, and other neoplasms. *Science* 250:1233–1238, 1990.

44. Hockenbery DM: The bcl-2 oncogene and apoptosis. *Semin Immunol* 4:413–420, 1992.

45. McDonnell TJ, Korsmeyer SJ: Progression from lymphoid hyperplasia to high-grade malignant lymphoma in mice transgenic for the t(14; 18). *Nature* 349:254–256, 1991.

46. Reed JC: Regulation of apoptosis by bcl-2 family proteins and its role in cancer and chemoresistance. *Curr Opin Oncol* 7:541–546, 1995.

47. Southern EM: Detection of specific sequences among DNA fragments separated by gel electrophoresis. *J Mol Biol* 98:503–517, 1975.

48. Woods WG: The use and significance of biologic markers in the evaluation and staging of a child with cancer. *Cancer* 58:442–448, 1986.

49. Jacobs EL, Haskell CM: Clinical use of tumor markers in oncology. *Curr Probl Cancer* 15:299–360, 1991.

50. Deutsch HF: Chemistry and biology of α-fetoprotein. *Adv Cancer Res* 56:253–312, 1991.

51. Brewer JA, Tank ES: Yolk sac tumors and alpha-fetoprotein in first year of life. *Urology* 42:79–80, 1993.

52. Wu JT, Book L, Sudar K: Serum alpha-fetoprotein (AFP) levels in normal infants. *Pediatr Res* 15:50–52, 1981.

53. Weissbach L, Altwein JE, Steins R: Germinal testicular tumors in childhood—Report of observations and literature review. *Eur Urol* 10:73–85, 1984.

54. Chen WJ, Lee JC, Hung WT: Primary malignant tumor of liver in infants and children in Taiwan. *J Pediatr Surg* 23:457–461, 1988.

55. Tsuchida Y, Kaneko M, Saito S, Endo Y: Differences in the structure of alpha-fetoprotein and its clinical use in pediatric surgery. *J Pediatr Surg* 20:260–265, 1985.

56. Heyward WL, Lanier AP, McMahon BJ, et al: Early detection of primary hepatocellular carcinoma. Screening for primary hepatocellular carcinoma among persons infected with hepatitis B virus. *JAMA* 254:3052–3054, 1985.

57. Kelstein ML, Chan DW, Bruzek DJ, Rock RC: Monitoring hepatocellular carcinoma by using a monoclonal immunoenzymometric assay for alpha-fetoprotein. *Clin Chem* 34:76–81, 1988.

58. Civantos F, Rywlin AM: Carcinoma with trophoblastic differentiation and secretion of chorionic gonadotropin. *Cancer* 29:789–798, 1972.

59. Eastham JA, Wilson TG, Russell C, et al: Surgical resection in patients with nonseminomatous germ cell tumors who fail to normalize tumor markers after chemotherapy. *Urology* 443:74–80, 1994.

60. O'Brien WJ, Finlay JL, Gilbert-Barness EF: Patterns of antigen expression in hepatocellular carcinoma in children. *Pediatr Hem Oncol* 6:361–365, 1989.

61. Watanabe I, Yamaguchi M, Kasai M: Histologic characteristics of gonadotropin-producing hepatoblastoma: A survey of seven cases from Japan. *J Pediatr Surg* 22:406–411, 1987.

62. Chisholm JC, Darmady JM, Kohler JA: Dysgerminoma in mother and daughter: Use of lactate dehydrogenase as a tumor marker in the child. *Pediatr Hem Oncol* 12:305–308, 1995.

63. Joshi VV, Cantor AB, Brodeur GM, et al: Correlation between morphology and the prognostic markers of neuroblastoma. A study of histologic grade, DNA index, N-*myc* gene copy number, and lactic dehydrogenase in patients in the Pediatric Oncology Group. *Cancer* 71:3171–3181, 1993.

64. Hisamitsu S, Shibuya H, Hoshima M, Horiuchi J: Prognostic factors in head and neck non-Hodgkin's lymphoma with special references to serum lactic dehydrogenase and serum copper. *Acta Oncol* 29:879–883, 1990.

65. Quinn JJ, Altman AJ, Frantz CN: Serum lactic

dehydrogenase, an indicator of tumor activity in neuroblastoma. *J Pediatr* 97:89–91, 1980.

66. Ito M, Taki T, Mitsuoka A, Miyake M: LDH isoenzyme-1 in the mediastinal yolk sac tumor. *Jpn J Surg* 18:419–422, 1988.

67. Sacks SS, Muligan G: Increase in lactate dehydrogenase isoenzyme-1 in plasma in pediatric malignancy. *Clin Chem* 36:1683–1685, 1990.

68. Cooper EH: Neuron-specific enolase. *Int J Biol Markers* 9:205–210, 1994.

69. Laug WE, Siegel SE, Shaw KN, et al: Initial urinary catecholamine metabolites and prognosis in neuroblastoma. *Pediatrics* 62:77–83, 1978.

70. Hann HW, Levy HM, Evans AE: Serum ferritin as a guide to therapy in neuroblastoma. *Cancer Res* 40:1411–1413, 1980.

71. Lin RY, Argenta PA, Sullivan KM, et al: Urinary hyaluronic acid is a Wilms' tumor marker. *J Pediatr Surg* 30:304–308, 1995.

72. Hiyama E, Hiyama K, Yokoyama T, Ishii T: Immunohistochemical analysis of N-*myc* protein expression in neuroblastoma: Correlation with with prognosis of patients. *J Pediatr Surg* 26:838–843, 1991.

73. Hurwitz M, Sawicki M, Samara G, Passaro E: Diagnostic and prognostic molecular markers in cancer. *Am J Surg* 164:299–306, 1992.

Chapter

7

Minimally Invasive Surgery

• *George W. Holcomb, III, M.D.*

Following the report by Reddick and Olsen in 1989 on a series of 25 adults undergoing laparoscopic cholecystectomy,[1] a revolution in minimally invasive surgery (MIS) was initiated. Since that time, many have detailed their experiences with MIS not only for gallbladder removal but also for laparoscopic appendectomy, herniorrhaphy, fundoplication, and even colectomy.[2–11] During the last few years others have documented the use of MIS in children for laparoscopic cholecystectomy, appendectomy, fundoplication, splenectomy, and even pull-through procedures.[12–22] A resurgence also has occurred in the use of thoracoscopy in children.[23–26]

Along with the laparoscopic and thoracoscopic approach for benign disease, the endoscopic approach has been applied to adult patients with cancer. In adults, diagnostic laparoscopy has gained acceptance for evaluation of metastatic peritoneal implants prior to open laparotomy.[27] Moreover, laparoscopy is beneficial for staging purposes in women with primary malignancy in the ovary or endometrium[28, 29] and in the staging assessment of pancreatic cancer.[30–32] The main reason for using laparoscopy in patients with this latter disease is to help decide on a curative or a palliative procedure. The ability to provide endoscopic palliation of the pancreatic and biliary tree through stents or other drainage devices supports the need for complete staging in adults, as some will fail to benefit from conventional surgical bypass. Moreover, conventional imaging may underestimate the stage of abdominal malignancy, thus prompting an open procedure that may not be beneficial.[27]

In adults, laparoscopy has also been useful as a second-look procedure to evaluate the possibility of a recurrent or residual tumor. This has been especially advantageous in patients with ovarian malignancies.[28] Laparoscopic staging of abdominal lymphomas has been reported as well. In one adult study, routine laparoscopic staging for Hodgkin's disease showed unsuspected hepatic involvement in 6% of patients, occult splenic involvement in 13%, and evidence of progression to another stage of disease in 23%.[33] Laparoscopic staging of gastric and esophageal cancer and laparoscopic resection of colorectal cancers also have been reported.[34–37] Laparoscopic pelvic lymph node dissection for patients with carcinomas of the prostate and bladder has been described.[38–40]

Video-assisted thoracoscopic surgery has been employed for tumors within the lung parenchyma as well as for pleural-based lesions in adults; both staging of these tumors and formal lobectomies by means of thoracoscopy have been described.[41–45] In addition, thoracoscopic lymph node staging and resection of metastatic disease in patients with esophageal cancer have been detailed.[46–47]

Although historically most of the literature on MIS and cancer has been derived from adult studies, this modality can be effectively employed in children, as described in the remainder of this chapter.

PATIENT SELECTION

When participating in the care of a child with cancer, it is important to consider the overall plan for this patient as determined by a team approach. The goal of complete surgical removal of the malignant disease is often not possible in children. Therefore, in many instances, chemotherapy and radiation therapy play an integral part in eradicating the malignancy. Because of the nature of pediatric malignancies, the surgical operation is usually only one aspect of a combined protocol involving surgical extirpation, chemotherapy, and radiotherapy. With continuing advances in adjuvant therapy, the role of the surgeon in the management of these malignancies is becoming more and more cooperative with other cancer specialists.

Although laparoscopy and thoracoscopy have been performed utilizing local infiltration with intravenous sedation in adults, they are rarely so performed in children. Most children undergoing MIS procedures require general anesthesia. It is important to remember this requirement and to select only patients who will tolerate a pneumoperitoneum or one-lung ventilation. As much information as possible must be obtained prior to the endoscopic evaluation. Imaging techniques such as computed tomography (CT) or magnetic resonance imaging (MRI) may be very helpful in identifying specific areas within solid organs for biopsy or lymph nodes for excision. Such studies may be especially useful when a second-look operation is required for assessment of possible residual or recurrent disease.

Lesions deep within solid organs, such as tumors within the liver or nodules within the lung parenchyma, are not easily palpable. Therefore it may be difficult to obtain a biopsy using either the laparoscopic or the thoracoscopic approach. Consequently, endoscopic operations for these and similar lesions may result in a high incidence of conversion to the open procedure, the possibility of which should be explained thoroughly to the family prior to the MIS procedure. Three contraindications to attempting either laparoscopic or thoracoscopic procedures are (1) a clotting disorder that cannot be corrected, (2) an inability to gain access to either the abdomen or thorax, usually as a result of previous operations or inflammation; and (3) an infection within the abdominal or thoracic wall at the site of the proposed cannula insertion. This last contraindication is usually not absolute as alternate sites are often available. Still another contraindication, as previously mentioned, is the patient's inability to tolerate either a pneumoperitoneum or single-lung ventilation.

A preoperative conference should be held with the parents and, if age appropriate, with the child. The MIS procedure may at any time need to be converted to an open operation. The most notable indication for such conversion is the inability to define the anatomy accurately for a safe endoscopic procedure. Other reasons are excessive and uncontrollable bleeding, inability to gain access to the thoracic or abdominal cavity (because of either previous inflammation or inability to collapse the ipsilateral lung), and various technical difficulties.

LAPAROSCOPY
Technique

The patient is prepared as for an open procedure and is positioned supine on the operating table.

Placement of the video monitors depends on the nature of the procedure and location of the target lesion. In general, for lesions within the upper abdominal cavity, two video screens are usually placed on either side of the head of the operating table (Fig. 7–1). For a procedure in the lower abdomen or pelvis, one or two video monitors are situated at the foot of the table (Fig. 7–2).

Intravenous access is established and general anesthesia administered. Following anesthetic induction, an orogastric tube is inserted for decompression. In older patients a Foley catheter may be used for a prolonged procedure, but in small children a Credé's maneuver is usually adequate for bladder decompression. The patient is then prepared and draped while special attention is given to cleansing the umbilicus thoroughly, as this is the site for placement of the initial cannula. An umbilical cutdown technique is preferred for introduction of this first cannula rather than utilizing the Veress needle procedure for abdominal insufflation followed by blind insertion of the cannula. A vertical incision is made within the umbilicus and extended through the fascia and peritoneum. Once the abdominal viscera are visualized, a 5-mm or 10-mm cannula with a blunt trocar is gently rotated through the fascia and peritoneum into the abdominal cavity. The insufflation tubing is then connected to the stopcock and pneumoperitoneum quickly established.

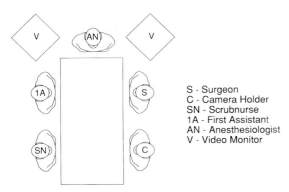

Figure 7–1 • This diagram depicts placement of two video monitors and personnel for upper abdominal procedures such as splenectomy. (From Holcomb GW III: Diagnostic laparoscopy: Equipment, technique, and special concerns in children. In Holcomb GW III (ed): *Pediatric Endoscopic Surgery.* Norwalk, CT: Appleton & Lange, 1994, with permission.)

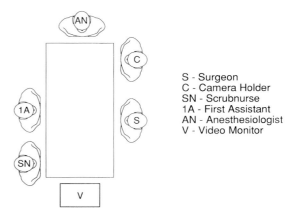

Figure 7–2 • A single video monitor is often employed for procedures in the lower abdominal cavity such as appendectomy and pelvic lymph node dissection. In addition, the personnel are arranged differently for these procedures as compared with Figure 7–1. (From Holcomb GW III: Diagnostic laparoscopy: Equipment, technique, and special concerns in children. In Holcomb GW III (ed): *Pediatric Endoscopic Surgery.* Norwalk, CT: Appleton & Lange, 1994, with permission.)

The first step in performing any laparoscopic procedure is diagnostic laparoscopy. The entire abdominal cavity is visualized and then specific attention turned to the target organ. Accessory cannulas likely will need to be introduced through which instruments can be inserted for biopsy, retraction, lymphadenectomy, or excision of the neoplasm. The typical laparoscopic instrumentation is usually adequate for the cancer patient. Grasping forceps for exposure, electrocautery, scissors connected to electrocautery, and suction equipment should be available. A True-Cut needle may also be utilized for biopsies of specific lesions such as liver nodules. Exposure may be enhanced by tilting the table either in the reverse Trendelenburg or Trendelenburg position and to the right or left. With these manipulations, adjacent viscera often will fall away from the target organ and exposure will be improved. If another small accessory cannula would be beneficial for insertion of another instrument for exposure, this should be done without hesitation.

Many of the same operations performed in children for cancer have also been performed for benign disease. Included in this list would be liver biopsies under laparoscopic visualization, splenectomy in association with staging laparoscopy, and lymph node biopsy for Hodgkin's disease, as well as appendectomy in patients undergoing adjuvant therapy for malignancy.[16–18, 48, 49] Lymph node dissections are not routinely indicated for children but have been performed extensively in adults with pelvic cancer.[38–40]

Children's Cancer Group Experience

The Children's Cancer Group (CCG) experience with laparoscopy for cancer in children reported on 25 patients who underwent a single laparoscopic operation between December 1, 1991, and October 1, 1993 (Table 7–1).[49] In the 16 cases where biopsy was performed, diagnostic tissue was obtained in every case. In each of the other cases, the procedure accomplished its purpose. There was no mortality associated with the laparoscopic operation, and no complications occurred in this group.

• *Comment* •

The definitive diagnosis of an intracavitary neoplasm usually cannot be made without biopsy or excision. In this series, the laparoscopic approach was very useful for obtaining guided biopsies in patients with neuroblastoma, hepatoblastoma, choriocarcinoma, and sarcoidosis. Moreover, laparoscopy made it easier to determine whether certain masses were resectable.

Laparoscopy was also helpful in four patients with Hodgkin's disease. This finding may be important in the future, as indicated by a pediatric study (comparing CT scanning and lymphography with laparotomy) showing that staging laparotomy affected the stage of the disease in 37% of cases.[50] It follows that if the needed operative procedure for Hodgkin's disease, including splenectomy and lymph node biopsies, can be performed laparoscopically, this approach may be utilized to the patient's advantage.

A second-look procedure also is sometimes required following adjuvant therapy. Although difficulties with adhesions may limit such utilization in some instances after a prior laparotomy, the technique was effective in four patients from this series following treatment of intra-abdominal malignancies.

THORACOSCOPY

Although acceptance of laparoscopy in children has historically followed pioneering advances in adults, thoracoscopy has been utilized in children for two decades.[51–53] Adoption of thoracoscopy for mediastinal and parenchymal lesions gained extensive application only after advances in MIS techniques. Now the most frequent use of thoracoscopy in children is for biopsy or resection of mediastinal and hilar masses. In contrast, the most common indication in adults remains the diagnosis and treatment of idiopathic pleural effusions.[54] Other applications in children include biopsy of diffuse and localized pulmonary infiltrates, irrigation for empyema with debridement, limited decortication, and bleb resection with pleurodesis for pneumothorax.

While it is not uncommon to perform thoracoscopy in adults using local anesthesia, general anesthesia is usually required for children. In most cases, the procedure is more easily performed with the ipsilateral lung collapsed. In teenagers, this often is accomplished using a double-lumen endotracheal tube. In younger children and infants, selective intubation of the contralateral airway is usually necessary. A pediatric bronchoscope is passed through the lumen of the endotracheal tube to verify the proper tube position.

Another option for single-lung ventilation is the introduction of a Fogarty balloon catheter into the lumen of the ipsilateral airway under bronchoscopic visualization. Although this approach is technically possible, it can be time-consuming and is often not successful for the duration of the procedure. A final option is insufflation of carbon dioxide into the ipsilateral thoracic cavity to collapse the lung. This approach is often necessary for pediatric patients since complete ipsilateral bronchial obstruction is not always possible.

As with laparoscopy, exposure of the target lesion is improved for thoracoscopy by proper patient positioning. For an anterior mediastinal lesion, the patient should be placed relatively face up, as opposed to face down for posterior mediastinal lesions. For a lung biopsy, the decubitus position is usually satisfactory (Fig. 7–3). A wide preparation and draping area, as for an open thoracotomy, is needed. The initial access to the thoracic cavity is usually obtained through a cutdown approach. Through a 5-mm or 10-mm incision, the underlying soft tissue and muscles in the intercostal space are separated, and a blunt cannula is introduced directly into the thoracic

Table 7-1 • Laparoscopic Procedures in Children with Cancer

Indication	Age	Sex	Preoperative Diagnosis	Procedure	Result
Evaluation of new mass for suspected cancer	14 yrs	F	Ovarian mass	Laparoscopy, biopsy of mass	Retroperitoneal neuro-blastoma; resected open
	14 yrs	M	Abdominal mass	Laparoscopy, biopsy of mass	Choriocarcinoma
	16 yrs	M	Periportal mass	Laparoscopy, biopsy of mass	Sarcoid
	2 yrs	F	Liver mass	Laparoscopy, liver biopsy	Hepatoblastoma
	2 yrs	M	Liver mass	Laparoscopy, liver biopsy	Hemangioma
	19 yrs	M	Liver mass	Laparoscopy. liver biopsy	Diffuse lymphoid hyperplasia
	10 yrs	F	Ovarian mass	Laparoscopy, ovarian biopsy	Teratoma
	13 yrs	F	Ovarian mass	Laparoscopy, ovarian biopsy	Stromal tumor
	8 yrs	M	Adrenal mass	Laparoscopy, adrenal biopsy	Adenoma, resected open
Staging	12 yrs	M	Hodgkin's disease—recurrent	Laparoscopy	No recurrent abdominal disease seen
	14 yrs	F	Hodgkin's disease—stage III	Laparoscopy, liver biopsy, node biopsy	No abdominal disease identified
	13 yrs	M	Hodgkin's disease	Laparoscopy including splenectomy, node biopsy	Multifocal splenic involvement; node negative
	12 yrs	F	Hodgkin's disease	Laparoscopy including splenectomy and oophoropexy, node biopsy	No abdominal disease present
	10 mos	F	Vaginal germ-cell tumor	Laparoscopy, ovarian biopsy	No malignancy identified
	3 yrs	F	Vaginal rhabdomyosarcoma, pre-chemotherapy	Laparoscopy	No tumor identified
Second-look evaluation	14 yrs	F	Malignant stromal tumor of ovary	Laparoscopy, fluid aspiration	Cytology negative
	1 yr	F	Endodermal sinus tumor of ovary	Laparoscopy, ovarian biopsy	Biopsy negative
	6 yrs	M	Burkitt's lymphoma	Laparoscopy, nodal biopsies	No malignancy
	3 yrs	F	Rhabdomyosarcoma, bladder	Laparoscopy	No malignancy
Evaluation of mass for resectability	2 yrs	M	Hepatoblastoma	Laparoscopy	Resectable; resected open
	1 yr	F	Hepatoblastoma	Laparoscopy	Resectable; resected open
Evaluation for suspected infection in patient with cancer	13 yrs	F	Leukemia, candidemia	Laparoscopy, liver biopsy	Resolving inflammation of liver and spleen
	13 yrs	M	Leukemia, fever of unknown origin	Laparoscopy, liver biopsy	Fungal abscess of liver
Evaluation for recurrent tumor	18 yrs	F	History of Hodgkin's disease—S/P staging laparotomy	Laparoscopy	No malignancy
Evaluation for metastatic tumor	17 yrs	F	ALL, liver mass	Laparoscopy, liver biopsy	No malignancy

From Holcomb GW III, Tomita SS, Hasse GM, et al: Minimally invasive surgery in children with cancer. *Cancer* 76:121–127, 1995, with permission.

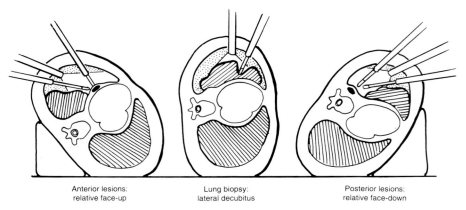

Anterior lesions:
relative face-up

Lung biopsy:
lateral decubitus

Posterior lesions:
relative face-down

Figure 7–3 • Patient positioning for the thoracoscopic approach to mediastinal and pulmonary lesions is important. The relative positions of the three cannulas are also illustrated for these lesions. (From Rodgers BM: Thoracoscopy. In Holcomb GW III (ed): *Pediatric Endoscopic Surgery.* Norwalk, CT: Appleton & Lange, 1994, with permission.)

space. The initial cannula for introduction of the telescope should be inserted slightly posterior to the midaxillary line for access to the anterior mediastinal and hilar masses (Fig. 7–4). For a posterior lesion, it should be situated slightly anterior to the midaxillary line (Fig. 7–5). The

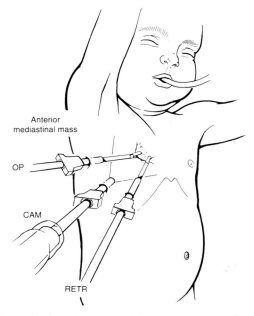

Anterior mediastinal mass

OP

CAM

RETR

Figure 7–4 • Placement of the instruments and camera for the approach to anterior mediastinal lesions in children is shown. (From Rodgers BM: Thoracoscopy. In Holcomb GW III (ed): *Pediatric Endoscopic Surgery.* Norwalk, CT: Appleton & Lange, 1994, with permission.)

camera is then inserted, and diagnostic thoracoscopy performed.

At this time, if the lung is not completely collapsed, carbon dioxide is introduced at a pressure of 4 mmHg to 8 mmHg. Accessory cannulas are then introduced in similar fashion to a laparoscopic operation, although a cutdown technique is also often necessary because of the resistance of the chest wall muscles. If the Endo GIA (US Surgical Corporation, Norwalk, CT) is employed, a 12-mm port is required. This instrument can be very useful for lung biopsies and wedge biopsies of pulmonary nodules. It may be cumbersome in small children, because 5 cm of the distal instrument must be within the chest to open the anvil. It is important to insert this cannula into the thoracic cavity as far caudally as possible to allow maximum space for intrathoracic manipulation (Fig. 7–6).

At the conclusion of the procedure, an appropriate chest tube is inserted through one of the cannula tracts. In addition, a small epidural catheter may be inserted through one of the posterior cannula sites for postoperative pain relief.

Children's Cancer Group Experience

Between December 1, 1991, and October 1, 1993, 60 children underwent 63 thoracoscopic operations at 15 CCG institutions (Table 7–2).[49] Two of them underwent bilateral thoracoscopy at separate sittings for evaluation of a new mass for suspected cancer. One patient with osteogenic

inability to obtain a positive biopsy for Hodgkin's disease (although the biopsy performed at subsequent thoracotomy was also negative for Hodgkin's disease), and, in a patient undergoing lung biopsy, severe hypercarbia at the time of single-lung ventilation. The seventh complication was a case of actelectasis that developed postoperatively.

• *Comment* •

In the future the diagnosis and management of pulmonary metastatic disease may become the primary indication for MIS in children with certain lesions. Resection of pulmonary metastases appears to favorably influence long-term survival in specific childhood cancers such as hepatoblastoma and osteosarcoma. Access to these lesions is usually accomplished easily by MIS as most disease is found in the periphery of the lung or in the pleura. In this review, metastatic tumors from osteosarcoma, Wilms' tumor,

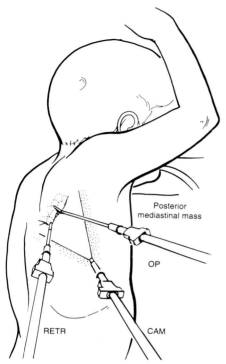

Figure 7–5 • Placement of the instruments and camera for the approach to posterior mediastinal lesions in children is shown. (From Rodgers BM: Thoracoscopy. In Holcomb GW III (ed): *Pediatric Endoscopic Surgery.* Norwalk, CT: Appleton & Lange, 1994, with permission.)

sarcoma had bilateral thoracoscopic wedge excisions of pulmonary nodules using one anesthethic. The three most common indications for thoracoscopy in this series were evaluation of metastatic disease (28 cases), suspected malignancy in a new mass (11 cases), and the need for lung biopsy in cancer patients with respiratory failure or pulmonary infiltrates (9 cases).

Of 51 thoracoscopic operations in which either a wedge resection or a biopsy was possible thoracoscopically, diagnostic tissue was obtained in all but one case. In contrast to the lack of complications in the children undergoing laparoscopy mentioned previously, seven complications were noted in this group of children undergoing thoracoscopic procedures. Six of the complications necessitated conversion to an open thoracotomy. In two cases the reason for conversion was extensive adhesions. In one case each the reasons were bleeding from the lung edge following dissection, inability to clearly visualize a nodular infiltrate,

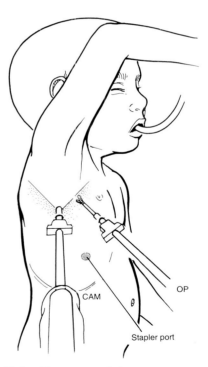

Figure 7–6 • Placement of the camera and biopsy forceps for biopsy of diffuse parenchymal infiltrates or specific lesions is shown. The location of the optional port for the endoscopic stapler is also depicted. (From Rodgers BM: Thoracoscopy. In Holcomb GW III (ed): *Pediatric Endoscopic Surgery.* Norwalk, CT: Appleton & Lange, 1994, with permission.)

Table 7–2 • Thoracoscopic Operations in Children with Cancer

Indication	Age	Sex	Preoperative Diagnosis	Procedure	Result
Evaluation for metastatic tumor	14 yrs	F	Osteogenic sarcoma, lung mass	Thoracoscopy, wedge resection	Metastatic osteogenic sarcoma
	12 yrs	M	Osteogenic sarcoma, bilateral lung masses	Bilateral thoracoscopy, wedge resection (one anesthesia)	Metastatic osteogenic sarcoma, bilateral
	14 yrs	F	Osteogenic sarcoma, lung mass	Thoracoscopy, wedge resection	Metastatic osteogenic sarcoma
	13 yrs	F	Osteogenic sarcoma, lung mass	Thoacoscopy, wedge resection	Metastatic osteogenic sarcoma
	6 yrs	F	Osteogenic sarcoma, lung mass	Thoracoscopy, wedge resection	Metastatic osteogenic sarcoma
	6 yrs	F	Osteogenic sarcoma, lung mass	Thoacoscopy, wedge resection	Metastatic osteogenic sarcoma
	12 yrs	M	Osteogenic sarcoma, lung mass	Thoracoscopy, wedge resection	Metastatic osteogenic sarcoma
	12 yrs	F	Osteogenic sarcoma, lung mass	Thoacoscopy, wedge resection	No malignancy
	16 yrs	M	Osteogenic sarcoma, pleural effusion	Thoracoscopy, pleural resection	No malignancy
	8 yrs	M	Wilms' tumor, lung mass	Thoracoscopy, wedge resection	Metastatic Wilms' tumor
	14 yrs	M	Wilms' tumor, lung mass	Thoracoscopy, wedge resection	No malignancy
	10 yrs	F	Wilms' tumor, pleural mass	Thoracoscopy, biopsy of mass	No malignancy
	14 yrs	M	Ewing's tumor, lung mass	Thoracoscopy, wedge resection	Metastatic Ewing's tumor
	14 yrs	M	PNET chest wall, lung mass	Thoracoscopy, wedge resection	Metastatic PNET
	16 yrs	M	Chondrosarcoma extremity, lung mass	Thoracoscopy, wedge resection	Metastatic chondrosarcoma
	6 yrs	F	Hepatoblastoma, lung mass	Thoracoscopy, wedge resection	Metastatic hepatoblastoma
	17 yrs	M	Germ-cell tumor testis, lung mass	Thoracoscopy, wedge resection	No malignancy
	10 yrs	M	Parapharyngeal rhabdomyosarcoma, lung mass	Thoracoscopy, wedge resection	No malignancy; converted to open procedure because of adhesions from previous thoracotomy
	6 yrs	F	Chest wall rhabdomyosarcoma, lung mass	Thoracoscopy, wedge resection	No malignancy
	15 yrs	F	Paravertebral rhabdomyosarcoma, pleural mass	Thoracoscopy, wedge resection	Metastatic rhabdomyosarcoma
	18 yrs	F	Chondrosarcoma extrremity, mediastinal mass	Thoracoscopy, biopsy of mass	No malignancy
	16 yrs	M	Paratesticular rhabdomyosarcoma, mediastinal mass	Thoracoscopy, biopsy of mass	No malignancy
	18 yrs	F	Rhabdomyosarcoma extremity, mediastinal mass	Thoracoscopy, biopsy of mass	Rhabdomyosarcoma
	16 yrs	F	Rhabdomyosarcoma extremity, mediastinal mass	Thoracoscopy, biopsy of mass	No malignancy

Table 7–2 • Thoracoscopic Operations in Children with Cancer *Continued*

Indication	Age	Sex	Preoperative Diagnosis	Procedure	Result
	4 yrs	F	Abdominal neuroblastoma, pleural mass	Thoracoscopy, biopsy of mass	No malignancy
	16 yrs	M	Malignant fibrous histiocytoma right maxillary sinus, pleural mass	Thoracoscopy, biopsy mass	Malignant fibrous histiocytoma
	5 yrs	F	PNET tumor, chest wall	Thoracoscopy, wedge resection	No malignancy
	14 yrs	M	Abdominal neuroblastoma, pulmonary nodules	Thoracoscopy, wedge resection	No malignancy
	6 yrs	F	Pulmonary rhabdomyosarcoma, s/p excision; pleural mass	Thoracoscopy, biopsy of mass	Rhabdomyosarcoma
Evaluation for recurrence of persistent mass	12 yrs	M	Hodgkin's disease s/p chemotherapy, mediastinal mass	Thoracoscopy, biopsy of mass	Recurrent Hodgkin's disease, converted because of adhesions
	16 yrs	M	Hodgkin's disease s/p chemotherapy, mediastinal mass	Thoracoscopy, biopsy of mass	No malignancy; converted to open procedure because a positive biopsy was not obtained but subsequent biopsy was negative
	15 yrs	M	Cervicothoracic lymphoma s/p chemotherapy, hilar mass	Thoracoscopy, biopsy of mass	No malignancy
Evaluation of new mass for suspected cancer	2 yrs	M	Right pleural mass	Right throacoscopy, biopsy of mass	Rhabdomyosarcoma
			Left lung mass	Left thoracoscopy, wedge excision	No malignancy
	15 yrs	M	Left pulmonary nodules	Left thoracoscopy, wedge excision	Kaposi's sarcoma
			Right pulmonary nodules	Right thoracoscopy, wedge excision	*Rhotococcus equii* infection
	12 yrs	F	Anterior mediastinal mass	Thoracoscopy, biopsy of mass	Hodgkin's disease
	15 yrs	F	Anterior mediastinal mass	Thoracoscopy, biopsy of mass	Hodgkin's disease
	11 yrs	M	Anterior mediastinal mass	Thoracoscopy, biopsy of mass	Hodgkin's disease
	14 yrs	F	Anterior mediastinal mass	Thoracoscopy, biopsy of mass	Hodgkin's disease; converted to open procedudre because of bleeding following separation of adherent left upper lobe from mass
	12 yrs	M	Anterior mediastinal mass	Thoracoscopy, biopsy of mass	No malignancy
	15 yrs	M	Anterior mediastinal mass	Thoracoscopy, biopsy of mass	Hodgkin's disease
	4 yrs	M	Posterior mediastinal mass and cervical mass	Thoracoscopy and cervical exploration, excision of mass	Ganglioneuroblastoma
	13 yrs	F	Anterior mediastinal mass	Thoracoscopy, biopsy of mass	Hodgkin's disease
	15 yrs	M	Anterior mediastinal mass	Thoracoscopy, biopsy of mass	No malignancy

Table continued on following page

Table 7–2 • Thoracoscopic Operations in Children with Cancer *Continued*

Indication	Age	Sex	Preoperative Diagnosis	Procedure	Result
	15 yrs	M	Anterior mediastinal mass	Thoracoscopy, biopsy of mass	Lymphoma
	3 yrs	F	Posterior mediastinal mass	Thoracoscopy, resection of tumor	Ganglioneuroma
Evaluate mass for resectability	18 yrs	M	Primary mediastinal germinoma, s/p chemotherapy	Thoracoscopy	No invasion of sternum; resected open
	3 yrs	F	Mediastinal mass	Thoracoscopy	No adherence to aorta; resected open; neurofibroma
	15 yrs	F	Chest wall tumor	Thoracoscopy	Lung involvement; resected open (PNET)
	10 yrs	F	Chest wall tumor	Thoracoscopy	No invasion of lung; resected open; malignant fibrous histiocytoma
Evaluate for suspected infection in patient with cancer	11 yrs	M	S/P bone marrow transplant, infiltrate	Thoracoscopy, lung biopsy	Obliterative bronchiolitis
	5 yrs	M	S/P bone marrow transplant, infiltrate	Thoracoscopy, lung biopsy	Pulmonary microemboli
	5 yrs	M	S/P bone marrow transplant, infiltrate	Thoracoscopy, lung biopsy	Interstitial pneumonitis; vasculopathy
	11 yrs	M	S/P bone marrow transplant, infiltrate	Thoracoscopy, lung biopsy	Interstitial fibrosis; lymphocytic infiltrates
	9 yrs	F	S/P bone marrow transplant, respiratory failure	Thoracoscopy, lung biopsy	Nonspecific pulmonary changes
	14 yrs	F	Leukemia, infiltrate	Thoracoscopy, lung biopsy	Bronchiolitis
	17 yrs	M	Leukemia, infiltrate	Thoracoscopy, lung biopsy	Leukemia, not identified
	18 yrs	F	Neuroblastoma, nodular infiltrate	Thoracoscopy, lung biopsy	*Pneumocystis carinii*; converted to open procedudre because nodule not identified at thoracoscopy
	2 yrs	M	Astrocytoma, respiratory failure	Thoracoscopy, lung biopsy	Interstitial pneumonia, converted to open procedure because $PCO_2 > 100$ on single-lung ventilation
Pleurolysis for intrapleural chemotherapy	14 yrs	M	S/P right middle lobectomy for undifferentiated sarcoma	Thoracoscopy, pleurodesis	N/A
Pleurodesis for pneumothorax	15 yrs	M	Histiocytosis X, spontaneous pneumothorax	Pleurodesis	N/A

From Holcomb GW III, Tomita SS, Hasse GM, et al: Minimally invasive surgery in children with cancer. *Cancer* 76:121–127, 1995, with permission.

Ewing's tumor, rhabdomyosarcoma, and hepatoblastoma were diagnosed and successfully resected by means of thoracoscopy.

Despite this success, one disadvantage of thoracoscopy is the inability to palpate lesions that cannot be visualized. It is unclear, however, whether resection of disease that is too small to visualize will alter prognosis. Whether the disease is found by CT scan, at thoracoscopy, or during thoracotomy, the patient will likely need to undergo additional chemotherapy to treat micrometastatic disease.

Thoracoscopic biopsy of mediastinal masses, reported as successful in adults, is likely to be used more frequently in children. Evaluation of mediastinal masses is readily accomplished this way, and biopsy usually can be successfully performed. The diagnostic accuracy of thoracoscopic evaluation for mediastinal masses has been reported to vary from 86% to 100%.[55-57]

Still another application of thoracoscopy in children is lung biopsy. Often immunocompromised children develop parenchymal infiltrates, and biopsy is required for diagnosis. In this series of patients from CCG institutions, nine children with fungal, bacterial, or viral infections of the lung underwent thoracoscopy for biopsy.[49]

SUMMARY

The advantages to the patient undergoing a laparoscopic or thoracoscopic procedure include reduced discomfort, shorter hospitalization stay with possibly earlier initiation of adjuvant therapy, improved cosmesis, and faster return to routine activities. In one study in adults, 45% of patients monitored for more than 2 years after traditional lateral thoracotomy reported residual post-thoracotomy pain.[58] In contrast, 12% to 23% of patients in another review, followed for at least 1 year after laparotomy, reported painful scars.[59]

Although MIS will not completely replace standard open operations for every aspect of pediatric surgical oncology, it does appear ideally suited in some instances. The ability to visualize very small lesions makes it a superior diagnostic tool compared with CT and ultrasonography for the detection of metastatic disease. It provides the topographic assessment of pleural and peritoneal surfaces that is needed in second-look procedures and staging operations. Biopsies and limited resections are accomplished more easily with improved instrumentation and advanced video technology. Moreover, as technology further improves, more extensive resections may be possible, and newer modalities, such as endoscopic ultrasonography, will be refined. These advances should enlarge the role of MIS in children with cancer. To evaluate that role, the Children's Cancer Group and Pediatric Oncology Group have initiated a prospective randomized multi-institutional trial.

References

1. Reddick EJ, Olsen DO: Laparoscopic laser cholecystectomy: A comparison with mini-lap cholecystectomy. *Surg Endosc* 3:131–133, 1989.
2. Schirmer BD, Edge SB, Dix J, et al: Laparoscopic cholecystectomy: Treatment of choice for symptomatic cholelithiasis. *Ann Surg* 213:665–677, 1991.
3. Graves HA Jr, Ballinger JF, Anderson WJ: Appraisal of laparoscopic cholecystectomy. *Ann Surg* 213:655–664, 1991.
4. The Southern Surgeons Club: A prospective analysis of 1518 laparoscopic cholecystectomies. *New Eng J Med* 324:1073–1078, 1991.
5. Lointier PH, Lautard M, Massoni C, et al: Laparoscopically assisted subtotal colectomy. *J Laparoendosc Surg* 3:439–453, 1993.
6. Nowzaradan Y, Barnes P: Laparoscopic Nissen fundoplication. *J Laparoendosc Surg* 3:429–438, 1993.
7. Scott-Conner CEH, Hall TJ, Anglin BL, et al: Laparoscopic appendectomy: Initial experience in a teaching program. *Ann Surg* 215:660–668, 1992.
8. Sosa JL, Sleeman D, McKenney MG, et al: A comparison of laparoscopic and traditional appendectomy. *J Laparoendosc Surg* 3(2):129–131, 1993.
9. MacFadyen BV, Arregui ME, Corbitt JD, et al: Complications of laparoscopic herniorrhaphy. *Surg Endosc* 7:155–158, 1993.
10. Senagore AJ, Luchtefeld MA, MacKeigan JM, et al: Open colectomy versus laparoscopic colectomy: Are there differences? *Am Surg* 8:549–554, 1993.
11. Wheeler KH: Laparoscopic inguinal herniorrhaphy with mesh: An 18-month experience. *J Laparoendosc Surg* 3:345–350, 1993.
12. Holzman MD, Sharp KW, Holcomb GW III, et al: An alternative technique for laparoscopic cholangiography. *Surg Endosc* 8:927–930, 1994.
13. Holcomb GW III: Laparoscopic cholecystectomy. *Semin Pediatr Surg* 2:159–167, 1993.
14. Newman KD, Marmon LM, Attori R, et al: Laparoscopic cholecystectomy in pediatric patients. *J Pediatr Surg* 26:1184–1185, 1991.
15. Davidoff AM, Branum GD, Murray EA, et al: The technique of laparoscopic cholecystectomy in children. *Ann Surg* 215:186–191, 1992.
16. Holcomb GW III: Laparoscopic appendectomy in children. *Laparosc Surg* 1(3):145–153, 1993.
17. Valla JS, Limonne B, Valla V, et al: Laparoscopic appendectomy in children: Report of 465 cases. *Surg Laparosc Endosc* 1:166–172, 1991.
18. Gilchrist BF, Lobe TE, Schropp KP, et al: Is there a role for laparoscopic appendectomy in pediatric surgery. *J Pediatr Surg* 27:209–214, 1992.
19. Tulman S, Holcomb GW III, Karamanoukian HL, et al: Pediatric laparoscopic splenectomy. *J Pediatr Surg* 28:689–692, 1993.

20. Lobe TE, Schropp KP, Lunsford K: Laparoscopic Nissen fundoplication in childhood. *J Pediatr Surg* 28:358–361, 1993.

21. Collins JB III, Georgeson KE, Vicente Y, et al: Comparison of open and laparoscopic gastrostomy and fundoplication in 120 patients. *J Pediatric Surg* 30(7):1065–1071, 1995.

22. Georgeson KE, Fuenfer MM, Hardin WD: Primary laparoscopic pull-through for Hirschsprung's disease in infants and children. *J Pediatric Surg* 30(7):1017–1022, 1995.

23. Janik JS, Nagaraj HS, Groff DB: Thoracoscopic evaluation of intrathoracic lesions in children. *J Thorac Cardiovasc Surg* 83:408–413, 1982.

24. Rodgers BM: Thoracoscopic procedures in children. *Semin Pediatr Surg* 2:182–189, 1993.

25. Laborde F, Noirhomme P, Karam J, et al: A new video-assisted thoracoscopic surgical technique for interruption of patent ductus arteriosus in infants and children. *J Thorac Cardiovasc Surg* 105:278–280, 1993.

26. Kern JA, Rodgers BM: Thoracoscopy in the management of empyema in children. *J Pediatr Surg* 28:1128–1132, 1993.

27. Greene FL: Laparoscopic surgery in cancer treatment. In DeVita VT, Hellman S, Rosenberg SA (eds): *Important Advances in Oncology.* Philadelphia: JB Lippincott Co, 1993.

28. Marti-Vincente A, Sainz S, Soriano G, et al: *Utilidad de la laparoscopia como metodo de second-look en las neoplasias de ovario. Rev Esp Enferm Apar Dig* 77:275–278, 1990.

29. Buchsbaum HJ, Lifshitz S: Staging and surgical evaluation of ovarian cancer. *Semin in Oncol* 11:(3)227–237, 1984.

30. Warshaw AL, Gu Z, Wittenberg J, et al: Preoperative staging and assessment of resectability of pancreatic cancer. *Arch Surg* 125:230–233, 1990.

31. Cuschieri A: Laparoscopy for pancreatic cancer: Does it benefit the patient? *Euro J Surg Oncol* 14:41–44, 1988.

32. Fockens P, Huibregtse K: Staging of pancreatic and ampullary cancer by endoscopy. *Endosc* 25:52–57, 1993.

33. Spinelli P, Difelice G: Laparoscopy in abdominal malignancies. *Probl Gen Surg* 8:329–347, 1991.

34. Watt I, Stewart I, Anderson D, et al: Laparoscopy, ultrasound and computed tomography in cancer of the oesophagus and gastric cardia: A prospective comparison for detecting intra-abdominal metastases. *Br J Surg* 76:1036–1039, 1989.

35. Colin-Jones DG, Rosch T, Dittler HJ: Staging of gastric cancer by endoscopy. *Endosc* 25:34–38, 1993.

36. Phillips EH, Franklin M, Carroll BJ, et al: Laparoscopic colectomy. *Ann Surg* 216:703–707, 1992.

37. Bleday R, Babineau T, Forse RA: Laparoscopic surgery for colon and rectal cancer. *Semin in Surg Oncol* 9:59–64, 1993.

38. Schuessler WW, Pharand D, Vancaillie TG: Laparoscopic standard pelvic node dissection for carcinoma of the prostate: Is it accurate? *J Urol* 150:898–901, 1993.

39. Kerbl K, Clayman RV, Petros JA, et al: Staging pelvic lymphadenectomy for prostate cancer: A comparison of laparoscopic and open techniques. *J Urol* 150:396–399, 1993.

40. Bowsher WG, Clark A, Clark DG, et al: Laparoscopic pelvic lymph node dissection for carcinoma of the prostate and bladder. *Aust N Z J Surg.* 62:634–637, 1992.

41. Sisler GE: Malignant tumors of the lung: Role of video-assisted thoracic surgery. *Chest Surg Clin North Am* 3:307–317, 1993.

42. Kirby TJ, Rice TW: Thoracoscopic lobectomy. *Ann Thorac Surg* 56:784–786, 1993.

43. Naruke T, Asamura H, Kondo H, et al: Thoracoscopy for staging of lung cancer. *Ann Thorac Surg* 56:661–663, 1993.

44. Shennib HAF, Landreneau R, Mulder DS, et al: Video-assisted thoracoscopic wedge resection of T1 lung cancer in high-risk patients. *Ann Surg* 218:555–560, 1993.

45. Lewis RJ, Caccavale RJ, Sisler GE, et al: Video-assisted thoracic surgical resection of malignant lung tumors. *J Thorac Cardiovasc Surg* 104:1679–1687, 1992.

46. Krasna MJ, McLaughlin JS: Thorascopic lymph node staging for esophageal cancer. *Ann Thorac Surg* 56:671–674, 1993.

47. Dowling RD, Ferson PF, Landreneau RJ. Thoracoscopic resection of pulmonary metastases. *Chest* 102:1450–1454, 1992.

48. GW Holcomb III (ed): *Pediatric Endoscopic Surgery.* Norwalk, CT: Appleton & Lange, 1994.

49. Holcomb GW, Tomita SS, Haase GM, et al: Minimally invasive surgery in children with cancer. *Cancer* 76:121–128, 1995.

50. Baker LL, Parker BR, Donaldson SS, et al: Staging of Hodgkin's disease in children: Comparison of CT and lymphography with laparotomy. AJR *Am J Roentgenol* 154:1251–1255, 1990.

51. Rodgers BM, Talbert JL. Thoracoscopy for diagnosis of intrathoracic lesions in children. *J Pediatr Surg* 11:703, 1976.

52. Rodgers BM, Moazam F, Talbert JL: Thoracoscopy in children. *Ann Surg* 189:176, 1979.

53. Rodgers BM, Ryckman FC, Moazam F, et al: Thoracoscopy for intrathoracic tumors. *Ann Thorac Surg* 31:414–420, 1981.

54. Rodgers BM: (title of chapter?). In GW Holcomb III (ed): *Thoracoscopy. Pediatric Endoscopic Surgery.* Norwalk, CT: Appleton & Lange, 1994.

55. Rogers DA, Philippe PG, Lobe TE, et al: Thoracoscopy in children: An initial experience with an evolving technique. *J Laparoendosc Surg* 2:7–13, 1992.

56. Ryckman FC, Rodgers BM: Thoracoscopy for

intrathoracic neoplasia in children. *J Pediatr Surg* 17:521–524, 1982.

57. Kern JA, Daniel TM, Tribble CG, et al: Thoracoscopic diagnosis and treatment of mediastinal masses. *Ann Thorac Surg* 56:92–96, 1993.

58. Dajczman E, Gordon A, Kreisman H, et al: Long-term post-thoracotomy pain. *Chest* 99:270–274, 1991.

59. Cameron AE, Parker CJ, Field ES, et al: A randomized comparison of polydioxanone (PDS) and polypropylene (prolene) for abdominal wound closure. *Ann Royal Coll Surg Engl* 69:113–115, 1987.

Vascular Access

• *Jeffrey R. Horwitz, M.D.* • *Kevin P. Lally, M.D., F.A.A.P., F.A.C.S.*

The treatment of childhood malignancies has become increasingly complex and sophisticated with multiagent therapies. Repeated venipunctures quickly deplete usable peripheral sites and lead to significant duress for the child and parents, making dependable, long-lasting vascular access one of the essential requirements for success in such treatment. Consequently, centrally placed, long-term venous catheters have gained widespread acceptance as an important adjunct in the modern care of pediatric cancer patients. These devices provide reliable avenues for delivering repeated and prolonged courses of chemotherapeutic drugs, nutritional support, antibiotics, fluids, and blood components. They also allow routine blood sampling without subjecting the patient to painful, repeated intravenous procedures.

Currently the two main types of catheters used in clinical practice are the tunneled external catheter and the totally implantable access device, or *port*. Insertion of these catheters has become one of the most common procedures performed by pediatric surgeons. A multicenter study from the Children's Cancer Study Group (CCSG) reported the placement of 1141 vascular access devices in pediatric oncology patients over a 2-year period.[1] Despite their general acceptance, these devices are not without risks, sometimes of even life-threatening complications. This chapter reviews the different types of devices currently available, the techniques of operative insertion, and the possible complications of using this increasingly important component in the care of children with cancer.

EXTERNAL CATHETERS

In 1968 Dudrick and coworkers reported the initial experience with providing long-term parenteral nutrition via a polyvinyl catheter inserted in the external jugular vein and threaded into the superior vena cava.[2] The catheter was stiff and created significant thrombotic and infectious complications. In 1973 Broviac and coworkers, after searching for an improved method to deliver home parenteral nutrition, reported on the use of a more flexible catheter made of silicone rubber.[3] Silicone rubber was chosen because it is less thrombogenic and chemically inert.[4] The catheter was 90 cm in length and had an attached Dacron cuff 30 cm from the catheter hub, similar to the design of a peritoneal dialysis catheter. The extravascular segment was tunneled subcutaneously from the site of vascular access (usually a cephalic vein cutdown) to a point on the anterior chest wall, where the cuff was placed just proximal to the exit site. The cuff promoted tissue ingrowth, which was thought to decrease the risk of catheter-related infection and to prevent inadvertent displacement.[3]

In 1979 Hickman and colleagues reported on a modification of this design for use in patients undergoing bone marrow transplantation.[5] The catheter had a slightly thicker wall and an internal diameter 0.10 mm larger to allow for blood sampling as well as infusion of chemotherapeutic agents and blood products. In addition, there was an extra Dacron cuff near the venous entrance site. Today *external tunneled catheters (ECs)* are the most common *vascular access devices (VADs)* in children, and their success is well documented.[6–10] Sizes in single- and multiple-lumen catheters range from 2.7 French for premature neonates to 14 French for older children. The main advantage of ECs is painless access. Disadvantages include a disturbed body image, an exposed catheter exit site that requires regular dressing changes, and a need for frequent catheter irrigation. In addition, the exposed catheter certainly limits some of the normal physical activities that young children enjoy (e.g., swimming).

TOTALLY IMPLANTED DEVICES

Totally implanted devices (TIDs), or *ports*, consist of a subcutaneous reservoir connected to a silicone rubber catheter. Their origin can be traced to attempts at using existing devices from other medical specialties to provide intermittent vascular access. Belin and coworkers used a hydrocephalic shunt to provide central venous nutrition for an infant over a 22-month period.[11] Use of an Ommaya reservoir to deliver long-term intrahepatic chemotherapy in a patient with an unresectable hepatic tumor was described by Fortner and Pahnke.[12] These efforts led to the development and clinical application of the modern implanted VADs.[13–15]

Following catheter insertion, the reservoir—available in stainless steel, titanium, or hard plastic—is placed in a subcutaneous pocket. The port is secured to the underlying fascia with two or three permanent sutures to prevent movement within the pocket. The skin side of the port has a thick silicone-rubber diaphragm roof that overlies the reservoir. Access to the reservoir is accomplished with a special (Huber) needle (Fig. 8–1). The needle's opening is on the side rather than the tip, which avoids coring of the silicone with repeated use. An upper limit of 2000 system

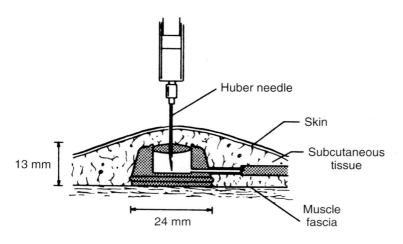

13 mm

24 mm

Huber needle

Skin

Subcutaneous tissue

Muscle fascia

Figure 8–1 • Cross-sectional view of a totally implantable venous access device. (From Bothe A, Jr, Piccione W, Ambrosino JJ, Benotti PN, Lokich JJ: Implantable central venous access system. *Am J Surg* 147:565–569, 1984, with permission.)

punctures before port failure has been reported.[16]

One addition to the VAD inventory is the low-profile PAS port, which is placed subcutaneously in the forearm following central access via a basilic or cephalic venous tributary.[17] This system has all the advantages of the other implanted devices but is much smaller and thus less noticeable. The disadvantage of this device is that because of its small size it may be difficult to access in children with larger amounts of overlying soft tissue.

Implanted ports have gained wide popularity among physicians caring for children with cancer.[18–25] The main advantages of these devices are that no local care is necessary, flushings are required less frequently, and body image is preserved. The main disadvantages are that needle access to the reservoir must occur through the skin, which can be painful, and that removal usually requires a separate operative procedure. A summary of the advantages of both ECs and TIDs is presented in Table 8–1.

COMPARISON OF EXTERNAL CATHETERS WITH TOTALLY IMPLANTED DEVICES

Totally implanted catheters (TIDs) require less manipulation for daily cleaning of the insertion site and less frequent flushing with heparin and are totally subcutaneous. These factors might be

Table 8–2 • Incidence of Catheter-Related Infections in Children with External, Tunneled Catheters

First Author and Reference Number	Catheter Days	Infectious Complications/100 Catheter Days
Severien[26]	6570	0.22
Ross[27]	11,808	0.16
Ingram[30]	19,383	0.29
King[109]	33,394	0.23
van Hoff[140]	12,982	0.23
Johnson[139]	17,581	0.28
Shapiro[110]	5224	0.27
Mulloy[138]	17,861	0.17
Kumar[111]	6463	0.37
Hartman[112]	15,214	0.25
Darbyshire[137]	4290	0.67
Cairo[9]	7650	0.30
Cameron[8]	32,481	0.57
Dawson[7]	83,000	0.21
Mueller[31]	10,592	0.16
Wacker[33]	15,245	0.09
Wurzell[32]	6610	0.21

Table 8–1 • Advantages of External, Tunneled Catheters versus Totally Implanted Devices

External, Tunneled Catheters

Easier to access.
Less expensive than ports.
Pose less risk for extravasation into subcutaneous tissue.
Allow more rapid infusion.
Can be removed at bedside with local anesthesia.

Totally Implanted Ports

Improved cosmetic result.
Less restriction in normal physical activities (e.g., swimming).
Less maintenance care.
Well protected; less chance for damage.
Lower risk of infection.

expected to be associated with a lower rate of infection compared with external, tunneled catheters (ECs), and indeed several retrospective and prospective nonrandomized studies have reported a significant reduction in infectious complications in pediatric oncology cases with TIDs compared with those with ECs.[26–30] These findings were contested by Mueller and coworkers, who performed a prospective randomized trial in adult cancer patients and found no statistical difference in infectious complications between the two types of VAD.[31]

The CCSG review found that ECs were removed more frequently than TIDs for infection, but no data comparing the number of infectious complications per catheter day of use were given.[1] Reports from two other investigators examining pediatric oncology patients reported similar infection rates for ECs and TIDs.[32, 33] Each of these studies, however, was retrospective and nonrandomized in nature. A summary of reports on this subject is shown in Tables 8–2 and 8–3.

Comparisons of these two groups are difficult. Although the majority of data on children suggest that TIDs are associated with a lower risk for infection, ECs are placed far more frequently,

Table 8–3 • Incidence of Catheter-Related Infections in Children with Subcutaneous Ports

First Author and Reference Number	Catheter Days	Infectious Complications/100 Catheter Days
Severien[26]	9611	0.05
Ross[27]	10,478	0.06
Ingram[30]	27,433	0.06
Hockenberry[23]	18,812	0.05
McGovern[18]	6724	0.0001
Golladay[22]	2927	0.034
Pegelow[19]	4094	0.05
Becton[20]	16,101	0.14
Shulman[24]	7558	0.05
Lokich[136]	12,797	0.06
Mueller[31]	14,634	0.12
Wacker[33]	10,356	0.05
Wurzell[32]	9163	0.14

which may contribute to the higher rate of infection sometimes associated with them. In addition, the definition of a catheter-related infection may vary from one institution to another. A prospective randomized investigation is ultimately needed to make a true comparison. However, in view of the possible benefit of fewer infectious complications plus the numerous other advantages of TIDs—allowing normal activity, requiring less maintenance, preserving body image—these devices should be preferred for pediatric oncology patients.

SINGLE- VERSUS MULTIPLE-LUMEN CATHETERS

Multiple-lumen catheters were developed because of a need for repeated central venous access in some patients and to reduce the potential for incompatibility between simultaneously delivered medications. But concern has been raised that use of these multiple-lumen catheters may increase the risk for catheter-related infection.[34] Shulman and colleagues conducted a prospective nonrandomized study of pediatric oncology patients that revealed, in spite of the greater number of catheter manipulations in the double-lumen group, no difference in the incidence of catheter infection.[35] Other investigators have also found no increased risk for infection with multi-

ple- versus single-lumen catheters.[1, 26] Still others have found up to a twofold increase in infection rates with multiple-lumen catheters.[36]

Each case must be judged on an individual basis, and the benefits of additional lumens must be weighed against the possible increased risk of infection. Certainly, since some evidence does exist of an increased risk of infection, the use of multiple-lumen catheters should be limited to patients requiring long-term access for simultaneous administration of two or more solutions.

PATIENT AND FAMILY ACCEPTANCE

There are numerous proponents for both ECs and TIDs. Satisfaction of the patient and family with these VADs is a key factor in deciding which to use. In a prospective study of patient and family acceptance of both ECs and TIDs reported by Poole and coworkers,[37] questionnaires were obtained at 3 and 12 months following catheter placement. The overall response to both devices was positive. The only uniformly negative replies had to do with the daily care required for the ECs and the pain associated with accessing the TIDs. Yet, even those patients who reported pain with the TIDs strongly recommended the devices. Moreover, the authors of that study admit that topical anesthesia was not routinely used and might well have increased the satisfaction with the implantable ports. Eutectic mixture of local anesthetics (EMLA), a new topical anesthetic ointment, has been shown in a placebo-controlled, double-blind study to significantly reduce pain reported by children following subcutaneous drug reservoir punctures.[38] For maximal effect the cream must be applied at least 1 hour prior to accessing the port. For outpatients the cream can be applied at home just before the child's clinic visit. If the negative factor of painful needle sticks is removed, TIDs will likely become the most desirable type of VAD for long-term use in terms of patient and parent satisfaction.

INSERTION TECHNIQUES

The vein selected for catheter insertion varies according to the preference of the individual surgeon. The most common sites for vascular access are the subclavian, external jugular, and internal jugular veins. Less common alternative sites include the common femoral vein[39] and the saphenous vein.[40] The inferior epigastric vein,[41] the inferior vena cava through translumbar and transhepatic approaches,[42, 43] the intercostal veins,[44] and the azygos vein[45, 46] have been used when other sites are not available. Alaish and coworkers have shown that a portion of splenic tissue placed subcutaneously can also function as an effective method of long-term venous access.[47]

Insertion in Subclavian Vein

Historically, subclavian venous access was obtained indirectly by utilizing the cephalic vein via a cutdown method in the deltopectoral groove.[48] This approach was often hindered by the small diameter of the cephalic vein.[49] The advantages of the percutaneous technique are a decreased operative time and the capability of repeated access in the same site with complication rates no greater than for cutdowns.[50] The early experience of Butts and Glass (1970)[51] with this technique in five children was followed by much larger studies documenting excellent results even in infants weighing less than 1000 g.[52-60]

Procedures are normally performed in the operating room with general endotracheal anesthesia but can be done with local anesthesia and conscious sedation in very cooperative older patients. Fluoroscopy at the time of catheter insertion is a very helpful adjunct for ensuring proper final catheter position. A roll is placed between the patient's shoulder blades, and the neck is extended and turned toward the contralateral side. The neck and chest are prepared and draped. A modified Seldinger technique is used, similar to that described for adults.[61, 62] With the patient in the Trendelenburg position, the subclavian vein is accessed via an infraclavicular approach with an 18-gauge needle positioned just below the medial one third of the clavicle (Fig. 8–2). In an infant, the right and left subclavian veins enter the central circulation at acute angles and are located in a more cephalad position. These angulations become less acute after 1 year of age.[63]

A flexible guidewire is introduced through the needle and advanced. The needle is removed, leaving the guidewire in position. A skin incision is made over the anterior chest wall just lateral to the xiphoid, being careful to avoid any breast tissue in females. A subcutaneous tunnel is created between this incision and the exit site of the guidewire, and the Silastic catheter is brought

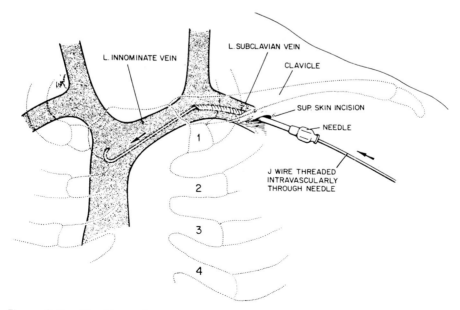

Figure 8–2 • Flexible guidewire is passed into the superior vena cava. (From Cohen AM, Wood WC: Simplified technique for placement of long-term central venous silicone catheters. *Surg Gynecol Obstet* 154:721–724, 1982. By permission of Surgery, Gynecology, and Obstetrics, now known as the Journal of the American College of Surgeons.)

through the tunnel (Fig. 8–3).[64, 65] The catheter is advanced until the Dacron cuff is positioned within the tunnel approximately 2 cm from the lower incision.[1]

The length of catheter necessary to position the tip at the superior vena cava–right atrium junction is estimated. The catheter is trimmed to an appropriate length and flushed with heparinized saline. For port insertion, a subcutaneous pocket is created either by extending the incision at the guidewire exit site or by using a separate incision slightly inferior to the guidewire. It is important to make the pocket large enough so that subsequent needle sticks will not traverse the area of the skin incision. The port is anchored in place with two to four nonabsorbable sutures and is flushed with heparinized saline. The attached catheter is measured for the appropriate length and trimmed.

A vein dilator and peel-away sheath are advanced over the guidewire only enough to enter the subclavian vein (Fig. 8–4). The wire and vein dilator are removed, and the catheter is introduced into the vein through the peel-away sheath (Fig. 8–5). After the catheter is fully ad-

vanced, the sheath is gently peeled apart while the catheter is securely held in place (Fig. 8–6). It may be necessary to slowly advance the catheter at times as the sheath is removed. Catheter position is confirmed by fluoroscopy at the time of insertion or by a chest radiograph postoperatively. Some have reported confirmation of catheter position with electrocardiographic techniques.[66, 67] After proper position is confirmed, the skin incisions are closed with absorbable subcuticular sutures (Fig. 8–7). A nylon suture is placed at the exit site to help prevent catheter dislodgement. An absorbable suture can also be placed just caudal to the Dacron cuff within the tunnel to provide extra protection against unintentional removal.[68]

Because of the acute angle formed at the junction of the subclavian and innominate veins, kinking of the peel-away sheath can create problems with catheter insertion. If this occurs, the guidewire can be reinserted through the catheter and beyond the end of the kinked sheath.[69] The sheath is then backed out slightly to remove the kink, and the catheter is advanced over the guidewire. The most common technical compli-

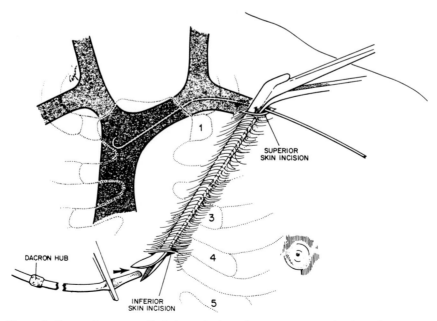

Figure 8–3 • Catheter is pulled through the subcutaneous tunnel. The subcutaneous cuff is positioned approximately 2 cm from the inferior skin incision. (From Cohen AM, Wood WC: Simplified technique for placement of long-term central venous silicone catheters. *Surg Gynecol Obstet* 154:721–724, 1982. By permission of Surgery, Gynecology, and Obstetrics, now known as the Journal of the American College of Surgeons.)

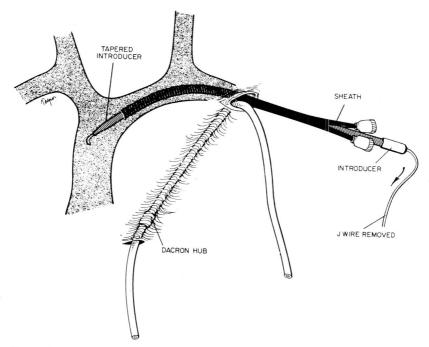

Figure 8–4 • The sheath and tapered introducer are passed over the guidewire. (From Cohen AM, Wood WC: Simplified technique for placement of long-term central venous silicone catheters. *Surg Gynecol Obstet* 154:721–724, 1982. By permission of Surgery, Gynecology, and Obstetrics, now known as the Journal of the American College of Surgeons.)

cations associated with this technique are pneumo- or hemothorax and subclavian artery puncture.[70] Incorrect positioning of the catheter may occur if during insertion fluoroscopy is not used. The reported incidence of aberrant catheter locations following a subclavian approach has been as high as 32%, with the innominate and jugular veins being the most common.[71] If fluoroscopy is available, this problem can be corrected at the time of the original procedure.

Techniques to reposition malpositioned catheters recognized on the post-procedure chest radiograph include burst-fluid injections through the existing catheter,[72] insertion of a Fogarty balloon catheter through the existing catheter,[73] and catheter repositioning with a separate pigtail catheter, inserted by way of a femoral venipuncture.[74] Extreme care must be taken to confirm proper placement of a lower-extremity catheter because there have been reports of accidental lumbar vein cannulation with infusion into the spinal venous plexus and subsequent quadriplegia.[75, 76]

Insertion in Internal/External Jugular Vein

The internal jugular vein (IJV) lies immediately deep to the sternocleidomastoid (SCM) muscle, favoring the lateral side of the triangle created by the two heads of the SCM and the clavicle.[77] The right IJV follows a straight course, entering the innominate vein before ending in the right atrium. Conversely, the left IVJ enters the junction of the confluence of the subclavian and innominate veins at almost a 90° angle. Each external jugular vein (EJV) enters the subclavian vein just lateral to the IJV at a nearly 90° angle, which means that any catheter must make an acute angle to enter the subclavian vein. This angulation may limit the success of the EJV approach in some patients.

Studies on percutaneous cannulation of the internal and external jugular veins in children reported greater success with the IJV compared with the EJV (86% versus 65%), although there was an 8% incidence of carotid artery punc-

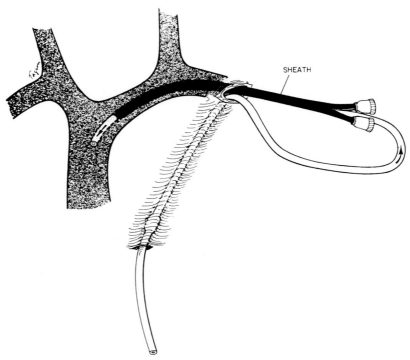

SHEATH

Figure 8–5 • The guidewire and introducer are removed, and the catheter is threaded through the sheath. (From Cohen AM, Wood WC: Simplified technique for placement of long-term central venous silicone catheters. *Surg Gynecol Obstet* 154:721–724, 1982. By permission of Surgery, Gynecology, and Obstetrics, now known as the Journal of the American College of Surgeons.)

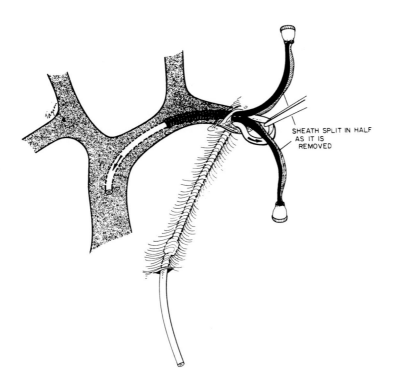

SHEATH SPLIT IN HALF
AS IT IS
REMOVED

Figure 8–6 • The sheath is gradually split and removed while the catheter is slowly advanced. (From Cohen AM, Wood WC: Simplified technique for placement of long-term central venous silicone catheters. *Surg Gynecol Obstet* 154:721–724, 1982. By permission of Surgery, Gynecology, and Obstetrics, now known as the Journal of the American College of Surgeons.)

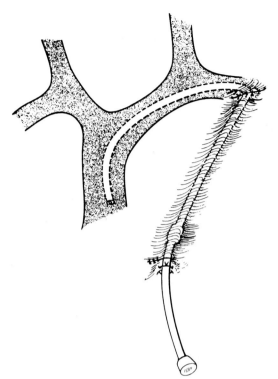

Figure 8–7 • Final position of the catheter. (From Cohen AM, Wood WC: Simplified technique for placement of long-term central venous silicone catheters. *Surg Gynecol Obstet* 154:721–724, 1982. By permission of Surgery, Gynecology, and Obstetrics, now known as the Journal of the American College of Surgeons.)

tures.[78] Hall and Geefhuysen[79] achieved a 90% success rate for IJV cannulation in 100 infants and children. The technique for percutaneous catheterization of both the IJV and EJV is similar to that described for the subclavian vein.

If percutaneous cannulation is not possible, a cutdown on either the EJV or the IJV can be performed. An incision midway between the clavicle and the ramus of the mandible should allow equal access to both the EJV and the IJV.[80] Either vein can be ligated proximally and cannulated directly, or a sizable branch (facial vein, middle thyroid vein) can be accessed, which may preserve main vessel integrity and allow repeated use.[81, 82] Alternatively, if the IJV approach is used, a purse-string suture can be placed around the proposed venotomy site and secured after placement of the catheter. Since the vein does not have to be ligated, this technique may provide

the additional advantage of repeated access via the same site.

COMPLICATIONS

The most common complications reported following placement of long-term central venous catheters are infection and occlusion.[83] Less common but equally serious complications include catheter extravasation,[84] hydrothorax,[85, 86] and cardiac perforation.[87, 88]

Catheter-Related Infection

Catheter-related infection is the most common complication following placement of a long-term central VAD. Infection rates and definitions of catheter-related infection in different institutions are variable. The CCSG study of over 1100 central access devices found that infection was responsible for nearly 20% of all catheter removals.[1] Catheter-related bacteremia is a diagnosis based on the isolation of the same organism from a catheter and a peripheral blood sample.[89] Raucher and coworkers studied patients with suspected catheter-related infection and found an increase in bacterial concentration in blood obtained from the catheter compared with peripheral blood.[90] In each of the nine patients with positive catheter blood cultures the concentration of pathogens was ten times greater than the concentration measured in a peripheral blood sample. This criterion at times can create inaccuracy, however, because blood traveling through the central circulation must traverse the lungs prior to reaching the periphery, and the lungs, as part of the reticuloendothelial system, are capable of removing bacteria from circulation.[91] Flynn and coworkers, therefore, recommend using a fivefold or greater bacterial concentration difference in catheter versus peripheral blood as a means of distinguishing catheter-related from non-catheter-related bacteremia.[92]

Coagulase-negative staphylococci (CONS) are the bacteria most commonly isolated in cases of catheter-related infection.[90, 92] Scanning electron microscopy of intravenous catheters has demonstrated a progressive adherence of CONS to catheter surfaces and has shown their ability to grow and proliferate on both the inner and outer surfaces in the absence of nutrients.[93] In addition, CONS produce a slimelike material, glycocalyx, which enhances their adhesion to the catheter and which may offer protection from the host's natural immune mechanisms. In vitro studies have also shown the ability of CONS to degrade and metabolize superficial catheter components, possibly improving their ability to colonize catheter surfaces.[93]

Modifications in the construction of central venous catheters may be one way to inhibit bacterial colonization. Antibiotic bonding to the catheters has been shown to reduce rates of bacterial adherence and colonization in a rat model following bacterial challenge at the exit site.[94] Unfortunately, 95% of the bound antibiotic became dissociated from the catheter within the first 24 hours, raising the question of whether the antibiotics were truly responsible for the reduced rates of bacteral adherence and colonization.

Greenfeld and coworkers reported that central venous catheters impregnated with chlorhexidine and sulfadiazine silver had significantly less tightly adhering bacteria on their outer and luminal surfaces 7 days following placement.[95] No biofilm (glycocalyx) was detected on any of the treated catheters. Neither of these studies, however, examined the long-term effects of these treatments. Gilsdorf and colleagues[96] found no association between the in vitro bacterial adherence and the tendency of in vitro catheters to become colonized but studied the effects for only 48 hours following catheter placement.

Controversy exists on the origin of catheter-related infections. The skin-entrance site theory is most often proposed.[97] Bacteria are believed to multiply and advance distally along the catheter, through the subcutaneous tissue, and ultimately gain access to the bloodstream. Supporting this theory, a study of 19 positive catheter-segment cultures found the same organism on subcutaneous and intravascular catheter segments as on the catheter exit site. In addition, a greater number of colonies measured from the subcutaneous segment than from the intravascular segment suggested that the infection had begun at the skin level.[97] The success of attachable subcutaneous silver-ion–impregnated cuffs in reducing catheter-related infection is also in agreement with the skin-flora theory.[98, 99] But critics of this hypothesis note that efforts to move the skin-insertion site farther away from the vascular system by tunneling catheters have failed to lower overall infection rates.[100, 101]

An alternative theory suggests that improper technique at the catheter hub may introduce intraluminal infection and may lead to catheter-related bacteremia.[102] A study of suspected catheter-related bacteremia examined 11 patients with positive blood and catheter-tip cultures for CONS. Only three patients had positive CONS skin cultures, and none were of the same species found on the catheter. Cultures of the subcutaneous catheter segments always agreed with the catheter hub, tip, and blood cultures but never with the skin flora.[102] These results were corroborated clinically by studies that showed a reduction in infectious complications obtained by minimizing the risk of catheter-hub contamination and improving staff education.[103, 104] Cooper and Hopkins,[105] using light microscopy and Gram's stain, found microorganisms more often on the outer surface of infected catheters rather than in the lumens, suggesting that the infectious origin was not the catheter hub. Efforts to reduce the incidence of intraluminal colonization of central venous catheters by flushing with a dilute vancomycin solution have not been uniformly successful.[106, 107]

Because of the limited access in a large number of oncology patients and the prolonged length of therapy, preservation of all available long-term venous access sites becomes a priority. Controversy exists about the need for catheter removal following the diagnosis of catheter-related infection. The traditional management of CONS bacteremia has specified catheter removal,[108] but some report successful treatment in 74% to 95% of cases with the catheter left in place.[109–112] Hence, current recommendations include in situ catheter management with antibiotics delivered via the catheter (or port) and repeat blood cultures, both peripheral and central, in 24–48 hours. Patients who respond then continue therapy for 14–21 days.[113] Persistent bacteremia or clinical evidence of sepsis, of course, necessitates expeditious catheter removal.[113–115]

King and coworkers reported that 48% of CONS species were nafcillin-resistant and recommended that administration of vancomycin and an aminoglycoside be the initial therapy for suspected catheter-associated sepsis.[109] Catheter-tunnel and port-pocket infections usually require removal of the device.[30] Careful follow-up is important because the risk of recurrent bacteremia is six times greater in patients when the catheter remains in place.[108]

Some patients with catheter-related sepsis fail to respond to antibiotic therapy unless the catheter is removed, and others are subject to multiple recurrent episodes after a presumed cure, possibly because of an infected thrombus in or along the catheter. Bacteria or fungus may reside deep within this thrombus and thus be unaffected by systemic therapy. Dissolution of the thrombus with urokinase (UK) in combination with antibiotics may improve catheter-salvage rates as well as reduce the incidence of recurrent infections. It did so in one large prospective nonrandomized study,[34] although results from the only randomized prospective study failed to confirm the findings of the nonrandomized study.[116] Unfortunately, the significance of this latter study was limited by a smaller patient enrollment and hemodynamic instability in some patients following UK infusion. Neither study evaluated patients for the presence of a catheter-tip thrombus either before or after UK therapy to better define the responses seen.

The major risk with UK therapy is hemorrhage. UK is a thrombolytic enzyme that converts plasminogen to activated plasmin, which lyses fibrin and results in clot breakdown. If this sequence occurs systemically, significant morbidity and mortality are possible. If a catheter-related infection fails to respond to appropriate antibiotic therapy, the presence of a thrombus at the catheter tip should be suspected. If a thrombus is identified, a bolus of UK in normal saline should be infused through the catheter and repeated 24 hours later. Close observation for signs of systemic fibrinolysis must be maintained. Concurrently, a full course of antibiotic therapy (10–14 days) is given via the catheter.[34] Patients who fail to respond to this protocol should have the catheters removed. A large prospective randomized trial is still necessary to define the benefit of thrombolytic therapy in cases of catheter-related infection.

The incidence of catheter-related fungal infections ranges from 0.3% to 8%.[117] In vitro studies have demonstrated that both *Candida albicans* and *Candida tropicalis* adhere more extensively to polyvinyl chloride (PVC), which is used for manufacturing central venous catheters, than to Teflon, which is generally used for peripheral catheters.[118] Contrary to the case of CONS cathe-

ter-related bacteremia, current information suggests that catheter removal may be required to achieve a successful cure in most cases of fungal catheter infection.

A retrospective review of 71 combined cases of catheter-related *Candida* sepsis found the greatest cure rate occurred with both catheter removal and amphotericin B therapy.[117] Patients who had catheters retained along with amphotericin B therapy had significantly poorer cure rates than those who had catheters removed. The conclusion was that catheter retention in cases of *Candida* infection decreased the chances for cure. Similar results were reported from a single institution reviewing eight cases of *Candida* infections in children treated without catheter removal.[119] Five of the eight patients who had retained catheters and amphotericin B therapy had persistence of *Candida* in the bloodstream. Only one patient was cured with the catheter left in place. One must conclude that catheter removal is necessary in most cases of *Candida* infection.

Occlusion

Occlusion of central venous catheters is a common mechanical problem that typically occurs consequent to thrombus formation in or around the catheter tip.[120] Other, less common causes include a precipitation of poorly soluble fluid components[121] or an anatomic obstruction, most commonly seen in subclavian catheters near the level of the first rib.[122] The formation of a well-organized thrombus around a catheter positioned near the right atrium not only creates a problem with catheter function but places the patient at risk for clot dislodgement, pulmonary embolus,[123, 124] and eventual vessel thrombosis.[125–128] Regular heparinized saline flushes are performed to reduce the incidence of thrombus formation.[129] Studies have documented that flushing with normal saline alone is equally effective.[130]

The incidence of catheter occlusion secondary to a fibrin-sheath or catheter-tip thrombus has been reported to be as high as 31%.[131] UK has been used to treat catheter occlusion resulting from thrombus in a variety of dosing regimens, with low morbidity. Winthrop and Wesson[120] used a bolus injection of 5000 U maintained in the catheter for 2 hours and achieved success in 17 of 21 pediatric cases. Continuous infusions in infants and children with dosages ranging from

100 U/kg/hr up to 10,000 U/kg/hr have been reported, with success rates of 50% to 92%.[131-133]

A pilot study used *tissue plasminogen activator (TPA)*, which may pose less risk for hemorrhagic complications, in children with occluded central catheters.[134] In six patients in whom UK had failed to clear the obstruction, 2 mg/2 ml of TPA were administered, and the obstruction cleared in all but one. No coagulation abnormalities or bleeding was observed.

Simple, noninvasive measurements of catheter resistance may provide earlier identification of poorly functioning catheters in addition to reducing the number of radiographic studies necessary to evaluate catheter patency.[135] The benefit of prompt recognition of catheter occlusion may be to increase the effectiveness of thrombolytic agents.

CONCLUSION

Maintaining long-lasting venous access is a critical concern in treating children with cancer. Less than 25 years ago, chemotherapeutic agents were delivered via peripheral intravenous catheters or temporary central lines, and accidental drug extravasation often led to cellulitis and significant soft-tissue loss. With the development of Silastic catheters and implantable access devices, dependable, long-term vascular access became possible. This approach has produced significant improvements in the quality of life for many patients.

Both tunneled ECs and totally implanted ports provide excellent routes for delivery of chemotherapy and other required infusions. Usually catheters should be inserted using general anesthesia in the operating room. Percutaneous placement via the subclavian or internal jugular vein is safe and effective in most children. Intraoperative fluoroscopy is a useful adjunct for proper placement. Implanted ports are recommended based upon data suggesting a reduced risk for infection, less required maintenance, and superior preservation of body image, which is very important in a young child. Although it may be possible to leave many of these devices in place throughout the completion of therapy, serious complications can occur that require removal. Most catheter-related infections can be treated with the catheter in situ. An exception is *Candida* infections. Occlusion secondary to thrombus formation, if recognized in a timely fashion, can usually be successfully managed with thrombolytic therapy.

References

1. Wiener ES, McGuire P, Stolar CJH, et al: The CCSG prospective study of venous access devices: An analysis of insertions and causes for removal. *J Pediatr Surg* 27:155–164, 1992.
2. Dudrick SJ, Wilmore DW, Vars HM, Rhoads JE: Long-term total parenteral nutrition with growth, development, and positive nitrogen balance. *Surgery* 64:134–142, 1968.
3. Broviac JW, Cole JJ, Scribner BH: A silicone rubber atrial catheter for prolonged parenteral alimentation. *Surg Gynecol Obstet* 136:602–606, 1973.
4. Atkins RC, Vizzo JE, Cole JJ, Blagg CR, Scribner BH: The artificial gut in hospital and home: Technical improvements. *Trans Am Soc Artif Intern Organs* 16:260–268, 1970.
5. Hickman RO, Buckner CD, Clift RA, et al: A modified right atrial catheter for access to the venous system in marrow transplant recipients. *Surg Gynecol Obstet* 148:871–875, 1979.
6. Weber TR, West KW, Grosfeld JL: Broviac central venous catheterization in infants and children. *Am J Surg* 145:202–204, 1983.
7. Dawson S, Pai MKR, Smith S, Rothney M, Ahmed K, Barr RD: Right atrial catheters in children with cancer: A decade of experience in the use of tunneled, exteriorized devices at a single institution. *Am J Pediatr Hematol Oncol* 13:126–129, 1991.
8. Cameron GS: Central venous catheters for children with malignant disease: Surgical Issues. *J Pediatr Surg* 22:702–704, 1987.
9. Cairo MS, Spooner S, Sowden L, Bennetts GA, Towne B, Hodder F: Long-term use of indwelling multipurpose Silastic catheters in pediatric cancer patients treated with aggressive chemotherapy. *J Clin Oncol* 4:784–788, 1986.
10. Merritt RJ, Ennis CE, Andrassy RJ, et al: Use of Hickman right atrial catheter in pediatric oncology patients. *JPEN* 5:83–85, 1981.
11. Belin RP, Koster JK, Bryant LJ, Griffen WO: Implantable subcutaneous feeding chamber for noncontinuous central venous alimentation. *Surg Gynecol Obstet* 174:491–493, 1972.
12. Fortner JG, Pahnke LD: A new method for long term intrahepatic chemotherapy. *Surg Gynecol Obstet* 143:979–980, 1976.
13. Gyves JW, Ensminger W, Niederhuber JE, et al: Totally implanted system for intravenous chemotherapy in patients with cancer. *Am J Med* 73:841–845, 1982.
14. Niederhuber JE, Ensminger W, Gyves JW, et al: Totally implanted venous and arterial access system to replace external catheters in cancer treatment. *Surgery* 92:706–712, 1982.

15. Bothe A Jr, Piccione W, Ambrosino JJ, Benotti PN, Lokich JJ: Implantable central venous access system. *Am J Surg* 147:565–569, 1984.

16. Soucy P: Experiences with the use of the port-a-cath in children. *J Pediatr Surg* 22:767–769, 1987.

17. Pearl JM, Goldstein L, Ciresi KF: Improved methods in long-term venous access using the P.A.S. port. *Surg Gynecol Obstet* 173:313–315, 1991.

18. McGovern B, Solenberger R, Reed K: A totally implantable venous access system for long-term chemotherapy in children. *J Pediatr Surg* 20:725–727, 1985.

19. Pegelow CH, Narvaez M, Toledano SR, et al: Experience with a totally implantable venous device in children. *Am J Dis Child* 140:69–71, 1986.

20. Becton DL, Kletzel M, Golladay ES, Hathaway G, Berry DH: An experience with an implanted port system in 66 children with cancer. *Cancer* 61:376–378, 1988.

21. Krul EJ, van Leeuwen EF, Vos A, Voute PA: Continuous venous access in children for long-term chemotherapy by means of an implantable system. *J Pediatr Surg* 21:689–690, 1986.

22. Golladay ES, Mollitt DL: Percutaneous placement of a venous access port in a pediatric patient population. *J Pediatr Surg* 21:683–684, 1986.

23. Hockenberry MJ, Schultz WH, Bennett B, Bryant R, Falletta JM: Experience with minimal complications in implanted catheters in children. *Am J Pediatr Hematol Oncol* 11:295–299, 1989.

24. Shulman RJ, Rahman S, Mahoney D, Pokorny WJ, Bloss R: A totally implanted venous access system used in pediatric patients with cancer. *J Clin Oncol* 5:137–140, 1987.

25. Essex-Cater A, Gilbert J, Robinson T, Littlewood JM: Totally implantable venous access systems in paediatric practice. *Arch Dis Child* 64:119–123, 1989.

26. Severien C, Nelson JD: Frequency of infections associated with implanted systems vs cuffed, tunneled Silastic venous catheters in patients with acute leukemia. *Am J Dis Child* 145:1433–1438, 1991.

27. Ross MN, Haase GM, Poole MA, Burrington JD, Odom LF: Comparison of totally implanted reservoirs with external catheters as venous access devices in pediatric oncologic patients. *Surg Gynecol Obstet* 167:141–144, 1988.

28. Mirro J Jr, Rao BN, Stokes DC, et al: A prospective study of Hickman/Broviac catheters and implantable ports in pediatric oncology patients. *J Clin Oncol* 7:214–222, 1989.

29. Mirro J Jr, Rao BN, Kumar M, et al: A comparison of placement techniques and complications of externalized catheters and implantable port use in children with cancer. *J Pediatr Surg* 25:120–124, 1990.

30. Ingram J, Weitzman S, Greenberg ML, Parkin P, Filler R: Complications of indwelling venous access lines in the pediatric hematology patient: A prospective comparison of external venous catheters and subcutaneous ports. *Am J Pediatr Hematol Oncol* 13:130–136, 1991.

31. Mueller BU, Skelton J, Callender DPE, et al: A prospective randomized trial comparing the infectious and noninfectious complications of an externalized catheter versus a subcutaneously implanted device in cancer patients. *J Clin Oncol* 10:1943–1948, 1992.

32. Wurzel CL, Halom K, Feldman JG, Rubin LG: Infection rates of Broviac-Hickman catheters and implantable venous devices. *Am J Dis Child* 142:536–540, 1988.

33. Wacker P, Bugmann P, Halperin DS, Babel JF, Le Coultre C, Wyss M: Comparison of totally implanted and external catheters in paediatric oncology patients. *Eur J Cancer* 28A:841–844, 1992.

34. Jones GR, Konsler GK, Dunaway RP, Lacey SR, Azizkhan RG: Prospective analysis of urokinase in the treatment of catheter sepsis in pediatric hematology-oncology patients. *J Pediatr Surg* 28:350–357, 1993.

35. Shulman RJ, O'Brian Smith E, Rahman S, Gardner P, Reed T, Mahoney D: Single- vs double-lumen central venous catheters in pediatric oncology patients. *Am J Dis Child* 142:893–895, 1988.

36. Vane DW, Ong B, Rescorla FJ, West KW, Grosfeld JL: Complications of central venous access in children: A review of 2281 catheter insertions. *Pediatr Surg Int* 5:174–178, 1990.

37. Poole MA, Ross MN, Haase GM, Odom LF: Right atrial catheters in pediatric oncology: A patient/parent questionnaire study. *Am J Pediatr Hematol Oncol* 13:152–155, 1991.

38. Halperin DL, Koren G, Attias D, Pellegrini E, Greenberg ML, Wyss M: Topical skin anesthesia for venous, subcutaneous drug reservoir and lumbar punctures in children. *Pediatrics* 84:281–284, 1989.

39. Kanter RK, Zimmerman JJ, Strauss RH, Stoeckel KA: Central venous catheter insertion by femoral vein: Safety and effectiveness for the pediatric patient. *Pediatrics* 77:842–847, 1986.

40. Fonkalsrud EW, Berquist W, Burke M, Ament ME: Long-term hyperalimentation in children through saphenous central venous catheterization. *Am J Surg* 143:209–211, 1982.

41. Donahoe PK, Kim SH: The inferior epigastric vein as an alternative site for central venous hyperalimentation. *J Pediatr Surg* 15:737–738, 1980.

42. Azizkhan RG, Taylor LA, Jaques PF, Mauro MA, Lacey SR: Percutaneous translumbar and transhepatic inferior vena caval catheters for prolonged vascular access in children. *J Pediatr Surg* 27:165–169, 1992.

43. Robertson LJ, Jaques PF, Mauro MA, Azizkhan

RG, Robards J: Percutaneous inferior vena cava placement of tunneled Silastic catheters for prolonged vascular access in infants. *J Pediatr Surg* 25:596–598, 1990.

44. Newman BM, Cooney DR, Karp MP, Jewett TC Jr: The intercostal vein: An alternate route for central venous alimentation. *J Pediatr Surg* 18:732–733, 1983.

45. Silverman SH, Stringel G: Two techniques for central catheter placement in the hypogastric and azygos veins. *Pediatr Surg Int* 3:62–63, 1988.

46. Pokorny WJ, McGill CW, Harberg FJ: Use of the azygous vein for central catheter insertion. *Surgery* 97:362, 1984.

47. Alaish SM, Narla LD, Bagwell CE: Long-term venous access using endogenous splenic tissue: The "Spleen-O-Port." *J Pediatr Surg* 30:1198–1200, 1995.

48. Heimbach DM, Ivey TD: Technique for placement of a permanent home hyperalimentation catheter. *Surg Gynecol Obstet* 143:634–636, 1976.

49. Linos DA, Muncha P Jr: A simplified technique for the placement of permanent central venous catheters. *Surg Gynecol Obstet* 154:248–250, 1982.

50. Davis SJ, Thompson JS, Edney JA: Insertion of Hickman catheters: A comparison of cutdown and percutaneous techniques. *Am Surg* 50:673–676, 1984.

51. Butts DR, Glass HG: Percutaneous subclavian vein catheterization in children. *Tex Med* 66:46–48, 1970.

52. Morgan WW Jr, Harkins GA: Percutaneous introduction of long-term indwelling venous catheters in infants. *J Pediatr Surg* 7:538–541, 1972.

53. Groff DB, Ahmed N: Subclavian vein catheterization in the infant. *J Pediatr Surg* 9:171–174, 1974.

54. Filson HC, Grant JP: A safer system for percutaneous subclavian venous catheterization in newborn infants. *J Pediatr Surg* 14:564–570, 1979.

55. Eichelberger MR, Rous PG, Hoelzer DJ, Garcia VF, Koop CE: Percutaneous subclavian venous catheters in neonates and children. *J Pediatr Surg* 16:547–553, 1981.

56. Gauderer MWL, Stellato TA, Izant RJ Jr: Broviac Silastic catheter insertion in children: A simplified direct subclavian approach. *J Pediatr Surg* 17:580–584, 1982.

57. Gauderer MWL, Stellato TA: Subclavian Broviac catheters in children—Technical considerations in 146 consecutive patients. *J Pediatr Surg* 20:402–405, 1985.

58. Kron IL, Rheuban K, Miller ED, Lake CL, Nolan SP: Subclavian vein catheterization for central line placement in children under 2 years of age. *Am Surg* 51:272–273, 1985.

59. Newman BM, Jewett TC Jr, Karp MP, Cooney DR: Percutaneous central venous catheterization in children: First-line choice for venous access. *J Pediatr Surg* 21:685–688, 1986.

60. Bonventre EV, Lally KP, Chwals WJ, Hardin WD Jr, Atkinson JB: Percutaneous insertion of subclavian venous catheters in infants and children. *Surg Gynecol Obstet* 169:203–205, 1989.

61. Linos DA, Muncha P Jr: A simplified technique for the placement of permanent central venous catheters. *Surg Gynecol Obstet* 154:248–250, 1982.

62. Cohen AM, Wood WC: Simplified technique for placement of long-term central venous silicone catheters. *Surg Gynecol Obstet* 154:721–724, 1982.

63. Cobb LM, Vinocur CD, Wagner CW, Weintraub WH: The central venous anatomy in infants. *Surg Gynecol Obstet* 165:230–234, 1987.

64. Holt RW, Heres EK: Creation of a subcutaneous tunnel for Broviac and Hickman catheters. *JPEN* 9:225, 1985.

65. Klein MD, Coran AG: A technique for tunneling central venous catheters. *JPEN* 9:521–522, 1985.

66. Koscielniak-Nielsen ZJ, Otkjaer S, Hansen OB, Hemmingsen C: CVP catheter electrocardiography: An alternative to radiographic control after cannulation of central veins? *Acta Anaesthesiol Scand* 35:762–766, 1991.

67. Hoffman MA, Langer JC, Pearl RH, et al: Central venous catheters—No x-rays needed: A prospective study in 50 consecutive infants and children. *J Pediatr Surg* 12:1201–1203, 1988.

68. Vazquez RM, Racenstein MJ: A method to prevent unintentional removal of a Hickman catheter. *JPEN* 11:509–510, 1987.

69. Atkinson JB, Chamberlin KL, de Csepel J, Srikanth M: Overcoming a kinked peel-away sheath during central line implantation. *J Pediatr Surg* 29:379–380, 1994.

70. Feliciano D, Mattox K, Graham J, et al: Major complications of percutaneous subclavian vein catheters. *Am J Surg* 138:869–874, 1979.

71. Conces DJ Jr, Holden RW: Aberrant locations and complications in initial placement of subclavian vein catheters. *Arch Surg* 119:293–295, 1984.

72. Warner BW, Ryckman FC: A simple technique to redirect malpositioned Silastic central venous catheters. *JPEN* 16:473–476, 1992.

73. Schaefer CJ, Geelhoed GW: Redirection of misplaced central venous catheters. *Arch Surg* 115:789–791, 1980.

74. Walker TG, Geller SC, Waltman AC, Malt RA, Athanasoulis CA: A simple technique for redirection of malpositioned Broviac or Hickman catheters. *Surg Gynecol Obstet* 167:247–248, 1988.

75. Greenholz SK, Karrer FM, Lilly JR:

Quadriplegia complicating parenteral nutrition. *Pediatr Surg Int* 3:64–65, 1988.

76. Mah MP, Fain JS, Hall SL, Wood BP: Intravenous hyperalimentation fluid obtained with lumbar puncture: An unusual complication of a central venous catheter. *Am J Dis Child* 145:1439–1440, 1991.

77. Cobb LM, Goss JC, Gilsdorf RB: Regional anatomy regarding the placement of central venous cannulas. *Ariz Med* 38:33–36, 1981.

78. Nicolson SC, Sweeney MF, Moore RA, Jobes DR: Comparison of internal and external jugular cannulation of the central circulation in the pediatric patient. *Crit Care Med* 13:747–749, 1985.

79. Hall DMB, Geefhuysen J: Percutaneous catheterization of the internal jugular vein in infants and children. *J Pediatr Surg* 12:719–722, 1977.

80. Kosloske AM, Klein MD: Techniques of central venous access for long-term parenteral nutrition in infants. *Surg Gynecol Obstet* 154:395–399, 1982.

81. Zumbro GL Jr, Mullin MJ, Nelson TG: Catheter placement in infants needing total parenteral nutrition utilizing common facial vein. *Arch Surg* 102:71–73, 1971.

82. Toufanian A, Knight P: The middle thyroid vein: An alternative route for central venous catheter insertion. *J Pediatr Surg* 18:156–157, 1983.

83. Wesley JR: Permanent central venous access devices. *Semin Pediatr Surg* 1:188–201, 1992.

84. Krasna IH, Krause T: Life-threatening fluid extravasation of central venous catheters. *J Pediatr Surg* 26:1346–1348, 1991.

85. Ross P Jr, Seashore JH: Bilateral hydrothorax complicating central venous catheterization in a child. *J Pediatr Surg* 24:263–264, 1989.

86. Iberti TJ, Katz LB, Reiner MA, Brownie T, Kwun KB: Hydrothorax as a late complication of central venous indwelling catheters. *Surgery* 94:842–846, 1983.

87. Agarwal KC, Ali Khan MA, Falla A, Amato JJ: Cardiac perforation from central venous catheters: Survival after cardiac tamponade in an infant. *Pediatrics* 73:333–338, 1984.

88. Cathcart-Rake WF, Mowery WE: Intrapericardial infusion of 5-fluorouracil. *Cancer* 67:735–737, 1991.

89. Norwood S, Ruby Allan, Civetta J, Cortes V: Catheter-related infections and associated septicemia. *Chest* 99:968–975, 1991.

90. Raucher HS, Hyatt AC, Barzilai A, et al: *Quantitative* blood cultures in the evaluation of septicemia in children with Broviac catheters. *J Pediatr* 104:29–33, 1984.

91. Crocker SH, Lowery BD, Eddy DO, et al: Pulmonary clearance of blood-borne bacteria. *Surg Gynecol Obstet* 153:845–851, 1981.

92. Flynn PM, Shenep JL, Stokes DC, Barrett FF: In situ management of confirmed central venous catheter-related bacteremia. *Pediatr Infect Dis J* 6:729–734, 1987.

93. Peters G, Locci R, Pulverer G: Adherence and growth of coagulase-negative staphylococci on surfaces of intravenous catheters. *J Infect Dis* 146:479–482, 1982.

94. Trooskin SZ, Donetz AP, Harvey RA, Greco RS: Prevention of catheter sepsis by antibiotic bonding. *Surgery* 97:547–551, 1985.

95. Greenfeld JI, Sampath L, Popilskis SJ, Brunnert SR, Stylianos S, Modak S: Decreased bacterial adherence and biofilm formation on chlorhexidine and silver sulfadiazine-impregnated central venous catheters implanted in swine. *Crit Care Med* 23:894–900, 1995.

96. Gilsdorf JR, Wilson K, Beals TF: Bacterial colonization of intravenous catheter materials in vitro and in vivo. *Surgery* 106:37–44, 1989.

97. Bjornson HS, Colley R, Bower RH, Duty VP, Schwartz-Fulton JT, Fischer JE: Association between microorganism growth at the catheter insertion site and colonization of the catheter in patients receiving total parenteral nutrition. *Surgery* 92:720–727, 1982.

98. Flowers RH III, Schwenzer KJ, Kopel R, Fisch MJ, Tucker SI, Farr BM: Efficacy of an attachable subcutaneous cuff for the prevention of intravascular catheter-related infection: A randomized, controlled trial. *J Am Med Assoc* 261:878–883, 1989.

99. Maki DG, Cobb L, Garman JK, Shapiro JM, Ringer M, Helgerson RB: An attachable silver-impregnated cuff for prevention of infection with central venous catheters: A prospective randomized multicenter trial. *Am J Med* 85:307–314, 1988.

100. von Meyenfeldt MMF, Stapert J, de Jong PCM, et al: TPN catheter sepsis: Lack of effect of subcutaneous tunnelling of PVC catheters on sepsis rate. *JPEN* 4:514–517, 1980.

101. Sitges-Serra A, Linares J: Tunnels do not protect against venous-catheter-related sepsis. *Lancet* 1:459–460 (letter), 1984.

102. Sitges-Serra A, Linares J, Garau J: Catheter sepsis: The clue is the hub. *Surgery* 97:355–357, 1985.

103. Puntis JWL, Holden CE, Smallman S, Finkel Y, George RH, Booth IW: Staff training: A key factor in reducing intravascular catheter sepsis. *Arch Dis Child* 65:335–337, 1990.

104. Stotter AT, Ward H, Waterfield AH, Hilton J, Sim AJW: Junctional care: The key to prevention of catheter sepsis in intravenous feeding. *JPEN* 11:159–162, 1987.

105. Cooper GL, Hopkins CC: Rapid diagnosis of intravascular catheter-associated infection by direct Gram staining of catheter segments. *N Engl J Med* 312:1142–1147, 1985.

106. Rackoff WR, Weiman M, Jakobowski D, et al: A randomized, controlled trial of the efficacy of a heparin and vancomycin solution in preventing central venous catheter infections in children. *J Pediatr* 127:147–151, 1995.

107. Schwartz C, Henrickson KJ, Roghmann K, Powell K: Prevention of bacteremia attributed to luminal colonization of tunneled central venous catheters with vancomycin-susceptible organisms. *J Clin Oncol* 8:1591–1597, 1990.

108. Raad I, Davis S, Khan A, Tarrand J, Elting L, Bodey GP: Impact of central venous catheter removal on the recurrence of catheter-related coagulase-negative staphylococcal bacteremia. *Infect Control Hosp Epidemiol* 13:215–221, 1992.

109. King DR, Komer M, Hoffman J, Ginn-Pease ME, et al: Broviac catheter sepsis: The natural history of an iatrogenic infection. *J Pediatr Surg* 20:728–733, 1985.

110. Shapiro ED, Wald ER, Nelson KA, Spiegelman KN: Broviac catheter-related bacteremia in oncology patients. *Am J Dis Child* 136:679–681, 1982.

111. Kumar A, Brar SS, Murray DL, Leater I, Gera R, Kulkarni R: Central venous catheter infections in pediatric patients in a community hospital. *Infect* 16:86–90, 1988.

112. Hartman GE, Shochat SJ: Management of septic complications associated with Silastic catheters in childhood malignancy. *Pediatr Infect Dis J* 6:1042–1047, 1987.

113. Hiemenz J, Skelton J, Pizzo PA: Perspective on the management of catheter-related infections in cancer patients. *Pediatr Infect Dis J* 5:6–11, 1986.

114. Nahata MC, King DR, Powell DA, Marx SM, Ginn-Pease ME: Management of catheter-related infections in pediatric patients. *JPEN* 12:58–59, 1988.

115. Wang EEL, Prober CG, Ford-Jones L, Gold R: The management of central intravenous catheter infections. *Pediatr Infect Dis J* 3:110–113, 1984.

116. La Quaglia MP, Caldwell C, Lucas A, et al: A prospective randomized double-blind trial of bolus urokinase in the treatment of established Hickman catheter sepsis in children. *J Pediatr Surg* 29:742–745, 1994.

117. Dato VM, Dajani AS: Candidemia in children with central venous catheters: Role of catheter removal and amphotericin B therapy. *Pediatr Infect Dis J* 9:309–314, 1990.

118. Rotrosen D, Gibson TR, Edwards JE Jr: Adherence of *Candida* species to intravenous catheters. *J Infect Dis* 147:594, 1983.

119. Eppes SC, Troutman JL, Gutman LT: Outcome of treatment of candidemia in children whose central catheters were removed or retained. *Pediatr Infect Dis J* 8:99–104, 1989.

120. Winthrop AL, Wesson DE: Urokinase in the treatment of occluded central venous catheters in children. *J Pediatr Surg* 19:536–538, 1984.

121. Shulman RJ, Reed T, Pitre D, Laine L: Use of hydrochloric acid to clear obstructed central venous catheters. *JPEN* 12:509–510, 1988.

122. Aitken DR, Minton JP: The "pinch-off sign": A warning of impending problems with permanent subclavian catheters. *Am J Surg* 148:633–636, 1984.

123. Hassall E, Ulich T, Ament ME: Pulmonary embolus and *Malassezia* pulmonary infection related to urokinase therapy. *J Pediatr* 102:722–725, 1983.

124. Mahony L, Snider R, Silverman NH: Echocardiographic diagnosis of intracardiac thrombi complicating total parenteral nutrition. *J Pediatr* 98:469–471, 1981.

125. Belcastro S, Susa A, Pavanelli L, Guberti A, Buccoliero C: Thrombosis of the superior vena cava due to a central catheter for total parenteral nutrition. *JPEN* 14:31–33, 1990.

126. Fonkalsrud EW, Ament ME, Berquist WE, Burke M: Occlusion of the vena cava in infants receiving central venous hyperalimentation. *Surg Gynecol Obstet* 154:189–192, 1982.

127. Graham L Jr, Gumbiner CH: Right atrial thrombus and superior vena cava syndrome in a child. *Pediatrics* 73:225–229, 1984.

128. Berman W Jr, Fripp RR, Yabek SM, Wernly J, Corlew S: Great vein and right atrial thrombosis in critically ill infants and children with central venous lines. *Chest* 99:963–967, 1991.

129. Garrelts JC, LaRocca J, Ast D, Smith DF Jr, Sweet DE: Comparison of heparin and 0.9% sodium chloride injection in the maintenance of indwelling intermittent i.v. devices. *Clin Pharm* 8:34–39, 1989.

130. Smith S, Dawson S, Hennessey R, Andrew M: Maintenance of the patency of indwelling central venous catheters: Is heparin necessary? *Am J Pediatr Hematol Oncol* 13:141–143, 1991.

131. Bagnall HA, Gomperts E, Atkinson JB: Continuous infusion of low-dose urokinase in the treatment of central venous catheter thrombosis in infants and children. *Pediatrics* 83:963–966, 1989.

132. Ross P Jr, Ehrenkranz R, Kleinman CS, Seashore JH: Thrombus associated with central venous catheters in infants and children. *J Pediatr Surg* 24:253–256, 1989.

133. Curnow A, Idowu J, Behrens E, Toomey F, Georgeson K: Urokinase therapy for Silastic catheter-induced intravascular thrombi in infants and children. *Arch Surg* 120:1237–1240, 1985.

134. Atkinson JB, Bagnall HA, Gomperts E: Investigational use of tissue plasminogen activator (t-PA) for occluded central venous catheters. *JPEN* 14:310–311, 1990.

135. Stokes DC, Rao BN, Mirro J Jr, et al: Early detection and simplified management of obstructed Hickman and Broviac catheters. *J Pediatr Surg* 24:257–262, 1989.

136. Lokich JJ, Bothe A Jr, Benoti P, Moore C: Complications and management of implanted venous access catheters. *J Clin Oncol* 3:710–717, 1985.

137. Darbyshire PJ, Weightman NC, Speller DCE:

Problems associated with indwelling central venous catheters. *Arch Dis Child* 60:129–134, 1985.

138. Mulloy RH, Jadavji T, Russell ML: Tunneled central venous catheter sepsis: Risk factors in a pediatric hospital. *JPEN* 15:460–463, 1991.

139. Johnson PR, Decker MD, Edwards KM, Schaffner W, Wright PF: Frequency of Broviac catheter infections in pediatric oncology patients. *J Infect Dis* 154:570–578, 1986.

140. Van Hoff J, Berg AT, Seashore JH: The effect of right atrial catheters on infectious complications of chemotherapy in children. *J Clin Oncol* 8:1255–1262, 1990.

Chapter 9

Wilms' Tumor

• *Michael L. Ritchey, M.D.*

The first published reports of childhood renal tumors were in the early 1800s, but early histologic descriptions were incomplete. The earliest known specimen of Wilms' tumor is preserved in the Hunterian Museum of the Royal College of Surgeons in London.[1] The kidneys of a young child with bilateral renal masses were saved by John Hunter sometime before 1793. Microscopic sections have been prepared from these well-preserved specimens that confirm the diagnosis of Wilms' tumor. Numerous reports of renal tumors followed, and a variety of eponyms were ascribed to these lesions. In 1899 surgeon Max Wilms proposed that all the various elements of the tumor were derived from the same cell,[2] and his careful pathologic description of this tumor led to the association of his name with it.

The first successful removal of a renal tumor in a child was by Kocher in 1886, but most children still succumbed to this disease at the turn of the century. As anesthetic and surgical techniques improved, long-term survivors of Wilms' tumor were reported. Nevertheless, by the late 1930s only 30% of patients with organ-confined disease were being helped by surgery. Radiation was added to the treatment of these tumors when they were found to be radioresponsive,[3] but it was the introduction of effective chemotherapy in the 1950s that produced a dramatic improvement in outcome.[4] In the past few decades, randomized trials conducted by cooperative groups such as the National Wilms' Tumor Study Group (NWTSG) and the International Society of Pediatric Oncology have resulted in excellent survival rates for children with nephroblastoma. The focus is now on reducing the morbidity of treatment for low-risk patients. Survival remains poor for some high-risk patients, and new treatment strategies are needed for them.

EPIDEMIOLOGY

Wilms' tumor is the most common malignant renal tumor of childhood, representing 5% to 6% of childhood cancers in the United States.[5] About 450–500 new cases are diagnosed annually in the United States for an incidence of 1 in 10,000 children.[6] The peak incidence of nephroblastoma occurs at 36.5 months of age for males and 42.5 months for females with unilateral tumors. The disease occurs nearly equally in girls and boys worldwide.[7] There is some ethnic variation in the incidence of childhood kidney tumors, with slightly higher rates reported for the black populations relative to white populations and a lower incidence in Asian children.

A number of studies have examined environmental risk factors in the development of Wilms' tumor. Early reports suggested that paternal exposure to hydrocarbons and lead might play a role.[8] Later studies, however, failed to show a consistent association of Wilms' tumor with any parental environmental exposure.[9]

ASSOCIATED SYNDROMES

Nephroblastoma is known to be associated with a number of congenital abnormalities, including sporadic aniridia, hemihypertrophy, and genitourinary malformations.[10] The incidence of these conditions for children registered in the NWTSG is reported in Table 9–1.

The incidence of aniridia in Wilms' tumor patients is 1.1%. There are two forms of aniridia, sporadic and familial, and nephroblastoma almost always occurs in association with the nonfamilial, or sporadic, form. Aniridia is a rare malformation, occurring in 1 in 50,000 persons. Aniridia and Wilms' tumor are most commonly associated in patients with the WAGR syndrome. Up to 50% of such affected individuals develop Wilms' tumor.[11] This syndrome is characterized by aniridia, genital anomalies, and mental retardation.[12] Most affected individuals have a constitutional deletion on chromosome 11.

Hemihypertrophy occurs in 3% of patients with Wilms' tumor and may not become clinically apparent until after that diagnosis is made.[13, 14] Isolated involvement of the leg is the most common manifestation in these patients. It may be ipsilateral or contralateral to the tumor.[15] Hemi-

Table 9–1 • Incidence of Congenital Anomalies Associated with Wilms' Tumor Patients as Reported to the National Wilms' Tumor Study

Anomaly	Rate (per 1000)
Aniridia	7.6
Beckwith-Wiedemann Syndrome	8.4
Hemihypertrophy	33.8
Genitourinary anomalies	
Hypospadias	13.4
Cryptorchidism	37.3
Hypospadias and cryptorchidism	12.0

hypertrophy, usually idiopathic, occurs at a rate of 1:53,000 in the general population. The risk of Wilms' tumor development in patients with hemihypertrophy is estimated to be on the order of 3–5%.[16]

Beckwith-Wiedemann syndrome (BWS) is a rare disorder consisting of developmental anomalies characterized by excess growth at the cellular, tissue (renal, pancreatic), organ (macroglossia, hepatomegaly), or body-segment (hemihypertrophy) levels.[17, 18] The incidence of tumor development is 10% to 20% and includes Wilms' tumor, adrenocortical neoplasms, and hepatoblastoma. Most cases of BWS are sporadic, but 15% exhibit heritable characteristics with apparent autosomal dominant inheritance. The mean age at diagnosis of Wilms' tumor in patients with BWS and hemihypertrophy is similar to that of the general Wilms' tumor population.[19]

Genitourinary anomalies (hypospadias, cryptorchidism, renal fusion anomalies) are present in 4.5% of patients with Wilms' tumor.[15] Since many of these disorders are common in children, prospective evaluation for the development of Wilms' tumor is not carried out in most children with genital anomalies. Of particular interest is the association of nephroblastoma with male pseudohermaphroditism and renal mesangial sclerosis, the Denys-Drash syndrome.[20, 21] Over 60 cases have been reported in the literature, and genetic studies indicate that Denys-Drash syndrome is associated with a specific mutation on the 11 chromosome.[22] One should have a high index of suspicion, therefore, for the development of these conditions in patients with male pseudohermaphroditism.

GENETICS

The genetics of Wilms' tumor was once thought to be very similar to that of retinoblastoma. Both tumors can be bilateral, and familial cases have been reported. Nephroblastoma is generally diagnosed at an earlier age in patients with congenital anomalies and in children with bilateral tumors.[14] Analysis of these differences between groups of patients with regard to age at diagnosis and multicentricity of tumors led to the proposal of a two-hit mutation theory for Wilms' tumor formation similar to that proposed for retinoblastoma.[23] This model predicts that two genetic events are necessary for tumor formation. The first mutation was hypothesized to be either a constitutional (pre-zygotic) or somatic (post-zygotic) event, whereas the second mutation was always post-zygotic. When the first mutation was constitutional, involving all the person's cells, the tumor would be heritable, and these patients would be expected to have an earlier age of onset and a greater incidence of multiple tumors. But the heritable fraction of Wilms' tumor is less than 1%,[24] far short of the 30% incidence predicted by the Knudson-Strong model. This finding was once thought to be explained by the lower survival rate for nephroblastoma in comparison to retinoblastoma. It is now clear, however, that the genetics for Wilms' tumor development is more complex than for retinoblastoma, and more than one gene may be involved.

The first clue to the location of the gene involved in Wilms' tumor development was the detection of a cytogenetically visible chromosomal deletion at the short arm of chromosome 11 in patients with the WAGR syndrome.[25] Subsequently, deletions and mutations of 11p13 have been shown to occur in tumor DNA from sporadic Wilms' tumors, as well as in the germline of patients with a genetic predisposition to cancer. Approximately 50% of tumors show *loss of heterozygosity (LOH)* for DNA markers on 11p13,[26, 27] indicating that these tumors had only one copy of the 11p, or WT1, gene. Tumor formation occurred after inactivation of one allele of an 11p13 gene and the subsequent mutation or loss of the homologous allele. WT1 is expressed transiently in the developing kidney and in specific cells of the gonads. The genetic consequences of WT1 inactivation appear to be restricted to organs that normally express this tumor-suppressor gene. Mutations at the WT1 locus, particularly in males, may confer extensive genitourinary defects, most notably male pseudohermaphroditism.[22, 28]

A second Wilms' tumor locus distinct from WT1 has been identified, 11p15.5, or WT2,[29] which has been linked to the BWS.[30] Many types of tumors show LOH in the 11p15 region,[27] suggesting that the WT2 gene may be important in the development of many different tumor types. BWS is associated with other embryonal neoplasms in addition to Wilms' tumor.

Other molecular genetic abnormalities are being studied in Wilms' tumor cases. Of great interest is the finding of LOH for the long arm of chromosome 16q, noted in approximately 20% of tumors[31] and suspected of playing a role in tumor progression rather than initiation.[32] An attempt is now under way to correlate these different genetic events with histopathologic features and staging to determine if they are an additional indicator of clinical behavior and outcome.

CLINICAL PRESENTATION

Most children with nephroblastoma have an abdominal mass on physical examination, often found incidentally by a family member. The tumor is generally quite large relative to the size of the child. The mass frequently crosses the midline, and therefore this feature does not distinguish it from neuroblastoma. Less common presentations are abdominal pain mimicking appendicitis and acute abdominal pain resulting from rupture of the tumor with hemorrhage into the free peritoneal cavity. Hematuria occurs in one fourth of children at diagnosis.

Vascular extension of Wilms' tumor into the renal vein and inferior vena cava can produce atypical presentations. Varicocele, hepatomegaly due to hepatic vein obstruction, ascites, and congestive heart failure were found in fewer than 10% of patients with intracaval or atrial tumor extension in NWTS-3.[33] Very rarely the tumor can embolize to the pulmonary artery with catastrophic consequences.[34]

The incidence of hypertension ranges from 25% to 50%. Explanations proposed for hypertension include the production of renin due to ischemia produced by tumor compression, arteriovenous fistula formation, or the release of renin by the tumor. Elevated plasma renin levels have been reported in Wilms' tumor cases, but they are not always associated with hypertension.[35]

PREOPERATIVE EVALUATION

Imaging studies are ordered with the intent of obtaining the correct diagnosis before surgery (Fig. 9–1). It is important for the surgeons to know that a solid tumor is present in order to plan for a major cancer operation. An increased incidence of surgical complications has been reported for Wilms' tumor cases where an incorrect preoperative diagnosis was made; that is, the child had Wilms' tumor, but there was an erroneous diagnosis prior to surgical exploration.[36] The majority of these children did not have any preoperative imaging studies performed, a fact that underscores the importance of such studies. An equally important goal is to establish that there is a contralateral functioning kidney prior to performing a nephrectomy.

Although relegated to a lesser role due to advances in modern imaging, the intravenous pyelogram (IVP) will reveal distortion of the renal contour with splaying of the collecting system. Nonopacification of the kidney is also common when there is tumor obstruction of the collecting system, complete replacement of the renal parenchyma with neoplasm, or intravascular tumor extension.[37] A review of NWTSG patients found that 28% of patients with inferior vena cava (IVC) or atrial extension had a nonfunctioning kidney on IVP.[33] If vascular invasion is not present, cystoscopy with retrograde pyelography is

warranted to exclude ureteral extension in children with a nonfunctioning kidney, particularly if hematuria is present.

Ultrasonography is now the favored initial imaging modality for children with abdominal masses. It allows one to distinguish between solid and cystic lesions and often to determine if the mass is of renal origin. An important role for ultrasound is to exclude the possibility of tumor extension into the IVC, which occurs in 4% of Wilms' tumor cases.[33] Color Doppler ultrasonography can assess flow and identify compression of the IVC. A free-floating thrombus within the lumen of the IVC can be readily documented (Fig. 9–2). Computed tomography (CT) visualization of the IVC is often hindered by unopacified blood due to an inadequate bolus injection of contrast. Inferior venacavography is now used sparingly, although there are few false-negative findings.[33] Magnetic resonance imaging (MRI) may be the best imaging modality for evaluating the extent of tumor within the IVC.[38] Although there are a limited number of reports, MRI is recommended in cases in which ultrasound findings were inconclusive.

The role of CT and MRI scans in the preoperative staging evaluation is controversial.[39, 40] Accurate staging of children with Wilms' tumors is crucial where outcome is highly correlated with stage and histology.[41] Yet current staging systems depend on data derived from findings at surgery as confirmed by pathologic examination. Preoperative CT can indicate whether there might be extension into the adjacent perirenal fat and regional adenopathy, although these possibilities

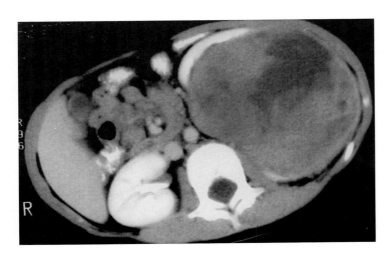

Figure 9–1 • Computed tomographic scan of a large left Wilms' tumor with a small rim of functioning renal parenchyma.

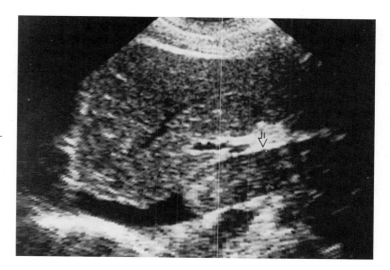

Figure 9–2 • Ultrasound depicting intracaval thrombus (arrow).

must also be confirmed at surgical exploration. Enlarged retroperitoneal benign lymph nodes are common in children, which can lead to significant diagnostic error. Correlation studies between intraoperative lymph node evaluation and pathologic findings in Wilms' tumor cases have found significant false-positive and false-negative rates.[42]

If the preoperative imaging evaluation can predict which tumors will be inoperable at surgical exploration, that information will greatly benefit the surgeon. Visceral involvement is uncommon with Wilms' tumor, but primary surgical resection is associated with increased surgical morbidity.[33] Infiltration of the bowel or liver invasion by right-sided tumors is particularly difficult to assess by CT. Dynamic scanning of the liver after bolus injection is recommended, but Ng and coworkers noted that the majority of children identified as having probable or possible invasion of the liver on CT later proved to have none at surgical exploration.[43] CT did have a 100% predictive value for absence of liver invasion, but deep-seated liver metastases that are not visible at surgery are uncommon.[44]

Therapeutic recommendations are different for patients with bilateral nephroblastoma, so it is important to identify these children.[45, 46] Historically, their recognition has relied on formal exploration of the contralateral kidney, but some reports have suggested that ultrasound and CT can adequately evaluate the contralateral kidney.[47, 48] Contradicting those reports was a review of 122 patients with synchronous bilateral Wilms'

tumor enrolled in NWTS-4 in whom 7% of bilateral lesions were missed by the preoperative imaging studies.[49] CT was more sensitive than ultrasound in detecting bilaterality, but neither technique was able to show more than 50% of lesions less than 1 cm in diameter. The NWTSG recommends formal exploration of the contralateral kidney with both palpation and inspection of all surfaces.

Metastases to the lungs are present in 8% of Wilms' tumor cases at the time of diagnosis. The majority of these lesions can be identified on routine chest radiographs. When this is the case, chest CT will add little to the evaluation. Additional smaller metastases will often be discovered, but CT findings will not alter the adjuvant treatment required.

There is controversy regarding the need for a chest CT in children with normal chest radiographs.[50, 51] Green and coworkers reviewed 32 cases of children enrolled in NWTS-3 who had normal chest radiographs but were shown to have metastatic lesions on chest CT.[50] The survival rate for those patients treated according to the local extent of the abdominal disease alone was equivalent to that for those receiving pulmonary irradiation. A different conclusion was reached by Wilimas and colleagues,[52] who reported that 40% of patients with favorable histology and pulmonary densities detected on CT alone developed recurrent disease when pulmonary irradiation was omitted.

Uncommon sites of metastases can occur in selected cases of renal tumors with unfavorable histology. *Clear-cell sarcoma of the kidney (CCSK)* and renal-cell carcinoma have a propensity to metastasize to the skeleton.[40] Skeletal surveys and bone scans are both recommended after the histologic diagnosis is confirmed. *Rhabdoid tumor of the kidney (RTK)* and CCSK are associated with brain metastases, so that an MRI of the brain should be obtained in the early postoperative period.

DIFFERENTIAL DIAGNOSIS

Nephroblastoma accounts for over 90% of renal tumors in children. RTK and CCSK are separate entities from Wilms' tumor that comprise 5% of pediatric renal tumors. The latter tumors are also known as the "bone-metastasizing renal tumours of childhood."[61] CCSK accounts for 3% of renal tumors reported to the NWTSG. Although it is not currently considered a variant of Wilms' tumor, the patient's age at time of diagnosis and the location of the tumor are the same as for nephroblastoma. Since CCSK is associated with a much higher rate of relapse and death, its recognition is quite important in order that the appropriate therapy be instituted. Studies have demonstrated that doxorubicin use is associated with a significant improvement in outcome for these children.[41]

RTK is a highly malignant tumor of the kidney that accounts for 2% of renal tumors registered to the NWTSG. RTK is now considered a sarcoma of the kidney and not of metanephric origin.[41] This tumor is typically seen in infants and very young children with a mean age of 13 months. RTK metastasizes to the brain, an exceedingly uncommon event in patients with Wilms' tumor. The prognosis for patients with RTK remains dismal with conventional chemotherapeutic regimens, and new treatment strategies are being developed for management of these children.

Congenital mesoblastic nephroma (CMN) is found predominantly in infants and is generally a benign lesion, although reports exist of local recurrence and occasional metastases.[62–64] CMN is found in approximately 2% of cases of childhood renal tumors. The typical patient is a newborn with an abdominal mass, but in recent years a number of patients have been recognized prenatally.[65] Complete excision is curative for most patients with CMN.[66] Local recurrence has been reported in several who had a cellular variant of CMN. Adequacy of surgical resection and the age at diagnosis in these patients appear to be more important predictors of relapse than histology.[67] The risk of recurrence is thought to be less in children who are younger than 3 months at the time of diagnosis, but metastases have been reported.[64]

Renal-cell carcinoma is the most common non-Wilms' renal tumor of childhood. Only 5% of such carcinomas occur in children.[53, 54] These patients generally present symptoms after the age of 5 years, and it is the most common renal malignancy in the second decade of life. The signs and symptoms are similar to those of other solid renal tumors, but hematuria is more common with renal-cell carcinoma than with Wilms' tumor.[54] Survival of children with renal-cell carcinoma depends on whether the tumor can be completely resected. Raney and coworkers found that all children with Stage I lesions survived, and others have reported 64% to 80% survival for Stage I and II tumors.[55–57] Overall survival rate is about 50%.

Renal *angiomyolipoma* is a hamartomatous lesion that is rarely seen in children. When it is, there is a clear association with tuberous sclerosis, and it is more often than not bilateral.[58] This tumor should be suspected preoperatively if CT demonstrates fat within the lesion.

Imaging studies cannot reliably establish the correct preoperative diagnosis in a child with a renal mass. One clinical parameter that aids the clinician in narrowing the diagnostic possibilities is patient age, since congenital mesoblastic nephroma is far more common in children younger than 6 months at the time of diagnosis.[59] Yet, patients with favorable histology along with Wilms' tumor or rhabdoid tumor of the kidney can also present in the first few months of life.[60] A renal mass in a child with aniridia, hemihypertrophy, or BWS is probably a Wilms' tumor. Bilateral or multicentric tumors are also typical of Wilms' tumor, but renal lymphoma can produce similar findings.

PATHOLOGY

The microscopic features of Wilms' tumor are variable. The classic triphasic pattern includes blastemal, stromal, and epithelial cells. The proportion of the three components varies greatly.

Tumors that consist predominantly of one or two of these elements are commonly encountered. Blastemal-predominant tumors behave more aggressively and indicate more advanced disease at time of presentation. The primitive blastemal cells usually show distinctive patterns that allow their recognition by experienced pathologists. The stromal component can differentiate into striated muscle, cartilage, or fat.

The most important determinants of outcome in children with Wilms' tumor are the histopathology and tumor stage. The current staging system employed by the NWTSG is summarized in Table 9–2. For NWTS-3, the distribution by stage of favorable-histology tumors was 47% for Stage, I 22% for Stage II, 22% for Stage III, and 9% for Stage IV.[41] Both surgeon and pathologist have responsibility for determining local tumor stage. Stage I tumors are limited to the kidney and completely resected. The first signs of spread outside the kidney are in the renal sinus and lymphatic vessels. Penetration through the renal capsule is the next most common site of extrarenal spread. Tumors that penetrate the renal capsule are considered Stage II lesions. Tumor extension into the soft tissues of the sinus or the presence of tumor cells in blood or lymphatic vessels of the renal sinus is also now considered Stage II.

The presence of lymph node metastases has an adverse outcome on survival, so it is important that adequate lymph node sampling be performed during the course of removal of a nephroblastoma. Local tumor extension is another important factor in identifying risk of tumor relapse. Patients with diffuse tumor spill are at increased risk of abdominal relapse and therefore considered to be in Stage III and given whole-abdominal irradiation.

Identification of unfavorable-histology tumors is more important than even stage assignment, since these tumors are responsible for 50% of tumor deaths although they account for only 10% of patients.[68, 69] Characteristics include tumors of extreme nuclear atypia (anaplasia) and monomorphic sarcomatous-appearing tumors. These latter tumors have been reclassified as the rhabdoid tumor and CCSK and are now considered to be distinct entities from Wilms' tumors.

Anaplasia was present in 4% of cases enrolled in NWTS-3. Unaplasia is rare in the first 2 years of life, but the incidence increases to 13% in children age 5 years or older.[70] Anaplastic Wilms' tumors are further stratified into focal and diffuse anaplasia.[71] The definition of focal anaplasia is based upon a topographical principle. It requires that the anaplastic nuclear changes be confined to a specified region of the primary tumor and be absent from the surrounding portions of the lesion. Diffuse anaplasia is diagnosed when anaplasia is present in more than one portion of the tumor or is found in any extrarenal or metastatic site.

Precursor Lesions of Wilms' Tumor

Lesions apparently representing Wilms' tumor precursors are found in 30% to 40% of kidneys

Table 9–2 • Staging System of the National Wilms' Tumor Study

Stage	
I	Tumor is limited to the kidney and can be completely excised. The renal capsule is intact, and the tumor was not ruptured prior to removal. There is no residual tumor.
II	Tumor extends through the perirenal capsule but can be completely excised. There may be local spillage of tumor confined to the flank, or a biopsy may have been taken of the tumor. Extrarenal vessels may contain tumor thrombus or be infiltrated by tumor.
III	A residual nonhematogenous tumor is confined to the abdomen. There may be lymph node involvement, diffuse peritoneal spillage, peritoneal implants, tumor existing beyond the surgical margin either grossly or microscopically, or the tumor not completely removed.
IV	Hematogenous metastases to lung, liver, bone, brain, and so forth.
V	Bilateral renal involvement is found on diagnosis.

removed for Wilms' tumor.[72] They have been found in 1% of kidneys in infants on postmortem examination.[73] The current preferred term for these lesions is *nephrogenic rests*, defined as foci of abnormally persistent nephrogenic cells that can form a Wilms' tumor.[74] Two distinct categories of nephrogenic rests have been identified, *perilobar nephrogenic rest (PLNR)* and *intralobar nephrogenic rest (ILNR)*. This classification is based upon the position of these lesions within the renal lobe. PLNR is found in the periphery (Fig. 9–3), whereas ILNR can be found anywhere within the renal lobe. The presence of multiple or diffuse nephrogenic rests will lead to the diagnosis of nephroblastomatosis. Hyperplastic nephrogenic rests can be mistaken for Wilms' tumor, and the exact criteria for distinguishing between these two lesions remain to be defined.

Multiple nephrogenic rests in one kidney usually imply that nephrogenic rests are present in the other kidney. Therefore, this is an extremely important pathologic feature that can identify patients at risk for metachronous Wilms' tumor. The patients need careful imaging follow-up to detect contralateral recurrence (Table 9–3). Both types of nephrogenic rests are associated with bilateral Wilms' tumor, and the incidence of nephrogenic rests is much higher in patients with bilateral Wilms' tumor than in those with unilateral Wilms' tumor. There are differences in the epidemiologic characteristics of ILNR and PLNR, and there is a higher prevalence of PLNR in children with hemihypertrophy and the Beckwith-Wiedemann syndrome. Children with WAGR and Denys-Drash syndromes are more likely to have ILNR.

Biologic Parameters

Prior randomized trials that evaluate different treatment protocols for patients with Wilms' tumor have stratified patients by stage and histologic parameters. Now that children with favorable-histology Wilms' tumor have an excellent survival rate, however, it is difficult to find any particular histologic feature that will predict the risk of relapse. If we could further stratify favorable-histology Wilms' tumor patients into low- and high-risk groups for relapse, this would allow a further reduction in treatment intensity for some patients while indicating the need for an intensification of treatment in others.

Flow cytometry is used to measure DNA content and to estimate the proliferative rate of populations of cells constituting solid malignancies. Flow cytometry attempts to identify aggressive populations of tumor cells that may predict which low-stage tumors are at risk for metastatic disease. Normal somatic cells have a diploid DNA content, cells in mitosis are tetraploid, and tumor cells with gross karyotypic abnormalities in number are labeled aneuploid. An analysis of 47 patients with Wilms' tumors found that those with a diploid or aneuploid DNA histogram had a 100% survival rate at 5 years.[75] Stage III and IV patients with tetraploid patterns fared significantly worse, with a 25% five-year survival. Others have found DNA ploidy no more accurate a predictor of survival than histology and stage.[76]

The ability of nuclear morphometric techniques to predict clinical outcome has been evaluated in cases of Wilms' tumor and other urologic solid tumors.[77, 78] In an initial review of 27 cases of favorable-histology Wilms' tumor, multivariate analysis found that nuclear morphometry could be employed to identify those having a poor prognosis. A subsequent review of 108 such cases found the same.[79]

As noted previously, LOH for a portion of chromosome 16q has been found in 20% of Wilms' tumor cases.[31] The 16q locus may play a

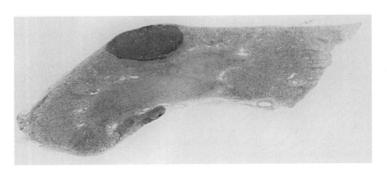

Figure 9–3 • Perilobar nephrogenic rest composed of blastemal cells just beneath the renal capsule (hematoxylin and eosin, ×40).

Table 9–3 • Recommended Imaging Studies for Follow-up of Children with Renal Neoplasms of Proven Histology and Who Were Free of Metastases at Time of Diagnosis

Tumor Type	Study	Schedule Following Primary Therapy
Favorable-histology Wilms' tumor Stage I anaplastic Wilms' tumor	Chest films	6 wks and 3 mos postop; then q. 3 mos × 5, q. 6 mos. × 3, yearly × 2
Irradiated patients only	Irradiated bony structures[a]	Yearly to full growth, then q. 5 yrs indefinitely[b]
Without NRs, Stages I and II	Abdominal ultrasound	Yearly × 3
Without NRs, Stage III	Abdominal ultrasound	Same as for chest films
With NRs, any stage[c]	Abdominal ultrasound	q. 3 mos × 10, q. 6 mos × 5, yearly × 5
Stage II and III anaplastic	Chest films Abdominal ultrasound	Same as for favorable-histology tumors q. 3 mos × 4; q. 6 mos × 4
Renal-cell carcinoma	Chest films Skeletal survey and bone scan	Same as for favorable-histology tumors Same as for CCSK
Clear-cell sarcoma (CCSK)	Brain MRI and/or opacified CT Skeletal survey and bone scan Chest films	When CCSK is established; then q. 6 mos × 10 Same as for favorable-histology tumors
Rhabdoid tumor	Brain MRI and/or opacified CT Chest films	Same as for CCSK Same as for favorable-histology tumors
Mesoblastic nephroma[d]	Abdominal ultrasound	q. 3 mos × 6

[a]To include any irradiated osseous structures.
[b]To detect second neoplasms, benign (osteochondromas) or malignant.
[c]The panelists at the First International Conference on Molecular and Clinical Genetics of Childhood Renal Tumors, Albuquerque, New Mexico, May 1992, recommended a variation: q. 3 mos for 5 yrs or until age 7, whichever comes first.
[d]Data from the files of Dr. J. B. Beckwith reveal that 20 of 293 MN patients (7%) relapsed or had metastases at time of diagnosis; 4 of the 20 in the lungs, 1 of the 4 at diagnosis. All but one of the 19 relapses occurred within 1 year. Chest films for MN patients may be elected on a schedule such as q. 3 mos × 4, q. 6 mos × 2.
From D'Angio GJ, Rosenberg H, Sharples K, Kelalis P, Breslow N, Green DM: Imaging methods for primary renal tumors of childhood: Cost versus benefits. *Med Pediatr Oncol* 21:205–212, 1993, adapted with permission of Wiley-Liss, Inc., a division of John Wiley & Sons, Inc.

role in tumor progression. A prospective study of 232 patients registered on the NWTS found LOH for 16q in 17% of the tumors.[32] These patients had a statistically significantly higher rate of relapse after 2 years and lower rate of overall survival than those without LOH for chromosome 16q. This finding is the first evidence to suggest that molecular markers can be used to stratify patients for therapy. It will be tested in NWTS-5.

Several biologic markers for Wilms' tumor have been investigated, including serum renin, neuron-specific enolase, basic fibroblast growth factor, and hyaluronic acid.[80–82] Elevated levels of hyaluronic acid and basic fibroblast growth factor have been found in the urine of patients with

Wilms' tumor. Following surgical removal of the tumor, the levels returned to normal. Patients with persistent disease or relapse had significantly higher levels 1 to 6 months after surgery.

SURGICAL MANAGEMENT

Prior to the introduction of effective chemotherapy and radiotherapy, surgical resection of Wilms' tumor was the only means for cure. Safe and complete removal of the tumor continues to be an essential part of management, not only in terms of patient survival but also to determine the intensity of adjuvant treatment necessary. The preoperative evaluation of a child discovered to have an abdominal mass can generally be completed in 48 hours in most medical centers. Emergency operation is not necessary unless there is evidence of active bleeding.

Thorough exploration of the abdominal cavity is carried out via a generous transperitoneal incision. It is important to exclude liver metastases, lymph node involvement, or other evidence of tumor spread. Exploration of the contralateral kidney should be performed prior to nephrectomy. As noted earlier, one cannot rely entirely on the preoperative imaging studies to exclude bilateral disease.[49] Patients with bilateral tumors are managed with biopsy followed by chemotherapy, without attempts at primary resection.[46] The colon is reflected, and Gerota's fascia opened so that the kidney can be palpated and inspected on all surfaces. Biopsies should be taken of any abnormalities of the opposite kidney to exclude the possibility of occult Wilms' tumor or nephrogenic rests.

Radical nephrectomy is performed with sampling of regional lymph nodes, but formal lymph node dissection is not required.[42] Gentle handling of the tumor throughout the procedure is mandatory to avoid tumor spillage as these cases have a sixfold increase in local abdominal relapse.[41] Ligation of the renal vessels is performed prior to mobilization of the tumor, but only if exposure is adequate. It is more important that the surgeon be sure not to ligate contralateral renal vessels, aorta, iliac, or superior mesenteric arteries by mistake.[83]

Palpation of the renal vein and IVC should be performed to exclude the possibility of intravascular tumor extension prior to vessel ligation. Identification of intracaval extension on the preoperative imaging studies will allow the surgical team to adequately prepare for the operative procedure. For vena caval involvement below the level of the hepatic veins, the caval thrombus can be removed via cavotomy after proximal and distal vascular control is obtained. Generally the thrombus will be free-floating, but if it adheres to the caval wall, it can often be delivered with the passage of a Fogarty or Foley balloon catheter. Patients with atrial extension may require cardiopulmonary bypass for thrombus removal.[84] Certain operative findings may suggest intravascular extension when it has not been correctly diagnosed preoperatively. For example, excessive bleeding from dilated superficial and retroperitoneal collaterals is a clue to the existence of obstruction of the vena cava. More ominous is the finding of sudden unexplained hypotension, which can result from embolization of the tumor thrombus.

Patients with extension of intracaval tumor thrombus above the level of the hepatic veins or into the right atrium should be managed with preoperative chemotherapy to shrink the tumor and thrombus.[85–87] This approach will facilitate the complete removal of the tumor with decreased morbidity. There has been one report of tumor embolus during chemotherapy,[88] but this complication can also occur prior to or during surgical removal of the tumor.[34, 89]

If the tumor is found to be unresectable, biopsy of the tumor can be followed by chemotherapy or radiation therapy, or both. This approach will generally result in a significant reduction of the tumor burden, allowing subsequent tumor resection.[90, 91] Radical en bloc resection of the tumor is probably not justified in most children as this is associated with increased surgical morbidity. Wilms' tumors are generally very large, and the gross appearance of the tumor at the time of surgery can be misleading in interpreting tumor extent. These tumors often compress and adhere to adjacent structures without frank invasion, and in the majority of cases tumor invasion is not confirmed after the adjacent visceral organs are removed.[36] There may still be circumstances, however, when removal of other organs is justified. In a patient known to have extracapsular extension, resection of a small portion of liver or tail of the pancreas to avoid leaving residual tumor, for example, may eliminate the need for radiation therapy and allow a reduction in the amount of chemotherapy. Even if the tumor is confined to the kidney, en bloc resection of nonessential structures may also prevent violation of the tumor capsule and obviate tumor rupture or spill during nephrectomy. Therefore, it is a tradeoff between the added surgical morbidity of en bloc resection versus a potential reduction in long-term complications of adjuvant treatment if this can be limited by complete tumor removal.

Surgery should not be overlooked as a cause of morbidity in children with Wilms' tumor. A review of NWTS-3 patients undergoing primary nephrectomy found a 20% incidence of surgical complications.[36] The most common complications were intestinal obstruction[92] and hemorrhage. Factors associated with increased surgical complications were higher local tumor stage, intravascular extension, en bloc resection of other visceral organs, and incorrect preoperative diagnosis. One factor that could contribute to increased bleeding is acquired von Willebrand's disease, which is found in 8% of newly diagnosed Wilms' tumor cases.[93]

COOPERATIVE TRIALS (NWTSG AND SIOP)

Many early accomplishments in the treatment of children with Wilms' tumor were made by individuals or large single institutions. These include the introduction of dactinomycin and vincristine for the treatment of children with Wilms' tumors.[4, 94] Even the largest institutions, however, do not treat enough patients to conduct prospective randomized trials to answer therapeutic questions. For this reason, the pediatric cooperative groups, Children's Cancer Group and the Pediatric Oncology Group, began clinical trials[95] and later formed the intergroup National Wilms' Tumor Study Group (NWTSG). The International Society of Pediatric Oncology, or (SIOP), has also conducted large clinical trials in the treatment of nephroblastoma.

There were many important findings in the early clinical trials. Combination chemotherapy of vincristine and dactinomycin was more effective than single agents alone.[96] Later it was found that the addition of doxorubicin improved survival rates for higher-stage patients.[41] Even more important findings were the identification of unfavorable histologic features of Wilms' tumor and of prognostic factors that allowed refinement of the staging system, stratifying patients into high-risk and low-risk treatment groups.[97] After the completion of NWTS-1 and NWTS-2, it was recognized that the presence of lymph node metastases had an adverse outcome on survival. This finding underscores the importance of adequate lymph node sampling during the course of removal of a nephroblastoma. Local tumor extension is another important factor in identifying risk of tumor relapse. Patients with diffuse tumor spill were found to be at increased risk of abdominal relapse and therefore considered to be in Stage III and given whole-abdominal irradiation. These findings were what allowed stratification of patients into low- and high-risk treatment

groups and thus allowed a reduction in the intensity of therapy for the majority of patients, maintaining overall survival rates.

For NWTS-3, the distribution by stage of favorable-histology tumors was 47% for Stage I, 22% for Stage II, 22% for Stage III, and 9% for Stage IV.[41] Patients with Stage I favorable-histology Wilms' tumor can be treated successfully with a 10-week regimen of vincristine (VCR) and dactinomycin (AMD). The 4-year relapse-free survival rate in NWTS-3 was 89%, and the overall survival was 95.6%. NWTS-3 patients with Stage II favorable-histology Wilms' tumors treated with AMD and VCR but no postoperative radiation therapy had an equivalent survival rate, 91.1%, for 4 years, to that of patients who received doxorubicin and radiation therapy. Patients with Stage III favorable-histology Wilms' tumors continued to receive abdominal radiation therapy, but the dose was reduced to 1000 cGy. This approach was shown to be as effective as 2000 cGy in preventing abdominal relapse if doxorubicin (DOX) was also given in addition to VCR and AMD. The 4-year relapse-free survival rate was 82% in NWTS-3 patients, and the 4-year overall survival rate was 90.9%. Currently, only 24% of children with favorable-histology tumors entered on NWTS-4 receive postoperative abdominal irradiation.[98] Patients with Stage IV favorable-histology tumors receive abdominal irradiation based on the local tumor stage and receive 1200 cGy to both lungs. In NWTS-3, the combination of VCR, AMD, and DOX produced a 4-year relapse-free survival rate of 71.9%, and the overall survival was 78.4%.

Radiation therapy is usually begun within the first week after surgery. The radiation fields vary according to the extent of disease. Except in patients with diffuse intra-abdominal spill, the radiation portals are confined to the tumor bed. If there is bulky residual disease, additional boosts of radiation are given to these areas. All metastatic sites also receive irradiation. The doses are adjusted according to age since radiation injury to normal tissues is greater in younger children.

NWTS-4 was closed for patient entry in September 1994. Its goals were to decrease treatment intensity for patients with a favorable prognosis while maintaining the excellent overall survival rate already established. In addition, this was the first clinical pediatric cancer trial to evaluate the economic impact of two different treatment approaches. Pulse-intensive regimens utilize simultaneous administration of agents at more frequent intervals to decrease the number of days of hospitalization required for administration of chemotherapy and hence the cost of cancer treatment. The pulse-intensive regimens were found to produce less hematological toxicity than the standard regimens, and the administered drug dose intensity is greater on the pulse-intensive regimens.[99] Patients treated with this regimen also have equivalent survival rates compared with patients treated with the standard chemotherapy regimen[100] A Brazilian Wilms' tumor study has confirmed these findings.[101] The 4-year survival rate of patients with favorable-histology Wilms' tumor now approaches 90%.

In NWTS-4, children with Stage I anaplastic tumors were treated in a similar fashion to those with favorable histology. Patients with Stage II-IV and focal anaplasia were treated with AMD, VCR, and ADR, while receiving irradiation to the tumor bed. If there was evidence of diffuse anaplasia, Stage II-III patients also received cyclophosphamide.

Current recommendations for treatment to be utilized in NWTS-5 cases are outlined in Table 9-4. Patients with a Stage I or II favorable-histology Wilms' tumor are treated with a pulse-intensive regimen of VCR and AMD for 18 weeks. Stage III favorable-histology patients receive AMD, VCR, and DOX, plus 1080 cGy abdominal irradiation. Patients with Stage IV favorable-histology tumors receive abdominal irra-

diation based on the local tumor stage and also receive 1200 cGy to both lungs.

One group of Stage I patients will be selected for management with surgery alone in NWTS-5. Omission of postoperative adjuvant therapy has been proposed for small Stage I tumors of favorable histology that occur in children less than 2 years of age (Cassady tumor).[102, 103] A study of NWTS-4 favorable-histology Stage I cases found that the 2-year relapse-free survival rate for patients younger than 2 years and with tumors weighing less than under 550 g was 95.5%.[104]

One of the most important features of NWTS-5 is that it is a single-arm therapeutic trial. Patients are not randomized for therapy, but instead biologic features of the tumors are assessed. If these variables are found to be predictive of clinical behavior, this information will then be used in subsequent clinical trials to further stratify patients for therapy. In addition, a retrieval study will be conducted to try to improve survival rates for those children who experience relapse.

BILATERAL WILMS' TUMORS

Synchronous bilateral nephroblastoma occurs in about 5% of children, with metachronous lesions developing in only 1%.[45, 46] The importance of intraoperative examination of the contralateral kidney is addressed earlier in this chapter. In the past, bilateral Wilms' tumor cases were managed primarily by surgery, but several investigators have found that survival rates are comparable for patients treated with preoperative chemother-

Table 9-4 • Protocol for National Wilms' Tumor Study-5

Stage of Tumor	Radiotherapy	Chemotherapy
Stage I, II FH and anaplasia	None	EE-4A—pulse-intensive AMD plus VCR (18 weeks)
Stage III, IV FH and focal anaplasia II–IV	1080 cGy	DD-4A—pulse-intensive AMD, VCR, and DOX (24 weeks)
Stage II–IV diffuse anaplasia and CCSK	Yes[a]	Regimen I[b]
Stage I–IV rhabdoid tumor of the kidney	Yes[a]	Regimen RTK[c]

[a]Radiation therapy is given to all clear-cell sarcoma patients. Stage IV FH patients are given radiation based on the local tumor stage. Consult protocol for specific treatment.
[b]Regimen I: AMD, VCR, DOX, cyclophosphamide, and etoposide.
[c]Regimen RTK: carboplatin, etoposide, and cyclophosphamide.
AMD = actinomycin-D; VCR = vincristine; DOX = doxorubicin; FH = favorable histology.

apy.[45, 105] One advantage of the latter approach is that more renal units will be spared if surgery is deferred until after the tumor burden is reduced.[46, 106] Failure has been reported in as many as 5% of patients with bilateral tumors.[107]

The NWTS-5 protocol recommends initial biopsy followed by preoperative chemotherapy for patients with bilateral Wilms' tumors. Radical excision of the tumor should not be performed at the initial operation. Rather, partial nephrectomy or wedge excision should be employed, provided that all the tumor can be removed with *preservation of two thirds or more of the renal parenchyma on both sides.* Bilateral biopsies should be obtained to confirm the presence of Wilms' tumor in both kidneys and to define the histologic type. Patients having lymph nodes suspected of harboring metastases should undergo biopsy and be assigned a surgical stage. Patients with favorable histology and Stage I or II disease are given dactinomycin and vincristine. Those with favorable histology and Stage III or IV disease are given dactinomycin, vincristine, and doxorubicin. The response to chemotherapy is assessed by serial imaging studies. Surgical exploration with definitive resection is deferred until there has been a significant reduction in tumor burden.

A second-look procedure is performed at the completion of chemotherapy. At that time, partial nephrectomies or wedge excisions of the tumors are performed. These should be done only if it will not compromise tumor resection and if negative margins can be obtained. If there is extensive tumor involvement precluding partial resection, complete excision of tumor from the least involved kidney is performed. If this approach leaves a viable kidney, then nephrectomy of the other kidney is carried out.

Some patients may not have a measurable response to preoperative chemotherapy. Patients with persistent viable tumor should be changed to a different chemotherapeutic regimen. The patient should be reassessed after an additional 12 weeks to assess feasibility of resection. Bilateral nephrectomy and dialysis may be required if the tumors fail to respond to chemotherapy and radiation therapy. The most common cause of renal failure in NWTS patients is bilateral nephrectomy for persistent tumor.[107] If transplantation is later considered, a waiting period of

2 years is recommended to ensure that the patient does not develop metastatic disease.[108]

PREOPERATIVE THERAPY

The most common indications for preoperative chemotherapy in NWTSG patients are bilateral Wilms' tumors and massive Wilms' tumors judged to be unresectable or involving vital structures that preclude primary excision.[90] Preoperative treatment can produce dramatic reduction in the size of the primary tumor, facilitating surgical excision (Fig. 9–4). The SIOP trials have utilized preoperative treatment for Wilms' tumor since the early 1970s, and their studies have demonstrated that the incidence of tumor rupture is lower after preoperative therapy.[109, 110] No survival advantage has been demonstrated over the primary surgical approach.

One notable difference between SIOP and the NWTSG is that SIOP investigators use the post-chemotherapy stage to determine the amount of postoperative therapy. A significant number of patients are "downstaged" after chemotherapy. This post-chemotherapy stage, however, may inadequately define the risk of intra-abdominal recurrence in patients who receive no radiation therapy. In SIOP-6, patients who were "post-chemotherapy Stage II" were randomized to receive or not receive abdominal irradiation. There was an unacceptable increase in the number of intra-abdominal recurrences in nonirradiated patients.[111] As a result, such patients are now given an anthracycline as part of the chemotherapy regimen,[112] which has the potential of increasing late complications, particularly congestive heart failure.

Occasionally patients present with massive tumors that are surgically unresectable. Pretreatment with chemotherapy almost always reduces the bulk of the tumor and renders it resectable.[91, 111] Unfortunately, this method does not result in improved survival rates, and there is loss of important staging information. Patients with unresectable tumors treated by preoperative therapy should be considered Stage III and treated accordingly.[91] In general, there is usually adequate reduction in the size of the tumor within 6 weeks to facilitate definitive resection. Serial imaging evaluation is helpful to assess response. Patients who fail to respond can be considered for preoperative irradiation, as this may

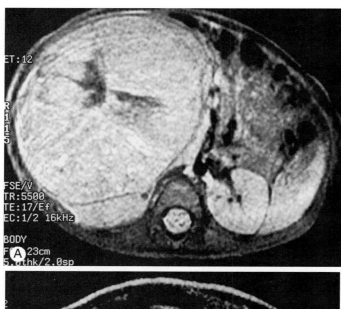

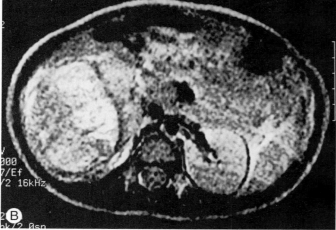

Figure 9–4 • *A*, Magnetic resonance imaging scan of a large inoperable Wilms' tumor. *B*, After six weeks of chemotherapy the same tumor has dramatically decreased in size.

produce enough shrinkage to facilitate nephrectomy. If the tumor remains inoperable, then biopsy of both the primary tumor and accessible metastatic lesions should be performed. Prognosis is very poor for patients with progressive disease, who will require treatment with a different chemotherapeutic regimen.[91]

The NWTSG continues to recommend primary surgical treatment of Wilms' tumor. This approach will allow precise staging of patients, providing modulation of treatment for each individual and thus a decrease in the intensity of treatment when possible while maintaining an excellent overall survival rate. The current recommendations from the NWTSG are for preoperative chemotherapy in patients with bilateral involvement,[45] tumors inoperable at surgical ex-

ploration,[91] or IVC extension above the hepatic veins.[86] All other patients should undergo primary nephrectomy.

TREATMENT OF RELAPSES

Children with relapsed Wilms' tumor have a variable prognosis depending on the initial stage, site of relapse, time from initial diagnosis to relapse, and prior therapy. Adverse prognostic factors include previous treatment that included doxorubicin, relapse less than 12 months after diagnosis, and intra-abdominal relapse in patients who received abdominal radiation therapy.[113] Results from NWTS-3 demonstrate that the risk of tumor relapse after 3 years is 9.6% for Stage I, 11.8% for Stage II, 22% for Stage III, and 22%

for Stage IV. Relapses occurred in 36% of cases with unfavorable-histology Stage I–III and IV.[41]

LATE EFFECTS OF CANCER TREATMENT

Children treated for Wilms' tumor are at increased risk for second malignant neoplasms. Alkylating agents have been implicated in chemotherapy-induced second tumors.[114] Investigators from the NWTSG have noted a 1.6% cumulative incidence of second tumors 15 years after treatment.[68] The amount of abdominal irradiation, use of doxorubicin, and treatment for relapse all were associated with an increased incidence of these tumors.

Numerous organ systems are subject to the late sequelae of anticancer therapy. An early report on NWTSG patients found that musculoskeletal problems such as scoliosis were seven times more common in children treated with radiation.[115] These were NWTS-1 and NWTS-2 cases, in which treatment intensity was much greater than is currently recommended. Damage to reproductive systems can lead to problems with hormonal dysfunction or infertility. Gonadal radiation in male patients can result in temporary azoospermia and hypogonadism.[116] The severity of damage to the testes is dependent on the dose. Female patients with Wilms' tumor who received abdominal radiation had a 12% incidence of ovarian failure.[117] In addition, women with prior abdominal radiation had the potential for adverse pregnancy outcomes. Perinatal mortality rates were higher and low birth weights more likely.[118]

Congestive heart failure is a well-known complication of treatment with anthracycline, and the incidence is dose-related.[119] In addition to the reports of acute cardiotoxicity, others are surfacing of cardiac failure up to 20 years after treatment.[120] In a preliminary review of patients entered on NWTS-1, NWTS-2, and NWTS-3, the frequency of congestive heart failure was 1.7% among doxorubicin-treated patients.[121] The risk was increased if the patient received whole-lung irradiation. In light of these findings, all children who undergo treatment with these modalities should undergo periodic reevaluation.

Concern has been expressed about the late occurrence of renal dysfunction in children who have undergone nephrectomy. There is both clinical and experimental evidence of hyperfiltration damage of remnant nephrons after a loss of renal mass.[122] Most experimental studies show a loss of greater than three fourths of the total renal mass, but there are only limited data assessing renal long-term function in children following unilateral nephrectomy.[123, 124]

This concern about renal dysfunction has led some surgeons to recommend parenchymal-sparing procedures for unilateral tumors.[125] The majority of Wilms' tumors are too large for a partial nephrectomy at initial presentation. After preoperative chemotherapy, 10% of patients may be amenable to partial nephrectomy. Disadvantages of such an approach include the potential for increased surgical complications and the possibility of local recurrence. The use of partial nephrectomy is probably a sound idea for those with solitary kidneys, renal insufficiency, or a genetic predisposition to bilateral tumors, as in Beckwith-Wiedemann syndrome, but for the majority of patients with unilateral Wilms' tumor the indication is less clear. The incidence of renal failure in patients with unilateral Wilms' tumor as reported to the NWTSG is less than 0.2%, and the majority of these had the Denys-Drash syndrome that is associated with end-stage renal disease.[107]

References

1. Beckwith JB: Wilms' tumor and other renal tumors of childhood: An update. *J Urol* 136:320–324, 1986.
2. Zantiga AR, Coppes MJ: Max Wilms (1867–1918): The man behind the eponym. *Med Pediatr Oncol* 20:515–518, 1992.
3. Priestly JT, Schulte TL: The treatment of Wilms' tumor. *Urology* 47:7–10, 1942.
4. Farber S: Chemotherapy in the treatment of leukemia and Wilms' tumor. *JAMA* 198:826–836, 1966.
5. Breslow N, Olshan A, Beckwith JB, Green DM: Epidemiology of Wilms' tumor. *Med Pediatr Oncol* 21:172–181, 1993.
6. Young JL and Miller RW: Incidence of malignant tumors in U.S. children. *J Pediatr* 86:254–258, 1975.
7. Breslow N, Olshan A, Beckwith JB, et al: Ethnic variation in the incidence, diagnosis, prognosis and follow-up of children with Wilms' tumor. *J Natl Cancer Inst* 86:49–51, 1994.
8. Birch JM, Breslow N: Epidemiologic features of Wilms' tumor. *Hematol Oncol Clin North Am* 9:1157–1178, 1995.
9. Olshan AF, Breslow NE, Daling JR, et al:

Wilms' tumor and paternal occupation. *Cancer Res* 50:3212–3217, 1990.

10. Clericuzio CL: Clinical phenotypes and Wilms' tumor. *Med Pediatr Oncol* 21:182–187, 1993.

11. Hittner HM, Riccardi VM, Ferrell RE, Strobel RJ, Ledbetter DH, Strong L, Lebo R: Genetic heterogeneity of aniridia: Negative linkage data. *Metab Pediatr Syst Ophthalmol* 4:179–182, 1980.

12. Haicken BN, Miller DR: Simultaneous occurrences of congenital aniridia, hamartoma, and Wilms' tumor. *J Pediatr* 78:497–502, 1971.

13. Boxer LA, Smith DL: Wilms' tumor prior to onset of hemihypertrophy. *Am J Dis Child* 120:564–565, 1970.

14. Breslow NE, Beckwith JB: Epidemiological features of Wilms' tumor: Results of the National Wilms' Tumor Study. *J Natl Cancer Inst* 68:429–436, 1982.

15. Green DM, Breslow NE, Beckwith JB, Norkool P: Screening of children with hemihypertrophy, aniridia, and Beckwith-Wiedemann syndrome in patients with Wilms' tumor: A report from the National Wilms' Tumor Study. *Med Pediatr Oncol* 21:188–192, 1993.

16. Tank ES, Kay R: Neoplasms associated with hemihypertrophy, Beckwith-Wiedemann syndrome and aniridia. *J Urol* 124:266–268, 1980.

17. Sotelo-Avila C, Gonzalez-Crussi F, Fowler JW: Complete and incomplete forms of Beckwith-Wiedemann syndrome: Their oncogenic potential. *J Pediatr* 96:47–50, 1980.

18. Beckwith JB: Macroglossia, omphalocele, adrenal cytomegaly, gigantism and hyperplastic visceromegaly: Birth Defects. *Orig Article Series* 5:188–196, 1969.

19. Breslow N, Beckwith JB, Ciol M, Sharples K: Age distribution of Wilms' tumor: Report from the National Wilms' Tumor Study. *Cancer Res* 48:1653–1657, 1988.

20. Drash A, Sherman F, Hartmann WH, Blizzard RM: A syndrome of pseudohermaphroditism, Wilms' tumor, hypertension and degenerative renal disease. *J Pediatr* 76:585–593, 1970.

21. Denys P, Malvaux P, Van Den Berghe H, et al: Association d'un syndrome anatomo-pathologique de pseudohermaphrodisitism masculin, d'une tumeur de Wilms, d'une nephropathie parenchymateuse et d'un mosaicism XX/XY. *Arch Fr Pediatr* 24:729–39, 1967.

22. Coppes MJ, Huff V, Pelletier J: Denys-Drash syndrome: Relating a clinical disorder to genetic alterations in the tumor suppressor gene WT1. *J Pediatr* 123:673–678, 1993.

23. Knudson AG, Strong LC: Mutation and cancer: A model for Wilms' tumor of the kidney. *J Natl Cancer Inst* 48:313–324, 1972.

24. Green DM, Fine NE, Li FP: Offspring of patients treated for unilateral Wilms' tumor in childhood. *Cancer* 49:2285–2288, 1982.

25. Riccardi VM, Sujansky E, Smith AC, Francke U: Chromosomal imbalance in the aniridia–Wilms' tumor association: 11p interstitial deletion. *Pediatrics* 61:604–610, 1978.

26. Koufos A, Hansen MF, Lampkin BC, et al: Loss of alleles at loci on human chromosome 11 during genesis of Wilms' tumor. *Nature* 309:170–172, 1984.

27. Huff V: Inheritance and functionality of Wilms' tumor genes. *The Cancer Bulletin* 46:255–259, 1994.

28. Pelletier J, Bruening W, Kashtan CE, et al: Germline mutations in the Wilms' tumor suppressor gene are associated with abnormal urogenital development in Denys-Drash syndrome. *Cell* 67:437–447, 1991.

29. Reeve AE, Sih SA, Raizis AM, Feinberg AP: Loss of allelic heterozygosity at a second locus on chromosome 11 in sporadic Wilms' tumor cells. *Mol Cell Biol* 44:711–719, 1989.

30. Koufos A, Grundy P, Morgan K, et al: Familial Wiedemann-Beckwith syndrome and a second Wilms' tumor locus both map to 11p15.5. *Am J Hum Genet* 44:711–719, 1989.

31. Maw MA, Grundy PE, Millow LJ, et al: A third Wilms' tumor locus on chromosome 16q. *Cancer Res* 52:3094–3098, 1992.

32. Grundy PE, Telzerow PE, Breslow N, et al: Loss of heterozygosity for chromosomes 16q and 1p in Wilms' tumor predicts an adverse outcome. *Cancer Res* 54:2331–2333, 1994.

33. Ritchey ML, Kelalis PP, Breslow N, et al: Intracaval and atrial involvement with nephroblastoma: Review of National Wilms' Tumor Study-3. *J Urol* 140:1113–1118, 1988.

34. Zakowski MF, Edwards RH, McDonough ET: Wilms' tumor presenting as sudden death due to tumor embolism. *Arch Pathol Lab Med* 114:605–608, 1990.

35. Voute PA, Van Der Meer J, Staugaard-Kloosterziel W: Plasma renin activity in Wilms' tumour. *Acta Endocrinol* 67:197–202, 1971.

36. Ritchey ML, Kelalis PP, Breslow N, et al: Surgical complications following nephrectomy for Wilms' tumor: A report of National Wilms' Tumor Study-3. *Surg Gynecol Obstet* 175:507–514, 1992.

37. Nakayama DK, Ortega W, D'Angio GJ, O'Neill JA: The nonopacified kidney with Wilms' tumor. *J Pediatr Surg* 23:152–155, 1988.

38. Weese DL, Applebaum H, Taber P: Mapping intravascular extension of Wilms' tumor with magnetic resonance imaging. *J Pediatr Surg* 26:64–67, 1991.

39. Cohen MD: Staging of Wilms' tumor. *Clin Radiol* 47:77–81, 1993.

40. D'Angio GJ, Rosenberg H, Sharples K, et al: Position paper: Imaging methods for primary renal tumors of childhood: Cost versus benefits. *Med Pediatr Oncol* 21:205–212, 1993.

41. D'Angio GJ, Breslow N, Beckwith JB, et al:

Treatment of Wilms' tumor: Results of the Third National Wilms' Tumor Study. *Cancer* 64:349–360, 1989.

42. Othersen HB, Jr, DeLorimer A, Hrabovsky E, et al: Surgical evaluation of lymph node metastases in Wilms' tumor. *J Pediatr Surg* 25:3:1–2, 1990.

43. Ng YY, Hall-Craggs MA, Dicks-Mireaux C, Pritchard J: Wilms' tumour: Pre- and post-chemotherapy CT appearances. *Clin Radiol* 43:255–259, 1991.

44. Thomas PRM, Shochat SJ, Norkool P, et al: Prognostic implications of hepatic adhesion, invasion, and metastases at diagnosis of Wilms' tumor. *Cancer* 68:2486–2488, 1991.

45. Blute ML, Kelalis PP, Offord KP, et al: Bilateral Wilms' Tumor. *J Urol* 138:968–973, 1987.

46. Montgomery BT, Kelalis PP, Blute ML, et al: Extended follow-up of bilateral Wilms' tumor: Results of the National Wilms' Tumor Study. *J Urol* 146:514–518, 1991.

47. Koo AS, Koyle MA, Hurwitz RS, et al: The necessity of contralateral surgical exploration in Wilms' tumor with modern noninvasive imaging technique: A reassessment. *J Urol* 144:416–417, 1990.

48. Goleta-Dy A, Shaw PJ, Stevens MM: Re: The necessity of contralateral surgical exploration in Wilms' tumor with modern noninvasive imaging technique: A reassessment. *J Urol* 147:171 (letter), 1992.

49. Ritchey ML, Green DM, Breslow NE, Norkool P: Accuracy of current imaging modalities in the diagnosis of synchronous bilateral Wilms' tumor. *Cancer* 75:600–604, 1995.

50. Green DM, Fernbach DJ, Norkool P, et al: The treatment of Wilms' tumor patients with pulmonary metastases detected only with computed tomography: A report from the National Wilms' Tumor Study. *J Clin Oncol* 9:1776–1781, 1991.

51. Cohen MD: Current controversey: Is CT scan of the chest needed in patients with Wilms' tumor? *J Pediatr Hematol Oncol* 16:191, 1994.

52. Wilimas J, Douglass EC, Magill HL, et al: Significance of pulmonary computed tomography at diagnosis in Wilms' tumor. *J Clin Oncol* 6:1144–1146, 1988.

53. Hartman D, Davis C, Madewell J, Friedman A: Primary malignant tumors in the second decade of life: Wilms' tumor versus renal cell carcinoma. *J Urol* 127:888–891, 1982.

54. Broecker B: Renal cell carcinoma in children. *Urology* 38:54–56, 1991.

55. Raney RB, Jr, Palmer N, Sutow WW, et al: Renal cell carcinoma in children. *Med Pediatr Oncol* 11:91–98, 1983.

56. Dehner LP, Leestma JE, Price EB Jr: Renal cell carcinoma in children: A clinicopathologic study of 15 cases and review of the literature. *J Pediatr* 76:358–368, 1970.

57. Castellanos RD, Aron BS, Evans AT: Renal adenocarcinoma in children: Incidence, therapy and prognosis. *J Urol* 111:534–537, 1974.

58. Blute ML, Malek RS, Segura JW: Angiomyolipoma: A clinical metamorphosis and concepts for management. *J Urol* 139:20–24, 1988.

59. Beckwith B: A pathologist's perspective on biopsies in pediatric renal tumor Management. *Dial Pediatr Urol* 14(12):2–5, 1991.

60. Ritchey ML, Azizkhan RG, Beckwith JB: Neonatal Wilms' tumors. *J Pediatr Surg* 30:856–859, 1995.

61. Marsden HB, Lawler W: Bone-metastasizing renal tumour of childhood: Histopathological and clinical review of 38 cases. *Virchows Arch* 387:341–351, 1980.

62. Joshi VV, Kasznica J, Walters TR: Atypical mesoblastic nephroma: Pathologic characterization of a potentially aggressive variant of conventional congenital mesoblastic nephroma. *Arch Pathol Lab Med* 110:100–106, 1986.

63. Gormley TS, Skoog SJ, Jones RV, Maybee D: Cellular congenital mesoblastic nephroma: What are the options? *J Urol* 142:479–483, 1989.

64. Heidelberger KP, Ritchey ML, Dauser RC, et al: Congenital mesoblastic nephroma metastatic to the brain. *Cancer* 72:2499–502, 1993.

65. Ohmichi M, Tasaka K, Sugita N, et al: Hydramnios associated with congenital mesoblastic nephroma: A case report. *Obstet Gynecol* 74:469–471, 1989.

66. Howell CJ, Othersen HB, Kiviat NE, et al: Therapy and outcome in 51 children with mesoblastic nephroma: A report of the National Wilms' Tumor Study. *J Pediatr Surg* 17:826–830, 1982.

67. Beckwith JB: Congenital mesoblastic nephroma: When should we worry? *Arch Pathol Lab Med* 110:98–99, 1986.

68. Breslow NE, Takashima JR, Whitton JA, et al: Second malignant neoplasms following treatment for Wilms' tumor: A report from the National Wilms' Tumor Study Group. *J Clin Oncol* 13:1851–1859, 1995.

69. Beckwith JB, Palmer NF: Histopathology and prognosis of Wilms' tumor: Results from the National Wilms' Tumor Study. *Cancer* 41:1937–1948, 1978.

70. Bonadio JF, Storer B, Norkool P, et al: Anaplastic Wilms' tumor: Clinical and pathological studies. *J Clin Oncol* 3:513–520, 1985.

71. Faria P, Beckwith JB, Mishra K, et al: Focal versus diffuse anaplasia in Wilms' tumor: New definitions with prognostic significance. A Report from the National Wilms' Tumor Study Group. *Am J Surg Pathol* (In press).

72. Bove KE, McAdams AJ: The nephroblastomatosis complex and its relationship to Wilms' tumor: A clinicopathologic treatise. *Perspect Pediatr Pathol* 3:185–223, 1976.

73. Bennington JL, Beckwith JB: Tumors of the kidney, renal pelvis, and ureter. In *Atlas of Tumor Pathology, Second Series, Fasicle 12.* Bethesda: Armed Forces Institute of Pathology, 1975.

74. Beckwith JB, Kiviat NB, Bonadio JF: Nephrogenic rests, nephroblastomatosis, and the pathogenesis of Wilms' tumor. *Pediatr Path* 10:1–36, 1990.

75. Rainwater LM, Hosaka Y, Farrow GM, et al: Wilms' tumors: Relationship of nuclear deoxyribonucleic acid ploidy to patient survival. *J Urol* 138:974–977, 1987.

76. Layfield LJ, Ritchie AWS, Ehrlich R: The relationship of deoxyribonucleic acid content to conventional prognostic factors in Wilms' tumor. *J Urol* 142:1040–1043, 1989.

77. Mohler JL, Partin AW, Epstein JI, et al: Nuclear roundness factor measurement for assessment of prognosis of patients with prostate carcinoma. *J Urol* 139:1080–1084, 1988.

78. Partin AW, Walsh AC, Epstein JI, et al: Nuclear morphometry as a predictor of response to therapy in Wilms' tumor: A preliminary report. *J Urol* 144:1222–1226, 1990.

79. Partin AW, Gearhart JP, Leonard MP, et al: The use of nuclear morphometry to predict prognosis in pediatric urologic malignancies: A review. *Med Pediatr Oncol* 21:222–229, 1993.

80. Coppes MJ: Serum biological markers and paraneoplastic syndromes in Wilms' tumor. *Med Pediatr Oncol* 21:213–221, 1993.

81. Lin RY, Argent PA, Sullivan KM, et al: Urinary hyaluronic acid is a Wilms' tumor marker. *J Pediatr Surg* 30:304–308, 1995.

82. Lin RY, Argent PA, Sullivan KM, Stern R, Adzick NS: Basic fibroblast growth factor as a Wilms' tumor marker. *Clin Cancer Res* 1:327–331, 1995.

83. Ritchey ML, Lally KP, Haase GM, et al: Superior mesenteric artery injury during nephrectomy for Wilms' tumor. *J Pediatr Surg* 27:612–615, 1992.

84. Nakayama DK, deLorimier AA, O'Neill JA Jr, et al: Intracardiac extension of Wilms' tumor: A report of the National Wilms' Tumor Study. *Ann Surg* 204:693–697, 1986.

85. Dykes EH, Marwaha RK, Dicks-Mireaux C, et al: Risks and benefits of percutaneous biopsy and primary chemotherapy in advanced Wilms' tumour. *J Pediatr Surg* 26:610–612, 1991.

86. Ritchey ML, Kelalis PP, Haase GM, et al: Preoperative therapy for intracaval and atrial extension of Wilms' tumor. *Cancer* 71:4104–4110, 1993.

87. Oberholzer HF, Falkson G, DeJager LC: Successful management of inferior vena cava and right atrial nephroblastoma tumor thrombus with preoperative chemotherapy. *Med Pediatr Oncol* 20:61–613, 1992.

88. Borden TA: Wilms' tumor and pulmonary embolism. *Soc Pediatr Urol Newsletter* (August): 27–29, 1992.

89. Shurin SB, Gauderer MWL, Dahms BB, Conrad WG: Fatal intraoperative pulmonary embolization of Wilms tumor. *J Pediatr* 101:559–562, 1982.

90. Bracken RB, Sutow WW, Jaffe N, et al: Preoperative chemotherapy for Wilms' tumor. *Urology* 19:55–60, 1982.

91. Ritchey ML, Pringle K, Breslow N, et al: Management and outcome of inoperable Wilms' tumor: A report of National Wilms' Tumor Study. *Ann Surg* 220:683–690, 1994.

92. Ritchey ML, Kelalis P, Breslow N, et al: Small bowel obstruction following nephrectomy for Wilms' tumor. *Ann Surg* 218:654–659, 1993.

93. Coppes MJ, Zandvoort SWH, Sparling CR, et al: Acquired von Willebrand disease in Wilms' tumor patients. *J Clin Oncol* 10:1–7, 1993.

94. Sutow WW: Chemotherapy in childhood cancer (except leukemia): An appraisal. *Cancer* 18:1585, 1965.

95. Wolff JA, Krivit W, Newton WA, D'Angio GJ: Single versus multiple dose dactinomycin therapy of Wilms' tumor: A controlled co-operative study conducted by the Children's Cancer Study Group A (formerly Acute Leukemia Co-operative Chemotherapy Group A). *New Engl J Med* 279:290, 1968.

96. D'Angio GJ, Evans A, Breslow N, et al: The treatment of Wilms' tumor: Results of the Second National Wilms' Tumor Study. *Cancer* 47:2302–2311, 1981.

97. Farewell VT, D'Angio GJ, Breslow N, Norkool P: Retrospective validation of a new staging system for Wilms' tumor. *Cancer Clin Trials* 4:167–171, 1981.

98. Green DM, D'Angio GJ, Kelalis PP, et al: The risks associated with prenephrectomy chemotherapy for unilateral Wilms' tumor patients. *Dial Pediatr Urol* 15:7–8, 1992.

99. Green DM, Breslow NE, Evan I, et al: Effect of dose intensity of chemotherapy on the hematological toxicity of the treatment of Wilms' tumor: A report from the National Wilms' Tumor Study. *Am J Pediatr Hematol Oncol* 16:207–212, 1994.

100. Green DM, Breslow N, Beckwith JB, et al: A comparison between single-dose and divided-dose administration of dactinomycin and doxorubicin: A report from the National Wilms' Tumor Study Group. *Med Pediatr Oncol* 27:218, 1996.

101. de Camargo B, Franco EL: A randomized clinical trial of single-dose versus fractionated-dose dactinomycin in the treatment of Wilms' Tumor: Results after extended follow-up. *Cancer* 73:3081–3086, 1993.

102. Larsen E, Perez-Atayde A, Green DM, et al: Surgery only for the treatment of patients with stage I (Cassady) Wilms' tumor. *Cancer* 66:264–266, 1990.

103. Green DM, Jaffe N: The role of chemotherapy in the treatment of Wilms' tumor. *Cancer* 4:52–57, 1979.

104. Green DM, Beckwith JB, Weeks DA, et al: The relationship between microsubstaging variables, tumor weight and age at diagnosis of children with stage I/favorable-histology Wilms' tumor: A report from the National Wilms Tumor Study. *Cancer* 74:1817–1820, 1994.

105. Coppes MJ, deKraker J, vanKijken PJ, et al: Bilateral Wilms' tumor: Long-term survival and some epidemiological features. *J Clin Oncol* 7:310–315, 1989.

106. Shaul DB, Srikanth MM, Ortega JA, Mahour GH: Treatment of bilateral Wilms' tumor: Comparison of initial biopsy and chemotherapy to initial surgical resection in the preservation of renal mass and function. *J Pediatr Surg* 27:1009–1015, 1992.

107. Ritchey ML, Green DM, Thomas P, et al: Renal failure in Wilms' tumor. A report from the National Wilms' Tumor Study Group. *Med Pediatr Oncol* 26:75–80, 1996.

108. Penn I: Renal transplantation for Wilms' tumor: Report of 20 cases. *J Urol* 122:793–794, 1979.

109. Lemerle J, Voute PA, Tournade MF, et al: Preoperative versus postoperative radiotherapy, single versus multiple courses of actinomycin D, in the treatment of Wilms' tumor: Preliminary results of a controlled clinical trial conducted by the International Society of Paediatric Oncology (SIOP). *Cancer* 38:647–654, 1976.

110. Lemerle J, Voute PA, Tournade MF, et al: Effectiveness of preoperative chemotherapy in Wilms' tumor: Results of an International Society of Paediatric Oncology (SIOP) clinical trial. *J Clin Oncol* 1:604–609, 1983.

111. Tournade MF, Com-Nougue C, Voute PA, et al: Results of the sixth International Society of Pediatric Oncology Wilms' tumor trial and study: A risk-adapted therapeutic approach in Wilms' tumor. *J Clin Oncol* 11:1014–1023, 1993.

112. Green DM, Breslow NE, D'Angio GJ: The treatment of children with unilateral Wilms' tumor. *J Clin Oncol* 11:1009–1010, 1993.

113. Grundy P, Breslow N, Green DM, et al: Prognostic factors for children with recurrent Wilms' tumor: Results from the Second and Third National Wilms Tumor Study. *J Clin Oncol* 7:638–647, 1989.

114. Harris CC: The carcinogenicity of anticancer drugs: A hazard in man. *Cancer* 37:1014–1023, 1976.

115. Evans AE, Norkool P, Evans I, et al: Late effects of treatment for Wilms' tumor: A report from the National Wilms' Tumor Study Group. *Cancer* 67:331–336, 1991.

116. Kinsella TJ, Trivette G, Rowland J, et al: Long-term follow-up of testicular function following radiation for early-stage Hodgkin's disease. *J Clin Oncol* 7:718–724, 1989.

117. Stillman RJ, Schinfeld JS, Schiff I, et al: Ovarian failure in long term survivors of childhood malignancy. *Am J Obstet Gynecol* 139:62–66, 1987.

118. Li FP, Gimbrere K, Gelber RD, et al: Outcome of pregnancy in survivors of Wilms' tumors. *JAMA* 257:216–219, 1987.

119. Gilladoga AC, Manuel C, Tan CT, et al: The cardiotoxicity of Adriamycin and daunomycin in children. *Cancer* 37:1070–1078, 1976.

120. Steinherz LJ, Steinherz PG, Tan CTC, et al: Cardiac toxicity 4 to 20 years after anthracycline therapy. *JAMA* 266:1672–1677, 1991.

121. Green DM, Breslow NE, Moksness J, D'Angio GJ: Congestive failure following initial therapy for Wilms' tumor. A report from the National Wilms' Tumor Study. *Pediatr Res* 35:161A (abstract), 1994.

122. Anderson S, Meyer TW, Brenner BM: The role of hemodynamic factors in the initiation and progression of renal disease. *J Urol* 363–368, 1985.

123. Argueso, LR, Ritchey, ML, Boyle, ET, Jr, et al: Prognosis of the solitary kidney after unilateral nephrectomy in childhood. *J Urol* 148:747–751, 1992.

124. Robitaille P, Mongeau JG, Lortie L, Sinnassamy P: Long-term follow-up of patients who underwent nephrectomy in childhood. *Lancet* 1:1297–1299, 1985.

125. McLorie GA, McKenna PH, Greenburg M, et al: Reduction in tumor burden allowing partial nephrectomy following preoperative chemotherapy in biopsy-proved Wilms' tumor. *J Urol* 146:509–513, 1991.

Neuroblastoma

• *C. Thomas Black, M.D.*

Neuroblastic tumors arise from primordial neural crest cells, the progenitors of the sympathetic nervous system. These cells migrate during embryogenesis to form the adrenal medulla and the sympathetic ganglia. Neuroblastic tumors occur, therefore, in diverse but predictable locations. Aside from tumors of the central nervous system, which are a much more heterogeneous group, neuroblastic tumors are the most common solid tumors in children.

The nomenclature of neuroblastic tumors is based upon cellular differentiation, which varies widely from (1) the neuroblastoma that is poorly differentiated and highly malignant to (2) the ganglioneuroma that is completely differentiated and benign. The ganglioneuroblastoma is a partially differentiated tumor displaying features of both the neuroblastoma and the ganglioneuroma and possibly representing an intermediary form along a continuum of spontaneous differentiation from malignant to benign.[1] A wide variety of other factors, particularly the patient's age,[2] are relevant both to the behavior of the tumor and to the prognosis for the patient. The admixture of location, degree of tumor differentiation, patient age, and other factors results in a wide spectrum of tumor types based upon clinical, genetic, and biologic characteristics.[3] This chapter discusses the neuroblastoma, the most malignant of the neuroblastic tumors.

Newer treatment regimens have improved the overall prognosis for children with neuroblastoma, but the prognosis for the subgroup of children with metastatic disease who were older than 1 year of age at the time of diagnosis remains quite dismal.[4, 5] Twenty years ago a child's age and the clinical stage of disease were the sole factors employed in determining treatment and prognosis for neuroblastoma. Today the identification of certain clinical, genetic, and biologic characteristics allows a more precise stratification of treatment and hence a more favorable outlook for the highest-risk patients. In addition, screening programs based upon certain of these characteristics have been devised in an effort to identify patients with neuroblastoma earlier in the course of the disease. Innovative modalities of treating neuroblastoma are being explored. These screening programs and treatment modalities are discussed in this chapter.

INCIDENCE

Epidemiology

Between 8% and 10% of all childhood cancers and more than 15% of cancer-related deaths in childhood are due to neuroblastoma. Just over 500 new cases of neuroblastoma are diagnosed in the United States annually. Young and coworkers[6] estimate the prevalence at about 1 case per 8000–10,000 live births. The incidence in children under 15 years of age is about 10.5 cases per million per year for white children and 8.8 cases per million per year for black children.[6] The overall male-to-female ratio is about 1.2:1 in combined series.[7] In one large series of children with high-risk neuroblastoma, the ratio was 1.5:1.[7] The incidence seems to be uniform across countries for which data are available. A biphasic incidence with peaks between birth and 12 months and between 24 and 48 months of age has been inconsistently reported.[8]

ETIOLOGY

Environmental Factors

Epidemiologic studies have failed to demonstrate a conclusive association between environmental factors and neuroblastoma development. Several reports exist of neuroblastoma occurring in association with fetal hydantoin and fetal alcohol syndromes,[9–13] maternal ingestion of sex hormones or diuretics, and maternal usage of hair coloring products.[14] An association between neuroblastoma and paternal exposure to electromagnetic fields has been reported,[15, 16] but another study failed to confirm this association.[17] To this point, no other environmental and behavioral factors, such as maternal usage of coffee or tobacco, have been implicated in the development of neuroblastoma.

Genetic Factors

Familial occurrence of neuroblastoma has occasionally been noted; one review chronicled 55 patients in 23 families.[18] Eight patients had multiple primary tumors. The majority were younger than 12 months of age, in contrast to the general population, in which 22 months is the median age for the detection of neuroblastoma. Kushner and Helson[19] have suggested that the fact of monozygotic siblings both developing neuroblastoma during infancy may mean hereditary factors are more important in the infantile form, whereas the lack of this finding in older twins may mean that a random mutation is more important in the later childhood form. Other familial cohorts have since been identified.[20, 21]

These differences suggest that the mechanism of tumorigenesis in familial neuroblastoma may involve the deactivation of a recessive tumor suppressor gene or an autosomal dominant pattern of inheritance. Knudson and Strong[22] estimated that up to 22% of all neuroblastomas may result from a germinal mutation. Knudson's[23] hypothesis that two mutations within a single cell are required to cause a malignant transformation may be applicable to neuroblastoma. According to that hypothesis, the hereditary form of neuroblastoma would result from the combination of an inherited first mutation and a single additional mutation within any cell. Conversely, the nonhereditary form would require both mutations to occur within a single cell, most likely resulting in a single tumor. Infants who inherit a first mutation, then, should have a higher risk of neuroblastoma of multifocal primary tumors, and of disease occurring at an earlier age. Because of the dominant inheritance, one half of a survivor's offspring would carry the mutation and have a 63% likelihood of neuroblastoma eventually developing.[24, 25]

Chromosomal analysis of neuroblastoma specimens has verified that abnormalities are frequently found on the short arm of chromosome 1 (1p36) (see the discussion under Pathologic Features Having Diagnostic and Prognostic Significance later in this chapter).

Association with Other Syndromes

The term *neurocristopathy* has been applied to disorders affecting cells of neural crest origin, including neuroblastoma. Colonic aganglionosis (Hirschsprung's disease) and central hypoventilation syndrome (Ondine's curse) have both occurred in conjunction with congenital neuroblastoma.[25] Although each of these conditions involves a disorder of neural crest cells, how they are associated with congenital neuroblastoma is unclear.[26] An apparent association between neuroblastoma and neurofibromatosis (Recklinghausen's disease) has been made.[27–30] Bellah and coworkers[31] and Beckwith[32] have suggested a link between neuroblastoma and congenital heart disease. Sirinelli and coworkers[33] found two patients with the Beckwith-Wiedemann syndrome who later had neuroblastic tumors. Whereas Horner's syndrome resulting from cervical neuroblastoma is a well-known phenomenon, the interesting association of Horner's syndrome with a distant neuroblastoma indicates a possible common neural crest cell dysfunction.[34] Other associations include the DiGeorge syndrome,[35] the Sotos syndrome (cerebral gigantism),[36] and the Simpson-Golabi-Behmel syndrome.[37] It is likely, however, that some of these disorders will eventually be shown to occur in patients with neuroblastoma at no higher a rate than in the general population.

PATHOGENESIS

Because neuroblastoma is the malignancy most likely to undergo spontaneous differentiation, continuing investigation into the molecular biology of this tumor may yield information that would enable the ultimate regulation of other tumor systems and the development of more effective and less toxic prophylactic or therapeutic techniques.[38–42]

Embryology

Many internal organs, including the liver, pancreas and kidney, are initially populated by organ-specific blast cells that differentiate into the mature cell types found in normal organs. Microscopic foci of neuroblastic cells with the appearance of neuroblastoma in situ are frequently found at autopsy in the adrenal glands of infants less than 3 months old who have died of unrelated causes.[43] It was initially presumed that this finding indicated a high incidence both of actual congenital neuroblastoma and of spontaneous tumor regression. Subsequent studies indicated

that these neuroblastic rests are simply the precursors of normal adrenal medullary cells and that most neuroblastic tissue found in normal adrenal glands regresses by the time of or soon after birth.[44, 45] It is likely, however, that neuroblastomas do arise from persistent rests of these neuroblastic cells.

Fetal neuroblastoma was detected by prenatal ultrasonography in 21 cases. An additional 71 cases were diagnosed within 1 month of birth, and these had features that could have been detected prenatally had ultrasonography been performed.[46]

Although regression of neuroblastoma, even of metastatic disease, has been well documented (see the section on Spontaneous Regression later in this chapter),[47–49] it probably occurs no more often than in 2% to 5% of all patients with documented disease.[50] As the diagnosis and true incidence of neuroblastoma in situ are quite difficult to determine, the overall incidence of regression of congenital tumors remains unknown.

PATHOLOGY

Neuroblastic tumors originate in neural crest cells, more specifically the primitive, pluripotential sympathogonia derived from the neural crest that give rise to the various normal tissues of the sympathetic nervous system, such as the paraspinal sympathetic chains and the adrenal medulla cells. The histopathology of neuroblastoma, ganglioneuroblastoma, and ganglioneuroma displays a variety of maturation and differentiation patterns that appear to correlate with differentiation patterns normally seen during the development of the sympathetic nervous system.[51]

Microscopically, a typical neuroblastoma consists of small, uniform cells (neuroblasts) composed of dense, hyperchromatic nuclei with very little cytoplasm (Fig. 10–1). Neuropil, or neuritic process, is a distinctive feature. Homer-Wright pseudorosettes are also diagnostic but are seen in less than half of all cases[52]; these pseudorosettes consist of eosinophilic neuropil surrounded by neuroblasts (Fig. 10–2). Other similar-appearing small-, blue-, round-cell neoplasms of childhood include Ewing's sarcoma, non-Hodgkin's lymphoma, primitive neuroectodermal tumors (PNET), and undifferentiated soft-tissue sarcomas (such as rhabdomyosarcomas).

On the opposite end of the spectrum from the neuroblastoma is the ganglioneuroma. Com-

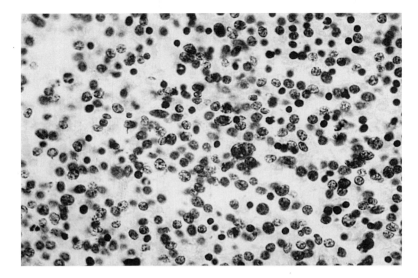

Figure 10-1 • Photomicrograph of a neuroblastoma showing small, uniform cells composed of dense, hyperchromatic nuclei and scanty cytoplasm.

pletely differentiated and benign, it is composed primarily of mature ganglion cells, Schwann's cells, and neuropil (Fig. 10–3).

Ganglioneuroblastomas are a disparate group of tumors ranging histopathologically from a neuroblastoma with a few islands of ganglioneuroma within it to a ganglioneuroma with a few rests of neuroblastoma.[53] Areas of ganglioneuroma within a neuroblastoma may be focal or diffuse; a diffuse pattern is associated with a more indolent form of disease. Variations in tumor composition may occur within a single tumor, so that multiple sections must be examined to obtain an accurate diagnosis. The term "maturing neuroblastoma" has been applied to tumors containing relatively more immature neuroblasts than mature ganglion cells, whereas "ganglioneuroblastoma" has been applied to tumors with more extensive maturation.

To distinguish neuroblastoma from the other small-, blue-, round-cell tumors of childhood requires special staining. Helpful stains include S-100, vimentin, and neuron-specific enolase (NSE).[54, 55] Electron microscopy reveals dense membrane-bound neurosecretory granules with microtubules and microfilaments in the neuropil.[56]

Pathologic Features with Diagnostic and Prognostic Significance

Several biologic variables have been studied, including histology, genetic features, serum mark-

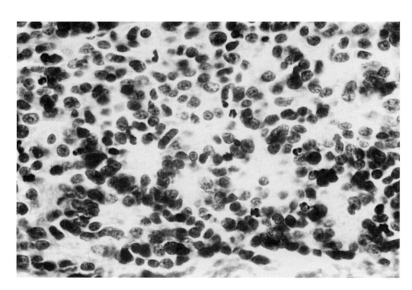

Figure 10-2 • Photomicrograph of a neuroblastoma showing Homer-Wright pseudorosette formation.

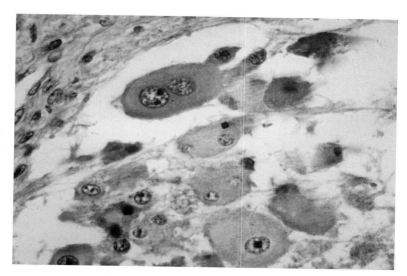

Figure 10–3 • Photomicrograph of a ganglioneuroma showing large ganglion cells and Schwann's cells.

ers, and cellular markers of neuronal differentiation, that appear to have value as independent prognostic markers in patients with neuroblastomas.

Histology

A histologic pattern of some differentiation, such as in ganglioneuroblastoma, generally is associated with localized tumors but does not have prognostic value that adds to age and stage.

Several investigators have classified neuroblastoma based on histopathologic findings,[57–60] but the system developed by Shimada and coworkers[61] has gained the widest acceptance. The Shimada classification incorporates the patient's age with histologic features that include the presence or absence of schwannian stroma, the degree of cellular differentiation, and the mitosis-karyorrhexis index (MKI). This system has been verified prospectively to be highly predictive of outcome. The Children's Cancer Group (CCG) evaluated the Shimada method in a retrospective review of 295 patients, and favorable and unfavorable subsets of patients could be identified.[62] The anatomical stage was less important than the histologic grade in predicting outcome.[63, 64]

Joshi and coworkers[65] analyzed 211 Pediatric Oncology Group (POG) patients with neuroblastoma in an attempt to simplify the Shimada classification while preserving accuracy. Tumors with calcification and a low mitotic rate (≤10 mitoses/10 high-power fields) were associated with a favorable prognosis regardless of stage or age. A grading system based on these features, the patient's age (<1 year versus >1 year), and the anatomical stage of disease defined low- and high-risk groups comparable to the Shimada groups of "favorable" and "unfavorable," but calcifications and mitotic rates are factors more assessable than Shimada histology.

Increased tumor vascularity assessed histologically appears to correlate strongly with the propensity of a tumor to disseminate widely. This feature has also been associated with unfavorable histology and N-*myc* amplification (discussed later).[66]

Chromosomal Features

Allelic Deletion or Translocation. A comparison between tumor DNA and autologous lymphocyte DNA demonstrates a *loss of heterozygosity* (LOH) on chromosome 1, indicating a deletion of the short arm (lp), in 70% to 80% of near-diploid tumors.[67–78] Rather than being completely deleted, chromosome lp is occasionally translocated.[79] Furthermore, lower-stage tumors are more likely to display a hyperdiploid or triploid karyotype and few deletions or translocations. An lp deletion reliably identifies high-risk patients in Stages 1, 2, and 4s who might otherwise be considered to have a favorable prognosis. Similarly, among patients with Stage 3 or 4 disease, those with lp LOH are in a high-risk category, whereas those not displaying the LOH are in an intermediate-risk category.[80, 81] Although the deleted segments of chromosome lp vary in length, common to all deletions is that of the lp36 region,[82, 83] which may code for a suppressor gene—the absence or translocation of which permits the development of malignant disease.[84] A strong correlation between a chromosome lp36 deletion and an amplification of the N-*myc* proto-oncogene (discussed later) implies a cause-and-effect association.[76, 83]

Van Roy and coworkers[85, 86] studied seven neuroblastoma cell lines and found a 1;17 translocation in three. Moreover, they found extra copies of 17q in all seven cell lines they examined, suggesting a role for certain genes on 17q in the development of neuroblastoma. A region of LOH on the long arm of chromosome 14 (14q) has been shown to be present in as many as half of all cases of neuroblastoma,[87] evidence for loss of another suppressor gene contributing to the development of the tumor. Srivatsan and coworkers[88] found deletions of chromosome 11 sequences (p or q or both p and q) in 12 of 37 (32%) cases of neuroblastoma and deletions of 14q in 6 of 27 (22%) cases, suggesting their possible importance.

Double-minute chromatin bodies (dmins) and *homogeneously staining regions* (HSRs) are also found in neuroblastoma and may represent the genetic basis of gene product amplification (see the discussion under Oncogene Expression).[89–92]

DNA Index (Ploidy). Although tumor karyotypic analysis has prognostic significance, it is labor-intensive and has a low success rate. DNA-flow cytometry is a simpler process than tumor karyotyping, and the results of measuring total cell DNA are consistent with those obtained by karyotyping. The *DNA index* (DI) of neuroblastomas tends to correlate well with their response to certain chemotherapeutic agents and to correlate well with general outcome.[93–99] A DI greater than 1 (hyperdiploid karyotype or increased DNA content) correlates with low-stage disease, a positive response to cyclophosphamide and doxorubicin, and a favorable outcome, whereas a DI equal to 1 (diploid state) correlates with an advanced-stage disease and a poor response to these agents.[100, 101]

Oncogene Expression

N-*myc* Amplification. Extrachromosomal DMINs and chromosomal HSRs are cytogenetic evidence of gene amplification.[89, 92] These amplified areas originate in the distal short arm of chromosome 2 (2p), which contains the N-*myc* proto-oncogene. The protein product of N-*myc* consists of, beginning at the C-terminal, a nuclear localization signal (N), a basic region (BR) that binds DNA, a helix-loop-helix (HLH), and a leucine zipper (Zip) domain that is critical for binding to another HLH-Zip protein called *max*. Apparently, N-*myc*/*max* dimers activate while *max*/*max* dimers repress the transcription of certain target genes that are as yet unidentified. When N-*myc* is unregulated, as in neuroblastoma, genes controlled by N-*myc* may be abnormally expressed, resulting in tumorigenesis.[102]

About 30% of all untreated primary neuroblastomas display N-*myc* amplification[92, 103] that correlates strongly with advanced-stage disease, and with rapid tumor progression, and poor prognosis, regardless of the age of the patient or the stage of the disease.[104–106] One study showed that N-*myc* activated angiogenesis, tumor dissemination, and PGY1 promoter.[107] N-*myc*, like *BCL2*, may be involved in apoptosis. Although not all patients with a poor outcome have N-*myc* amplification, virtually all patients with such amplification treated with conventional therapy experience rapid progression of disease and die as a result. Only about 5% to 10% of lesser-stage or Stage 4s neuroblastomas display N-*myc* amplification, as opposed to 40% of advanced-stage tumors.[78, 92] The factors of DI and N-*myc* amplification seem to be additive—the poor prognosis associated with a low DI is even worse when N-*myc* amplification is also present.[108] The presence or absence of N-*myc* amplification rarely changes over the course of the disease, allowing the early identification of an aggressive type of tumor with a predictably poor prognosis.[109] Tumors displaying N-*myc* amplification generally also have a higher level of expression than do tumors with a single copy; however, a tumor with a single N-*myc* copy and a high level of expression is not an ominous finding.[110–116]

Neuroblastomas with N-*myc* amplification have been found to be associated with high levels of expression of the gene for the *multidrug resistance protein* (MRP).[117] When MRP and N-*myc* were analyzed separately, MRP retained significant prognostic value for survival, but N-*myc* lost any prognostic value, suggesting that the expression of the gene for MRP accounts for the association between N-*myc* amplification and poor outcome.[118]

The c-src Proto-oncogene. The proto-oncogene c-*src* is expressed both by its neuronal product, pp60[c-srcN], and its fibroblast product, pp60[c-src]. The neuronal product pp60[c-srcN] may be a diagnostic marker specific for neuroblastoma, whereas pp60[c-src] levels greater than pp60[c-srcN] seem to characterize a highly aggressive form of neuroblastoma from a more favorable form found in infants.[119] High expression of pp60[c-srcN] may predict long-term survival in infants with high-risk disease.[120]

The pattern of c-*src* proto-oncogene expression distinguishes neuroblastomas from other histologically similar tumors such as Askin's tumor and esthesioneuroblastoma, both of which may be classified as neuroepitheliomas.[121] The ultimate clinical utility of the analysis of oncogene expression in neuroblastomas remains to be determined.

The p53 Gene. The p53 gene was expressed by four of five neuroblastoma-derived cell lines as opposed to neither of two neuroepithelioma-derived cell lines.[122] In another study, 30 of 31 undifferentiated neuroblastomas had high levels of cytoplasmic p53 protein but no detectable p53 protein within the nucleus, implying an inability of protein transport from cytoplasm to nucleus that resulted in poor growth suppression. By contrast, no p53 abnormalities were noted in any of 14 differentiated ganglioneuroblastomas studied or in the single ganglioneuroma.[123, 124]

The ret Proto-oncogene. Staining by an antibody to the *ret* proto-oncogene product has been correlated with ganglionic differentiation and maturation. The *ret* product may be a new marker for evaluating the degree of neuronal differentiation in neuroblastic tumors.[125]

The ras Proto-oncogene. The *ras* family gene has not been associated with neuroblastoma often enough to implicate it in the disease process.[126–130]

The genetic features of neuroblastoma that have been proposed as prognostic markers include tumor cell DI, N-*myc* oncogene copy number, and deletion or LOH involving lp. An analysis of DI, lp abnormalities (LOH and allelic deletion), N-*myc* amplification, and CD44 expression as prognostic factors in 377 cases of neuroblastoma found that all but DI and LOH at lp were significantly predictive of prognosis. Because of associations among the variables, N-*myc* amplification was the only relevant factor by multivariate analysis.[131] No study at the time of this writing has examined all variables in a large set of patients.

Serum Markers

The serum markers include ferritin, NSE, cell-membrane ganglioside (GD2), and lactic dehydrogenase (LDH).

Ferritin. Many patients with neuroblastoma have elevated serum ferritin levels.[132, 133] The degree of elevation seems to correlate with the stage of disease; serum ferritin is rarely elevated in patients with low-stage disease, but as many as half of patients with advanced-stage disease have levels greater than 142 ng/ml. Increased ferritin levels are also associated with lower rates of progression-free survival ($p = <.01$).[134] Increased ferritin levels may be a sign of tumor growth, or the tumor cells may produce ferritin,[135] or elevated ferritin or iron may potentiate the growth of neuroblastoma.

Neuron-Specific Enolase. Neuron-specific enolase (NSE) is a cytoplasmic protein found in neural cells. Poor survival rates in advanced-stage patients with neuroblastoma are associated with serum NSE levels of more than 100 ng/ml ($p = <.01$).[136–139] NSE is probably not really "neuron specific" as elevated levels are seen in association with other pediatric tumors. NSE levels are, however, widely obtained in clinical trials, and studies regarding its prognostic significance continue.

Lactic Dehydrogenase. The serum LDH level is a nonspecific marker for neuroblastoma. Increased levels are associated with rapid cellular turnovers or with large tumors. Infants with neuroblastomas whose LDH levels are over 1500 U/ml have a poorer prognosis.[140–142]

Cellular Markers of Neuronal Differentiation

Cellular markers must be assayed from tumor tissue obtained during the initial diagnostic evaluation.

Nerve Growth Factor and TRK-A. Neuroblastoma cells are known to differentiate occasionally into ganglioneuroblastoma or even to ganglioneuroma; thus, the malignant tendency of the neuroblastoma may represent either a lack of the stimulus to initiate cellular differentiation or a failure of the cell to respond to such a stimulus. Certain cell markers associated with neural cell differentiation seem to have prognostic significance in neuroblastoma. These markers include nerve growth factor (NGF) and its associated high-affinity receptor (gp140[TRK-A]), a transmembrane glycoprotein tyrosine kinase receptor.[143] The TRK tyrosine kinase receptor seems to be critical in allowing the differentiation and regression of neuroblastoma.[144] In one study, transfection of TRK-deficient neuroblastoma cell lines with the exogenous TRK-A gene restored the NGF-dependent ability to differentiate.[145] An association between high levels of expression of the TRK gene and favorable outcome in patients with neuroblastomas has been observed.[146, 147] Defects in the TRK receptor correlate with both a lack of N-*myc* amplification and a favorable prognosis, whereas lack of the receptor correlates with both multiple copies of N-*myc* and an unfavorable prognosis.[146–149]

Chromogranin A. Chromogranin A is probably another marker of neuronal differentiation.[150] Chromogranin A is an acidic protein present in the neurosecretory granules of neuroendocrine tumor cells, including those of the adrenal medulla.[151–153] It may prove to be an accurate serum marker indicating the level of activity of undifferentiated cells and the degree of response to treatment.[154]

Neuropeptide Y. Neuropeptide Y (NPY), another neurosecretory protein, appears to be an additional marker of neuronal differentiation. Levels vary with the degree of cellular differentiation.[155, 156] NPY was studied as a marker for neuroblastoma in 12 children. All but one patient with neuroblastoma had elevated plasma NPY concentrations at diagnosis. During treatment, NPY values returned to normal in 9 of the 12 children. All three children without normalization of plasma NPY values died; two of them had a relapse, and the third died of toxic effects. Plasma NPY appears to be a sensitive marker of neuroblastoma.[157]

Somatostatin Receptors. Somatostatin receptors, which are known to be expressed on other tumors of neural crest origin, were found to be expressed in a subgroup of patients with neuroblastoma. The expression of somatostatin receptors was found to be a favorable prognostic factor.[158]

Ganglioside GD2. Several independently derived monoclonal antibodies against neuroblastoma cells recognize gangliosides, which are sialic acid–containing glycosphingolipids. The most characteristic ganglioside on human neuroblastoma cell membranes is GD2. Not only is the presence of this ganglioside useful for identifying neuroblastoma cells, but also increased levels have been found in the plasma of patients with neuroblastoma. Measurement of circulating GD2 may serve as another useful marker of disease activity or response to treatment.[159–162] Indeed, gangliosides shed by tumor cells may play a role in accelerating tumor progression.[163, 164] The administration of monoclonal antibodies against GD2 has shown some promise in the treatment of neuroblastoma in a phase I study.[165] The combination of 14.G2a, a murine antiganglioside GD2 monoclonal antibody, and interleukin-2 has been shown to induce cytotoxicity against neuroblastoma in a murine model.[166]

CD44. CD44, a cell-surface glycoprotein marker indicating aggressiveness in other neoplasms, may be another significant marker in neuroblastoma.[167] Interestingly, the expression of CD44 in all other models correlates with more aggressive behavior, but in the neuroblastoma model, expression correlates with less aggressive behavior.[168] In a study comparing the prognostic value of CD44 expression with that of tumor stage, patient age, tumor histology, and degree of N-*myc* amplification, the expression of CD44 and the absence of N-*myc* amplification were the most predictive of favorable outcome.[168]

Proliferating Cell Nuclear Antigen. The proliferating cell nuclear antigen (PCNA) is a marker of cell proliferation and is expressed as the *PCNA index* (percent of cells staining positive for PCNA). The index has been predictive of outcome for patients with neuroblastoma and closely related to N-*myc* amplification.[169]

VGF. VGF is a gene regulated by NGF; the function of the VGF protein is not known, but it is present in human neuroblastomas, probably as a result of the effect of NGF.[170]

In summary, increasing evidence exists for at least two or three genetic subsets of neuroblastomas that are highly predictive of clinical behavior. One proposed classification takes into account abnormalities of 1p, N-*myc* copy number, and assessment of DNA content.[171] Three distinct genetic subsets of neuroblastomas can be identified by this classification. The first genetic subtype is characterized by a hyperdiploid or near-triploid modal karyotype with few if any cytogenetic rearrangements. Patients with this characteristic are generally less than 1 year of age and have a localized disease and a very good prognosis (>95% survival). The second genetic subset has a near-diploid karyotype with no consistent abnormality identified to date. Patients with this characteristic are generally older with more advanced-stage disease that progresses slowly and is often fatal (~50% survival). The third group has a near-diploid or tetraploid karyotype with deletions or LOH for 1p36, amplification of N-*myc*, or both. Patients with this characteristic are generally older with advanced-stage disease that progresses rapidly and is almost always fatal (<5% survival). Thus, genetic analysis of neuroblastoma cells may provide prognostic information that could direct more appropriate choice of treatment.

DIAGNOSTIC FEATURES AND METASTATIC PATTERNS

Clinical Presentation

The locations of the primary tumor of neuroblastoma are as diverse as the locations where sympathetic nervous tissue is found and vary somewhat with patient age. Although two thirds of primary tumors are intra-abdominal in patients of all ages, adrenal tumors are somewhat more frequent in children older than 12 months of age compared with those younger, in whom thoracic and cervical primaries are more common. An unknown primary tumor is a rare occurrence. Although cases are reported even in adults, the incidence of neuroblastoma declines after the age of 2.

Fullness and discomfort and a fixed, hard mass are typical symptoms and signs of a primary abdominal neuroblastoma (Fig. 10–4). The symptoms may be more dramatic when spontaneous hemorrhage into the tumor has occurred. Pelvic tumors may cause bowel or bladder dysfunction, generally because of compression of these organs. Respiratory compromise is a potentially life-threatening sign of massive involvement of the liver in Stage 4s disease. Tumor compression of a renal artery may cause renovascular hypertension.[172, 173] Gastrointestinal obstruction is uncommon.

A paraspinal tumor anywhere along the length of the spinal column may extend through the foramina of the vertebrae, causing neurologic symptoms ranging from radiculopathy to paraplegia to bladder or bowel dysfunction. Apical thoracic or cervical tumors may involve the stellate ganglion, resulting in Horner's syndrome. Ophthalmic heterochromia is a sign associated with congenital cervical neuroblastoma.[174] A thoracic neuroblastoma is generally diagnosed serendipitously when a chest radiograph is obtained for unrelated reasons. It is rare for a thoracic neuroblastoma to cause superior vena cava syndrome.

Lymphatic metastases are present at the time of diagnosis in about one third of patients with tumors that appear to be localized. A patient with lymphatic spread appears to have a more favorable prognosis than one with hematogenous spread,[175] which most frequently involves bone marrow and bone but occasionally involves liver and skin in Stage 4s disease. Further dissemination to lung or brain generally indicates recurrent or end-stage disease. Older children have a greater likelihood of having metastatic disease at the time of diagnosis than infants.

Symptoms of metastatic disease include weight loss, malaise, anorexia, and occasionally fever. More than half of all patients have hematogenous metastases at diagnosis, the majority of which are in cortical bones and are painful, causing irritability in the younger child and limping in those old enough to walk. Neuroblastoma has a propensity to metastasize hematogenously to the retrobulbar and periorbital regions, giving an appearance of facial trauma.[176] Painless subcutaneous nodules with a distinct bluish discoloration that occur in infants with Stage 4s disease are termed blueberry muffin–like spots and indicate metastatic deposits of neuroblastoma. Cervical lymphadenopathy unresponsive to antibiotics

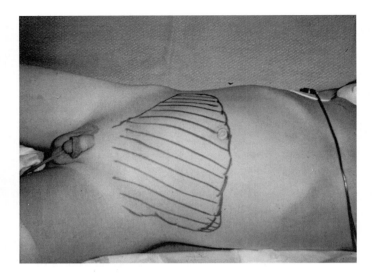

Figure 10–4 • A firm mass is outlined that proved to be a neuroblastoma of pelvic origin.

may be the harbinger of primary or metastatic neuroblastoma.

A group of signs and symptoms accompany certain paraneoplastic syndromes associated with neuroblastomas. Opsomyoclonus—characterized by involuntary jerking muscular contractions and random eye movements—ataxia, and dementia are associated with acute cerebellar encephalopathy, which affects up to 4% of patients with neuroblastoma.[177, 178] Although these symptoms may be related to the response of the cerebellum to antibodies formed against the neural tissue of the tumor,[179] they do not necessarily disappear following successful therapy. Because these symptoms are more common in low-stage disease, they may be associated with a more favorable outcome.[178] Hypokalemia and dehydration secondary to intractable secretory diarrhea may be the result of tumor secretion of vasoactive intestinal peptide (VIP).[180] Resection of the tumor generally leads to resolution of the symptoms. Levels of VIP and somatostatin (SOM) assayed by immunoreactivity are transiently elevated during tumor manipulation.[181]

Methods of Diagnosis

To confirm the diagnosis of neuroblastoma, one of several criteria is required, although these may vary from institution to institution. A demonstration of neural origin by microscopic or by immunohistochemical studies of a biopsy specimen is most certain. Increased urinary catecholamine metabolites are also considered to be diagnostic when accompanied by positive results of bone marrow biopsy, meaning that cells compatible with neuroblastoma were found. Alternatively, increased urinary catecholamine metabolites accompanied by a compatible appearance on radiography or nuclear scan may also be diagnostic.

Laboratory Studies

Catecholamine Metabolism. Up to 95% of neuroblastomas produce detectable urinary catecholamine metabolites that aid not only in diagnosis but in detecting recurrent disease.[182–185] Normal catecholamine synthesis requires phenylalanine, which is converted to tyrosine; tyrosine is then converted to 3,4-dihydroxyphenylalanine (DOPA), which is converted to dopamine; and dopamine is converted to norepinephrine, which is converted to epinephrine. Homovanillic acid (HVA) is a major metabolite of DOPA and dopamine. Vanillylmandelic acid (VMA) is the major metabolite of norepinephrine and epinephrine. Urinary HVA and VMA are generally routinely measured when neuroblastoma is suspected.

Imaging Studies

Imaging modalities employed in the diagnosis and staging of neuroblastoma include plain radiography, nuclear scintigraphy,[186–189] ultrasonography[190, 191] (including prenatal ultrasonography,[192–194] computed tomography (CT), [190, 195] and magnetic resonance imaging (MRI).[190] Plain radi-

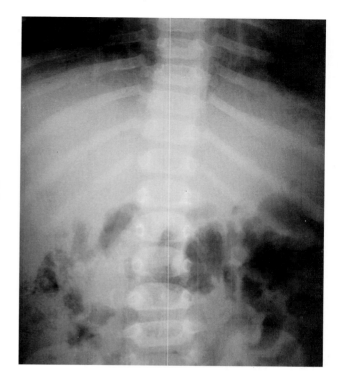

Figure 10–5 • A plain abdominal radiograph showing faint stippled calcifications suggestive of neuroblastoma.

ography may reveal stippled calcification in an abdominal mass (Fig. 10–5), posterior mediastinal mass (Fig. 10–6), or cortical bone lesion, each of which is suspect in neuroblastoma. Nuclear scintigraphy (bone scan) has been an important tool in the detection of cortical bone metastases.[186] Ultrasonography may aid in localizing an extrathoracic tumor to a particular organ or detecting a plane between a tumor and adjacent organs. CT and MRI may reveal the extent of lymph node involvement, the presence of tumor extension within the spinal canal, and the presence of metastatic deposits on either side of the diaphragm or within the head and neck.

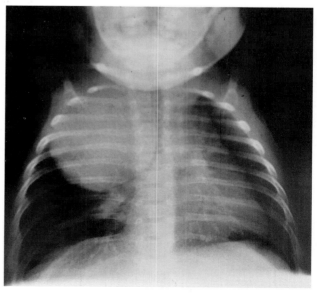

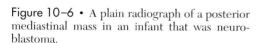

Figure 10–6 • A plain radiograph of a posterior mediastinal mass in an infant that was neuroblastoma.

Ultrasonography of 25 cases of abdominal neuroblastoma detected by a urinary mass screening program revealed the primary site in 24. Estimation of tumor weight based on ultrasonographic measurements was performed and, when combined with the presence or absence of distant metastases, allowed ultrasonographic grading that corresponded closely to the surgical staging (in 84% of cases). The cases of neuroblastoma of adrenal origin with a mass volume of less than 16 mL were all found to be Stage 1, which presents the highest possibility for spontaneous regression.[196]

MRI was compared with ^{131}I-labeled monoclonal antibody scanning for the ability to detect bone marrow metastases in the spine, pelvis, and femurs of five children with disseminated neuroblastoma following extensive treatment. The two modalities were equally able to identify marrow abnormalities; however, MRI was likely to be less specific than monoclonal antibody imaging. Both methods were more useful than conventional radiography, CT, and ^{99m}Tc-diphosphonate bone scans for identifying sites of marrow involvement by neuroblastoma.[197]

Meta-iodobenzylguaninine (MIBG) is assimilated by most neuroblastomas but not by normal bone, allowing identification of primary disease and differentiation of cortical disease from normal bone.[198, 199] Radiolabeled MIBG scintigraphy is a very specific and sensitive method of assessing primary and metastatic neuroblastoma (Fig. 10–7).[200] MIBG scintigraphy is being utilized increasingly with ^{99m}Tc-diphosphonate scintigraphy for evaluating bone disease and with CT or MRI for evaluating soft-tissue disease.

A radiolabeled somatostatin congener, [^{123}I-Tyr[3]]-octreotide, which binds to somatostatin receptors, has been used to detect areas of primary and metastatic neuroblastoma. After a seemingly complete surgical resection or ablative radiochemotherapy, any residual neuroblastoma may be localized by a [^{123}I-Tyr[3]]-octreotide and a gamma-sensitive probe, allowing more complete surgical extirpation if necessary. As noted earlier, however, the presence of somatostatin receptors correlates with biologically favorable disease, so that the most unfavorable tumors remain undetected by this technique.[201]

Surgical Biopsy

A bone marrow aspiration or biopsy is perhaps the least invasive means of securing both a histologic diagnosis of neuroblastoma and determination of stage. Generally, bone marrow aspiration and biopsy from both anterior or posterior iliac crests is required for an adequate sample size.

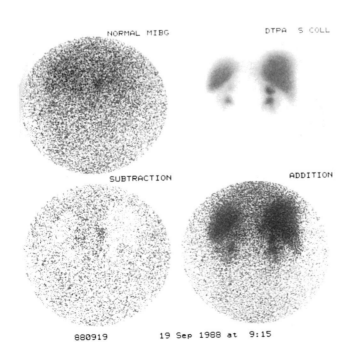

Figure 10–7 • The MIBG scan (upper left) is suggestive of an area of increased uptake. After the pattern obtained on the DTPA sulfur colloid scan (upper right) was subtracted, the subtraction image (lower left) shows a definite "hot" area indicative of a neuroendocrine tumor.

Occasionally metastatic deposits in skin, lymph nodes, or other locations may also be amenable to biopsy.

Should biopsy of the primary tumor be necessary, percutaneous fine needle aspiration (FNA) can decrease the necessity for open biopsy.[202] In a large study of children with advanced-stage neuroblastoma, resection of the primary tumor was accompanied by less morbidity when diagnostic biopsy of the primary had been performed by means other than laparotomy and open biopsy.[7] Although FNA is reliably diagnostic, the volume of tumor recovered is far too small to permit the battery of histologic and cytogenetic tests currently thought to be of prognostic value. Less controversial is FNA in the assessment of possibly recurrent disease. When available testing has been narrowed to only a few key prognostic approaches, and the minimum volume required to perform them has been decreased, the practicality of FNA in biopsy of the primary tumor will be reassessed.

It is unclear whether the techniques of minimally invasive surgery (MIS), which are less invasive than laparotomy but more so than FNA, will have a positive impact on the ease, accuracy, and morbidity associated with surgical biopsy of the abdominal and thoracic cavities. Although the size of the biopsy is not limited with MIS as it is with FNA, the MIS procedures are much more invasive and require general anesthesia in the operating room. At the time of this writing, a cooperative trial is being conducted by the CCG and POG to investigate the effect of MIS on later tumor resection.

Guidelines for biopsy of other organs at the time of laparotomy have not been standardized. A reasonable approach would be to perform a biopsy on an organ if (1) it is safe, (2) the stage of the tumor would be affected, and (3) the inspection, palpation, or preoperative studies have indicated that the presence of tumor is probable.

Diagnostic Criteria

By convention, neuroblastoma is diagnosed if (1) results of histologic testing of biopsied tumor tissue are unequivocal and (2) tumor cells are detected in the bone marrow *and* urinary catecholamine metabolite levels (VMA or HVA) are elevated.[203] A third criterion accepted by many clinicians is the clear radiographic or scintigraphic evidence of neuroblastoma coupled with elevated urinary catecholamine metabolite levels. On occasion a neurogenic tumor other than neuroblastoma will satisfy this criterion, and inappropriate treatment might therefore be delivered.[204]

Either the VMA or HVA or both will be elevated in the majority of patients with neuroblastoma. Spot urine testing may be as reliable if collected every 12–24 hours.[205]

Differential Diagnosis

A typical adrenal neuroblastoma is indistinguishable on palpation from other upper abdominal flank masses, particularly nephroblastomas, which such masses are statistically somewhat more likely to be. Because just 90% of neuroblastic tumors occur within the abdominal cavity, nephroblastoma occurs slightly more frequently in that location.

Rarely, hepatoblastomas or a variety of nonmalignant masses may appear similarly. Calcifications resulting from adrenal hemorrhage may be difficult to distinguish from a neuroblastoma.[206, 207] Testing for urinary catecholamine metabolites offers no assistance in identifying the 5% to 10% of neuroblastomas that do not produce them.[208, 209] Periorbital metastases causing proptosis and ecchymoses may cause a child to be mistakenly suspected of being the victim of physical abuse.[176] Symptomatic metastases in cortical bones may cause symptoms resembling osteomyelitis or rheumatoid arthritis. In approximately 1% of children with metastatic neuroblastoma, no primary tumor is found. Cervical lymphadenopathy in such a patient may resemble that of infectious origin. The nonspecific diarrhea of the VIP syndrome resembles diarrhea from a variety of causes.[210] Symptoms of opsomyoclonus or ataxia may be confused with several neurologic diseases.[211, 212]

Neuroblastoma is one of the classic small-, blue-, round-cell tumors whose differential diagnosis includes rhabdomyosarcoma, Ewing's sarcoma, leukemia, and lymphoma. When detected, circulating neuroblasts may also resemble leukemia.[213]

Anatomical Staging

The four anatomical systems of staging neuroblastoma (Table 10–1) are (1) the Evans classifi-

Table 10–1 · Comparison of the Evans, St. Jude, and International Staging System Classifications

Evans Classification	St. Jude Classification	International Staging System Classification
Stage I. Tumor confined to the organ or structure of origin.	*Stage A.* Complete gross resection of the primary tumor with or without microscopic residual disease. Intracavitary lymph nodes not adhered to the primary tumor. Nodes adhered to the surface of or within the primary may be positive. Liver free of tumor.	*Stage 1.* Localized tumor confined to the area of origin. Complete gross excision with or without microscopic residual disease. Identifiable ipsilateral and contralateral lymph nodes are microscopically negative.
Stage II. Tumor extending in continuity beyond the organ or structure of origin but not crossing the midline. Regional lymph nodes on the ipsilateral side may be involved.	*Stage B.* Grossly unresected primary tumor. Nodes and liver the same as in Stage A.	*Stage 2a.* Unilateral tumor with incomplete gross excision. Identifiable ipsilateral and contralateral lymph nodes are microscopically negative. *Stage 2b.* Unilateral tumor with complete or incomplete gross excision, with positive ipsilateral regional lymph nodes. Identifiable contralateral lymph nodes are microscopically negative.
Stage III. Tumor extending in continuity beyond the midline. Regional lymph nodes may be involved bilaterally.	*Stage C.* Complete or incomplete resection of primary. Intracavitary nodes not adhered to primary must be histologically positive for tumor. Liver same as in Stage A.	*Stage 3.* Tumor infiltrating across the midline with or without regional lymph node involvement. Or unilateral tumor with contralateral regional lymph node involvement. Or midline tumor with bilateral lymph node involvement.
Stage IV. Remote disease involving the skeleton, bone marrow, soft tissue, and distant lymph node groups. *Stage IV-S.* As defined in Stage I or II, except for the presence of remote disease confined to the liver, skin, or bone marrow (without cortical bone metastases).	*Stage D.* Dissemination of disease beyond intracavitary nodes (e.g., extracavitary nodes, liver, skin, bone marrow, bone, etc.). *Stage DS.* Infants younger than 1 year with Evans Stage IV-S disease.	*Stage 4.* Dissemination of tumor to bone, bone marrow, liver, distant lymph nodes, or other organs (except as defined in Stage 4s). *Stage 4s.* Localized primary tumor as defined for Stage 1 or 2 with dissemination limited to liver, skin, and/or bone marrow.

From Evans AE, D'Angio GJ, Randolph J: A proposed staging for children with neuroblastoma. Children's Cancer Study Group A. *Cancer* 27:374–378, 1971; Hayes FA, Green A, Hustu HO, et al: Surgicopathologic staging of neuroblastoma: Prognostic significance of regional lymph node metastases. *J Pediatr* 102:59–62, 1983; Brodeur GM, Seeger RC, Barrett A, et al: International criteria for diagnosis, staging, and response to treatment in patients with neuroblastoma. *J Clin Oncol* 6:1874–1881, 1988.

cation used by CCG-affiliated institutions and others,[214] (2) the St. Jude system used at the St. Jude Children's Research Hospital and other POG-affiliated centers,[215] (3) the variations of the tumor-node-metastasis (TNM) classification,[216] and the International Neuroblastoma Staging System (INSS).[217]

INSS

In contradistinction to the two systems most widely used in the past—the Evans classification, which uses Roman numerals, and the POG classification, which uses English letters—the INSS uses Arabic numbers. The INSS has resolved some of the discrepancies between the two earlier systems.

Stages 1, I, and A are similar except concerning the resectability of localized tumors (Fig. 10–8).

Because of disagreement regarding the significance of ipsilateral versus contralateral lymph node involvement with tumor,[218] both Stage 2a (incompletely excised tumor) and 2b (ipsilateral lymph node involvement) have been defined. A tumor defined as Stage 3 demonstrates contiguous infiltration across the midline or contralateral lymph node involvement. Tumors arising from the organs of Zuckerkandl or from midline pelvic structures without lymph node involvement are classified as Stage 1 if resectable and 2a if not. Tumors with ipsilateral lymph nodes involved are classified as Stage 2b. Those with bilateral unresectable disease or lymph node involvement are classified as Stage 3.

Stage 4s is similar to IV-S or DS and carries a reasonably favorable outcome (Fig. 10–9).[219-221] Metastasis to bone marrow alone does not alter the staging of a case otherwise considered to be 4s.

Stages 4, IV, and D are equivalent and are defined by disease involving distant lymph nodes, bone cortex or marrow, or liver or other organs (Fig. 10–10). Although Stage 4 disease is not subclassified, cortical bone involvement, particularly in infants, may be associated with a worse prognosis than metastatic spread to other areas.

If the identification of optimal treatment and the accurate prediction of outcome are the goals of staging malignant disease, it is apparent that any system based solely upon clinical, radiographic, and surgical criteria will, in this day and age of molecular biology, prove inadequate. Eventually, the macroscopic evaluation will simply be one of many criteria, including tumor markers and imaging studies, that are used in a biologically based risk-grouping system (discussed next).

Risk Groupings

Matching outcomes with conventional clinical staging allows patients to be stratified into groups based on the risk of developing recurrent disease. Patients with similar risks may then be treated similarly. Generally, three distinct risk groups (low, intermediate, and high) have been developed; however, the existence of several systems based on different clinical and biologic factors can make the grouping of patients by risk confus-

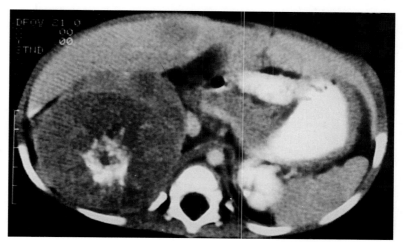

Figure 10–8 • CT scan of Stage 1 neuroblastoma.

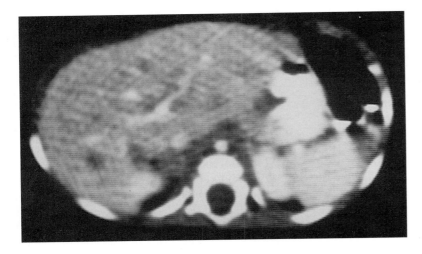

Figure 10–9 • CT scan of Stage 4s tumor.

ing. As additional biologic markers with prognostic value are incorporated into the staging process and improved treatment protocols emerge, further revision and stratification will undoubtedly take place.

Risk Groups Based Solely upon INSS

Based solely upon the INSS classification, patients with low-risk disease are infants and children with Stage 1 or 2a tumors or infants with Stage 2b, 3, or 4s disease. Patients with intermediate-risk disease are children with disease metastatic only to regional lymph nodes (Stages 2b or 3) or infants with Stage 4 tumors. Older children

with metastatic or Stage 4 disease are at highest risk.

Biologically Based Risk Groupings

Certain methods of risk grouping for neuroblastoma are beginning to incorporate biologic features with clinical stage and age of the patient in an effort to predict those who will fail treatment (Table 10–2). A variety of serum and cell markers have been identified (see preceding discussion), and others will likely be identified in the future. Currently, the most important factors seem to be serum ferritin, NSE, LDH, tumor

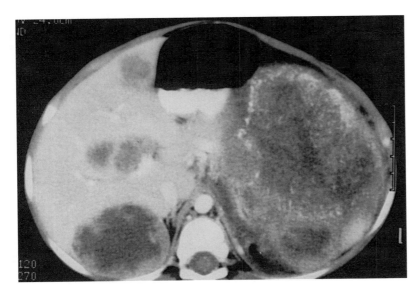

Figure 10–10 • CT scan of Stage 4 tumor.

Table 10–2 · Comparison of CCG and Brodeur Risk-Grouping Classifications

Risk Group	CCG	Brodeur
Low Risk	Stage 1: No N-*myc* amplification Stage 2: No N-*myc* amplification	INSS Stage 1, 2, or 4s Age usually <1 year No N-*myc* amplification Hyperdiploid/triploid with DI >1.25 No 1p LOH High TRK >90% cure
Intermediate Risk	Stage 3: Age <1 year *or* no N-*myc* amplification, low serum ferritin, low neuron-specific enolase, bone marrow negative, favorable Shimada Stage 4: Age <1 year, no N-*myc* amplification, low serum ferritin, low neuron-specific enolase, bone marrow negative, hyperdiploid, favorable Shimada Stage 4s: No N-*myc* amplification	INSS Stage 3 or 4 Age usually >1 year No N-*myc* amplification Near-diploid or tetraploid Low TRK Presence of 1p allelic loss or other structural change >25–50% cure
High Risk	Stage 2: N-*myc* amplification Stage 3: Age >1 year, N-*myc* amplification, and unfavorable Shimada, *or* age >1 year and high serum ferritin Stage 4: Age >1 year *or* age <1 year and N-*myc* amplification	INSS Stage 3 or 4 Age 1–5 years N-*myc* amplified Near-diploid or tetraploid Presence of 1p allelic loss Low TRK <5% cure

From Matthay KK: Neuroblastoma: A clinical challenge and a biologic puzzle. *CA Cancer J Clin* 45:179–192, 1995; Brodeur GM: Molecular basis for heterogeneity in human neuroblastomas. *Eur J Cancer* 31A:505–510, 1995.

histology, DI, N-*myc* copy number, 1p deletion, and TRK-A.[203]

One such grouping employed by the CCG places into the low-risk group all Stage 1 and 2 patients without N-*myc* amplification.[222] The intermediate-risk group includes all 4s patients without N-*myc* amplification, all Stage 4 patients younger than a year of age without N-*myc* amplification, and all Stage 3 patients either younger than 1 year of age or with favorable Shimada pathology, single-copy N-*myc* amplification, and low serum ferritin. High-risk patients are (1) those who have Stage 2 disease, are older than 1 year of age, and have N-*myc* amplification; (2) those who have Stage 4 disease, are older than 1 year of age, or are younger than 1 year of age and have N-*myc* amplification; and (3) those who have Stage 3 disease, are older than 1 year of age, and have either unfavorable Shimada pathology, N-*myc* amplification, or high serum ferritin.

Based upon both clinical and additional biologic characteristics, Brodeur[223] has classified neu-

roblastomas into one of three subtypes. The first group consists of tumors with a hyperdiploid or triploid karyotype or with a DI of greater than 1.25 on flow cytometry. Additionally, 1p LOH and N-*myc* amplification are absent, and expression of TRK-A is high. These patients are generally less than 1 year of age and usually have a low stage of disease (1, 2, or 4s). Their predicted survival rate is at least 90%.

Tumors belonging to the second group do not have an amplified N-*myc*, but the karyotype is near diploid or tetraploid, TRK-A expression is low, and structural changes such as an allelic loss at 1p or 14q are usually present. The patients are usually over 1 year old and have Stage 3 or 4 disease. Their predicted survival rate is 25% to 50%.

The final group of tumors have an amplified N-*myc*. They are usually near diploid or tetraploid, have a 1p allelic loss, and low TRK-A expression. The patients are usually 1 to 5 years old, have Stage 3 or 4 disease, and their predicted survival rate is less than 5%. As other markers are assayed for prognostic significance, further refinements in classification may be anticipated in accordance with the ultimate goal of delivering the most effective therapy and the least morbidity.

TREATMENT

Surgery, chemotherapy, and radiotherapy are the modalities in the treatment of neuroblastoma. Current therapy is based primarily on the stage of the disease with some consideration given to the child's age and certain biologic features of the tumor.

Surgery

Initial surgical intervention may be therapeutic, by resecting the tumor if possible; diagnostic, by procuring representative tissue for laboratory studies or information for more precise staging; or both. If resection of the primary tumor is not possible initially, it may be possible after a period of chemotherapy. After initial resection and chemotherapy, evaluation and excision of residual disease by second-look surgery may be indicated.

The initial goals of surgery are (1) resection if possible and (2) staging by inspection, palpation, and biopsy as indicated.

The resectability of a primary tumor depends upon its adherence to adjacent organs, including the fixation to musculoskeletal structures and major vessels, the ability of the surgeon to control blood loss, and the overall likelihood of cure. A large CCG review of patients with advanced disease at diagnosis showed a significant increase in operative morbidity (including loss of healthy organs and hemorrhage) with no increase in survival for patients undergoing initial resection as compared with patients in whom excision was delayed until chemotherapy had reduced the size of the primary tumor and lymph node metastases.[7] The efficacy of resecting the primary tumor or metastatic deposits in patients with Stage 4 disease remains controversial.

Factors influencing staging, such as adherence of the tumor to surrounding structures and lymph node involvement, should be assessed. Routine liver biopsy is often performed and is of low risk, but its value, particularly for older children, is questionable, both because of sam-

pling error and because of a lack of demonstrable ability to detect metastases in the biopsy specimen that are not already apparent on radiographic or other imaging studies.[224]

In patients with localized low-risk or intermediate-risk disease—that is, Stages 1, 2a, or 2b—surgery is the primary therapeutic modality. In a controversial report, Haase and coworkers[225] espoused the view that excision of the primary tumor in patients with Stage III disease improves patient survival. Of 26 patients with a primary tumor that was resectable at or subsequent to diagnosis, 20 survived disease-free for a median of more than 3 years. Only 9 of 32 patients with a tumor that could not be entirely removed survived that long. Unfortunately, this study has several weaknesses and is not conclusive. Others have also inconclusively addressed this issue.[226] DeCou and coworkers,[227] however, found improved survival rates with resection of the primary tumor in metastatic disease in infants.

The role of surgery in treating patients with high-risk disease—that is, older children with Stage 4 disease—is not yet well-defined. Shorter and coworkers[228] have reviewed the evidence for and against the efficacy of resection of the primary tumor in patients with Evans Stage IV neuroblastoma, as well as the timing and extent of surgery that should be performed, without reaching any conclusion other than that of recommending further definitive studies. Chamberlain and coworkers[229] found a significant prolongation of both mean and progression-free survival rates in a group of children with Evans Stage IV disease who underwent complete surgical resection of the primary tumor and metastases versus a similar group who underwent only partial resection. The study, however, was retrospective and nonrandomized. Data from a CCG study just completed at the time of this writing may yield some valuable information about the results of resection of the primary tumor in patients with high-risk disease.[7]

Chemotherapy

Although surgery alone may be curative in patients with low- or even intermediate-risk disease, chemotherapy is the mainstay of treating patients with advanced disease. Several agents used singly or in combination are effective against neuroblastoma, including cyclophosphamide, vincristine, doxorubicin, cisplatin, carboplatin, and etoposide. Devising combinations of potentially effective chemotherapeutic agents is based upon a knowledge of where in the tumor cell cycle the agent exerts its effect, what the toxicities and side effects of the agent are, whether any drug-drug synergies may occur, and what the potential is for the tumor to develop resistance to a particular agent. Many studies have shown that response to a chemotherapeutic regimen is frequently dose-related; a high dose delivered over a short period of time yields a greater response rate and hence a higher survival rate. Such regimens are limited by dose-related toxicities and side effects, although much effort is being directed toward developing means of increasing dosages to improve response while controlling toxicity to survivable levels. Peripheral blood stem-cell infusion, augmented by hematopoietic agents such as granulocyte colony-stimulating factor and granulocyte macrophage colony-stimulating factor (discussed later), or the reinfusion of purged *autologous bone marrow cells* (ABMT) (discussed later), may allow increased delivery of chemotherapeutic agents while controlling potentially lethal neutropenia.

The goal of the induction phase of chemotherapy is to deplete rapidly the number of tumor cells, arrest tumor growth, and impede further tumor dissemination. The CCG induction regimen consists of two cycles of cyclophosphamide, vincristine, and doxorubicin administered over a 3-day period with the cycles 21 days apart. The reduction of tumor burden and an eradication of metastatic deposits may lead to a much more easily resectable tumor. Furthermore, intensive induction may clear the bone marrow of tumor, allowing harvesting and preservation of a tumor-free specimen in preparation for future ABMT. Histologic changes due to chemotherapeutic effects may be seen in the resected primary tumor.

Following the induction phase, the consolidation phase is administered to eradicate residual disease. The CCG consolidation regimen consists of three cycles of cyclophosphamide, carboplatin, and etoposide, each cycle given over 3-day periods, 21 days apart.

Kushner and coworkers[230] have suggested that chemotherapy for non-Stage 4 patients without N-*myc* amplification is unnecessary because (1) such biologically favorable disease rarely evolves into biologically unfavorable or metastatic disease

and (2) the presence of tumor in lymph nodes has no prognostic significance.

Bone Marrow Transplantation

The search for methods to intensify treatment while decreasing the adverse effects has led to marrow-ablative chemotherapy followed by bone marrow transplant for patients with high-risk disease. ABMT may be augmented by purging the infusate of tumor cells.[231, 232] Allogeneic transplantation requires matching graft to host for immunologic compatibility. Bone marrow transplantation in patients with advanced-stage neuroblastoma has been increasing.

Numerous nonrandomized trials of ABMT to treat neuroblastoma have been conducted. Using a VAMP-TBI (vincristine, amethopterin, mercaptopurine, and prednisone plus total body irradiation) protocol, the CCG reported an estimated disease-free survival rate of 45% over 29 months in a highly selected group of patients, and this estimated disease-free survival rate was increased to 68% by adding courses of cisplatin and etoposide.[233] A POG study of selected patients reported a 2-year disease-free survival rate of 34% if ABMT was performed at the time of the first response, the rate was just 8% if ABMT was performed after the second response.[234]

A nonrandomized trial of 22 children conducted in Japan utilized high-dose chemotherapy, complete resection of all primary tumor and regional lymph nodes, intraoperative irradiation, intensive conditioning, ABMT, and post-transplant administration of *cis*-retinoic acid. A 70% 3-year disease-free survival was reported, but possible selection bias prevents definitive conclusions from being drawn.[235]

In another nonrandomized CCG study, Stage IV neuroblastoma patients older than 1 year at the time of diagnosis received ABMT and had a 3-year event-free survival of 49% thereafter, compared with 19% for similar patients who received chemotherapy instead of ABMT. Patients appearing to benefit the most from ABMT were those older than 2 years at the time of diagnosis, those with bone marrow metastases at the time of diagnosis, and those with only a partial response to multiple courses of chemotherapy.[236]

Still another nonrandomized study of older patients with Stage IV neuroblastoma who received ABMT reported that 17 of 28 experienced remission after intensive chemotherapy, primary tumor resection, and radiotherapy to the tumor bed. Despite manageable toxicity, 15 of the 17 patients remained disease-free with no toxic deaths between 1 and 4 years later.[237]

The only randomized marrow transplant study published at the time of this writing was conducted by the European Neuroblastoma Study Group. Patients received either ABMT (unpurged marrow infusate) or no additional therapy. No significant difference in disease-free survival could be demonstrated between the groups.[238]

Although the relative benefits of high-dose nonmyeloablative versus myeloablative treatment with ABMT have not been conclusively determined,[239] it is clear that patients given high-dose myeloablative chemotherapy and ABMT are more likely to survive if the treatment begins before disease progression has occurred.[240, 241]

Improved techniques for purging residual tumor cells from harvested marrow are being investigated. Important future concerns will include the patient selection criteria for optimizing outcome, the role of marrow purging, the ideal technique of marrow purging, and the management of late effects of transplantation.

Radiotherapy

Neuroblastoma is a variably radiosensitive tumor.[242] Radiotherapy of 2500–3000 cGy delivered to the site of a primary high-risk neuroblastoma has been found to decrease the local relapse rate, particularly when combined with low doses of cyclophosphamide and doxorubicin.[240] Doses delivered to the thorax or abdomen are limited to 2000 cGy unless *total body irradiation* (TBI) is planned, in which case the dose is decreased such that the overall dosage totals 2000 cGy. For patients with Stage 4s disease in whom liver metastases are causing significant clinical problems, such as respiratory distress, local irradiation to the liver (450 cGy) can be beneficial.[243]

After adequate bone marrow is harvested, TBI is given to prepare a patient for ABMT. Irradiation of symptomatic intraspinal extensions of tumor may be effective treatment but is associated with vertebral body damage, including growth arrest and instability that result in scoliosis. When such treatment is necessary, the entire width of the spine should be included. Chemo-therapy alone may be as efficacious as irradiation in managing intraspinal tumor extension.[244, 245] Palliation of pain from cortical bone metastases may be achieved by irradiation at 2000 cGy.

MIBG

Both ^{125}I and ^{131}I-MIBG have been shown to have therapeutic benefit against advanced-stage neuroblastoma.[246–249] One complete response and 18 partial responses were noted among 33 previously untreated patients with advanced-stage neuroblastoma treated with ^{131}I-MIBG alone.[250] In one study, treatment by ^{131}I-MIBG of children with recurrent Evans Stage IV disease was enhanced by concurrent administration of hyperbaric oxygen.[251]

De Kraker and coworkers[252] administered MIBG preoperatively instead of chemotherapy. They found minimal toxicity with significant response, just over half of evaluable patients had a 95% reduction in tumor size, and only 20% had no appreciable change.

Despite widespread use in Europe and elsewhere, MIBG has not yet been as accepted in the United States.

Therapy and Prognosis by INSS Stage

Low-Risk Disease

The disease-free survival rate of infants and children of any age who have an INSS Stage 1 tumor treated by surgery alone is greater than 90%.[6, 253] Neither radio- nor chemotherapy is employed in the initial treatment of Stage 1 disease, but chemotherapy has a high rate of inducing remission and extending disease-free survival rates in those patients with Stage 1 tumors who experience relapse following excision.[6]

Patients with INSS Stage 2a and infants with INSS Stage 2b or 3 disease who undergo surgery and a shortened course of postoperative chemotherapy have a 2-year survival rate of nearly 90%. Furthermore, relapses are often counteracted with the administration of additional chemotherapeutic agents or radiation. Matthay and coworkers[253] suggested, following a review of comparable CCG patients, that neither postoperative chemotherapy nor radiotherapy is necessary as survival rates were excellent regardless.[253]

The management of infants with 4s tumors

remains individualized, with the threat of respiratory compromise resulting from hepatomegaly requiring close assessment. Minimal chemotherapy, hepatic irradiation, or temporary abdominal wall augmentation by surgical placement of a prosthetic patch will decrease intra-abdominal pressure.[220] Stephenson and coworkers[254] found that infants who were younger than 6 weeks and had no skin metastases had a survival rate of 38%, inexplicably much poorer than the mean survival of 86% in a comparable group with skin involvement, or all infants in the group older than 6 weeks. In a review of infants with Stage 4s neuroblastoma, Martinez and colleagues[255] concluded that resection of the primary tumor was safe and effective. Only one of 24 patients who underwent resection died, whereas 7 of 13 who did not undergo resection died. The study was, however, retrospective and nonrandomized.

Intermediate-Risk Disease

The risk for children with INSS Stage 2b or 3 disease is low. In a study of similar patients (POG Stage B), Nitschke and coworkers[4] found a 3-year disease-free survival rate after initial or salvage therapy of 84%. Furthermore, Castleberry and coworkers[220] reported that infants with POG Stage C neuroblastoma have a survival rate similar to that of infants with POG Stage B disease.

De Bernardi and coworkers[256] in the Italian Cooperative Group on Neuroblastoma and others suggest that infants under 6 months of age with disseminated disease have a quite favorable prognosis compared with those over 6 months of age. In one study, infants with INSS Stage 4 tumors treated aggressively with chemotherapy, and occasionally with irradiation to metastatic sites, had a survival rate of 75%.[257]

High-Risk Disease

Chemotherapy dosages are generally maximized in treating high-risk patients.[258] Regardless of the regimen, however, overall survival of Stage 4 patients of 20% to 30% has only modestly increased. Survival time itself has increased since the institution of therapy. In an effort to avoid the toxicity of high doses of myelotoxic agents, cytokines such as granulocyte colony-stimulating factor (G-CSF) and granulocyte-macrophage colony-stimulating factor (GM-CSF) have been employed as well as purged ABMT harvesting and reinfusion or allogenic bone marrow transplantation. At the time of this writing, the CCG had just closed a large study of high-risk patients comparing results of ABMT with those of high-dose chemotherapy alone. Data are forthcoming.

Newer Treatment Strategies

GM-CSF has been shown to reduce neutropenia and infectious episodes in neuroblastoma patients but at the cost of mild thrombocytopenia.[259] Similarly, G-CSF administration has reduced the duration of neutropenia, allowed an increase in chemotherapeutic dose intensity, and reduced the cost of treatment.[260]

Immunotherapy

Monoclonal Antibodies

Because tumor regression may occur spontaneously, immune factors have been theorized to play a role. Monoclonal antibodies directed against various cellular antigens have shown some promise in phase II trials.[261–263]

Retinoic Acid

The retinoids, including 9- and 13-*cis*-, and *trans*-retinoic acids, have been shown to induce differentiation in neuroblastoma cells in culture.[264–266] A phase I trial has shown that serum levels corresponding to those effective against neuroblastoma in vitro are safely achievable in vivo,[267] and 13-*cis*-retinoic acid is, at the time of this writing, being utilized in a CCG clinical trial. Evidence exists that retinoic acid exerts its effect by regulating the TRK receptors.[268]

Virotherapy

After a single intralesional injection of live *Newcastle disease virus* (NDV) strain 73-T, 17 of 18 human neuroblastoma xenografts growing subcutaneously in live mice regressed completely; the 18th showed a partial response and regressed completely after a second injection. No side effects occurred, even after 500 times the therapeutic dose was administered. All animals not receiving NDV or receiving UV-inactivated virus died.[269] The same investigators report that retinoic acid enhanced this phenomenon.[270]

Neuroblastoma transduced in vitro with interleukin-2 gene was found to induce systemic immunity and eradicate minimal residual disease.[271]

PROGNOSTIC CONSIDERATIONS

Definitions of Terminology

Care must be taken in interpreting reports on responses to treatment because definitions of commonly used terms are not standardized. The terms "CR" and "PR" may indicate "complete response" and "partial response," respectively, in communications dealing primarily with chemotherapeutic regimens but may denote "complete resection" and "partial resection," respectively, in surgical communications. Likewise, "MR" may mean "maximum response" or even "minimum response" but in surgical writings generally means "microscopic residual." The distinction between complete resection and microscopic residual is indeterminate to the surgeon, as the results of both procedures have an identical appearance following resection. Many surgeons have begun using the term "no gross residual disease" to indicate either complete resection or microscopic residual. It is important to remember that "complete" or "partial" "resection" or "residual" refers not only to the primary tumor but also to the sites of metastases unless specifically stated otherwise.

Site-Specific Considerations

Neuroblastomas originating within the adrenal gland have more serious implications than those originating elsewhere. The prognosis for thoracic neuroblastoma (see Fig. 10–6) seems much more favorable than that for its abdominal counterpart, but whether that is due to a difference in the age of presentation or to actual biologic factors is unclear. Although complete surgical resection, if possible, is recommended, aggressive attempts at complete resection are probably not indicated as the prognosis is favorable.[272]

Neuroblastoma in the Older Patient

Neuroblastomas are diagnosed before age 10 in 97% of all cases. In a retrospective review of 46 patients with neuroblastic tumors diagnosed after age 10, 43 had neuroblastomas and 3 had ganglioneuroblastomas. The tumors were retroperitoneal or abdominal in 29 patients (63%), thoracic in 6 (13%), pelvic in 7 (15%), and cervical in 4 (9%). VMA was elevated in 6 of the 16 patients in whom it was measured. In 16 patients the disease was localized or regional, in 30 the disease was disseminated. Although ages ranged from 10 through 68 years, no difference in survival by age was seen in patients with the same stage of disease. One of the three patients with ganglioneuroblastomas died. Of the 43 patients with neuroblastomas, 34 died. The estimated 5-year survival rate was 62% for patients with Stage 1 disease, 75% for those with Stage 2, 25% for those with Stage 3, and 13% for those with Stage 4.[273]

Older-onset neuroblastomas tended to occur more frequently than expected in the pelvis and neck but less frequently in the abdomen. Survival rates for infants with lower-stage disease, particularly Stage 1, were lower than expected.[273]

Adult Neuroblastoma

At the University of Texas MD Anderson Cancer Center, 11 patients have been diagnosed with what has been termed "adult neuroblastoma." The tumor of adult neuroblastoma tends to occur in the extremities or the face. Histologically it is indistinguishable from the infantile form of neuroblastoma. Of 11 patients with adult neuroblastomas, 6 died of the disease.[273]

Spontaneous Regression

Nishi and coworkers[274] attempted to differentiate between those cases of neuroblastoma found during mass screening that would spontaneously regress versus those that would not, based upon the urinary HVA/VMA ratio (<1, 1–2, or ≥ 2) and the primary tumor site (adrenal or extra-adrenal). Extra-adrenal tumors had a likelihood of spontaneous regression of 80% to 100%, but the prognosis was particularly favorable when the HVA/VMA ratio was <1 or ≥ 2. A tumor of adrenal origin whose HVA/VMA ratio was <1 had a spontaneous regression rate of zero to 4%.

The concept of apoptosis suggests that cells are programmed to die unless prevented from doing so by trophic factors such as NGF. When

NGF supply is limited, most of it binds to the TRK high-affinity receptors, leaving the low-affinity receptors (p75[NGFR]) unbound, promoting apoptosis.[275]

Apoptosis is also prevented by expression of genes such as *BCL2*, an oncoprotein that prevents neuronal cell death[276]; the lack of *BCL2* has been associated with regression of neuroblastoma.[277] The effect of *BCL2* seems to be nonspecific for certain stages of disease.[278] *BCL-2* oncoprotein was detected much less frequently in ganglioneuromas than in neuroblastomas. Furthermore, the oncoprotein was detected more frequently around calcifications in patients under 1 year of age, and apoptotic cells tended to be distributed in areas where the oncoprotein was not found.[279]

BCL2 is also associated with and may induce inhibition of chemotherapy-induced apoptosis in neuroblastoma, which may be an important mechanism of resistance in differentiated tumor cells.[280] When differentiation of neuroblastoma is induced by retinoic acid, loss of the apoptotic response and resistance to cytotoxic agents develop—effects accompanied by very high levels of *BCL2*, whereas *BCL2* is undetectable in cell lines not induced to differentiate.[281]

Gestblom and coworkers[282] showed that the karyorrhectic cells described in the Shimada classification were either proliferating or undergoing apoptosis. They described a prognostic index based upon the MKI (mitosis-karyorrhesis index): A high ratio signifies a large proportion of proliferating cells and a poor outcome, whereas a low ratio signifies a large proportion of apoptotic cells and a favorable outcome.

Ambros and colleagues[283] found data to suggest that intact lp36, the absence of N-*myc* amplification, and the presence of near-triploidy (at least in localized tumors) represent prerequisites for spontaneous regression or maturation.

Squire and coworkers[284] found evidence strongly suggestive of the theory that the spontaneous regression of Stage IV-S disease is an immunologically mediated event. Of eight neuroblastoma cell lines studied by Bolande and Mayer[285] for cytotoxicity following treatment with normal pregnancy serum, cell death and cytolysis occurred in four. Evidence suggested that these effects resulted from IgM and complement-mediated cell lysis, which may contribute to a cytolytic form of spontaneous regression of neuroblastoma.

Pritchard and Hickman[286] have theorized that the normal tendency to undergo apoptosis soon after birth may be inhibited in neuroblastoma. In Stage 4s disease in particular, apoptosis may be delayed, although it is later successfully initiated, allowing tumor regression. These investigators suggest further that tumorigenesis is dependent upon the survival of one or more mutant cells whose growth is promoted by the expression of genes that inhibit apoptosis or by the effect of trophic substances—or by both factors. Certain of these mutations or expressed genes, such as *BCL2*, may also confer an element of resistance to chemotherapeutic agents.

COMPLICATIONS OF NEUROBLASTOMA AND ITS TREATMENT

Nonspecific complications of neuroblastoma include those related to failure of the bone marrow to generate adequate erythrocytes, leukocytes, and thrombocytes, generally because of tumor replacement of the marrow. Anemia, leukopenia, and thrombocytopenia may present as pallor, lassitude, weight loss, increased susceptibility to infection, or unusual bleeding. Hypertension, resulting from hypersecretion of catecholamine, and hypercalcemia[287] have also been reported, as well as coagulopathy causing intravascular thrombosis.[288, 289]

Complications of Chemotherapy

Complications of chemotherapy are numerous and well-described for each agent and most combinations. These complications include neutropenia, which may be severe and result in life-threatening infections; nausea and vomiting; fever; alopecia; secondary malignancies; and damage to other organs and organ systems, including neuro-, cardio-, nephro-, or ototoxicity. Mechanisms for minimizing or avoiding certain complications have been devised, such as the concurrent administration of sodium 2-mercaptoethanesulfonate (MESNA) with cyclophosphamide to prevent the development of associated hemorrhagic cystitis.

Complications of Radiotherapy

That irradiation causes the death of osteoblasts and chondroblasts with resultant bone necrosis and growth arrest is well-known. These effects have been noted particularly in children who have suffered neurologic impairment and were found to have intraspinal neuroblastoma and were treated acutely. Hayes and coworkers[245] reported that such effects may be avoided with excellent results obtained with chemotherapy rather than irradiation.

To reduce the effects of external-beam irradiation on intervening radiosensitive tissues, radiotherapy has been administered intraoperatively after displacement of those tissues. The benefits of intraoperative radiotherapy have been reported in small series, but not as yet in numbers large enough and with follow-up periods long enough to demonstrate conclusive advantage.[290]

Chou and coworkers[291] reported that total body irradiation, even at a young age, does not cause severe, acute, or late toxicities. A risk of pulmonary and endocrine dysfunction and a small decrement in IQ, however, has been found on long-term follow-up.

Complications of Surgery

Surgical complications related to resection of a primary tumor of neuroblastoma vary depending on the primary site, the aggressiveness of the surgeon, and the timing of the procedure. For procedures leaving no gross residual tumor, the rate of complications of all types varies between 5% and 25%.[292, 293] The most common complications are those that lead to nephrectomy, resection of other normal organs, intraoperative hemorrhage, renovascular injury resulting in renal infarction and necrosis, nonspecific problems such as abdominal adhesions, wound infection, and pneumonia, and unusual site-specific complications of surgical treatment such as Horner's syndrome. The risk of complications is greatest when an abdominal tumor is aggressively resected at the time of diagnosis or at a second-look procedure following open biopsy of the primary tumor. Complications are significantly lower for patients undergoing delayed primary resections after the tumor has shrunk in size, lost much of its vascularity, and become less friable as a result of chemotherapy.[7, 294] Resection of abdominal tumors in patients with advanced-stage disease following control of metastases seems to be more advantageous than less aggressive attempts, but this approach is controversial.[295]

Neurologic Complications

Approximately 30% of all neuroblastomas originate in a ganglion along one of the two paraspinal sympathetic chains. Nerves enter and exit the spinal canal through the neural foramina adjacent to each ganglion. As a paraspinous neuroblastoma enlarges, it may grow along those nerves into the spinal canal, causing spinal cord compression at that level. Acute neurologic impairment, including paraplegia, neurogenic bladder, or fecal incontinence, may be the first sign of a paraspinous tumor. A variety of approaches to this emergent problem have been suggested, including immediate laminectomy and cord decompression, irradiation to the area, and chemotherapy. Each approach has advantages and disadvantages. Laminectomy or spinal irradiation in young patients may cause scoliosis later in life. Chemotherapy has been found by some to be a superior method of treatment as the likelihood of recovery is similar to that of other treatment methods but long-term morbidity is less.[244, 245]

The central nervous system may be compressed by enlarging metastases within the bones of the calvarium or by dissemination to the meninges.[296, 297]

Patients with neuroblastoma who present with acute cerebellar encephalopathy, an uncommon paraneoplastic syndrome (see preceding discussion), have a high survival rate. Despite resection of the tumor and administration of steroids, the majority of patients will likely have some persistent neurologic sequelae.[298]

Second Malignancies

Second malignant diseases reported to have arisen in patients who had undergone treatment for neuroblastoma include pheochromocytoma,[299] renal cell carcinoma,[299] acute leukemia,[300, 301] and brain tumor.[302] Smith and colleagues[303] at the MD Anderson Cancer Center found 5 cases of second malignancies among 202 cases of neuroblastoma. Of these 5 cases, 3 were bone cancer and 2 were thyroid cancer. Poustchi-Amin and coworkers[304] found a relationship between the development of both osteosarcoma and osteochondroma and the treatment of neuroblastoma with bone marrow transplantation. No specific relationship between neuroblastoma and any other neoplasm occurring as a second malignancy has been established.[305]

SCREENING STUDIES

Because the majority of neuroblastomas produce catecholamine metabolites (VMA and HVA) detectable in the urine, a program to detect abnormal levels early in life by screening the urine of all infants began in a manner similar to that of screening programs for phenylketonuria, galactosemia, and other congenital disorders. Japan was the first country to institute a screening program. Japan's program initially involved only a few prefectures but has now become a nationwide project.[306, 307]

It is certain from the Japanese experience that screening detects more cases of neuroblastoma than would otherwise be found, but there is no evidence that the actual incidence of neuroblastoma has changed in the population.[308]

Such a screening program assumes that all neuroblastomas begin as Stage 1 disease that, without intervention, will steadily progress to advanced-stage disease; this is as yet unproven. The majority of screened patients with neuroblastomas have low-stage disease, and nearly all tumors thus identified have a hyperdiploid or near-triploid DI, which is associated with a very favorable prognosis.[96, 99, 101]

Although the total incidence of cases of neuroblastoma found since screening began has increased from 1/12,000 to 1/8000,[309] the incidence in children over 1 year of age is unchanged. Thus, screening obviously identifies a number of children with tumors that never would have progressed to clinical disease. Apparently these tumors, which are associated with a favorable karyotype and prognosis, undergo spontaneous regression or maturation. Such patients, however, are likely to undergo unnecessary treatment, including surgery and possibly chemotherapy. Among cases of neuroblastoma identified by screening in which the tumors had unfavorable biologic features, the course of the disease was not ameliorated.

One study identified 82 neuroblastoma patients, 41 of them by mass screening (group A).[310] Tumors were found clinically in the other 41 patients, 12 of whom were younger than 1 year of age (group B) and 29 of whom were older (group C). All group A patients had favorable (hyperdiploid or near-triploid) karyotypes and were free of tumor between 4 and 84 months after diagnosis. Of group B patients, one had a Stage 4 tumor with a near-diploid karyotype and N-*myc* amplification and died 18 months after diagnosis. Another had a Stage 4s tumor with near-diploid karyotype and N-*myc* amplification and died 9 months after diagnosis. All other group B patients had tumors with hyperdiploid or near-triploid karyotypes and no N-*myc* amplification and were free of tumor 12–89 months after diagnosis. All but two of the group C patients had tumors with near-diploid or hypotetraploid karyotypes, and 21 of these 29 patients died within 18 months. A 13-month-old and a 7-year-old patient who were both found to have Stage 2 disease and near-triploid karyotypes were both alive more than 6 years after diagnosis.

An asymptomatic 7-month-old found to have neuroblastoma by screening was observed without receiving treatment of any sort for 11 months until the tumor had nearly disappeared, at which time it was resected and found to be a well-differentiated ganglioneuroblastoma.[311]

Such cases suggest that the course of the disease may depend much more upon the biologic features of the tumor than the time of either detection or institution of treatment.

Because some neuroblastomas do not become apparent until at least 6 months after the time of screening because of false-negative results on testing, and partly because tumors detected at such an early age have a high likelihood of regression, some suggest that a later screening time, such as 12 or 18 months of age, might be preferable.[312–314]

The future of neuroblastoma screening depends upon determining the optimal patient age to perform the test; developing methods to differentiate tumors requiring treatment from those that do not, sparing unnecessary treatment; and demonstrating an improvement in clinical course, particularly survival rate, in screened versus unscreened populations.[315] At the time of this writing, Japan, Canada, and the United States are all conducting localized screening programs in an effort to resolve these dilemmas.[316]

THE FUTURE

Screening of the general infant population for early detection of neuroblastoma may eventually prove to be quite beneficial, and if so, will undoubtedly be widely adopted. Unfortunately, most tumors detected thus far have had favorable biologic characteristics, and so it is unclear whether the course of the patients with unfavorable tumors could have been altered by earlier detection. Should the causes of neuroblastoma prove to be multifactorial, contributing environmental factors will be of significance. Chromosomal deletion or allelic loss associated with neuroblastoma may eventually be corrected using gene transfer technology. At-risk patients may someday be detected by identifying additional oncogenes associated specifically with neuroblastoma. As NGF, its associated high-affinity receptor TRK-A, and other factors important in the differentiation and regression of neuroblastoma are identified, agents such as retinoic acid that enhance this differentiation may be developed. Similarly, regulating the inhibition of apoptosis, a factor in uncontrolled cellular replication, by pharmacologic or genetic intervention at the level of NGF or *BCL2*, may allow unimpeded tumor death rather than unrestrained growth.

MIBG and certain serum markers may eventually prove invaluable in the diagnosis and follow-up of patients with neuroblastomas, eliminating the need for second-look procedures and rebiopsy. Radioactive agents are being developed for use in the operating room to assess the extent of resection necessary. It is very likely that the INSS will become the universal clinical staging system. The risks of many currently known and some as yet unknown biologic factors will eventually be quantitated. Together with the INSS, they will combine to form a staging system more precisely predictive of outcome than any system alone.

Less toxic chemotherapeutic agents await discovery as well as improved methods of bone marrow transplantation. Some investigators have associated immunologic factors with the regression of neuroblastoma, and immunotherapeutic methods, long sought for and as yet found, may finally be discovered. The fascinating findings of tumor regression in mice following treatment with Newcastle disease virus may someday usher in virotherapy as a new form of treatment against cancer. The role of surgery in advanced-stage neuroblastoma awaits a more clear definition. Furthermore, the risk of a patient developing a second malignancy following treatment for neuroblastoma must be more clearly delineated along with the operative factors in this process.

References

1. Everson TC, Cole WH: Spontaneous regression of neuroblastoma. In Everson TC, Cole WH (eds): *Spontaneous Regression of Cancer: A Study and Abstract of Reports in the World Medical Literature and of Personal Communications Concerning Spontaneous Regression of Malignant Disease*. Philadelphia: WB Saunders, 1966, p. 88.
2. Breslow N, McCann B: Statistical estimation of prognosis for children with neuroblastoma. *Cancer Res* 31:2098–2103, 1971.
3. Brodeur GM: Neuroblastoma and other peripheral neuroectodermal tumors. In Fernbach DJ, Vietti TJ (eds): *Clinical Pediatric Oncology*, 4th ed. St. Louis: Mosby Year Book, 1991, p. 337.
4. Nitschke R, Smith EI, Altshuler G, et al: Postoperative treatment of nonmetastatic visible residual neuroblastoma. A Pediatric Oncology Group study. *J Clin Oncol* 9:1181–1188, 1991.
5. Nitschke R, Smith EI, Shochat S, et al: Localized neuroblastoma treated by surgery: A Pediatric Oncology Group Study. *J Clin Oncol* 6:1271–1279, 1988.
6. Young JL Jr, Ries LG, Silverberg E, et al: Cancer incidence, survival, and mortality for children younger than age 15 years. *Cancer* 58:598–602, 1986.
7. Black CT, Haase GM, Azizkhan RG, et al: Optimal timing of primary tumor resection in high risk neuroblastoma. *Med Pediatr Oncol* 27:220, 1996.
8. Voute PA: Neuroblastoma. In Sutow WW, Fernbach DJ, Vietti TJ (eds): *Clinical Pediatric Oncology*, 3rd ed. St. Louis: CV Mosby, 1984, p. 559.
9. Allen RW, Ogden B, Bentley FL, et al: Fetal hydantoin syndrome, neuroblastoma, and hemorrhagic disease in a neonate. *JAMA* 244:1464–1465, 1980.
10. Kinney H, Faix R, Brazy J: The fetal alcohol syndrome and neuroblastoma. *Pediatrics* 66:130–132, 1980.
11. Koren G, Demitrakoudis D, Weksberg R, et al: Neuroblastoma after prenatal exposure to phenytoin: Cause and effect? *Teratology* 40:157–162, 1989.
12. Al-Shammri S, Guberman A, Hsu E: Neuroblastoma and fetal exposure to phenytoin in a child without dysmorphic features. *Can J Neurol Sci* 19:243–245, 1992.

13. Battisti L, Degani D, Rugolotto S, et al: Fetal alcohol syndrome and malignant disease: A case report. *Am J Pediatr Hematol Oncol* 15:136–137, 1993.

14. Kramer S, Ward E, Meadows AT, et al: Medical and drug risk factors associated with neuroblastoma: A case-control study. *J Natl Cancer Inst* 78:797–804, 1987.

15. Spitz MR, Johnson CC: Neuroblastoma and paternal occupation. A case-control analysis. *Am J Epidemiol* 121:924–929, 1985.

16. Wilkins JR III, Hundley VD: Paternal occupational exposure to electromagnetic fields and neuroblastoma in offspring. *Am J Epidemiol* 131:995–1008, 1990.

17. Bunin GR, Ward E, Kramer S, et al: Neuroblastoma and parental occupation. *Am J Epidemiol* 131:776–780, 1990.

18. Kushner BH, Gilbert F, Helson L: Familial neuroblastoma. Case reports, literature review, and etiologic considerations. *Cancer* 57:1887–1893, 1986.

19. Kushner BH, Helson L: Monozygotic siblings discordant for neuroblastoma: Etiologic implications. *J Pediatr* 107:405–409, 1985.

20. Clausen N, Andersson P, Tommerup N: Familial occurrence of neuroblastoma, von Recklinghausen's neurofibromatosis, Hirschsprung's agangliosis and jaw-winking syndrome. *Acta Paediatr Scand* 78:736–741, 1989.

21. Robertson CM, Tyrrell JC, Pritchard J: Familial neural crest tumours. *Eur J Pediatr* 150:789–792, 1991.

22. Knudson AG Jr, Strong LC: Mutation and cancer: Neuroblastoma and pheochromocytoma. *Am J Hum Genet* 24:514–532, 1972.

23. Knudson AG Jr: Mutation and cancer: statistical study of retinoblastoma. *Proc Natl Acad Sci U S A* 68:820–823, 1971.

24. Knudson AG Jr, Meadows AT: Developmental genetics of neuroblastoma. *J Natl Cancer Inst* 57:675–682, 1976.

25. Stovroff M, Dykes F, Teague WG: The complete spectrum of neurocristopathy in an infant with congenital hypoventilation, Hirschsprung's disease, and neuroblastoma. *J Pediatr Surg* 30:1218–1221, 1995.

26. Bolande RP: The neurocristopathies: A unifying concept of disease arising in neural crest development. *Hum Pathol* 5:409, 1974.

27. Knudson AG Jr, Amromin GD: Neuroblastoma and ganglioneuroma in a child with multiple neurofibromatosis. Implications for the mutational origin of neuroblastoma. *Cancer* 19:1032–1037, 1966.

28. Bolande RP, Towler WF: A possible relationship of neuroblastoma to von Recklinghausen's disease. *Cancer* 26:162–175, 1970.

29. Witzleben CL, Landy RA: Disseminated neuroblastoma in a child with von Recklinghausen's disease. *Cancer* 34:786–790, 1974.

30. Kushner BH, Hajdu SI, Helson L: Synchronous neuroblastoma and von Recklinghausen's disease: A review of the literature. *J Clin Oncol* 3:117–120, 1985.

31. Bellah R, D'Andrea A, Darillis E, et al: The association of congenital neuroblastoma and congenital heart disease. Is there a common embryologic basis? *Pediatr Radiol* 19:119–121, 1989.

32. Beckwith JB: Cardiovascular malformations and the neural crest. *Pediatr Radiol* 19:122–123, 1989.

33. Sirinelli D, Silberman B, Baudon JJ, et al: Beckwith-Wiedemann syndrome and neural crest tumors. A report of two cases. *Pediatr Radiol* 19:242–245, 1989.

34. Gibbs J, Appleton RE, Martin J, et al: Congenital Horner syndrome associated with non-cervical neuroblastoma. *Dev Med Child Neurol* 34:642–644, 1992.

35. Patrone PM, Chatten J, Weinberg P: Neuroblastoma and DiGeorge anomaly. *Pediatr Pathol* 10:425–430, 1990.

36. Nance MA, Neglia JP, Talwar D, et al: Neuroblastoma in a patient with Sotos' syndrome. *J Med Genet* 27:130–132, 1990.

37. Hughes-Benzie RM, Hunter AG, Allanson JE, et al: Simpson-Golabi-Behmel syndrome associated with renal dysplasia and embryonal tumor: localization of the gene to Xqcen-q21. *Am J Med Genet* 43:428–435, 1992.

38. Evans AE: *Advances in Neuroblastoma Research*. New York: Raven Press, 1980.

39. Evans AE, D'Angio GJ, Seeger RC: *Advances in Neuroblastoma Research*. New York: Alan R. Liss, 1985.

40. Evans AE, D'Angio GJ, Knudson AGJ, et al: *Advances in Neuroblastoma Research 2*. New York: Alan R. Liss, 1988.

41. Evans AE, D'Angio GJ, Knudson AGJ, et al: *Advances in Neuroblastoma Research 3*. New York: Wiley-Liss, 1991.

42. Evans AE, D'Angio GJ, Knudson AGJ, et al: *Advances in Neuroblastoma Research 4*. New York: Wiley-Liss, 1994.

43. Beckwith J, Perrin E: In situ neuroblastomas: A contribution to the natural history of neural crest tumors. *Am J Pathol* 43:1089, 1963.

44. Turkel SB, Itabashi HH: The natural history of neuroblastic cells in the fetal adrenal gland. *Am J Pathol* 76:225–244, 1975.

45. Ikeda Y, Lister J, Bouton JM, et al: Congenital neuroblastoma, neuroblastoma in situ, and the normal fetal development of the adrenal. *J Pediatr Surg* 16:636–644, 1981.

46. Jennings RW, LaQuaglia MP, Leong K et al: Fetal neuroblastoma: Prenatal diagnosis and natural history. *J Pediatr Surg* 28:1168–1174, 1993.

47. Schwartz AD, Dadash-Zadeh M, Lee H, et al: Spontaneous regression of disseminated neuroblastoma. *J Pediatr* 85:760–763, 1974.

48. Altman AC, Gross S: Progression from stage IVS to stage IV neuroblastoma with eventual spontaneous resolution. *Am J Pediatr Hematol Oncol* 3:441–444, 1981.

49. Haas D, Ablin AR, Miller C, et al: Complete pathologic maturation and regression of stage IVS neuroblastoma without treatment. *Cancer* 62:818–825, 1988.

50. Carlsen NL: Neuroblastoma: Epidemiology and spontaneous remission. Significance for evaluation of screening studies. *Ugeskr Laeger* 154:3742–3746, 1992.

51. Hicks MJ, Mackay B: Comparison of ultrastructural features among neuroblastic tumors: Maturation from neuroblastoma to ganglioneuroma. *Ultrastruct Pathol* 19:311–322, 1995.

52. Russell DS, Rubenstein LJ: Tumors of peripheral neuroblasts and ganglion cells. In Russell DS, Rubenstein LJ (eds): *Pathology of Tumors of the Nervous System*, 5th ed. Baltimore: Williams & Wilkins, 1989, p. 900.

53. Stout AP: Ganglioneuroma of the sympathetic nervous system. *Surg Gynecol Obstet* 84:101, 1947.

54. Dehner LP: Pathologic anatomy of classic neuroblastoma: Including prognostic features and differential diagnosis. In Pochedly C (ed): *Neuroblastoma: Tumor Biology and Therapy*, Boca Raton, FL: CRC Press, 1990, p. 111.

55. Triche TJ: Neuroblastoma and other childhood neural tumors: A review. *Pediatr Pathol* 10:175–193, 1990.

56. Triche TJ, Askin FB, Kissane JM: Neuroblastoma, Ewing's sarcoma, and the differential diagnosis of small-, round-, blue-cell tumors. In Finegold M (ed): *Pathology of Neoplasia in Children and Adolescents*, Philadelphia: Saunders, 1986, p. 145.

57. Hughes M, Marsden HB, Palmer MK: Histologic patterns of neuroblastoma related to prognosis and clinical staging. *Cancer* 34:1706–1711, 1974.

58. Hassenbusch S, Kaizer H, White JJ: Prognostic factors in neuroblastic tumors. *J Pediatr Surg* 11:287–297, 1976.

59. Sandstedt B, Jereb B, Eklund G: Prognostic factors in neuroblastomas. *Acta Pathol Microbiol Immunol Scand* 91:365–371, 1983.

60. Thomas PR, Lee LY, Fineberg BB, et al: An analysis of neuroblastoma at a single institution. *Cancer* 53:2079–2082, 1984.

61. Shimada H, Chatten J, Newton WA Jr, et al: Histopathologic prognostic factors in neuroblastic tumors: Definition of subtypes of ganglioneuroblastoma and an age-linked classification of neuroblastomas. *J Natl Cancer Inst* 73:405–416, 1984.

62. Chatten J, Shimada H, Sather HN, et al: Prognostic value of histopathology in advanced neuroblastoma: A report from the Children's Cancer Study Group. *Hum Pathol* 19:1187–1198, 1988.

63. O'Neill JA, Littman P, Blitzer P, et al: The role of surgery in localized neuroblastoma. *J Pediatr Surg* 20:708–712, 1985.

64. Evans AE, D'Angio GJ, Propert K, et al: Prognostic factors in neuroblastoma. *Cancer* 59:1853–1859, 1987.

65. Joshi V, Cantor A, Altshuler G, et al: Prognostic significance of histopathologic features of neuroblastoma: A grading system based on the review of 211 cases from the Pediatric Oncology Group. *Proc Am Soc Clin Oncol* 10:311, 1991.

66. Meitar D, Crawford SE, Rademaker AW, et al: Tumor angiogenesis correlates with metastatic disease, N-*myc* amplification, and poor outcome in human neuroblastoma. *J Clin Oncol* 14:405–414, 1996.

67. Brodeur GM, Sekhon G, Goldstein MN: Chromosomal aberrations in human neuroblastomas. *Cancer* 40:2256–2263, 1977.

68. Brodeur GM, Green AA, Hayes FA, et al: Cytogenetic features of human neuroblastomas and cell lines. *Cancer Res* 41:4678–4686, 1981.

69. Gilbert F, Balaban G, Moorhead P, et al: Abnormalities of chromosome lp in human neuroblastoma tumors and cell lines. *Cancer Genet Cytogenet* 7:33–42, 1982.

70. Gilbert F, Feder M, Balaban G, et al: Human neuroblastomas and abnormalities of chromosomes 1 and 17. *Cancer Res* 44:5444–5449, 1984.

71. Franke F, Rudolph B, Christiansen H, et al: Tumour karyotype may be important in the prognosis of human neuroblastoma. *J Cancer Res Clin Oncol* 111:266–272, 1986.

72. Hayashi Y, Hanada R, Yamamoto K, et al: Chromosome findings and prognosis in neuroblastoma. *Cancer Genet Cytogenet* 29:175–177, 1987.

73. Kaneko Y, Kanda N, Maseki N, et al: Different karyotypic patterns in early and advanced-stage neuroblastomas. *Cancer Res* 47:311–318, 1987.

74. Brodeur GM, Fong CT, Morita M, et al: Molecular analysis and clinical significance of N-*myc* amplification and chromosome 1 monosomy in human neuroblastomas. *Prog Clin Biol Res* 271:3–15, 1988.

75. Christiansen H, Lampert F: Tumour karyotype discriminates between good and bad prognostic outcome in neuroblastoma. *Br J Cancer* 57:121–126, 1988.

76. Fong CT, Dracopoli NC, White PS, et al: Loss of heterozygosity for the short arm of chromosome 1 in human neuroblastomas: Correlation with N-*myc* amplification. *Proc Natl Acad Sci U S A* 86:3753–3757, 1989.

77. Hayashi Y, Kanda N, Inaba T, et al: Cytogenetic findings and prognosis in neuroblastoma with emphasis on marker chromosome 1. *Cancer* 63:126, 1989.

78. Brodeur GM, Fong CT: Molecular biology and genetics of human neuroblastoma. *Cancer Genet Cytogenet* 41:153–174, 1989.

79. Caron H, Van Sluis P, Van Roy N, et al: Recurrent 1;17 translocations in human neuroblastoma reveal nonhomologous mitotic recombination during the S/G2 phase as a novel mechanism for loss of heterozygosity. *Am J Hum Genet* 5:341–347, 1994.

80. Maris JM, White PS, Beltinger CP et al: Significance of chromosome 1p loss of heterozygosity in neuroblastoma. *Cancer Res* 55:4664–4669, 1995.

81. Caron H, van Sluis P, de Kraker J, et al: Allelic loss of chromosome 1p as a predictor of unfavorable outcome in patients with neuroblastoma. *N Engl J Med* 334:225–230, 1996.

82. Weith A, Martinsson T, Cziepluch C, et al: Neuroblastoma consensus deletion maps to 1p36.1-2. *Genes Chromosom Cancer* 1:159–166, 1989.

83. Fong CT, White PS, Peterson K, et al: Loss of heterozygosity for chromosomes 1 or 14 defines subsets of advanced neuroblastomas. *Cancer Res* 52:1780–1785, 1992.

84. Oren M: The involvement of oncogenes and tumor suppressor genes in the control of apoptosis. *Can Metastasis Rev* 11:141–148, 1992.

85. Van Roy N, Laureys G, Cheng NC, et al: 1;17 translocations and other chromosome 17 rearrangements in human primary neuroblastoma tumors and cell lines. *Genes Chromosom Cancer* 10:103–114, 1994.

86. Van Roy N, Cheng NC, Laureys G, et al: Molecular cytogenetic analysis of 1;17 translocations in neuroblastoma. *Eur J Cancer* 31A:530–535, 1995.

87. Suzuki T, Yokota J, Mugishima H, et al: Frequent loss of heterozygosity on chromosome 14q in neuroblastoma. *Cancer Res* 49:1095–1098, 1989.

88. Srivatsan ES, Ying KL, Seeger RC: Deletion of chromosome 11 and of 14q sequences in neuroblastoma. *Genes Chromosom Cancer* 7:32–37, 1993.

89. Balaban-Malenbaum G, Gilbert F: Double-minute chromosomes and the homogeneously staining regions in chromosomes of a human neuroblastoma cell line. *Science* 198:739–741, 1977.

90. Cowell JK: Double minutes and homogeneously staining regions: Gene amplification in mammalian cells. *Ann Rev Gen* 16:21–59, 1982.

91. Bahr G, Gilbert F, Balaban G, et al: Homogeneously staining regions and double minutes in a human cell line: Chromatin organization and DNA content. *J Natl Cancer Inst* 71:657–661, 1983.

92. Brodeur GM: Neuroblastoma—Clinical applications of molecular parameters. *Brain Pathol* 1:47–54, 1990.

93. Look AT, Hayes FA, Nitschke R, et al: Cellular DNA content as a predictor of response to chemotherapy in infants with unresectable neuroblastoma. *N Engl J Med* 311:231–235, 1984.

94. Taylor SR, Blatt J, Costantino JP, et al: Flow cytometric DNA analysis of neuroblastoma and ganglioneuroma. A 10-year retrospective study. *Cancer* 62:749–754, 1988.

95. Cohn SL, Rademaker AW, Salwen HR, et al: Analysis of DNA ploidy and proliferative activity in relation to histology and N-*myc* amplification in neuroblastoma. *Am J Pathol* 136:1043–1052, 1990.

96. Look AT, Hayes FA, Shuster JJ, et al: Clinical relevance of tumor cell ploidy and N-*myc* gene amplification in childhood neuroblastoma: A Pediatric Oncology Group Study. *J Clin Oncol* 9:581–591, 1991.

97. Naito M, Iwafuchi M, Ohsawa Y, et al: Flow cytometric DNA analysis of neuroblastoma: prognostic significance of DNA ploidy in unfavorable group. *J Pediatr Surg* 26:834–837, 1991.

98. Huddart SN, Muir KR, Parkes SE, et al: Retrospective study of prognostic value of DNA ploidy and proliferative activity in neuroblastoma. *J Clin Pathol* 46:1101–1104, 1993.

99. Naito M, Iwafuchi M, Hirota M: Flow cytometric DNA analysis of neuroblastoma—Clinical significance of DNA tetraploidy. *Prog Clin Biol Res* 385:87–93, 1994.

100. Hayashi Y, Habu Y, Fujii Y, et al: Chromosome abnormalities in neuroblastomas found by VMA mass screening. *Cancer Genet Cytogenet* 22:363–364, 1986.

101. Hayashi Y, Inaba T, Hanada R, et al: Chromosome findings and prognosis in 15 patients with neuroblastoma found by VMA mass screening. *J Pediatr* 112:567–571, 1988.

102. Wenzel A, Schwab M: The *myc*N/*max* protein complex in neuroblastoma. Short review. *Eur J Cancer* 31A:516–519, 1995.

103. Brodeur GM, Seeger RC, Schwab M, et al: Amplification of N-*myc* in untreated human neuroblastomas correlates with advanced disease stage. *Science* 224:1121–1124, 1984.

104. Seeger RC, Brodeur GM, Sather H, et al: Association of multiple copies of the N-*myc* oncogene with rapid progression of neuroblastomas. *N Engl J Med* 313:1111–1116, 1985.

105. Brodeur GM, Seeger RC, Sather H, et al: Clinical implications of oncogene activation in human neuroblastomas. *Cancer* 58:541–545, 1986.

106. Seeger RC, Wada R, Brodeur GM, et al: Expression of N-*myc* by neuroblastomas with one or multiple copies of the oncogene. *Prog Clin Biol Res* 271:41–49, 1988.

107. Benard J: Genetic alterations associated with metastatic dissemination and chemoresistance in neuroblastoma. *Eur J Cancer* 31A:560–564, 1995.

108. Bourhis J, DeVathaire F, Wilson GD, et al: Combined analysis of DNA ploidy index and N-*myc* genomic content in neuroblastoma. *Cancer Res* 51:33–36, 1991.

109. Brodeur GM, Hayes FA, Green AA, et al: Consistent N-*myc* copy number in simultaneous or consecutive neuroblastoma samples from sixty individual patients. *Cancer Res* 47:4248–4253, 1987.

110. Schwab M, Ellison J, Busch M, et al: Enhanced expression of the human gene N-*myc* consequent to amplification of DNA may contribute to malignant progression of neuroblastoma. *Proc Natl Acad Sci U S A* 81:4940–4044, 1984.

111. Grady-Leopardi EF, Schwab M, Ablin AR, et al: Detection of N-*myc* oncogene expression in human neuroblastoma by in situ hybridization and blot analysis: Relationship to clinical outcome. *Cancer Res* 46:3196–3199, 1986.

112. Rosen N, Reynolds CP, Thiele CJ, et al: Increased N-*myc* expression following progressive growth of human neuroblastoma. *Cancer Res* 46:4139–4142, 1986.

113. Bartram CR, Berthold F: Amplification and expression of the N-*myc* gene in neuroblastoma. *Eur J Pediatr* 146:162–165, 1987.

114. Nisen PD, Waber PG, Rich MA, et al: N-*myc* oncogene RNA expression in neuroblastoma. *J Natl Cancer Inst* 80:1633–1637, 1988.

115. Zaizen Y, Taniguchi S, Noguchi S, et al: The effect of N-*myc* amplification and expression on invasiveness of neuroblastoma cells. *J Pediatr Surg* 28:766–769, 1993.

116. Benard J, Bourhis J, de Vathaire F, et al: Prognostic value of *MDR1* gene expression in neuroblastoma: Results of a multivariate analysis. *Prog Clin Biol Res* 385:111–116, 1994.

117. Bordow SB, Haber M, Madafiglio J, et al: Expression of the multidrug resistance-associated protein (MRP) gene correlates with amplification and overexpression of the N-*myc* oncogene in childhood neuroblastoma. *Cancer Res* 54:5036–5040, 1994.

118. Norris MD, Bordow SB, Marshall GM, et al: Expression of the gene for multidrug-resistance-associated protein and outcome in patients with neuroblastoma. *N Engl J Med* 334:231–238, 1996.

119. Bjelfman C, Hedborg F, Johansson I, et al: Expression of the neuronal form of pp60C-src in neuroblastoma in relation to clinical stage and prognosis. *Cancer Res* 50:6908–6914, 1990.

120. Hedborg F, Bjelfman C, Sparen P, et al: Biochemical evidence for a mature phenotype in morphologically poorly differentiated neuroblastomas with a favorable outcome. *Eur J Cancer* 31A:435–443, 1995.

121. Thiele CJ, McKeon C, Triche TJ, et al: Differential proto-oncogene expression characterizes histopathologically indistinguishable tumors of the peripheral nervous system. *J Clin Invest* 80:804–811, 1987.

122. Davidoff AM, Pence JA, Shorter NA, et al: Expression of p53 in human neuroblastoma- and neuroepithelioma-derived cell lines. *Oncogene* 7:127–133, 1992.

123. Imamura J, Bartram CR, Berthold F, et al: Mutation of the p53 gene in neuroblastoma and its relationship with N-*myc* amplification. *Cancer Res* 53:4053–4058, 1993.

124. Moll UM, LaQuaglia M, Benard J, et al: Wild-type p53 protein undergoes cytoplasmic sequestration in undifferentiated neuroblastomas but not in differentiated tumors. *Proc Natl Acad Sci U S A* 92:4407–4411, 1995.

125. Ikuno N, Shimokawa I, Nakamura T, et al: *Ret*-oncogene expression correlates with neuronal differentiation of neuroblastic tumors. *Pathol Res Pract* 191:92–99, 1995.

126. Tanaka T, Slamon DJ, Shimoda H, et al: Ha-*ras* p21 in neuroblastoma: A new marker in prediction of patient outcome. *Prog Clin Biol Res* 385:275–280, 1994.

127. Ireland CM: Activated N-*ras* oncogenes in human neuroblastoma. *Cancer Res* 49:5530–5533, 1989.

128. Tanaka T, Slamon DJ, Shimada H, et al: A significant association of Ha-*ras* p21 in neuroblastoma cells with patient prognosis. A retrospective study of 103 cases. *Cancer* 68:1296–1302, 1991.

129. Nakada K, Fujioka T, Kitagawa H, et al: Expressions of N-*myc* and *ras* oncogene products in neuroblastoma and their correlations with prognosis. *Jpn J Clin Oncol* 23:149–155, 1993.

130. Tanaka T, Seeger RC, Tanabe M, et al: Prognostic prediction in neuroblastomas: Clinical significance of combined analysis for Ha-*ras* p21 expression and N-*myc* gene amplification. *Cancer Detect Prev* 18:283–289, 1994.

131. Christiansen H, Sahin K, Berthold F, et al: Comparison of DNA aneuploidy, chromosome 1 abnormalities, *MYCN* amplification and CD44 expression as prognostic factors in neuroblastoma. *Eur J Canc* 31A:541–544, 1995.

132. Blatt J, Wharton V: Stimulation of growth of neuroblastoma cells by ferritin in vitro. *J Lab Clin Med* 119:139–143, 1992.

133. Selig RA, Madafiglio J, Haber M, et al: Ferritin production and desferrioxamine cytotoxicity in human neuroblastoma cell lines. *Anticancer Res* 13:721–725, 1993.

134. Hann HW, Evans AE, Siegel SE, et al: Prognostic importance of serum ferritin in patients with stages III and IV neuroblastoma: The Children's Cancer Study Group Experience. *Cancer Res* 45:2843–2848, 1985.

135. Silber JH, Evans AE, Fridman M: Models to predict outcome from childhood neuroblastoma: The role of serum ferritin and tumor histology. *Cancer Res* 51:1426–1433, 1991.

136. Berthold F, Engelhardt-Fahrner U, Schneider A, et al: Age dependence and prognostic impact of neuron-specific enolase (NSE) in children with neuroblastoma. *In Vivo* 5:245–247, 1991.

137. Crary GS, Singleton TP, Neglia JP, et al: Detection of metastatic neuroblastoma in bone marrow biopsy specimens with an antibody to neuron-specific enolase. *Mod Pathol* 5:308–311, 1992.

138. Carter RL, al-Sams SZ, Corbett RP, et al: A comparative study of immunohistochemical staining for neuron-specific enolase, protein gene product 9.5 and S-100 protein in neuroblastoma, Ewing's sarcoma and other round cell tumours in children. *Histopathology* 16:461–467, 1990.

139. Ishiwata I, Ishiwata C, Soma M, et al: N-*myc* amplification and neuron-specific enolase production of a neuroblastoma cell line and germ cell tumor cell lines. *Gyn Oncol* 33:356–359, 1989.

140. Quinn JJ, Altman AJ, Frantz CN: Serum lactic dehydrogenase, an indicator of tumor activity in neuroblastoma. *J Pediatr* 97:89, 1980.

141. Woods WG: The use and significance of biologic markers in the evaluation and staging of a child with cancer. *Cancer* 58:442–448, 1986.

142. Joshi VV, Cantor AB, Brodeur GM, et al: Correlation between morphologic and other prognostic markers of neuroblastoma. A study of histologic grade, DNA index, N-*myc* gene copy number, and lactic dehydrogenase in patients in the Pediatric Oncology Group. *Cancer* 71:3173–3181, 1993.

143. Parada LF, Tsoulfas P, Tessarollo L, et al: The Trk family of tyrosine kinases: Receptors for NGF-related neurotrophins. *Cold Spring Harb Symp Quant Biol* 57:43–51, 1992.

144. Matsushima H, Bogenmann E: Expression of trkA cDNA in neuroblastoma mediates differentiation in vitro and in vivo. *Mol Cell Biol* 13:7447–7456, 1993.

145. Lavenius E, Gestblom, C, Johansson I, et al: Transfection of TRK-A into human neuroblastoma cells restores their ability to differentiate in response to nerve growth factor. *Cell Growth Differ* 6:727–736, 1995.

146. Nakagawara A, Arima M, Azar C, et al: Inverse relationship between trk expression and N-*myc* amplification in human neuroblastomas. *Cancer Res* 52:1364–1368, 1992.

147. Nakagawara A, Arima-Nakagawara M, Scavarda NJ, et al: High expression of the TRK gene in human neuroblastoma is associated with favorable outcome: Possible role of tumor differentiation and regression. *N Engl J Med* 328:847–854, 1993.

148. Suzuki T, Bogenmann E, Shimada H, et al: Lack of high-affinity nerve growth factor receptors in aggressive neuroblastomas. *J Natl Cancer Inst* 85:377–384, 1993.

149. Borrello MG, Bongarzone I, Pierotti MA, et al: trk and ret proto-oncogene expression in human neuroblastoma specimens: High frequency of trk expression in non-advanced stages. *Int J Cancer* 54:540–545, 1993.

150. Gaetano C, Manni I, Bossi G, et al: Retinoic acid and cAMP differentially regulate human chromogranin A promoter activity during differentiation of neuroblastoma cells. *Eur J Cancer* 31A:447–452, 1995.

151. Schmid KW, Dockhorn-Dworniczak B, Fahrenkamp A: Chromogranin A, secretogranin II and vasoactive intestinal peptide in phaeochromocytomas and ganglioneuromas. *Histopathology* 22:527–533, 1993.

152. Helman LJ, Gazdar AF, Park JG, et al: Chromogranin A expression in normal and malignant human tissues. *J Clin Invest* 82:686–690, 1988.

153. Cooper MJ, Hutchins GM, Cohen PS, et al: Human neuroblastoma tumor cell lines correspond to the arrested differentiation of chromaffin adrenal medullary neuroblasts. *Cell Growth Differ* 1:149–159, 1990.

154. Hsiao RJ, Seeger RC, Yu AL, et al: Chromogranin A in children with neuroblastoma. Serum concentration parallels disease stage and predicts survival. *J Clin Invest* 85:1555–1559, 1990.

155. O'Hare MM, Schwartz TW: Expression and precursor processing of neuropeptide Y in human pheochromocytoma and neuroblastoma tumors. *Cancer Res* 49:7010–7014, 1989.

156. Mouri T, Sone M, Takahashi K, et al: Neuropeptide Y as a plasma marker for phaeochromocytoma, ganglioneuroblastoma and neuroblastoma. *Clin Sci* 83:205–211, 1992.

157. Rascher W, Kremens B, Wagner S, et al: Serial measurements of neuropeptide Y in plasma for monitoring neuroblastoma in children. *J Pediatr* 122:914–916, 1993.

158. Moertel CL, Reubi J-C, Scheithauer BS, et al: Expression of somatostatin receptors in childhood neuroblastoma. *Am J Clin Pathol* 102:752–756, 1994.

159. Schulz G, Cheresh DA, Varki NM, et al: Detection of ganglioside GD2 in tumor tissues and sera of neuroblastoma patients. *Cancer Res* 44:5914–5920, 1984.

160. Ladisch S, Wu Z-L: Detection of a tumour-associated ganglioside in plasma of patients with neuroblastoma. *Lancet* 1:136–138, 1985.

161. Sariola H, Terava H, Rapola J, et al: Cell-surface ganglioside GD2 in the immuno-histochemical detection and differential diagnosis of neuroblastoma. *Am J Clin Pathol* 96:248–252, 1991.

162. Sung CC, Pearl DK, Coons SW, et al: Gangliosides as diagnostic markers of human astrocytomas and primitive neuroectodermal tumors. *Cancer* 74:3010–3022, 1994.

163. Ladisch S, Wu ZL, Feig S, et al: Shedding of

GD2 ganglioside by human neuroblastoma. *Int J Cancer* 39:73–76, 1987.

164. Valentino L, Moss T, Olson E, et al: Shed tumor gangliosides and progression of human neuroblastoma. *Blood* 75:1564–1567, 1990.

165. Handgretinger R, Anderson K, Lang P, et al: A phase I study of human/mouse chimeric antiganglioside GD2 antibody ch14.18 in patients with neuroblastoma. *Eur J Cancer* 31A:261–267, 1995.

166. Hank JA, Surfus J, Gan J, et al: Treatment of neuroblastoma patients with antiganglioside GD2 antibody plus interleukin-2 induces antibody-dependent cellular cytotoxicity against neuroblastoma in vitro. *J Immunother* 15:29–37, 1994.

167. Gross N, Beretta C, Peruisseau G, et al: CD44H expression by human neuroblastoma cells: Relation to *MYCN* amplification and lineage differentiation. *Cancer Res* 54:4238–4242, 1994.

168. Combaret V, Lasset C, Frappaz D, et al: Evaluation of CD44 prognostic value in neuroblastoma: Comparison with the other prognostic factors. *Eur J Cancer* 31A:545–549, 1995.

169. Kawasaki H, Mukai K, Yajima S, et al: Prognostic value of proliferating cell nuclear antigen (PCNA) immunostaining in neuroblastoma. *Med Pediatr Oncol* 24:300–304, 1995.

170. Rossi A, Granata F, Augusti-Tocco G, et al: Expression in murine and human neuroblastoma cell lines of VGF, a tissue-specific protein. *Int J Dev Neurosci* 10:527–534, 1992.

171. Brodeur GM: Neuroblastoma: Clinical significance of genetic abnormalities. *Cancer Surv* 9:673–688, 1990.

172. Kedar A, Glassman M, Voorhess ML, et al: Severe hypertension in a child with ganglioneuroblastoma. *Cancer* 47:2077–2080, 1981.

173. Weinblatt ME, Heisel MA, Siegel SE: Hypertension in children with neurogenic tumors. *Pediatrics* 71:947–951, 1983.

174. Jaffe N, Cassady R, Petersen R, et al: Heterochromia and Horner syndrome associated with cervical and mediastinal neuroblastoma. *J Pediatr* 87:75–77, 1975.

175. Rosen EM, Cassady JR, Frantz CN, et al: Neuroblastoma: The Joint Center for Radiation Therapy/Dana-Farber Cancer Institute/Children's Hospital experience. *J Clin Oncol* 2:719–732, 1984.

176. Bohdiewicz PJ, Gallegos E, Fink-Bennett D: Raccoon eyes and the MIBG super scan: Scintigraphic signs of neuroblastoma in a case of suspected child abuse. *Pediatr Radiol* 25 (suppl. 1):S90–92, 1995.

177. Roberts KB: Cerebellar ataxia and "occult neuroblastoma" without opsoclonus. *Pediatrics* 56:464–465, 1975.

178. Altman AJ, Baehner RL: Favorable prognosis for survival in children with coincident opsomyoclonus and neuroblastoma. *Cancer* 37:846–852, 1976.

179. Fisher PG, Wechsler DS, Singer HS: Anti-Hu antibody in a neuroblastoma-associated paraneoplastic syndrome. *Pediatr Neurol* 10:309–312, 1994.

180. Kaplan SJ, Holbrook CT, McDaniel HG, et al: Vasoactive intestinal peptide secreting tumors of childhood. *Am J Dis Child* 134:21–24, 1980.

181. Bjellerup P, Theodorsson E, Kogner P: Somatostatin and vasoactive intestinal peptide (VIP) in neuroblastoma and ganglioneuroma: Chromatographic characterisation and release during surgery. *Eur J Cancer* 31A:481–485, 1995.

182. Itoh T, Ohmori K: Biosynthesis and storage of catecholamines in pheochromocytoma and neuroblastoma cells. *J Lab Clin Med* 81:889–896, 1973.

183. Laug WE, Siegel SE, Shaw KN, et al: Initial urinary catecholamine metabolite concentrations and prognosis in neuroblastoma. *Pediatrics* 62:77–83, 1978.

184. LaBrosse EH, Com-Nougue C, Zucker JM, et al: Urinary excretion of 3-methoxy-4-hydroxymandelic acid and 3-methoxy-4-hydroxyphenylacetic acid by 288 patients with neuroblastoma and related neural crest tumors. *Cancer Res* 40:1995–2001, 1980.

185. Graham-Pole J, Salmi T, Anton AH, et al: Tumor and urine catecholamines (CATS) in neurogenic tumors. Correlations with other prognostic factors and survival. *Cancer* 51:834–839, 1983.

186. Heisel MA, Miller JH, Reid BS, et al: Radionuclide bone scan in neuroblastoma. *Pediatrics* 71:206–209, 1983.

187. Podrasky AE, Stark DD, Hattner RS, et al: Radionuclide bone scanning in neuroblastoma: Skeletal metastases and primary tumor localization of 99mTc-MDP. *Am J Roentgenol* 141:469–472, 1983.

188. Daubenton JD, Fisher RM, Karabus CD, et al: The relationship between prognosis and scintigraphic evidence of bone metastases in neuroblastoma. *Cancer* 59:1586–1589, 1987.

189. MacDonald WB, Stevens MM, Dalla Pozza L, et al: Gallium-67 and technetium-99m-methylene diphosphonate skeletal scintigraphy in determining prognosis for children with stage IV neuroblastoma. *J Nucl Med* 34:1082–1086, 1993.

190. White SJ, Stuck KJ, Blane CE, et al: Sonography of neuroblastoma. *Am J Roentgenol* 141:465–468, 1983.

191. Berdon WE, Ruzal-Shapiro C, Abramson SJ, et al: The diagnosis of abdominal neuroblastoma: Relative roles of ultrasonography, CT, and MRI. *Urol Radiol* 14:252–262, 1992.

192. Gadwood KA, Reynes CJ: Prenatal sonography

of metastatic neuroblastoma. *J Clin Ultrasound* 11:512–515, 1983.

193. Janetschek G, Weitzel D, Stein W, et al: Prenatal diagnosis of neuroblastoma by sonography. *Urology* 24:397–402, 1984.

194. Toma P, Lucigrai G, Marzoli A, et al: Prenatal diagnosis of metastatic adrenal neuroblastoma with sonography and MR imaging. *Am J Roentgenol* 162:1183–1184, 1994.

195. Golding SJ, McElwain TJ, Husband JE: The role of computed tomography in the management of children with advanced neuroblastoma. *Br J Radiol* 57:661–666, 1984.

196. Hirata T, Tatara H, Zaizen Y, et al: Role of ultrasound in managing neuroblastoma detected by mass screening: A proposed ultrasonographic grading for children with neuroblastoma. *J Clin Ultrasound* 23:305–313, 1995.

197. Fletcher BD, Miraldi FD, Cheung NK: Comparison of radiolabeled monoclonal antibody and magnetic resonance imaging in the detection of metastatic neuroblastoma in bone marrow: Preliminary results. *Pediatr Radiol* 20:72–75, 1989.

198. Hadj-Djilani NL, Lebtahi NE, Delaloye AB, et al: Diagnosis and follow-up of neuroblastoma by means of iodine-123 metaiodobenzylguanidine scintigraphy and bone scan, and the influence of histology. *Eur J Nucl Med* 22:322–329, 1995.

199. Andrich MP, Shalaby-Rana E, Movassaghi N, et al: The role of [131]iodine-metaiodobenzyl-guanidine scanning in the correlative imaging of patients with neuroblastoma. *Pediatrics* 97:246–250, 1996.

200. Suc A, Lumbroso J, Rubie H, et al: Metastatic neuroblastoma in children older than one year: Prognostic significance of the initial metaiodobenzylguanidine scan and proposal for a scoring system. *Cancer* 77:805–811, 1996.

201. O'Dorisio MS, Hauger M, Cecalupo AJ: Somatostatin receptors in neuroblastoma: diagnostic and therapeutic implications. *Semin Oncol* 21:33–37, 1994.

202. Smith MB, Katz R, Black CT, et al: A rational approach to the use of fine needle aspiration biopsy in the evaluation of primary and recurrent neoplasms in children. *J Pediatr Surg* 28:1245–1247, 1993.

203. Brodeur GM, Pritchard J, Berthold F, et al: Revisions of the international criteria for neuroblastoma diagnosis, staging and response to treatment. *J Clin Oncol* 11:1466–1477, 1993.

204. Hayes FA, Green AA, Rao BN: Clinical manifestations of ganglioneuroma. *Cancer* 63:1211–1214, 1989.

205. Nishi M, Miyake H, Takeda T, et al: Can a patient with neuroblastoma be diagnosed by a single urine sample collected randomly? *Oncology* 48:31–33, 1991.

206. Murthy TV, Irving IM, Lister J: Massive adrenal hemorrhage in neonatal neuroblastoma. *J Pediatr Surg* 13:31–34, 1978.

207. Strouse PJ, Bowerman RA, Schlesinger AE: Antenatal sonographic findings of fetal adrenal hemorrhage. *J Clin Ultrasound* 23:442–446, 1995.

208. Tuchman M, Fisher EJ, Heisel MA, et al: Feasibility study for neonatal neuroblastoma screening in the United States. *Med Pediatr Oncol* 17:258–264, 1989.

209. Sawada T, Shikata T, Matsumura T: Analysis of 598 cases of neuroblastoma (NB) detected by screening and changes in the age distribution and incidence of NB patients after mass screening in infants in Japan. NB Screening Study Group. *Prog Clin Biol Res* 385:371–375, 1994.

210. El Shafie M, Samuel D, Klippel CH, et al: Intractable diarrhea in children with VIP-secreting ganglioneuroblastomas. *J Pediatr Surg* 18:34–36, 1983.

211. Mitchell WG, Snodgrass SR: Opsoclonus-ataxia due to childhood neural crest tumors: A chronic neurologic syndrome. *J Child Neurol* 5:153–158, 1990.

212. Hassan MM: Ganglioneuroblastoma presenting as myasthenia gravis. *Childs Brain* 3:65–68, 1977.

213. Moss TJ, Sanders DG: Detection of neuroblastoma cells in blood. *J Clin Oncol* 8:736–740, 1990.

214. Evans AE, D'Angio GJ, Randolph J: A proposed staging for children with neuroblastoma. Children's Cancer Study Group A. *Cancer* 27:374–378, 1971.

215. Hayes FA, Green A, Hustu HO, et al: Surgicopathologic staging of neuroblastoma: Prognostic significance of regional lymph node metastases. *J Pediatr* 102:59–62, 1983.

216. American Joint Committee on Cancer: Neuroblastoma. In Beahrs OH, Myers MH (eds): *Manual for Staging of Cancer*, 2nd ed. Philadelphia: JB Lippincott, 1983, p. 237.

217. Brodeur GM, Seeger RC, Barrett A, et al: International criteria for diagnosis, staging, and response to treatment in patients with neuroblastoma. *J Clin Oncol* 6:1874–1881, 1988.

218. Ninane J, Pritchard J, Jones PH, et al: Stage II neuroblastoma. Adverse prognostic significance of lymph node involvement. *Arch Dis Child* 57:438–442, 1982.

219. D'Angio GJ, Evans AE, Koop CE: Special pattern of widespread neuroblastoma with a favourable prognosis. *Lancet* 1:1046–1049, 1971.

220. Evans AE, Chatten J, D'Angio GJ, et al: A review of 17 IV-S neuroblastoma patients at the Children's Hospital of Philadelphia. *Cancer* 45:833–839, 1980.

221. Nickersen HJ, Nesbit ME, Grosfeld JL, et al: Comparison of stage IV and IV-S neuroblastoma in the first year of life. *Med Pediatr Oncol* 13:261–268, 1985.

222. Matthay KK: Neuroblastoma: A clinical challenge and a biologic puzzle. *CA Cancer J Clin* 45:179–192, 1995.

223. Brodeur GM: Molecular basis for heterogeneity in human neuroblastomas. *Eur J Cancer* 31A:505–510, 1995.

224. Castleberry RP, Shuster JJ, Altshuler G, et al: Infants with neuroblastoma and regional lymph node metastases have a favorable outlook after limited postoperative chemotherapy: A Pediatric Oncology Group study. *J Clin Oncol* 10:1299–1304, 1992.

225. Haase GM, Wong KY, DeLorimier AA, et al: Improvement in survival after excision of primary tumor in stage III neuroblastoma. *J Pediatr Surg* 24:194–200, 1989.

226. Shamberger RC, Allarde-Segundo A, Kozakewich HP, et al: Surgical management of stage III and IV neuroblastoma: Resection before or after chemotherapy? *J Pediatr Surg* 26:1113–1117, 1991.

227. DeCou JM, Bowman LC, Rao BN: Infants with metastatic neuroblastoma have improved survival with resection of the primary tumor. *J Pediatr Surg* 30:937–940, 1995.

228. Shorter NA, Davidoff AM, Evans AE, et al: The role of surgery in the management of stage IV neuroblastoma: A single-institution study. *Med Pediatr Oncol* 24:287–291, 1995.

229. Chamberlain RS, Quinones R, Dinndorf P, et al: Complete surgical resection combined with aggressive adjuvant chemotherapy and bone marrow transplantation prolongs survival in children with advanced neuroblastoma. *Ann Surg Oncol* 2:93–100, 1995.

230. Kushner BH, Cheung NK, LaQuaglia MP, et al: Survival from locally invasive or widespread neuroblastoma without cytotoxic therapy. *J Clin Oncol* 14:373–381, 1996

231. Robertson KA: Pediatric bone marrow transplantation. *Curr Opin Pediatr* 5:103–109, 1993.

232. Seeger RC, Reynolds CP: Treatment of high-risk solid tumors of childhood with intensive therapy and autologous bone marrow transplantation. *Pediatr Clin North Am* 38:393–424, 1991.

233. Seeger RC, Matthay KK, Villablanca JG, et al: Intensive chemoradiotherapy and autologous bone marrow transplantation (ABMT) for high-risk neuroblastoma. *Proc Am Soc Clin Oncol* 10:310, 1991.

234. Graham-Pole J, Casper J, Elfenbein G, et al: High-dose chemoradiotherapy supported by marrow infusions for advanced neuroblastoma: A Pediatric Oncology Group study. *J Clin Oncol* 9:152–158, 1991.

235. Mugishima H, Iwata M, Okabe I, et al: Autologous bone marrow transplantation in children with advanced neuroblastoma. *Cancer* 74:972–977, 1994.

236. Stram DO, Matthay KK, O'Leary MC, et al: Autologous bone marrow transplantation vs continued chemotherapy for stage IV neuroblastoma: A nonrandomized childrens' cancer group study. *Proc Annu Meet Am Soc Clin Oncol* 14:A1435, 1995.

237. Lockwood L, Mameghan H, Vowels MR, et al: Local irradiation followed by consolidation with modified VAMP-TBI and unpurged autologous rescue is effective therapy for Stage IV neuroblastoma. *Proc Annu Meet Am Soc Clin Oncol* 14:A1421, 1995.

238. Pinkerton CR: ENSG 1-randomised study of high-dose melphalan in neuroblastoma. *Bone Marrow Transplant* 7(suppl. 3):112–113, 1991.

239. Shuster JJ, Cantor AB, McWilliams N, et al: The prognostic significance of autologous bone marrow transplant in advanced neuroblastoma. *J Clin Oncol* 9:1045–1049, 1991.

240. Kushner BH, O'Reilly RJ, Mandell LR, et al: Myeloablative combination chemotherapy without total body irradiation for neuroblastoma. *J Clin Oncol* 9:274–279, 1991.

241. Seeger RC, Moss TJ, Feig SA, et al: Bone marrow transplantation for poor prognosis neuroblastoma. *Prog Clin Biol Res* 271:203–213, 1988.

242. Deacon JM, Wilson PA, Peckham MJ: The radiobiology of human neuroblastoma. *Radiother Oncol* 3:201–209, 1985.

243. Peschel RE, Chen M, Seashore J: The treatment of massive hepatomegaly in stage IV-S neuroblastoma. *Int J Radiat Oncol Biol Phys* 7:549–553, 1991.

244. Hayes FA, Thompson EI, Hvizdala E, et al: Chemotherapy as an alternative to laminectomy and radiation in the management of epidural tumor. *J Pediatr* 104:221–224, 1984.

245. Hayes FA, Green M, O'Connor DM: Chemotherapeutic management of epidural neuroblastoma. *Med Pediatr Oncol* 17:6–8, 1989.

246. Voute PA, Hoefnagel CA, de Kraker J, et al: Results of treatment with ^{131}I-metaiodobenzyl-guanidine (^{131}I-MIBG) in patients with neuroblastoma. Future prospects of zetotherapy. *Prog Clin Biol Res* 366:439–445, 1991.

247. Gaze MN, Wheldon TE: Radiolabelled mIBG in the treatment of neuroblastoma. *Eur J Cancer* 32A:93–96, 1996.

248. Sisson JC, Shapiro B, Hutchinson RJ, et al: Survival of patients with neuroblastoma treated with 125-I MIBG. *Am J Clin Oncol* 19:144–148, 1996.

249. Mastrangelo R, Tornesello A, Riccardi R, et al: A new approach in the treatment of stage IV neuroblastoma using a combination of ^{131}I]meta-iodobenzylguanidine (MIBG) and cisplatin. *Eur J Cancer* 31A:606–611, 1995.

250. DeKraker J, Hoefnagel CA, Caron RA, et al: First-line targeted radiotherapy, a new concept in the treatment of advanced-stage neuroblastoma. *Eur J Cancer* 31A:600–602, 1995.

251. Voute PA, van der Kleij, DeKraker J, et al: Clinical experience with radiation enhancement

by hyperbaric oxygen in children with recurrent neuroblastoma stage IV. *Eur J Cancer* 31A:596–600, 1995.

252. de Kraker J, Hoefnagel CA, Caron H, et al: Preoperative therapy with iodine-^{131}-meta-iodobenzylguanidine (MIBG), a new approach in newly diagnosed neuroblastoma patients. *Proc Annu Meet Am Soc Clin Oncol* 14:A1458, 1995.

253. Matthay KK, Sather HN, Seeger RC, et al: Excellent outcome of stage II neuroblastoma is independent of residual disease and radiation therapy. *J Clin Oncol* 7:236–244, 1989.

254. Stephenson SR, Cook BA, Mease AD, et al: The prognostic significance of age and pattern of metastases in stage IV-S neuroblastoma. *Cancer* 58:372–375, 1986.

255. Martinez DA, King DR, Ginn-Pease ME, et al: Resection of the primary tumor is appropriate for children with stage IV-S neuroblastoma: An analysis of 37 patients. *J Pediatr Surg* 27:1016–1021, 1992.

256. De Bernardi B, Pianca C, Boni L, et al: Disseminated neuroblastoma (stage IV and IV-S) in the first year of life. Outcome related to age and stage. *Cancer* 70:1625–1633, 1992.

257. Paul SR, Tarbell NJ, Korf B, et al: Stage IV neuroblastoma in infants. Long-term survival. *Cancer* 67:1493–1497, 1991.

258. Philip T: Overview of current treatment of neuroblastoma. *Am J Pediatr Hematol Oncol* 14:97–102, 1992.

259. Burdach SE, Muschenich M, Josephs W, et al: Granulocyte-macrophage-colony stimulating factor for prevention of neutropenia and infections in children and adolescents with solid tumors. Results of a prospective randomized study. *Cancer* 76:510–516, 1995.

260. Pelletier J, Laurier C, Poirier I, et al: The role of G-CSF in children with neuroblastoma treated with high-dose chemotherapy. Clinical and pharmacologic study. *Proc Annu Meet Am Soc Clin Oncol* 14:A723, 1995.

261. Bethge W, Holzer U, Dohlsten M, et al: Antibody-targeted superantigen induces T-dependent lysis of neuroblastoma cells. *Proc Annu Meet Am Assoc Cancer Res* 36:A2896, 1995.

262. Cheung NK, Burch L, Kushner BH, et al: Monoclonal antibody 3F8 can effect durable remissions in neuroblastoma patients refractory to chemotherapy: A phase II trial. *Prog Clin Biol Res* 366:395–400, 1991.

263. Hank JA, Surfus J, Gan J, et al: In vivo induction of immunologic conditions able to mediate antibody-dependent cell-mediated cytotoxicity (ADCC) in vitro. *Proc Annu Meet Am Assoc Cancer Res* 33:A1464, 1992.

264. Redfern CP. Lovat PE. Malcolm AJ: Gene expression and neuroblastoma cell differentiation in response to retinoic acid: Differential effects of 9-*cis* and all-*trans* retinoic acid. *Eur J Cancer* 31A:486–494, 1995.

265. Han G, Chang B, Connor MJ, et al: Enhanced potency of 9-*cis* versus all-*trans*-retinoic acid to induce the differentiation of human neuroblastoma cells. *Differentiation* 59:61–69, 1995.

266. Peverali FA, Orioli D, Tonon L, et al: Retinoic acid-induced growth arrest and differentiation of neuroblastoma cells are counteracted by N-*myc* and enhanced by *max* overexpressions. *Oncogene* 12:457–462, 1996.

267. Villablanca JG, Khan AA, Avramis VI, et al: Phase I trial of 13-*cis*-retinoic acid in children with neuroblastoma following bone marrow transplantation. *J Clin Onc* 13:894–901, 1995.

268. Lucarelli E, Kaplan DR, Thiele CJ: Selective regulation of trkA and trkB receptors by retinoic acid and interferon-gamma in human neuroblastoma cell lines. *J Biol Chem* 270:24725–24731, 1995.

269. Lorence RM, Reichard KW, Katubig BB, et al: Complete regression of human neuroblastoma xenografts in athymic mice after local Newcastle disease virus therapy. *J Natl Cancer Inst* 86:1228–1233, 1994.

270. Reichard KW, Lorence RM, Katubig BB, et al: Retinoic acid enhances killing of neuroblastoma cells by Newcastle disease virus. *J Pediatr Surg* 28:1221–1225, 1993.

271. Katsanis E, Orchard PJ, Bausero MA, et al: Interleukin-2 gene transfer into murine neuroblastoma decreases tumorigenicity and enhances systemic immunity causing regression of preestablished retroperitoneal tumors. *J Immunother* 15:81–90, 1994.

272. Adams GA, Shochat SJ, Smith EI, et al: Thoracic neuroblastoma: A Pediatric Oncology Group Study. *J Pediatr Surg* 28:372–378, 1993.

273. Corpron CA, Ater J, Burgess M, et al: Adolescent and adult neuroblastoma. *J Pediatr Surg* (in press).

274. Nishi M, Miyake H, Takeda T, et al: A trial to discriminate spontaneous regression from non-regression cases during mass screening for neuroblastoma. *Jpn J Clin Oncol* 24:247–251, 1994.

275. Rabizadeh S, Oh J, Zhong L, et al: Induction of apoptosis by the low-affinity NGF receptor. *Science* 261:345–348, 1993.

276. Korsmeyer SJ: Bcl-2 initiates a new category of oncogenes: Regulators of cell death. *Blood* 80:879–886, 1992.

277. Koizumi H, Wakisaka M, Nakada K, et al: Demonstration of apoptosis in neuroblastoma and its relationship to tumour regression. *Virchows Arch* 427:167–173, 1995.

278. Weinreb M, Day PJR, Niggli F, et al: BCL-2 oncoprotein in neuroblastoma. *Lancet* 345:992–993, 1995.

279. Ikeda H, Hirato J, Akami M, et al: Bcl-2 oncoprotein expression and apoptosis in neuroblastoma. *J Pediatr Surg* 30:805–808, 1995.

280. Dole M, Nunez G, Merchant AK, et al: Bcl-2 inhibits chemotherapy-induced apoptosis in neuroblastoma. *Cancer Res* 54:3253–3259, 1994.

281. Lasorella A, Iavarone A, Israel MA: Differentiation of neuroblastoma enhances Bcl-2 expression and induces alterations of apoptosis and drug resistance. *Cancer Res* 55:4711–4716, 1995.

282. Gestblom G, Hoehner JC, Pahlman S: Proliferation and apoptosis in neuroblastoma: Subdividing the mitosis-karyorrhexis index. *Eur J Cancer* 31A:458–463, 1995.

283. Ambros PF, Ambros IM, Strehl S, et al: Regression and progression in neuroblastoma. Does genetics predict tumour behaviour? *Eur J Cancer* 31A:510–515, 1995.

284. Squire R, Fowler CL, Brooks SP, et al: Relationship of Class I MHC antigen expression to stage IV-S disease and survival in neuroblastoma. *J Pediatr Surg* 25:381–386, 1990.

285. Bolande RP, Mayer DC: The cytolysis of human neuroblastoma cells by a natural IgM 'antibody'-complement system in pregnancy serum. *Cancer Invest* 8:603–611, 1990.

286. Pritchard J, Hickman JA: Why does stage 4s neuroblastoma regress spontaneously? *Lancet* 344:869–870, 1994.

287. Al-Rashid RA, Cress C: Hypercalcemia associated with neuroblastoma. *Am J Dis Child* 133:838–841, 1979.

288. Scott JP, Morgan E: Coagulopathy of disseminated neuroblastoma. *J Pediatr* 103:219–222, 1983.

289. Quinn JJ, Altman AJ: The multiple hematologic manifestations of neuroblastoma. *Am J Pediatr Hematol Oncol* 1:201–205, 1979.

290. Aitken DR, Hopkins GA, Archambeau JO, et al: Intraoperative radiotherapy in the treatment of neuroblastoma: Report of a pilot study. *Ann Surg Oncol* 2:343–350, 1995.

291. Chou RH, Wong GB, Swift PS, et al: Toxicities of total body irradiation (TBI) for pediatric neuroblastoma bone marrow transplantation (BMT). *Proc Annu Meet Am Soc Clin Oncol* 14:A1432, 1995.

292. Losty P, Quinn F, Breatnach F, et al: Neuroblastoma—A surgical perspective. *Eur J Surg Oncol* 19:33–36, 1993.

293. Azizkhan RG, Shaw A, Chandler JG: Surgical complications of neuroblastoma resection. *Surgery* 97:514–527, 1985.

294. Berthold F, Utsch S, Holschneider AM: The impact of preoperative chemotherapy on resectability of primary tumour and complication rate in metastatic neuroblastoma. *Zeitschr Kinderchir* 44:21–24, 1989.

295. Kiely EM: Radical surgery for abdominal neuroblastoma. *Semin Surg Oncol* 9:489–492, 1993.

296. Weyl-Ben Arush M, Stein M, Perez-Nachum M, et al: Neurologic complications in pediatric solid tumors. *Oncology* 52:89–92, 1995.

297. Aysun S. Topcu M, Gunay M, et al: Neurologic features as initial presentations of childhood malignancies. *Pediatr Neurol* 10:40–43, 1994.

298. Koh PS, Raffensperger JG, Berry S, et al: Long-term outcome in children with opsoclonus-myoclonus and ataxia and coincident neuroblastoma. *J Pediatr* 125:712–716, 1994.

299. Fairchild RS, Kyner JL, Hermreck A, et al: Neuroblastoma, pheochromocytoma and renal cell carcinoma. Occurrence in a single patient. *JAMA* 242:2210–2211, 1979.

300. Hunger SP, Sklar J, Link MP: Acute lymphoblastic leukemia occurring as a second malignant neoplasm in childhood: Report of three cases and review of the literature. *J Clin Oncol* 10:156–163, 1992.

301. Weh HJ, Kabisch H, Landbeck G, et al: Translocation (9;11)(p21;q23) in a child with acute monoblastic leukemia following 2½ years after successful chemotherapy for neuroblastoma. *J Clin Oncol* 4:1518–1520, 1986.

302. Ben-Arush MW, Doron Y, Braun J, et al: Brain tumor as a second malignant neoplasm following neuroblastoma stage IVS. *Med Pediatr Oncol* 18:240–245, 1990.

303. Smith MB, Xue H, Strong L, et al: Forty-year experience with second malignancies after treatment of childhood cancer: Analysis of outcome following the development of the second malignancy. *J Pediatr Surg* 28:1342–1348, 1993.

304. Poustchi-Amin M, Leonidas JC, Elkowitz SS: Simultaneous occurrence of osteosarcoma and osteochondroma following treatment of neuroblastoma with chemotherapy, radiotherapy, and bone marrow transplantation. *Pediatr Radiol* 26:155–157, 1996.

305. Meadows AT, Baum E, Fossati-Bellani F, et al: Second malignant neoplasms in children: An update from the Late Effects Study Group. *J Clin Oncol* 3:532–358, 1985.

306. Kodama K, Nakata T, Ishii J, et al: VMA mass screening program of neuroblastoma for infants in Nagoya City, Japan. *Am J Public Health* 75:173–175, 1985.

307. Sawada T, Todo S, Fujita K, et al: Mass screening of neuroblastoma in infancy. *Am J Dis Child* 136:710–712, 1982.

308. Kaneko Y, Kanda N, Maseki N, et al: Current urinary mass screening for catecholamine metabolites at 6 months of age may be detecting only a small portion of high-risk neuroblastomas: A chromosome and N-*myc* amplification study. *J Clin Oncol* 8:2005–2013, 1990.

309. Sawada T: Past and future of neuroblastoma screening in Japan. *Am J Pediatr Hematol Oncol* 14:320–326, 1992.

310. Hayashi Y, Hanada R, Yamamoto K: Biology of neuroblastomas in Japan found by screening. *Am J Pediatr Hematol Oncol* 14:342–347, 1992.

311. Matsumura M, Tsunoda A, Nishi T, et al:

Spontaneous regression of neuroblastoma detected by mass screening. *Lancet* 338:447–448, 1991.

312. Goodman SN: Neuroblastoma screening data: An epidemiologic analysis. *Am J Dis Child* 145:1415–1422, 1991.

313. Murphy SB, Cohn SL, Craft AW, et al: Do children benefit from mass screening for neuroblastoma? Concensus statement from the American Cancer Society Workshop on neuroblastoma screening. *Lancet* 337:344–346, 1991.

314. Ishimoto K, Kiyokawa N, Fujita H, et al: Problems of mass screening for neuroblastoma: Analysis of false-negative cases. *J Pediatr Surg* 25:398–401, 1990.

315. Treuner J, Schilling FH: Neuroblastoma mass screening: The arguments for and against. *Eur J Cancer* 31A:565–568, 1995.

316. Takeuchi LA, Hachitanda Y, Woods WG, et al: Screening for neuroblastoma in North America. Preliminary results of a pathology review from the Quebec Project. *Cancer* 76:2363–2371, 1995.

Hepatoblastoma

• *John C. Bleacher, M.D.* • *Kurt D. Newman, M.D.*

Primary liver tumors are uncommon in children but unfortunately are malignant in 60% to 67% of cases[1, 2] and present complex challenges in care. The two most common types of pediatric hepatic malignancy are hepatoblastoma and hepatocellular carcinoma. The ratios of incidence of these cancers range from 1.2:1 to 4:1.[1, 2] All other types of malignant tumors are even rarer than either hepatoblastoma or hepatocellular carcinoma (Table 11–1).[1–4]

Because of the rare nature of hepatoblastoma, multi-institutional, intergroup protocols between the Children's Cancer Group (CCG) and Pediatric Oncology Group (POG), which facilitate the study of large numbers of children, have been very valuable for producing advances in care.[5, 6] Largely because of these collaborative efforts, as well as the better understanding of how histology and staging can direct therapy, the overall survival rate for hepatoblastoma has been raised to 70%.[5–9] This rate is a tremendous improvement over the 33% survival reported less than 2 decades ago when resection was the only effective therapy.[2] In contrast, the cure rate for pediatric hepatocellular carcinoma is only 25%.[5, 10]

Future studies should produce further refinements of chemotherapeutic regimens to improve chances of survival yet minimize toxicity in pa-

---

Table 11–1 • Rare Pediatric Hepatic Malignancies

Mesenchymoma
Rhabdomyosarcoma
Angiosarcoma
Undifferentiated sarcomas
Teratocarcinoma
Cholangiocarcinoma
Malignant histiocytoma
Germ-cell tumors

---

tients with hepatoblastoma.[5] Another fundamental goal is to identify those children who are at higher risk for treatment failure.[5]

PRESENTATION

Most liver masses are discovered by the child's parent while the child is being held or bathed, or by the pediatrician during a routine physical examination.[1] By far the most common presentation is that of a child with an asymptomatic abdominal mass or abdominal enlargement.[1] Although less frequent, anorexia and weight loss are seen in about one quarter of children with a liver mass.[1] A more complete list of presenting signs and symptoms is given in Table 11–2. The less common manifestations often signify a more advanced tumor.

The presentation for hepatoblastoma is nearly always before 3 years of age.[1] Approximately one half of such cases are discovered by 18 months of age, 10% of these in the first 6 weeks of life.[1] In contrast, the age of presentation for hepatocellular carcinoma is bimodal.[1, 11] The first peak incidence is from age 0 to 4 years; the second from 12 to 15 years of age.[1, 11]

Hepatoblastoma affects males more frequently than females, at a ratio of 3:2.[1] For hepatocellular carcinoma the ratio between males and females

is nearly 1:1.[1] Overall, the incidence of hepatoblastoma is thought to be about 0.9 per million children.[12]

ETIOLOGY

Although the etiology of pediatric liver malignancy remains to be elucidated, there is a growing body of evidence establishing an association between hepatoblastoma and Beckwith-Wiedemann syndrome, hemihypertrophy, and other embryonal tumors such as Wilms' tumors and rhabdomyosarcomas. This association suggests a common etiology, namely a similar genetic mutation.[13–20] The most intensely studied of these genetic mutations involves the short arm of chromosome 11 (the 11p region), which is the same chromosomal region where mutations have been recognized in association with Wilms' tumors and Beckwith-Wiedemann syndrome.[13–15, 18–20] Specifically, loss of constitutive heterozygosity of one parental allele at the 11p15.5 gene locus is frequently identified in children with hepatoblastoma.[13, 18–20] Tumor expression with loss of heterozygosity at this gene locus suggests the presence of an onco-suppressor gene at 11p15.5.[18–20] This phenomenon also implies genomic imprinting at that chromosomal region.[18, 19] The 11p15.5 gene locus is distinct from the 11p13 locus for the onco-suppressor gene involved with the expression of Wilms' tumors.[19] Other chromosomal abnormalities and point genetic mutations have been seen in children with hepatoblastomas as well.[16, 17]

Environmental factors have also been investigated as a possible cause of hepatoblastoma. CCG distributed an epidemiological survey to assess in utero exposures to carcinogens by the fetus through maternal occupational factors.[21] The survey demonstrated a small but finite increased risk for hepatoblastoma associated with maternal occupational exposures to paints, pigments, oil products, and metals.[21] By contrast, the implication of environmental factors in the etiology of hepatocellular carcinoma is much stronger.[22] Hepatitis B virus increases the lifetime risk of hepatocellular carcinoma 200 times.[23]

DIAGNOSIS

When a child presents with an abdominal mass, the first priority is to define the organ of origin.

Table 11–2 • Presenting Signs and Symptoms for Hepatoblastoma

Sign/symptom	Frequency (%)
Upper abdominal mass	75
Abdominal enlargement	23
Anorexia	25
Weight loss	26
Pain	22
Vomiting	12
Jaundice	5
Weakness	Rare
Lethargy	Rare
Irritability	Rare
Diarrhea	Rare
Pruritis	Rare
Fever	Rare
Precocious puberty	Rare

Data from Exelby PR, Filler RM, Grosfeld JL: Liver tumors in children in the particular reference to hepatoblastoma and hepatocellular carcinoma. American Academy of Pediatrics Surgical Section Survey, 1974. *J Pediatr Surg* 10:329–337, 1975.

Tumors of the liver, kidney, adrenals, or retroperitoneum may all have a similar presentation. Imaging studies should be done immediately. Commonly, the first study obtained after plain radiographs is a computed tomography (CT) scan or an ultrasound. A contrast-enhanced CT scan is very reliable in determining the organ of origin and may also provide some guidance regarding the tumor's resectability.[24] Ultrasound is also useful in defining the origin of an abdominal mass. It is especially helpful in differentiating between a solid and cystic mass.[25] Ultrasound can be used, as well, to locate the tumor for a percutaneous needle biopsy if that is necessary and appropriate. Magnetic resonance imaging (MRI) has gained acceptance as an imaging modality equivalent to CT with respect to its usefulness in making a correct preoperative diagnosis of a liver tumor and in helping the surgeon determine resectability.[26, 27] MRI may even be superior to CT in identifying tumor recurrences postoperatively.[26]

Because of the accuracy of CT and MRI, plus the existence of magnetic resonance arteriography (MRA), with its ability to identify aberrant vessels and be reconstructed to several different views, the need to risk additional morbidity for a preoperative arteriogram has greatly diminished. Of course, if MRI is not available, or if the surgeons and radiologists are not comfortable with the MRI interpretation, arteriography can provide information about the nature of the liver mass (benign or malignant), its vascular anatomy, and its potential resectability.[28] After the operation, serial imaging studies are crucial in identifying residual or recurrent disease.

Serum tumor markers are useful in differentiating the various liver tumors, particularly hepatoblastoma. Alpha-fetoprotein (AFP), a product of embryonal endoderm, is elevated in 90% of children with hepatoblastomas.[29] In Germany an elevated AFP in a child between 6 months and 3 years of age with a liver mass documented on a CT scan is sufficient evidence for a tumor to be diagnosed and treated as a hepatoblastoma.[30] In North America this finding is insufficient evidence; a biopsy is recommended to confirm diagnosis. Other tumors can cause elevations in AFP, such as yolk-sac tumors. Pregnancy will also give a false-positive result. Nevertheless, serial AFP levels are important to measure the response of the tumor to chemotherapy or to assess the completeness of operative resection as well as to allow early recognition of tumor recurrence. A rising AFP level after therapy may indicate recurrence. The absolute value of the AFP level is not as important as the trend in the level over time, although levels greater than 500 ng/mL are suggestive of malignancy.[12]

STAGING

The stage of a hepatoblastoma is determined following surgical exploration. In most protocols, the staging system is based on the location and spread of the tumor and the completeness of resection. In many protocols, therefore, all patients undergo a staging laparotomy if their condition permits.[31] Adherence to this staging standard is important for individualizing therapy, conducting meaningful multi-institutional studies, and making a prognosis. For some protocols, such as CCG-8881, staging is done at the time of diagnosis so that "unresectable" tumors can undergo preoperative chemotherapy before an attempt at resection is made (Figure 11–1).[31] The shortcoming of staging by CT scan preoperatively is that the scan may be misleading with regard to resectability and thus lead to assignment of the incorrect stage. This approach could have a direct effect on reported outcomes by stage. Many centers rely on imaging modalities alone to determine the initial therapeutic approach.

Stage I tumors are confined to the liver and are completely resected at the initial operation. Stage II tumors are likewise confined to the liver and are grossly resected at the initial operation, but microscopic residual disease is present in the surgical margins as determined by histologic examination. Stage III tumors are unresectable or only partially resectable at the initial exploration because of the extent of hepatic disease or the presence of regional lymph node involvement. This stage also includes tumors that have ruptured from the liver capsule. Stage IV hepatoblastomas are those with distant metastases, most commonly to the lungs and brain and less commonly to the bone or bone marrow. The resectability of the primary tumor has no bearing on the staging of hepatoblastomas when distant metastases are present.

The staging for hepatocellular carcinoma is the same as that described for hepatoblastoma. It is

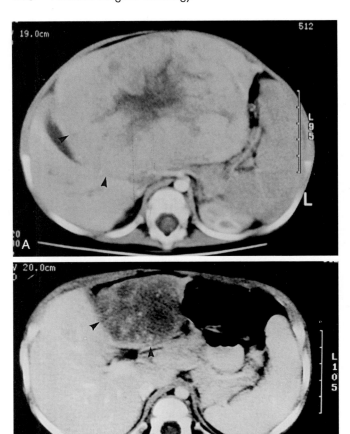

Figure 11-1 • *A,* This hepatoblastoma was thought to be too extensive to safely resect primarily based on the computed tomography scan. The arrows mark the border between the tumor and the normal liver parenchyma. *B,* The same tumor after preoperative chemotherapy has undergone volume reduction to the point where complete resection was safely performed. The tumor is marked by arrows.

based on the extent of resection of the tumor at initial laparotomy.

THERAPY

Complete resection of a liver tumor remains the best chance for long-term survival. Therefore, at the time of initial laparotomy if a tumor appears resectable, all reasonably safe attempts should be made to do so completely. Improvements in anesthesia, nutrition, and critical care have diminished the operative mortality and morbidity rates for children undergoing major hepatic resections.[32] If the tumor is unresectable, a generous biopsy should be taken, but 67% to 75% of hepatoblastomas are resectable at the initial exploration.[1, 2]

The difficulty in basing the staging system for hepatoblastoma on the resectability of the tumor is the variation of opinion among surgeons and institutions about what constitutes a resectable tumor. Especially in light of more effective chemotherapy to preoperatively shrink the tumor, some surgeons may deem a tumor "unresectable" if a resection would be technically formidable and preresection chemotherapy might make it technically less difficult. Thus, what might have been reported as a Stage I tumor if the difficult resection had been undertaken becomes an "unresectable" Stage III tumor.

Because hepatoblastomas occur three times more often in the right lobe than the left, a right hepatic lobectomy is often required for complete resection. Resection can be safely performed even if an extended right lobectomy or trisegmentectomy is required.[33] Intraoperative ultrasound can help clarify the extent of tumor and its proximity to major intrahepatic vascular and biliary structures.[34]

Technically successful hepatic resections require a thorough knowledge of liver and porta hepatis anatomy as well as the anatomic variants that may be encountered. Supra-umbilical transverse incisions offer excellent exposure and can readily be extended into the thorax if necessary. Exposure is key to safe hepatic resections. All suspensory ligaments to the liver should be divided. Proximal and distal control of the inferior vena cava should be attained with vessel loops in the infrahepatic and suprahepatic regions.

A careful, meticulous dissection of the portal vein, hepatic artery, and hepatic ducts and their branches is performed to ensure that the appropriate structures are preserved. The branches of the portal vein, hepatic artery, and bile ducts to the lobe that will be resected are ligated and divided. While the liver is compressed by an assistant, the parenchyma is divided 1 cm into the ischemic demarcation. This dissection is accomplished with finger fracture, electrocautery, ultrasonic dissector, or laser. The hepatic vein is ligated and the specimen removed. The cut surface of the remaining lobe is imbricated with sutures.

The parenchyma can be divided under total vascular occlusion to minimize blood loss. Deep hypothermic circulatory arrest has been described for extensive tumor resections.[35] Tumor margins are checked by taking frozen sections intraoperatively, and additional liver is resected when necessary.

The liver has tremendous regenerative capability.[36] It takes only about 20% of the original liver mass to maintain its synthetic and metabolic functions. Complete return to the original liver mass can be expected. Yet this regeneration is well-controlled as growth ceases when the liver attains its pre-resection mass.

Efforts to improve survival rates in patients with hepatoblastoma take the form of refinements in adjuvant chemotherapy. Prior to the consistent use of cisplatin-based combination chemotherapy, survival of patients with completely resected hepatoblastomas was only 44% to 58%.[1, 2] Now survival of children with Stage I or II disease is greater than 90%.[7, 8] An intergroup study comparing cisplatin/vincristine/5-fluorouracil with cisplatin/Adriamycin (doxorubicin) intravenous continuous infusion showed them to be equivalent therapies.[5] Less toxicity was found in the regimen of cisplatin/vincristine/5-fluorouracil.[6] Current standards for Stage I or II hepatoblastomas are to treat with four courses of postoperative cisplatin/vincristine/5-fluorouracil.[5–7] Furthermore, Stage I tumors with purely fetal histology may be treated with four courses of postoperative doxorubicin with virtually 100% survival expected.[5, 6]

For Stage III and IV disease, preoperative cisplatin-based chemotherapy allows complete resection of the tumor in more than 80% of patients at the time of a second-look laparotomy.[5] The patients should then receive two postoperative courses of the same chemotherapy. Disease-free survival rate and overall survival rate for patients with Stage III and IV hepatoblastomas were 62% and 69%, respectively, at 5 years after surgery in one study.[5]

For cases of Stage III and IV disease that are still unresectable at a second look after four courses of cisplatin-based chemotherapy, alternative therapy must be considered: (1) high-dose cisplatin/etoposide or continuous infusion or doxorubicin; (2) radiation therapy followed by reexploration; (3) direct hepatic artery infusion of chemotherapy; and (4) orthotopic liver transplantation if metastatic disease can be controlled.[37–43] For all of these modalities, the mortality is still high.

In recurrent disease, particularly isolated pulmonary metastases occurring in patients whose Stage I hepatoblastomas has been resected, disease-free survival can be extended with thoracotomy and wedge resection.[44–47] Survival may be prolonged even when repeated thoracotomies are required.[44]

Therapy for hepatocellular carcinoma is the same as for hepatoblastoma. Complete resection is the key to long-term survival. Adjuvant chemotherapeutic regimens are likewise the same for hepatocellular carcinoma: cisplatin-based combination chemotherapy. Hepatocellular carcinomas, however, do not respond to chemotherapy to the same extent as hepatoblastomas in general. For patients in Stages I through IV, the long-term survival is 100%, 36%, 12%, and 8%, respectively.[1, 9] Moreover, the prognosis for recurrent hepatocellular carcinomas is very poor.

PATHOLOGY

Most liver tumors are quite large. Over 50% are greater than 10 cm in diameter; however, it is the histologic subtype rather than the size of the

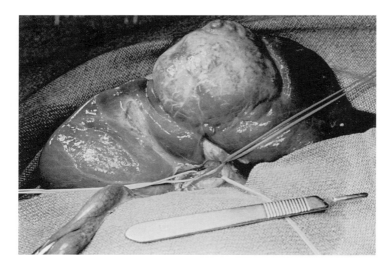

Figure 11-2 • Gross inspection of a hepatoblastoma at exploration shows a large tumor surrounded by an otherwise normal-appearing liver.

tumor that affects prognosis (Figure 11–2).[48–50] The tumor histology may be characterized as fetal, embryonal, undifferentiated, or some combination of these groups. The purely fetal tumors are less primitive, and such patients have the best prognosis.[9, 51–54] On histologic examination of these patients the fetal cells are less dense than in embryonal or undifferentiated tumors.[4] They have lower nuclear-to-cytoplasmic ratios and infrequent mitoses.[4] Unfortunately, most hepatoblastomas have some of the more primitive embryonal or undifferentiated components.[4, 9, 52–54] DNA analysis of hepatoblastomas with flow and image cytometry show a tendency toward better prognosis for patients with tumors that are diploid or have a low proliferation index (less than or equal to 7%), although the difference does not quite reach statistical significance.[55]

Hepatoblastomas are found in otherwise normal livers, whereas hepatocellular carcinomas generally are found in cirrhotic livers. Fibrolamellar carcinomas are a variant of hepatocellular carcinomas that occur in otherwise normal livers of older children and adolescents.[56–59] Prognosis for patients with this particular variant is better than for those with the typical hepatocellular carcinoma.[56–59]

CONCLUSION

Hepatoblastoma is the most common primary hepatic malignancy of childhood. This tumor remains a challenge for multiple disciplines of physicians and nurses. Although surgical resection remains the key to long-term survival, refinements in adjuvant therapy have further improved survival rates. Continued advancement requires cooperation with multi-institutional protocols and a better understanding of molecular biology, tumor-directed immunotherapy, genetics, and pharmacology.

References

1. Exelby PR, Filler RM, Grosfeld JL: Liver tumors in children in the particular reference to hepatoblastoma and hepatocellular carcinoma. American Academy of Pediatrics Surgical Section Survey, 1974. *J Pediatr Surg* 10:329–337, 1975.
2. Randolph JG, Altman RP, Arensman RM, et al: Liver resection in children with hepatic neoplasms. *Ann Surg* 187:599–605.
3. Newman KD, Schisgall R, Reaman G, et al: Malignant mesenchymoma of the liver in children. *J Pediatr Surg* 24:781–783, 1989.
4. Horwitz ME, Etcubanas E, Webber BL, et al: Hepatic undifferentiated carcinoma and rhabdomyosarcoma in children: Results of therapy. *Cancer* 59:396–402, 1987.
5. Ortega J: Intergroup protocol for the treatment of childhood hepatoblastoma and hepatocellular carcinoma. Study Committee Progress Report CCG 8881: 327–341, 1995.
6. Ortega JA, Douglass E, Feusner J, et al: A randomized trial of cisplatin (DDP)/vincristine (VCR)/5-fluorouracil (5FU) vs. DDP/doxorubicin (DOX) IV continuous infusion (CI) for the treatment of hepatoblastoma (HB): Results from the pediatric intergroup hepatoma study (CCG-8881/POG 8945). *Proc Am Soc Clin Oncol* 13:A–1421, 416, 1994.
7. Douglass EC, Reynolds M, Finegold M, et al:

Cisplatin, vincristine, and fluorouracil therapy for hepatoblastoma: A Pediatric Oncology Group Study. *J Clin Oncology* 11:96–99, 1993.

8. Ortega JA, Krailo MD, Haas JE, et al: Effective treatment of unresectable or metastatic hepatoblastoma with cisplatin and continuous-infusion doxorubicin chemotherapy: A report from the Childrens' Cancer Study Group. *J Clin Oncology* 9:2167–2176, 1991.

9. Haas JE, Muczynsky KA, Krailo M, et al: Histopathology and prognosis in childhood hepatoblastoma and hepatocarcinoma. *Cancer* 64:1982–1095, 1989.

10. Douglass E, Ortega J, Feusner J, et al: Hepatocellular carcinoma (HCA) in children and adolescents: Results from the Pediatric Intergroup Hepatoma Study (CCG 8881/POG 8945). *Proc Am Soc Clin Oncol* 13:A-1439, 420, 1994.

11. Dehner LP: Hepatic tumors in the pediatric age group: A distinctive clinical-pathologic spectrum. In Rosenberg HS, Bolande RP (eds): *Perspectives in Pediatric Pathology*, vol. 4. Chicago: Year Book, 1978, pp. 217–268.

12. Hays DM, Stanley P: Lesions of the liver. In Ashcraft KW and Holder TM (eds): *Pediatric Surgery*, 2nd ed. Philadelphia: WB Saunders Co., 1993, pp. 840–846.

13. Little MH, Thomson DB, Hayward NK, et al: Loss of alleles on the short arm of chromosome 11 and a hepatoblastoma from a child with Beckwith-Wiedemann syndrome. *Hum Genet* 79:186–189, 1988.

14. Sotelo-Avila C, Gonzalez-Crussi F, Fowler JW: Complete and incomplete forms of Beckwith-Wiedemann syndrome: Their oncogenic potential. *J Pediatr* 96:47–50, 1980.

15. Koufos A, Hansen MF, Lampkin BC, et al: Loss of alleles at loci on human chromosome 11 during genesis of Wilms' tumor. *Nature* 309:170–174, 1984.

16. Oda H, Nakatsuru Y, Imai Y, et al: A mutational hot spot in the p53 gene is associated with hepatoblastomas. *Int J Cancer* 60:786–790, 1995.

17. Saraswathi A, and Malati T: Trisomy 2, trisomy 20, and del (17p) as sole chromosomal abnormalities in three cases of hepatoblastoma. *Genes, Chromosomes and Cancer* 11:199–202, 1994.

18. Montagna M, Menin C, Chieco-Bianchi L, et al: Occasional loss of constitutive heterozygosity at 11p15.5 and imprinting relaxation of the IGFII maternal allele in hepatoblastoma. *J Cancer Res Clin Oncol* 120:732–736, 1994.

19. Albrecht S, von Schweinitz D, Waha A, et al: Loss of maternal alleles on chromosome arm 11p in hepatoblastoma. *Cancer Res* 54:5041–5044, 1994.

20. Byrne JA, Simms LA, Little MH, et al: Three non-overlapping regions of chromosome arm 11p allele loss identified in infantile tumors of adrenal and liver. *Genes, Chromosomes & Cancer* 8:104–111, 1993.

21. Buckley JD, Sather H, Ruccione K, et al: A case-control study of risk factors for hepatoblastoma. *Cancer* 64:1169–1176, 1989.

22. Fraumeni JF, Miller RW, Hill JA: Primary carcinoma of the liver in childhood: An epidemiologic study. *J Natl Cancer Inst* 40:1087–1099, 1968.

23. Oberfield RA, Steele G, Gollan JL, et al: Liver cancer. *CA* 39:206–218, 1989.

24. Korobkin M, Kurks DR, Sullivan DC, et al: Computed tomography of primary liver tumors in children. *Radiology* 139:431–435, 1981.

25. DeCampo M, DeCampo JF: Ultrasound of primary hepatic tumors in childhood. *Pediatr Radiol* 19:19–24, 1988.

26. Boechat MI, Kangarlooh H, Ortega J, et al: Primary liver tumors in children: Comparison of CT and MR imaging. *Radiology* 169:727–732, 1988.

27. Finn JP, Hall-Craggs MA, Dicks-Mireaux C, et al: Primary malignant liver tumors in childhood: Assessment of resectability with high-field MR and comparison with CT. *Pediatr Radiol* 21:34–38, 1990.

28. Ponkin IL, Wrenn EL, Hollebaugh RS: The continued value of angiography in planning surgical resection of benign and malignant hepatic tumors in children. *Pediatr Radiol* 18:35–44, 1988.

29. Weinberg AG, Finegold MJ: Primary hepatic tumors of childhood. *Hum Pathol* 14:512–537, 1983.

30. Von Schweinitz D, Burger D, Mildenberger H: Is laparotomy the first step in treatment of childhood liver tumors? The experience from the German Cooperative Pediatric Liver Tumor Study HB-89. *Eur J Pediatr Surg* 4:82–86, 1994.

31. Children's Cancer Study Group, Protocol CCG-8881 Hepatoma Study, Surgical Guidelines, pp 19–21.

32. Guzzetta PC, Randolph JG: Pediatric hepatic surgery. *Surg Clin North Am* 69:251–257, 1989.

33. Starzl TE, Bell RH, Beart RW, et al: Hepatic trisegmentectomy and other liver resections. *Surg Gynecol Obstet* 141:429–437, 1975.

34. Thomas BL, Krummel TM, Parker GA, et al: Use of intraoperative ultrasound during hepatic resection in pediatric patients. *J Pediatr Surg* 24:690–693, 1989.

35. Chang JG, Jarick JS, Burrington JD, et al: Extensive tumor resection under deep hypothermia and circulatory arrest. *J Pediatr Surg* 23:254–258, 1988.

36. Nagasue N, Yukaya H, Ogawa Y, et al: Human liver regeneration after major hepatic resection. *Ann Surg* 206:30–39, 1987.

37. Douglass EC, Pediatric Oncology Group: Phase II Study of CBDCA and CBDCA/5-FU/VCR in pediatric patients with unresectable or metastatic (stage III/IV) hepatoblastoma, with CDDP/VP-16 for those who remain unresectable following initial chemotherapy (summary last modified 09/93), POG-9345, clinical trial, closed, 02/15/95.

38. Habrand JL, Nehme D, Kalifa C, et al: Is there a place for radiation therapy in the management of hepatoblastomas and hepatocellular carcinomas in children? *Int J Radiat Oncol Biol Phys* 23:525–531, 1992.

39. Sue K, Ikeda K, Nadagawara A, et al: Intrahepatic arterial injections of cisplatin-phosphatidylcholine-Lipiodol suspension in two unresectable hepatoblastoma cases. *Med Pediatr Oncol* 17:496–500, 1989.

40. Takayama T, Makuuchi M, Takayasu K, et al: Resection after intra-arterial chemotherapy of a hepatoblastoma originating in the caudate lobe. *Surgery* 107:231–235, 1990.

41. Ogita S, Tokiwa K Taniguchi H, et al: Intra-arterial chemotherapy with lipid contrast medium for hepatic malignancies in infants. *Cancer* 60:2886–2890, 1987.

42. Venook AP, Stagg RJ, Lewis BJ, et al: Chemoembolization for hepatocellular carcinoma. *J Clin Oncol* 8:1108–1114, 1990.

43. Koneru B, Flye MW, Busettil RW, et al: Liver transplantation for hepatoblastoma: The American experience. *Ann Surg* 213:118–121, 1991.

44. Passmore SJ, Noblett HR, Wisheart JD, et al: Prolonged survival following multiple thoracotomies for metastatic hepatoblastoma. *Med Pediatr Oncol* 24:58–60, 1995.

45. Feusner JH, Krailo MD, Haas JE, et al: Treatment of pulmonary metastases of initial stage I hepatoblastoma in childhood: Report from the Childrens Cancer Group. *Cancer* 71:859–864, 1993.

46. Black CT, Juck SR, Musemeche CA, et al: Aggressive excision of pulmonary metastases is warranted in the management of childhod hepatic tumors. *J Pediatr Surg* 26:1082–1087, 1991.

47. Lembke J, Havers W, Doetsch N, et al: Long-term results following surgical removal of pulmonary metastases in children with malignomas. *J Thorac Cardiovasc Surg* 34:137–139, 1986.

48. Lack EE, Neav EC, Vawter GF: Hepatoblastoma: A clinical and pathologic study of 54 cases. *Am J Surg Pathol* 6:693–705, 1982.

49. Gonzalez-Crussi F, Upton MP, Maurer HS: Hepatoblastoma: Attempt at characterization of histologic subtypes. *Am J Surg Pathol* 6:599–612, 1982.

50. Dehner LP, Manivel JC: Hepatoblastoma: An analysis of the relationship between morphologic subtypes and prognosis. *Am J Pediatr Hematol Oncol* 10:301–307, 1988.

51. Evans AE, Land VJ, Newton WA, et al: Combination chemotherapy in the treatment of children with malignant hepatoma. *Cancer* 50:821–826, 1982.

52. Ishak KG, Glunz PR: Hepatoblastoma and hepatocarcinoma in infancy and childhood: Report of 47 cases. *Cancer* 20:396–422, 1967.

53. Fraumeni JF, Miller RW, Hill JA: Primary carcinoma of the liver in childhood: An epidemiologic study. *J Natl Cancer Inst* 40:1987–1099, 1968.

54. Weinberg AG, Finegold MJ: Primary hepatic tumors of childhood. *Hum Pathol* 14:512–537, 1983.

55. Schmidt D, Wischmeyer P, Leuschner I, et al: DNA analysis in hepatoblastoma by flow and image cytometry. *Cancer* 72:2914–2919, 1993.

56. Berman MM, Libbey NP, Foster JH: Hepatocellular carcinoma: Polygonal cell type with fibrous stroma—An atypical variant with a favorable prognosis. *Cancer* 46:1448–1455, 1980.

57. Lack EE, Neave C, Vawter GF: Hepatocellular carcinoma: Review of 32 cases in childhood and adolescence. *Cancer* 52:1510–1515, 1983.

58. Craig JR, Peters RL, Edmondson HA, et al: Fibrolamellar carcinoma of the liver: A tumor of adolescents and young adults with distinctive clinico-pathologic features. *Cancer* 46:372–379, 1980.

59. Farhi DC, Shikes RH, Murari PJ, et al: Hepatocellular carcinoma in young people. *Cancer* 52:1516–1525, 1983.

Rhabdomyosarcoma

• *Barry R. Cofer, M.D.* • *Eugene S. Wiener, M.D.*

Rhabdomyosarcoma (Greek *rhabdos*, "rod"; *mys*, "muscle"; *sarkos*, "flesh") is a primary malignancy in children and adolescents that arises from embryonic mesenchyme with the potential to differentiate into skeletal muscle. Its first description in the English literature was by Raycoff[1] in 1937. Horn and Enterline[2] later described a classification system that divided this tumor into major histologic types with differing prognoses, in 1958, and it is still used today. Before the development of effective chemotherapy and radiation therapy protocols, complete (and often mutilating) surgical excision was the only hope for cure. In 1972 the first prospective, multidisciplinary study of this disease began under the auspices of the Intergroup Rhabdomyosarcoma Study (IRS) group, and at the time of this writing the results of three comprehensive studies from this group have been published: IRS-I in 1972–1978, IRS-II in 1978–1984, and IRS-III in 1984–1989. IRS-IV was under way as of 1996. Although the trend has been toward more nonoperative treatment of these patients, complete tumor excision is still the primary treatment, and the surgeon continues to play an essential role in all aspects of management, including diagnosis, staging, and access for chemotherapy.

DEMOGRAPHICS

Rhabdomyosarcoma is the most common soft-tissue sarcoma in pediatric patients and represents the third most common solid malignancy in this age group, behind neuroblastoma and Wilms' tumor. Rhabdomyosarcoma accounts for 4% to 8% of all malignant disease and 5% to 15% of all solid malignancies of childhood. There is a slightly increased incidence in male compared with female patients (3:2) and in Caucasians compared with non-Caucasians.[3]

The peak age at presentation is bimodal, with the primary peak occurring between 2 and 5 years of age and the secondary peak between 15 and 19 years of age. As many as 50% of these sarcomas are discovered before 5 years of age and 6% during infancy (Fig. 12–1).[4]

Rhabdomyosarcoma is known to occur with increased frequency in patients with neurofibromatosis Type I and in patients with the Beckwith-Wiedemann syndrome. The Li-Fraumani syndrome is a cancer-family syndrome in which there is a significantly increased risk of rhabdomyosarcoma as well as nonrhabdomyosarcomatous soft-tissue sarcomas, premenopausal breast carcinomas, and other types of carcinomas in affected kindreds.[5] This risk has been associated with certain germline mutations in the tumor-suppressor gene p53, a phenomenon seen in a number of other malignancies.[6]

BIOLOGY

Rhabdomyosarcomas are a biologically diverse group of tumors displaying a variety of molecular genetic alterations. The two major histologic subtypes, embryonal and alveolar, have each been demonstrated to have characteristic genetic alterations that may in part explain their clinical behavior.

Embryonal rhabdomyosarcomas are known to demonstrate a loss of heterozygosity on the short arm of chromosome 11, a locus where the insulin-growth factor II (IGF-II) gene resides, leading to an overexpression of this gene.[7] IGF-II has been demonstrated to stimulate the growth of rhabdomyosarcoma cells, whereas the blockade of this factor using monoclonal antibodies will inhibit tumor growth both in vitro and in vivo.[8] Of interest are several other pediatric solid neoplasms associated with genomic deletions on the short arm of chromosome 11, including Wilms' tumor, hepatoblastoma, and neuroblastoma. These genomic deletions have also been demonstrated in the Beckwith-Wiedemann syndrome. It appears likely that overexpression of IGF-II plays a significant role in the growth and development of these tumors.[9]

Alveolar rhabdomyosarcomas have been demonstrated to have a characteristic translocation between the long arm of chromosome 2 and the long arm of chromosome 13 (t[2;13][q35;q14]). This translocation involves the juxtaposition of the PAX3 gene, believed to regulate transcription during early neuromuscular development, with the ALV gene, a member of the forkhead family of transcription factors.[10] Although the significance of this association has not been determined, a polymerase chain reaction (PCR) assay has been developed that may aid in the early diagnosis of alveolar rhabdomyosarcoma.[11]

The MyoD family of genes code for DNA-binding proteins that regulate the transcription of DNA sequences encoding myogenic proteins such as desmin, creatine kinase, and myosin.[12] In rhabdomyosarcoma, the down-regulation of this gene does not occur, so that MyoD1 expression stays at high levels in tumor cells.[13] The biologic significance of this overexpression is not clear; however, the detection of high levels of the MyoD1 gene product has been considered in making the diagnosis of rhabdomyosarcoma.[14]

The change in DNA content of a cell is a common occurrence in tumor cells and has some prognostic significance for different malignan-

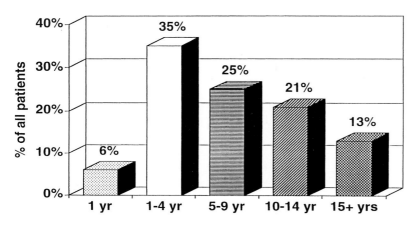

Figure 12–1 • Age distribution of patients with rhabdomyosarcoma in IRS-III. (From Crist W, Gehan EA, Ragab AH, et al: The third intergroup rhabdomyosarcoma study. *J Clin Oncol* 13:610–630, 1995, with permission.)

cies. The ploidy of rhabdomyosarcoma cells has been shown to have prognostic significance. Shapiro and colleagues[15] found that in patients with unresectable rhabdomyosarcoma the presence of a diploid tumor cell line was associated with a dismal prognosis (no survivors), whereas patients with hyperdiploid tumors had a good survival rate (83%). Hyperdiploid tumors were exclusively of the embryonal type. Near-tetraploidy was associated with alveolar histology.

PATHOLOGY

Rhabdomyosarcoma cells arise from undifferentiated mesodermal tissue and may appear in any part of the body, including tissues that do not ordinarily contain striated muscle. Rhabdomyosarcoma has been reported as a primary tumor in virtually every part of the body except the brain. Histologically, it is classified within the category of small, round, blue-cell tumors of childhood, a category that also includes neuroblastoma, Ewing's sarcoma, small-cell osteogenic sarcoma, non-Hodgkin's lymphoma, and leukemia. It may be difficult to distinguish among these tumors by light microscopy alone, necessitating more sophisticated microscopic and biochemical tools.[16]

Gross features of the rhabdomyosarcomatous tumor are not characteristic and are not particularly helpful in distinguishing it from other soft-tissue tumors, with the exception of sarcoma botryoides, which is a mass of grapelike clusters arising from within a hollow viscus. The rhabdomyosarcomatous tumors are usually firm, nodular, and of varying size. They have a tendency to form pseudocapsules, but microscopic evaluation will reveal that the tumor infiltrates tissue beyond the pseudocapsule, thus necessitating a wide resection for complete tumor removal. The ability to achieve complete removal helps determine clinical group staging and has prognostic and therapeutic significance.

The pathologic description of rhabdomyosarcoma as a tumor of myogenic lineage was first advanced in 1958 by Horn and Enterline.[2] These investigators proposed the first classification scheme, one that divided rhabdomyosarcoma into four different pathologic types—embryonal, botryoid, alveolar, and pleomorphic. This scheme has been the standard pathologic nomenclature for this tumor for several decades and has been used by the IRS since its inception. But, in addition, several different classification schemes have been proposed over the years, each with its own advantages and limitations.[17] The existence of these different methods of classification made necessary the development of a comprehensive, universal classification system. Just such a "universal" system was described in an international collaborative effort among pediatric pathologists in 1994, and it is currently used in most institutions (Table 12–1). Essentially a modification of the Horn and Enterline system, it furthermore ascribes prognostic significance to each histologic type by classifying them into favorable-, intermediate-, and poor-prognosis groups.[18]

Favorable-prognosis tumors include the botryoid and spindle-cell variants.[18] *Botryoid rhabdomyosarcoma* is best described as a "cluster of grapes" in gross appearance. The central mass of this tumor has a loosely cellular, myxoid appearance, with eosinophils scattered throughout the myxoid stroma; a cambium layer of condensed tumor cells is located directly under the overlying mucosa. Individual tumor cells of this type usually show evidence of myogenesis in their cytoplasm. The botryoid variant appears primarily in young children in visceral cavities such as the nasopharynx, vagina, and biliary tree and is associated with the best prognosis of all types of rhabdomyosarcoma.[16]

Spindle-cell rhabdomyosarcoma is a collagen-poor, leiomyosarcomatous form or a collagen-rich form with a storiform pattern. This variant has a

---

Table 12–1 • Histologic Variants of Childhood Rhabdomyosarcoma: International Rhabdomyosarcoma Pathologic Classification

I. Favorable Prognosis
   a. Botryoid
   b. Spindle-cell
II. Intermediate Prognosis
   a. Embryonal
   b. Pleomorphic (rare)
III. Poor Prognosis
   a. Alveolar (including solid variant)
   b. Undifferentiated

Data from Asmar L, Gehan EA, Newton WA, et al: Agreement among and within groups of pathologists in the classification of rhabdomyosarcoma and related childhood sarcomas: Report of an international study of four pathology classifications. *Cancer* 74:2579–2588, 1994.

predilection for paratesticular sites and, like the botryoid variant, is associated with a very favorable outcome; patients with nonparatesticular spindle-cell tumors have a prognosis similar to that of those with the embryonal variant of rhabdomyosarcoma.[19] Unfortunately, botryoid and spindle-cell rhabdomyosarcomas, both of which are associated with favorable prognoses, account for only 5% to 6% of all rhabdomyosarcomas (Fig. 12–2).

Intermediate-prognosis tumors are of the embryonal type.[18] Embryonal rhabdomyosarcoma is composed of small round or spindle-shaped cells with variable cellularity and myogenous differentiation; there is no evidence of an alveolar pattern. The cytoplasm is predominantly eosinophilic, and longitudinal cross-striations may be visible. Embryonal histology is the predominant type seen in infants and young children. The median age of the patient at diagnosis is 8 years. Embryonal rhabdomyosarcomas account for more than 50% of all newly diagnosed tumors, more than 80% of distal urinary tract tumors, 60% of head and neck tumors, and roughly 50% of tumors at other sites, not including the trunk and perineum.[16] Both the botryoid and spindle-cell variants are considered subvariants of embryonal rhabdomyosarcoma but are now classified in the favorable-prognosis category.

Unfavorable-prognosis tumors include alveolar and undifferentiated rhabdomyosarcomas.[18] The alveolar variant is characterized by a prominent alveolar arrangement of stroma and dense, small, round tumor cells resembling those of lung tissue. The degree of histologic differentiation is variable. A subtype of alveolar rhabdomyosar-coma is the "solid" alveolar rhabdomyosarcoma, characterized by an architecture of dense cellular sheets lacking any intercellular stroma but with cytologic features identical to those found in the classically alveolar tumors. It is not uncommon to have a mixture of histologic types of rhabdomyosarcoma within a given tumor; however, a tumor with any degree of alveolar component is designated and treated as an alveolar rhabdomyosarcoma. Alveolar tumors frequently arise from the extremities, trunk, or perineum; they account for roughly 20% of rhabdomyosarcomas seen in children. *Undifferentiated sarcoma* is a poorly defined category of sarcomatous tumors whose cells show no evidence of myogenesis or other differentiation. This sarcoma occurs most commonly in the extremity or head and neck sites and is associated with a very poor prognosis (see Fig. 12–2).[16, 17]

Pleomorphic sarcoma is characterized by large pleomorphic cells with multinucleated giant cells and is most often seen on the extremity or trunk; it is rare in children. A tumor variant with a cytology different from any of the more common subtypes of rhabdomyosarcoma has been designated as small, round-cell sarcoma, type indeterminate. This variant is thought to represent a mesenchymal tumor arising from a primitive cell type in which its line of differentiation could not be determined. It accounted for 13% of lesions seen in the IRS-III study (see Fig. 12–2).[16, 17]

Extraosseous Ewing's sarcoma (EOS) is composed of uniform, small, round cells with scanty cytoplasm. EOS has the same morphologic and cytologic features as osseous Ewing's sarcoma. Electron microscopy and immunohistochemi-

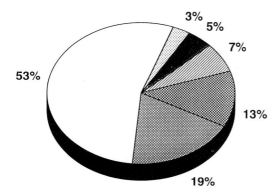

3% 5% 7% 53% 13% 19%

☐ **embryonal**
☒ **EOS**
■ **botryoid**
▨ **undifferentiated**
▩ **undetermined**
▩ **alveolar**

Figure 12–2 • Histologic distribution of patients with rhabdomyosarcoma in IRS-III

EOS: extra-osseous Ewing's sarcoma

cal analysis of tumors are rapidly emerging as useful tools for demonstrating characteristics of rhabdomyosarcomatous tumors that could not be clearly shown with classic light microscopy. The diagnostic ultrastructural features of rhabdomyosarcoma include the following: well-defined sarcomeres with visible Z-bands, Z-bands with or without insertion of thick and thin filaments, thick and thin filaments in a hexagonal array, and an "Indian file" arrangement of the ribosome/myosin complexes.[17, 20]

A number of monoclonal antibodies have been shown to react with elements of rhabdomyosarcomas and have been useful in their diagnosis. These include antibodies to desmin, muscle-specific actin, sarcomeric actin, and myoglobin. All have been used to confirm the myogenous lineage of cells and when used in combination have very good specificity and sensitivity.[17] Monoclonal antibodies have also been developed to the gene product of MyoD1, a lineage marker gene for rhabdomyosarcoma, and can be utilized in frozen section analysis.[14, 21] Other nonmyogenous protein products that can be identified in these tumors include cytokeratin, neuron-specific enolase, S-100 protein, and Leu-7. These are seen more frequently in nonsarcomatous tumors and lack the specificity of the previously mentioned markers.[17] The characteristic cytogenetic abnormality in alveolar tumors (the reciprocal t[2;13][q35;q14] translocation) has been identified using the reverse transcriptase-polymerase chain reaction (RT-PCR) technique. This has helped confirm the diagnosis of poorly differentiated tumors or the solid variant of alveolar rhabdomyosarcoma.[11, 22]

CLINICAL FEATURES

The clinical manifestations of rhabdomyosarcoma vary with the site of origin of the primary tumor, the age of the patient, and the presence or absence of metastatic disease. Not infrequently, the tumor is so large that determination of the exact location of its primary site is impossible, as in the case of massive pelvic tumors. The majority of symptoms will be related to the effects of tumor compression on adjacent organs, or the patient will present with an asymptomatic mass. There are no characteristic paraneoplastic syndromes associated with this malignancy.

The most common site of presentation is in the head and neck region, accounting for 35% of all primary tumors in IRS-III (Table 12–2).[23] The head and neck are divided into the orbits (10%), parameningeal tissues (middle ear, nasal cavity and paranasal sinuses, nasopharynx, and infratemporal fossa; 15%), and nonparameningeal tissues (scalp, face, oral cavity, oropharynx, hypopharynx, and neck; 10%). These tumors are most commonly embryonal and tend to appear in younger patients either as asymptomatic masses or as masses causing interruption of normal structural function (e.g., exophthalmos or strabismus in orbital rhabdomyosarcoma).[24] Extension to regional lymph nodes is uncommon, but parameningeal tumors may extend into the cranium with resultant cranial nerve palsy and meningeal symptoms.

Genitourinary rhabdomyosarcomas accounted for 26% of all primary tumors in the IRS-III study.[23] These tumors are considered as two distinct entities: bladder/prostate tumors (10%) and

Table 12–2 • Primary Tumor Site and Group Distribution for Patients with Rhabdomyosarcoma in IRS-III

Site	Total	Group I	Group II	Group III	Group IV
All Sites	*1062*	*213 (20%)*	*221 (21%)*	*478 (45%)*	*150 (14%)*
Head and Neck	*375 (35%)*	*31*	*94*	*222*	*28*
Orbit	109 (10%)	3	46	58	2
Parameningeal	155 (15%)	4	9	121	21
Nonparameningeal	111 (10%)	24	39	43	5
GU (non B/P)	167 (16%)	89	36	33	9
GU (B/P)	110 (10%)	9	7	88	6
Extremity	202 (19%)	64	53	39	46
Other	208 (20%)	20	31	96	61

GU = genitourinary; B/P = bladder/prostate.
Data from Crist W, Gehan EA, Ragab AH, et al: The third intergroup rhabdomyosarcoma study. J Clin Oncol 13:610–630, 1995.

non-bladder/prostate tumors, the latter occurring at paratesticular sites, the perineum, vulva, vagina, and uterus (16%) (see Table 12–2). The most common histologic type for these tumors is embryonal. Botryoid tumors may be seen at the vaginal site, although the overall incidence of vaginal botryoid tumors is quite low.[25] Spindle-cell tumors are associated with paratesticular rhabdomyosarcoma and with one of the best prognoses for all sites of primary tumor.[19] There is a propensity for early lymphatic spread from tumors in these locations, however.

Rhabdomyosarcoma of the extremity tends to occur more commonly on the lower than on the upper extremity. This was the location of 19% of all tumors in IRS-III (see Table 12–2). Tumors of the extremities typically occurred in adolescents and tended to behave more aggressively, with a higher incidence of regional nodal involvement and distant metastases, than other tumors. Usually they are first seen as a painless lump or as adenopathy, and most are of the alveolar variant, with its attendant poorer prognosis.[26]

Other sites that accounted for 20% of all primary tumor sites in IRS-III included the thorax, diaphragm, abdominal or pelvic wall, and intra-abdominal or intrapelvic organs (exclusive of those organs described earlier) (see Table 12–2).[23]

DIAGNOSTIC EVALUATION

The goal of the diagnostic evaluation for rhabdomyosarcoma is to determine the histologic variant of the tumor, its primary site, and the extent of disease (both local and distant). Each of these variables has an important influence on the choice of treatment and prognosis. Except for the usual preoperative blood counts and chemistries, there are no hematologic or serologic studies specifically useful for diagnosis of rhabdomyosarcoma. CT scan and magnetic resonance imaging (MRI) have proved essential to the evaluation of the primary tumor in that they allow an accurate assessment of its relationship to surrounding structures. The most common sites of metastatic spread include the lungs, the bone marrow, and the skeletal system, and each should be evaluated by CT scan, bone marrow aspirate or biopsy, and bone scan, respectively. As the metastatic pattern tends to be tumor site–specific, other tests may be indicated: an abdomi-

nal/pelvic CT scan for paratesticular tumors to look for retroperitoneal lymphadenopathy, a lumbar puncture with CSF sampling for paramenimgeal and paraspinal tumors, and an examination by CT or MRI of the draining nodal basins for any tumor of an extremity.[27]

The most important part of the diagnostic process is obtaining adequate tissue for histologic and cytologic diagnosis and classification. This procedure is usually accomplished by an open incisional biopsy using general anesthesia. Complete excisional biopsy is frequently impossible. The tissue should be given to the pathologist fresh so that the appropriate studies can be obtained. It is imperative that the surgeon obtain an amount adequate for diagnosis as well as for evaluation of cytologic and biologic markers. Percutaneous needle or core biopsies may have a role in the diagnostic process but may not provide adequate tissue for a complete evaluation, and they should probably be used only in special circumstances.

CLINICAL GROUPING AND STAGING

Staging for rhabdomyosarcoma is performed in order to allow (1) different treatment regimens for different extents of disease and (2) comparisons of treatment and outcome, both within and among institutions. The Clinical Grouping System developed by the IRS is based upon pretreatment and operative outcome (Table 12–3). Its premise is that total tumor extirpation at the original operation is the best hope for cure, hence tumors are stratified according to their resectability. This staging system has led to aggressive and often mutilating procedures in an effort to accomplish complete surgical removal of the primary tumor. The system does not take into account the biologic nature or natural history of the tumor or the experience and aggressiveness of the operating surgeon. Therefore, attempts have been made to supplant it with a system that takes those factors into account, including the site and histologic peculiarities of the tumor.[28] Table 12–4 presents the pretreatment clinical staging system that is a modification of the familiar tumor/node metastasis (TNM) classification used in the majority of malignancies and at the time of this writing being evaluated in the IRS-IV study. Both systems remain useful in the

Table 12-3 • IRS Clinical Groups of Rhabdomyosarcoma

Group I	Localized disease, completely removed a. Confined to muscle or organ of origin b. Infiltration outside organ or muscle of origin; regional nodes not involved
Group II	Total gross resection with evidence of regional spread a. Grossly resected tumor with microscopic residual b. Regional disease with involved nodes, completely resected with no microscopic residual c. Regional disease with involved nodes, grossly resected, but with evidence of microscopic residual and/or histologic involvement of the most distal regional node in the dissection
Group III	Incomplete resection, or biopsy with presence of gross disease
Group IV	Distant metastasis

management of children with rhabdomyosarcoma.

The stratification of cases by clinical group in IRS-III was as follows: I, 20%; II, 21%; III, 45%; and IV, 14%. There were more patients in clinical group III in the IRS-III study than in the IRS-II study, most likely because of a decrease in the rate of initial complete excision, especially in children with special pelvic-site primaries.[23] Clinical grouping by site in IRS-III is shown in Table 12-2.

GENERAL TREATMENT STRATEGY

The treatment strategy for rhabdomyosarcoma requires a multidisciplinary approach involving surgeons, oncologists, radiation-oncologists, and pathologists. As with most uncommon tumors, entry into a treatment protocol such as the IRS-IV study is advantageous.

General Surgical Principles

The surgical treatment of rhabdomyosarcoma is site-specific, and the nuances of the management of individual sites are discussed in a later section. The general principles include complete wide excision of the primary tumor and surrounding uninvolved tissues while preserving cosmesis and function where possible. Incomplete excision or tumor debulking is not beneficial and should not be performed, nor should severely mutilating or debilitating excisions.[29] Secondary excision after initial biopsy and neoadjuvant therapy has a better outcome than partial or incomplete resection and should be planned in cases in which primary excision is not possible. What was originally a massive soft-tissue tumor will often have a dramatic reduction in size after chemotherapy and/or radiation therapy, thereby allowing successful delayed resection. When initial excision is not possible, incisional biopsy only is employed, along with biopsy of clinically suspicious-looking lymph nodes as indicated. Pathologic evaluation

Table 12-4 • TNM Pretreatment Staging Classification of Patients with Rhabdomyosarcoma in IRS-IV Tumor Size Regional Nodes Metastasis

Stage	Sites	Tumor Size	Regional Nodes	Metastasis
I	Orbit Head and neck (superficial) Genitourinary (non B/P)	a or b	$N_0 N_1$ or N_x	M_0
II	Bladder/prostate Extremity, trunk Parameningeal Other	a	N_0 or N_x	M_0
III	Bladder/prostate Extremity, trunk Parameningeal Other	b	N_1 $N_0 N_1$ or N_x	M_0
IV	All	a or b	Any N	M_1

TNM = tumor/node/metastasis; a = ≤ 5cm in diameter; b = > 5cm in diameter; N_0 = not clinically involved; N_1 = clinically involved; N_x = clinical status unknown; M_0 = no distant metastasis; M_1 = distant metastasis present; head and neck = entire area excluding nonparameningeal tumors; B/P = bladder/prostate; other = all other sites.

of clinically uninvolved nodes is site-specific, as in cases of extremity lesions and incompletely resected paratesticular tumors. Needle biopsy or fine-needle aspiration may be safer in certain situations but may not provide adequate tissue for special histologic, cytologic, and biochemical studies.

Primary Re-excision

In some patients with extremity or trunk rhabdomyosarcoma, initial tumor resection is thought to be complete, but then histopathologic review reveals microscopic residual disease corresponding to clinical group IIa in the surgical margins. In many of these patients, *primary re-excision (PRE)* is possible, achieving wider and, it is hoped, disease-free surgical margins. The report by Hays and coworkers[30] demonstrates the benefit of PRE. In IRS-I and IRS-II, 154 patients with extremity or trunk rhabdomyosarcomas were initially placed in clinical group IIa; then 41 patients underwent successful PRE and were converted to clinical group I prior to the onset of adjuvant therapy. These patients were compared with 113 patients who had microscopic residual disease and did not undergo PRE and with 73 patients who were free of disease after the initial resection (clinical group I). Among the 41 PRE patients, the 3-year Kaplan-Meier survival estimate was 91%, compared with 74% for group IIa patients not undergoing PRE and 74% for clinical group I patients. This approach may be applicable to tumors of other locations as well. PRE should be considered, even if the margins are apparently normal, if the initial resection was not a "cancer" operation, that is, if malignancy was not suspected preoperatively.

Second-Look Operations

Second-look operations (SLO) have been used for several types of pediatric tumors to evaluate therapeutic response and to remove any residual tumor after completing initial therapy. The utility of SLO was evaluated in IRS-III and shown to be beneficial in clinical group III rhabdomyosarcoma patients. Wiener and coworkers[31] evaluated separately 257 patients from IRS-III in clinical group III (excluding special pelvic sites). SLO was performed in 21% of patients with *complete response (CR)*, 66% of patients with *partial re-*sponse (PR), and 52% of patients with *clinical nonresponse (NR)*. The performance of SLO significantly changed the response status in a significant number of patients: 12% of presumed CR patients were found to harbor residual tumor, whereas 74% of both PR and NR patients were recategorized as CR after operation. The survival of those recategorized PR and NR patients was similar to that of patients confirmed to be CR at reexploration; clinical NR patients who were reassigned to CR after SLO enjoyed a 73% survival compared with an 80% survival in all CR patients.[31] Of equal importance, those patients who became CR avoided the more toxic second-line treatment regimens.

Adjuvant Therapy

The management of rhabdomyosarcoma has been altered significantly by the use of more effective and less toxic chemotherapy regimens. Specific chemotherapy regimens are based upon the initial extent of disease and the site of origin of the primary tumor.

Nonalveolar clinical group I patients were treated with combination vincristine and actinomycin D (VA) without radiation therapy in the first three IRS studies. In IRS-IV, in which no distinction was made among histologic variants, VA therapy was reserved for clinical group I paratesticular or orbital tumors and all other group I patients randomized among three three-drug regimens: VAC (vincristine, actinomycin D, cyclophosphamide), VAI (vincristine, actinomycin D, ifosfamide), and VIE (vincristine, ifosfamide, etoposide).[8]

For clinical group II patients with nonalveolar tumors, VA administration alone resulted in an excellent outcome, although this appeared to be site-specific in regard to paratesticular and non-parameningeal head and neck tumors.[32, 33] In IRS-IV, VA was reserved for patients with clinical group II orbital tumors and all other group II patients randomized among VAC, VAI, or VAE regimens as in group I. Radiation therapy was given to all patients with microscopic residual disease.

There was a significant improvement in survival rates for clinical group III patients with gross residual disease between the early IRS studies and IRS-III.[23, 32, 33] In IRS-III, therapy for group III patients was based on the extent of disease as well as the histology and site of the primary tumor. Patients with nonparameningeal head and neck tumors received VA chemotherapy, whereas patients with special pelvic tumors received pulse VAdriaC (vincristine, doxorubicin [Adriamycin], cyclophosphamide)–VAC plus cisplatin. Patients with favorable-histology tumors from all other sites and patients with unfavorable-histology tumors from any site were randomized to one of three multiagent regimens consisting of various combinations of vincristine, Adriamycin (doxorubicin), cyclophosphamide, actinomycin D, cisplatin, and etoposide.[23] In IRS-IV all clinical group III patients were randomized between VAC, VAI, and VAE regimens, as were patients with more limited disease.[8]

Clinical group IV patients (metastatic disease) had a poor prognosis, as shown in the IRS-I study, with essentially no improvement in subsequent IRS studies despite more aggressive (and toxic) treatment regimens. Although most patients enjoyed an initial response to therapy, most experienced recurrences within 18 to 24 months[34]; the 5-year survival for group IV patients in IRS-III was 27%.[23] An interest in very-high-dose myeloablative chemoradiotherapy followed by autologous or allogeneic bone marrow transplant has emerged in the treatment of other solid tumors of childhood, most notably neuroblastoma, and has been applied to patients with metastatic rhabdomyosarcoma. No reports on its efficacy have been published to date.

Radiation therapy is primarily designed to achieve local control of residual microscopic or macroscopic tumor that has not been completely removed by surgery. In cases of microscopic residual disease, radiation doses of 40–45 Gy are adequate to achieve local control in the majority of patients; the dose is increased to 50–55 Gy in patients with larger tumors and gross residual disease.[33] Prophylactic irradiation of clinically uninvolved lymph nodes is unnecessary. Patients with clinical group I tumors of nonalveolar histology and patients with tumors of the vagina, uterus, and vulva that are completely excised on second-look operations may not require radiation therapy; virtually all other groups require radiation to achieve lasting local control.[8] Brachytherapy and intraoperative radiation therapy for some tumors, including vulvovaginal, bladder, prostate, retroperitoneal, and extremity primaries, is being studied.[35]

SPECIFIC TREATMENT STRATEGY AND OUTCOME

Head and Neck

The most common sites for primary rhabdomyosarcomas in children are in the head and neck region, including the orbit. Prior to the advent of effective chemotherapy and radiation therapy, radical excision of the tumor was the treatment of choice, with resulting major morbidity but little effect on outcome. Since then, the use of multimodality therapies has significantly reduced the necessity for mutilating treatment of such lesions as orbital rhabdomyosarcomas yet has improved overall outcomes.

The head and neck region is considered as three anatomic areas: the orbit, the parameningeal region (nasopharynx, paranasal sinuses, middle ear, mastoid, pterygopalatine, and infratemporal fossae), and the nonparameningeal region (parotid, cheek, masseter muscle, oral cavity, oropharynx, hypopharynx, scalp, face, pinna).[36] The orbit is the most common site of rhabdomyosarcoma in this region, and orbital tumors are usually diagnosed at an early stage due to their visibility. Historically, primary orbital exenteration was the treatment of choice, followed by radiation therapy. Abramson and coworkers[37] demonstrated that primary chemotherapy or chemotherapy plus irradiation without surgical removal resulted in a survival rate of over 90%.

In the IRS-III report, orbital tumors accounted for 10% of all cases and 29% of all head and neck rhabdomyosarcomas; most of these tumors were of the embryonal variant.[23] Since the treatment of orbital tumors (with the exception of tumors arising from the eyelid) is primarily nonsurgical, these tumors were assigned to clinical group III, but they are Stage I. In IRS-IV, patients with clinical group I tumors received VA without radiation, whereas clinical group II/III patients received cyclic VA chemotherapy combined with irradiation. Orbital exenteration is reserved for recurrences and treatment failures. The majority of orbital tumors are localized at the time of diagnosis, and patients with these tumors can be expected to have an overall survival rate higher than 90% after treatment.[38] Complications of treatment are significant, though; in a study of 50 patients with orbital rhabdomyosarcomas who received 50–60 Gy of radiation, cataract formation was seen in 34, corneal changes in 10, retinal damage in 3, ptosis in 13, exophthalmos in 10, and lacrimal duct stenosis in 7.[39]

Parameningeal rhabdomyosarcomas arise in relatively hidden areas of the head and neck region, and diagnosis is therefore frequently delayed. Tumors in these sites accounted for 15% of all cases in the IRS-III study. They represent 41% of all head and neck rhabdomyosarcomas in children.[23] Cranial nerve palsy is a particularly ominous presenting sign, as this implies invasion or compression along the area of the skull base and within the cranial vault. Although originating outside the central nervous system, parameningeal rhabdomyosarcomas can invade and penetrate through the bone and meninges; therefore, cytologic analysis of the cerebrospinal fluid should be included in the initial evaluation. Up to 15% of patients present with metastatic disease, so a general metastatic evaluation should be performed.[36] Treatment of parameningeal tumors involves intensive radiation therapy to the area of the lesion and the entire cranial neuraxis as well as intrathecal and systemic chemotherapy. IRS patients receiving this therapy had a 3-year tumor-free survival rate that was 24% higher than the survival rate for nonintensively treated patients.[40] The use of newer skull-base surgical techniques and reconstruction after chemotherapy and radiation therapy has resulted in an improved outcome and survival rate in other series.[41]

Patients with nonparameningeal rhabdomyosarcomas have a much better prognosis than those with parameningeal tumors because diagnosis is usually made earlier. Nonparameningeal tumors accounted for 30% of all head and neck rhabdomyosarcomas in IRS-III and 10% of all tumor sites.[23] Complete tumor excision is preferable, and it is often possible due to the relatively superficial location of these tumors, provided the cosmetic and functional results are acceptable. Like orbital tumors, tumors from these sites are usually considered Stage I/clinical group II or III unless total excision was possible prior to treatment. Occasionally a nonparameningeal tumor grows large enough to invade into an area considered "parameningeal" and in this case should be evaluated and treated as a parameningeal primary tumor.

Initial cervical node metastasis arising from these tumors is uncommon, and routine nodal biopsy is not indicated unless clinically suspicious-looking nodes are evident; formal cervical node dissection is never indicated.

Genitourinary Tract

Rhabdomyosarcoma is the most common malignancy of the pelvic structures seen in children. Tumors in these locations are considered in two different categories on account of their different prognoses according to site: bladder/prostate versus vulvovagina, uterus, and paratesticle. These sites accounted for approximately 25% of cases in the IRS-III report[23]; in 6% of those patients with pelvic tumors in the IRS-I and IRS-II studies the exact site of origin within the pelvis could not be defined.

Bladder and prostate rhabdomyosarcomas can be difficult to distinguish from one another because of their anatomical proximity and tendency to grow to large sizes prior to diagnosis. When this determination is possible, it becomes evident that patients with bladder primaries enjoy a somewhat better prognosis than those with tumors arising from the prostate.[42] The majority of tumors in these areas are of embryonal (71%) or botryoid (20%) variants; 2% are of alveolar histology.[43]

Bladder/prostate tumors commonly arise near the area of the trigone and produce symptoms of bladder outlet obstruction or hematuria. Diagnosis is usually made by cystoscopic evaluation and biopsy as well as CT or MRI scanning. Previously, the initial management of these tumors in children was usually anterior or total pelvic exenteration followed by chemotherapy and radiation; this treatment produced very good long-term survival rates, approaching 85% in some series, but it also necessitated the morbidity of permanent urinary conduit and, in rare cases, colostomy.[43] Now bladder salvage is emphasized and less aggressive surgical means employed. Neoadjuvant chemotherapy and radiation have decreased the rate of exenterative cystectomy from greater than 50% to approximately 30%.[44] In IRS-III, 50% of patients with bladder rhabdomyosarcoma received cisplatin in addition to VAdrC–VAC and irradiation. Of 171 children with primary bladder lesions enrolled in the IRS-I through IRS-III studies, 40 underwent partial cystectomy after receiving neoadjuvant chemotherapy and radiation. Relapse occurred in nine patients (seven locally). The Kaplan-Meier estimate of survival rate with a functioning bladder among all children with bladder/prostate tumors in IRS-III was 60%, long-term survival was in excess of 80%.[44]

Vulvovaginal and uterine rhabdomyosarcoma is the most common malignancy of the pediatric female genital system. Treatment for these areas has consisted of exenterative surgery in the past but now is more oriented toward preoperative neoadjuvant chemotherapy and radiation therapy; a more localized, less radical operation can then be performed, if necessary. The age of patients at the time of diagnosis varies according to the primary site of the tumor. The mean age of presentation for patients with uterine tumors is 14 years, and the mean age of presentation for patients with vaginal tumors is 1.8 years, with 90% of patients being younger than 5 years of age. The mean age of presentation for girls with vulvar tumors is 8 years.[43]

The majority of tumors arising from the uterus or vagina are of the embryonal variant, with the favorable-prognosis botryoid variant being seen somewhat frequently. Vulvar tumors are usually of the alveolar variety. Survival rates when neoadjuvant therapy is coupled with less radical resection have shown a gradual improvement compared with the early IRS experience. During IRS-III, 24 patients were on a preoperative chemotherapy protocol of Adriamycin (doxorubicin), cisplatin, vincristine, actinomycin D, and cyclophosphamide. Seven patients (29%) eventually required surgical resection (five hysterectomies and two vaginectomies). Bladder preservation was accomplished in all but one patient. There were no local recurrences, and the overall survival rate was 80%. Of note, six of the seven patients undergoing resection of a residual tumor mass were found to have no viable tumor within the resection specimen, and the other patient was shown to have only maturing rhabdomyoblast still present.[45]

Paratesticular rhabdomyosarcomas arise in the distal area of the spermatic cord, sometimes invading the testis or surrounding tissues. The majority of paratesticular tumors are of the embryonal subtype, with a high percentage being of the favorable-histology spindle-cell variant. These tumors account for 7% of childhood rhabdomyosarcomas and 12% of all childhood scrotal tumors.[42] Initial management includes inguinal orchiectomy with high ligation of the cord structures as in the case of any suspected scrotal tumor. Scrotal incisions for biopsy or orchiectomy should not be performed because they violate tissue planes and are associated with an increased risk of local recurrence and systemic lymphatic metastases.

Routine retroperitoneal lymph node dissection (RPLND) is controversial. Wiener[46] and coworkers reported on 121 patients in IRS-III with nonmetastatic paratesticular rhabdomyosarcoma who underwent RPLND. Of the patients who had clinically normal nodes, 14% were shown to have lymphatic metastases. Only two experienced regional nodal recurrence. The conclusions from this study were that routine RPLND is not warranted in patients with paratesticular rhabdomyosarcoma. Furthermore, systematic retroperitoneal node biopsies are unnecessary in children with clinically normal nodes, although they should be performed in patients with clinical suspicion of diseased nodes or incompletely resected paratesticular tumors.[46] In IRS-III the survival rate was 95% at 3 years and 91% at 5 years; children younger than 10 years of age had a better (97%) survival rate when compared with that of older children (84%). Late morbidity was reported in 86 children with paratesticular rhabdomyosarcoma enrolled in the IRS-I and IRS-II studies. Diminished contralateral testicular size was found in 30% of patients who received radiation and cyclophosphamide, and 50% demonstrated an elevated follicle-stimulating hormone level or azoospermia.[47]

Extremities

Rhabdomyosarcoma arising in the extremities accounted for 19% of all cases in the IRS-III study and was associated with a poorer long-term outcome than tumors arising in the other two major anatomic sites (head and neck region and genitourinary tract). A significant number of these tumors are of alveolar histology (45%), although this was not an independent prognostic factor. Distal involvement is more common than proximal involvement in rhabdomyosarcoma, and the lower extremities are involved more frequently than the upper extremities.

In IRS-I and IRS-II, 593 patients had histologic evaluation of lymph nodes, and 12% of all patients with extremity tumors had involvement of the regional nodes. The presence of these nodal metastases was a significant prognostic factor, lowering the 3-year survival rate from 80% to 46%.[26, 48] Incomplete resection of extremity lesions is not uncommon, and many patients benefit from primary re-excision in an attempt to achieve complete tumor eradication. Complete surgical removal with limb-sparing techniques should be attempted in all patients with extremity lesions, since clinical group I patients have a better outcome than patients with microscopic or gross evidence of tumor in surgical margins. In a review from IRS-I and IRS-II, 55 clinical group III patients with extremity tumors were evaluated for appropriateness of surgical resection. It was determined that 35 of these patients could have been group II had a more aggressive initial surgical therapy been employed. When these 35 cases of potentially resectable tumors were compared with cases of truly nonresectable group III and IV tumors, the 3-year survival rate was improved by 20%.[26] Amputation, however, should be rarely necessary except for very distal tumors such as those on the hand or foot.

Since regional node involvement has such an impact on survival, evaluation of regional nodal basins by biopsy or modified node dissection is necessary in order to direct further treatment. The overall survival rate of children with non-metastatic extremity rhabdomyosarcoma is poorer than that of patients with orbital or genitourinary primary tumors. The 5-year survival rate for nonmetastatic rhabdomyosarcoma of the extremity is 74%, with a local recurrence of 16% and a distant recurrence of 25%. Survival correlates with clinical group; in IRS-III, 5-year survival rate was 95% for group I patients, 67% for group II patients, 58% for group III patients, and only 33% group IV patients.[23]

Trunk

Truncal rhabdomyosarcoma includes tumors of the chest wall, paraspinal region, and abdominal wall and accounts for approximately 10% of all primary sites. There is a high incidence of the alveolar histologic variant—up to 40% of cases. Approximately one third of tumors in these sites are resectable, and prognosis is between that of the more favorable one for the genitourinary site and the less favorable one for extremity sites.[49]

Chest wall tumors occur more commonly in female patients, the mean age at diagnosis being 12.5 years. A number of these tumors have been classified in the past as being extraosseus Ewing's sarcoma or undifferentiated sarcoma, which are no longer considered rhabdomyosarcoma variants. In addition, *primitive neuroectodermal tumors (PNETs)* occur with some frequency in the chest wall and may be confused with rhabdomyosarcomas. The operative approach to these tumors is wide local incision, performed primarily or after neoadjuvant chemotherapy and radiation therapy.

The 76 patients with chest wall tumors in IRS-II and IRS-III were evaluated separately. Clinical grouping was as follows: group I, 15%; group II, 20%; group III, 40%; and group IV, 25%. Survival was 42% overall, and 59% for group I, 75% for group II, 44% for group III, and 0% for group IV.[50] The paradoxical improved survival rate for group II as compared with group I was not statistically significant and was probably due to the radiation therapy received by all group II patients.

Paraspinal rhabdomyosarcoma accounted for 3.5% of all tumor sites in IRS-I and IRS-II. Ortega and coworkers[51] reviewed these studies and found that 56 patients were treated for paraspinal tumors. These were located in the lumbar and lumbosacral region in 21 patients, the thorax or thoracolumbar area in 17 patients, and the cervical and cervicothoracic area in 5 patients; extraosseous Ewing's sarcoma and undifferentiated tumor accounted for 45% of cases. Patients with these tumors may present with acute neurologic deficits due to spinal cord compression, and they may require emergent laminectomy to preserve spinal function. In Ortega's series, 55% of patients developed clinical evidence of neurologic dysfunction, and 33% had tumor cells within the cerebrospinal fluid. Although 82% of patients with this site achieved complete remission, 46% subsequently relapsed. In IRS-II, survival did not correlate with clinical grouping; it was 50% for group I, 50% for group II, 57% for group III, and 33% for group IV.[52]

Miscellaneous Sites

Retroperitoneal rhabdomyosarcomas account for 10% of nongenitourinary tumors and are of either embryonal or alveolar histology. These lesions are large, extensive, and ordinarily unresectable at time of diagnosis; also, lymphatic and distant metastases are likely. Treatment is generally as outlined earlier and usually requires intensive chemotherapy and radiation therapy. Primary re-excision or second-look laparotomy procedures may occasionally convert a patient to complete-response status. Patients with retroperitoneal rhabdomyosarcoma had the poorest prognosis of all patients in IRS-II, with an overall 5-year survival rate of 48%.[53]

Perineal rhabdomyosarcoma is rare, accounting for less than 2% of primary sites. The majority are of the alveolar type. Although the initial response rate to treatment is favorable, there is a high relapse rate; the overall survival rate is in the range of 20%.

Pulmonary rhabdomyosarcoma is uncommon but appears to have an increased incidence in children with preexisting congenital lung disorders such as cystic adenomatoid malformation.[54] Treatment is by pulmonary resection, and the survival rate for completely resected lesions is high.

INFANT RHABDOMYOSARCOMA

Approximately 6% of patients entered into the IRS-III protocol were less than 1 year of age. There is a greater incidence of undifferentiated tumors, botryoid tumors, and primary lesions of the bladder, vagina, and prostate in children in this age group than in older children with rhabdomyosarcoma. They tend to undergo less radical surgical and nonsurgical treatment, and they also tend to develop more toxicity than older patients. Despite these factors their survival rate is similar.[55]

Rhabdomyosarcoma in the neonatal period (before 30 days of life) is very rare, occurring in 0.4% of all patients enrolled in the IRS studies. There is a slight predominance in males and the most common histology is embryonal or botryoid (64%) or undifferentiated (29%). Half of such tumors in the IRS studies in the caudal regions (buttocks/sacrococcygeal, genitourinary, perineal), sites associated with a favorable outcome. Cellular necrosis and small round cells were predictive of poor outcome, whereas the absence of necrosis and the presence of large spindle cells were associated with favorable outcome. In one series, 32% of patients with rhabdomyosarcoma in infancy were found to have other congenital anomalies.[56]

METASTATIC DISEASE

Metastatic disease most commonly involves the lung (58%), bone (33%), regional lymph nodes (33%), liver (22%), and brain (20%).[57–59] Of patients enrolled in the IRS-III,[23] 14% were clinical group IV at the time of diagnosis. Primary sites more likely to have metastases include the extremities (23%), parameningeal (13%), retroperitoneum, trunk, gastrointestinal, and intrathoracic sites. Primary sites with a low incidence of metastases include the orbit (1.8 %), nonparameningeal or nonorbital head and neck (4.5%), and genitourinary (5.4%) sites.[1] Although the overall survival rate of patients with metastatic disease is poor, there are certain favorable and unfavorable prognostic factors among clinical group IV patients. Favorable prognostic factors include younger age, genitourinary primary tumor rather than other types, and embryonal histology with metastases limited to the lymph nodes or lungs. Lymphatic metastases are present in approximately 10% of patients, with a frequency varying according to the primary site of tumor origin.[1] The relative frequency of nodal metastases by site is 32% for paratesticular, 12% for extremity, 7% for nonorbital head and neck, and 1% for orbit sites.[1] There are some uncommon clinical situations in which surgical resection of a metastatic lesion is appropriate—for example, when (1) the lung is the metastatic site, (2) the primary tumor site has been controlled, (3) no concurrent nonpulmonary metastases are evident, and (4) preoperative evaluation suggests that all the tumor can be removed.

OUTCOME

The overall trend has been an increase in survival for each subsequent IRS study. The survival rate depends on the clinical group, stage, and primary site at the time of diagnosis. The overall 5-year survival rate in the IRS-III study was 71%: 90% for clinical group I, 80% for clinical group II, 70% for clinical group III, and 30% for clinical group IV (Fig. 12–3).[3] The survival rate by pretreatment staging classification was 80% for Stage I, 68% for Stage II, 49% for Stage III, 21% for Stage IV.[3] Survival by primary tumor site is shown in Figure 12–4.

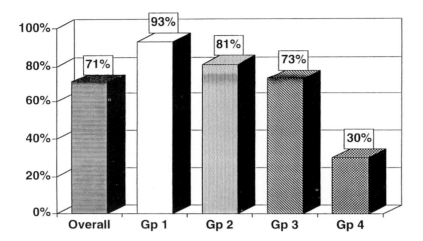

Figure 12–3 • Five-year survival of patients with rhabdomyosarcoma in IRS-III by clinical group IRS-III

Figure 12–4 • Five-year survival of patients with rhabdomyosarcoma in IRS-III by primary site for IRS III patients. (From Crist W, Gehan EA, Ragab AH, et al: The third intergroup rhabdomyosarcoma study. *J Clin Oncol* 13:610–630, 1995, with permission.)

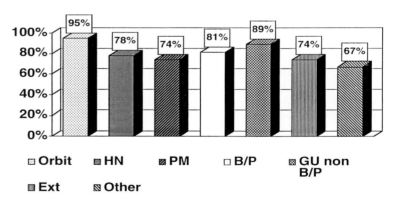

HN - Head and neck (non-parameningeal)
PM - Parameningeal head and neck
B/P - Bladder / prostate
GU - Genitourinary

References

1. Ruymann FB: Rhabdomyosarcoma in children and adolescents: A review. *Hematol Oncol Clin North Am* 1:621–654, 1987.
2. Horn RC, Enterline HT: Rhabdomyosarcoma: A clinicopathological study and classification of 39 cases. *Cancer* 11:181–199, 1958.
3. Young JL, Ries LG, Silverberg E, et al: Cancer incidence, survival, and mortality for children younger than 15 years. *Cancer* 58:598–602, 1986.
4. Malogolowkin MH, Ortega JA: Rhabdomyosarcoma of childhood. *Pediat Ann* 17:251–268, 1988.
5. Hartley AL, Birch JM, Blair V, et al: Patterns of cancer in the families of children with soft tissue sarcoma. *Cancer* 72:923–930, 1993.
6. Malkin D, Li FP, Strong LC, et al: Germ line p53 mutations in a familial syndrome of breast cancer, sarcomas, and other neoplasms. *Science* 250:1233–1238, 1990.
7. Yun K: A new marker for rhabdomyosarcoma: Insulin-like growth factor II. *Lab Invest* 67:653–664, 1992.
8. Wexler LH, Helman LJ: Pediatric soft tissue sarcomas. *CA* 44:211–247, 1994.
9. Garvin AJ, Gansler T, Gerald W, et al: Insulin-like growth factor production by childhood solid tumors. *Perspect Pediatr Pathol* 15:106–116, 1992.
10. Shapiro DN, Sublett JE, Li B, et al: Fusion of *PAX3* to a member of the forkhead family of transcription factors in human alveolar rhabdomyosarcoma. *Cancer Res* 53:5108–5112, 1993.
11. Downing JR, Head DR, Parham DM, et al: Detection of the (11;22)(q24;q12) translocation of Ewing's sarcoma and peripheral neuroectodermal tumor by reverse transcription polymerase chain reaction. *Am J Pathol* 143:1294–1300, 1993.
12. Weintraub H, Davis R, Tapscott S, et al: The *myoD* gene family: Nodal point during specification of the muscle cell lineage. *Science* 251:761–766, 1991.
13. Tapscott SJ, Thayer MJ, Weintraub H: Deficiency in rhabdomyosarcomas of a factor required for MyoD activity and myogenisis. *Science* 259:1450–1453, 1993.
14. Dias P, Parham DM, Shapiro DN, et al: Myogenic regulatory protein (MyoD1) expression in childhood solid tumors: Diagnostic utility in rhabdomyosarcoma. *Am J Pathol* 137:1283–1291, 1990.
15. Shapiro DN, Parham DM, Douglass EC, et al: Relationship of tumor-cell ploidy to histologic subtype and treatment outcome in children and adolescents with unresectable rhabdomyosarcoma. *J Clin Oncol* 9:159–166, 1991.
16. Newton WA, Hamoudi A, Weber B, Dickman PS: Pathology of rhabdomyosarcoma and related tumors: Experience of the intergroup rhabdomyosarcoma studies. In Maurer HM, Ruymann FB, Pochedly C (eds): *Rhabdomyosarcoma and Related Tumors in Children and Adolescents.* Boca Raton, FL: CRC Press, 1991, pp. 19–47.
17. Tsokos M: The diagnosis and classification of childhood rhabdomyosarcoma. *Semin Diag Pathol* 11:26–38, 1994.
18. Asmar L, Gehan EA, Newton WA, et al: Agreement among and within groups of pathologists in the classification of rhabdomyosarcoma and related childhood sarcomas: Report of an international study of four pathology classifications. *Cancer* 74:2579–2588, 1994.
19. Leuschner I, Newton WA, Schmidt D, et al: Spindle-cell variants of embryonal rhabdomyosarcoma in the paratesticular region: A report of the Intergroup Rhabdomyosarcoma Study. *Am J Surg Pathol* 17:221–230, 1993.
20. Schmidt D, Harms D, Pilin VA: Small-cell pediatric tumors: Histology, immunohistochemistry, and electron microscopy. *Clin Lab Med* 7:63–89, 1987.
21. Dias P, Parham DM, Shapiro DN, et al: Monoclonal antibodies to the myogenic regulatory protein MyoD1: Epitope mapping and diagnostic utility. *Cancer Res* 52:6431–6439, 1992.
22. Barr FG, Galili N, Holick J, et al: Rearrangement of the *PAX3* paired box gene in the paediatric solid tumour alveolar rhabdomyosarcoma. *Natl Genet* 3:113–117, 1993.
23. Crist W, Gehan EA, Ragab AH, et al: The third intergroup rhabdomyosarcoma study. *J Clin Oncol* 13:610–630, 1995.
24. Raney RB, Jr: Rhabdomyosarcoma and related tumors of the head and neck in childhood. In Maurer HM, Ruymann FB, Pochedly C (ed.): *Rhabdomyosarcoma and Related Tumors in Children and Adolescents.* Boca Raton, FL: CRC Press, 1991, pp. 319–331.
25. LaQuaglia M: Genitourinary rhabdomyosarcoma in children. *Urol Clin North Am* 18:575–580, 1991.
26. Lawrence W Jr, Hays DH, Heyn R, et al: Surgical lessons from the Intergroup Rhabdomyosarcoma Study (IRS) pertaining to extremity tumors. *World J Surg* 12:676–684, 1988.
27. Flamant F, Luboinski B, Couanet D, et al: Rhabdomyosarcoma in children: Clinical symptoms, diagnosis, and staging. In Maurer HM, Ruymann FB, Pochedly C (eds): *Rhabdomyosarcoma and Related Tumors in Children and Adolescents.* Boca Raton, FL: CRC Press, 1991, pp. 91–124.
28. Lawrence W Jr, Gehan EA, Hays DM, et al: Prognostic significance of staging factors of the UICC staging system in childhood rhabdomyosarcoma: A report from the

Intergroup Rhabdomyosarcoma Study (IRS-II). *J Clin Oncol* 5:46–54, 1987.

29. Lawrence W Jr: Surgical principles in the management of sarcomas of children. In Maurer HM, Ruymann FB, Pochedly C (eds): *Rhabdomyosarcoma and Related Tumors in Children and Adolescents.* Boca Raton, FL: CRC Press, 1991, pp. 171–179.

30. Hays DM, Lawrence W, Wharam M, et al: Primary re-excision for patients with "microscopic residual" tumor following initial excision of sarcomas of trunk and extremity sites. *J Pediatr Surg* 24:5–10, 1989.

31. Wiener E, Lawrence W, Hays D, et al: Survival is improved in clinical group III children with complete response established by second-look operations in the Intergroup Rhabdomyosarcoma Study (IRS) III. *Med Pediatr Oncol* 19:399 (abstract), 1991.

32. Maurer HM, Beltangady M, Gehan EA, et al: The Intergroup Rhabdomyosarcoma Study-I: A final report. *Cancer* 61:209–220, 1988.

33. Maurer HM, Gehan EA, Beltgandy M, et al: The Intergroup Rhabdomyosarcoma Study-II. *Cancer* 71:1904–1922, 1993.

34. Koscielniak E, Rodary C, Flamant F, et al: Metastatic rhabdomyosarcoma and histologically similar tumors in childhood: A retrospective European multi-center analysis. *Med Pediatr Oncol* 20:209–214, 1992.

35. Nag S, Grecula J, Ruymann FB: Aggressive chemotherapy, organ-preserving surgery, and high-dose-rate remote brachytherapy in the treatment of rhabdomyosarcoma in infants and young children. *Cancer* 72:2769–2776, 1993.

36. Wiener ES: Head and neck rhabdomyosarcoma. *Semin Pediatr Surg* 3:203–206, 1994.

37. Abramson DH, Ellsworth RM, Tretter P, et al: The treatment of orbital rhabdomyosarcoma with irradiation and chemotherapy. *Opthalmology* 86:1330–1335, 1979.

38. Fiorillo A, Migliorati R, Grimaldi M, et al: Multidisciplinary treatment of primary orbital rhabdomyosarcoma: A single-institution experience. *Cancer* 67:560–563, 1991.

39. Heyn R, Ragab AH, Raney RB, et al: Late effects of therapy in orbital rhabdomyosarcoma (RMS): A report from the Intergroup Rhabdomyosarcoma Study I (IRS-I). *Proc Am Soc Clin Oncol* 2:C–257, 1983.

40. Raney RB, Tefft M, Newton WA, et al: Improved prognosis with intensive treatment of children with cranial soft-tissue sarcomas arising in nonorbital parameningeal sites: A report from the Intergroup Rhabdomyosarcoma Study. *Cancer* 59:147–155, 1987.

41. Healy GB, Upton J, Black PM, et al: The role of surgery in rhabdomyosarcoma of the head and neck in children. *Arch Otolaryngol Head Neck Surg* 117:1185–1188, 1991.

42. Wiener ES: Rhabdomyosarcoma: New dimensions in management. *Semin Pediatr Surg* 2:47–58, 1993.

43. Ghavimi F: Genitourinary rhabdomyosarcoma. In Maurer HM, Ruymann RB, Pochedly C (eds): *Rhabdomyosarcoma and Related Tumors in Children and Adolescents.* Boca Raton, FL: CRC Press, 1991, pp. 347–362.

44. Hays DM, Raney RB, Wharam MD, et al: Children with vesical rhabdomyosarcoma (RMS) treated by partial cystectomy with neoadjuvant or adjuvant chemotherapy, with or without radiotherapy: A report from the Intergroup Rhabdomyosarcoma Study (IRS) Committee. *J Pediatr Hematol Oncol* 17:46–52, 1995.

45. Andrassy RJ, Hays DM, Raney RB, et al: Conservative surgical management of vaginal and vulvar pediatric rhabdomyosarcoma: A report from the Intergroup Rhabdomyosarcoma Study-III. *J Pediatr Surg* 30:1034–1037, 1995.

46. Wiener ES, Lawrence W, Hays D, et al: Retroperitoneal node biopsy in paratesticular rhabdomyosarcoma. *J Pediatr Surg* 29:171–178, 1994.

47. Heyn R, Raney B, Hays D, et al: Late effects of therapy in patients with paratesticular rhabdomyosarcoma. For the Intergroup Rhabdomyosarcoma Study Committee. *J Clin Oncol* 10:614–623, 1992.

48. Mandell L, Ghavimi F, LaQuaglia M, et al: Prognostic significance of regional lymph node involvement in childhood extremity rhabdomyosarcoma. *Med Pediatr Oncol* 18:466–471, 1990.

49. Raney RB, Ragab A, Ruymann F, et al: Soft tissue sarcoma of the trunk in childhood: Results of the Intergroup Rhabdomyosarcoma Study 1972–1976. *Cancer* 49:2612–2616, 1982.

50. Andrassy R, Corpron C, Wiener E, et al: Thoracic sarcomas in children. *Ann Surg* In press.

51. Ortega JA, Wharam M, Gehan EA, et al: Clinical features and end results of therapy for children with paraspinal rhabdomyosarcoma: A report of the Intergroup Rhabdomyosarcoma Study. *J Clin Oncol* 9:796–801, 1991.

52. Wiener ES, Hays DM: Rhabdomyosarcoma in extremity and trunk sites. In Maurer HM, Ruymann FB, Pochedly C (eds): *Rhabdomyosarcoma and Related Tumors in Children and Adolescents.* Boca Raton, FL: CRC Press, 1991, pp. 364–372.

53. Crist W, Raney RB, Tefft M, et al: Soft tissue sarcomas arising in the retroperitoneal space in children: A report from the Intergroup Rhabdomyosarcoma Study Committee. *Cancer* 56:2125–2132, 1985.

54. Murphy JJ, Blair GK, Fraser GC, et al: Rhabdomyosarcoma arising within congenital pulmonary cysts: Report of three cases. *J Pediatr Surg* 27:1364–1367, 1992.

55. Pias RC, Ragab AH: Rhabdomyosarcomas in infancy. In Maurer HM, Ruymann FB, Pochedly C (eds): *Rhabdomyosarcoma and Related Tumors in Children and Adolescents.* Boca Raton, FL: CRC Press, 1991, pp. 373–384.

56. Lobe T, Wiener E, Hays D, et al: Neonatal rhabdomyosarcoma (RMS): The IRS experience. *J Pediatr Surg* 29:1167–1170, 1994.

57. Raney RB, Tefft M, Maurer HM, et al: Disease pattern and survival rate in children with metastatic soft-tissue sarcoma: A report from the Intergroup Rhabdomyosarcoma Study (IRS-I). *Cancer* 62:1257–1266, 1988.

58. Shimada H, Newton W Jr, Soule E, et al: Pathology of fatal rhabdomyosarcoma: Report from the Intergroup Rhabdomyosarcoma Study (IRS-I and II). *Cancer* 59:459–465, 1987.

Chapter

13

Pediatric Germ-Cell Tumors

• *Frederick J. Rescorla, M.D.*

Malignant germ-cell tumors account for approximately 3% of childhood malignancies. The incidence is approximately 4 per million among children younger than 15 years, resulting in approximately 225 new cases per year in the United States. Girls are more likely than boys to develop these tumors. They occur in both gonadal and extragonadal sites, with extragonadal and testicular tumors predominating in children younger than 3 years of age and gonadal tumors in pubescent or post-pubescent patients.[1]

Germ-cell tumors are interesting for several reasons: (1) abnormal migration of primordial germ cells accounts for many of the childhood germ-cell tumors; (2) markers exist to allow evaluation of extent of resection in regard to development of recurrence for many of the tumors; and (3) introduction of cisplatin-based chemotherapy has markedly improved the survival rate for patients with germ-cell tumors as well as the salvage rate for those with recurrent or metastatic disease.

EMBRYOLOGY AND CLASSIFICATION

Primordial germ cells originate in the area of the allantois of the embryonic yolk-sac endoderm and migrate to the genital ridge on the posterior abdominal wall at 4 to 5 weeks of gestation. Arrested or aberrant migration of these germ cells is thought to account for the occurrence of germ-cell tumors in midline sites including the pineal, mediastinum, retroperitoneum, and sacrococcygeal region.[2–4] Gonadal outgrowths lined by a surface epithelial layer protrude from the genital ridges during the migratory phase. In the male, a layer of connective tissue, the tunica albuginea, separates the epithelium from the underlying germ cells and Sertoli cells.

Teilum[5] originally proposed the germ-cell origin of gonadal tumors, and although the germ-cell origin of seminoma was accepted, some doubted that it was the origin of other histologic types.[6, 7] Experimental studies from several groups, however, have provided strong support to Teilum's theory, and it is generally accepted at the present time.[8–10] According to this classification system (Fig. 13–1), seminoma or dysgerminoma is a primitive germ-cell neoplasm that lacks the capacity for further differentiation. *Embryonal carcinoma* is a germ-cell tumor composed of multipotential cells capable of further differentiation into embryonic (mature or immature teratomas) or extra-embryonic (choriocarcinoma and endodermal sinus or yolk-sac) tumors. The process of differentiation is dynamic. The appearance of histologically different tumor elements at different stages within the same tumor lends further support to the hypothesis of germ-cell origin. DNA studies have noted that mature cystic teratomas arise from germ cells arrested at various stages of meiosis whereas immature teratomas arise from postmeiotic germ cells. Dysgerminomas develop from premeiotic oogonia (primordial germ cells).[11]

In 1959 Teilum[12] and coworkers described the *yolk-sac tumor* or *endodermal sinus tumor* due to histologic similarities of the rat placenta. Although this tumor and *choriocarcinoma* are well differentiated, like mature teratomas, they differ from mature teratomas by being highly malignant. Common sites for endodermal sinus tumors are the testes, ovary, and sacrococcygeal region. They account for nearly all prepubertal testicular tumors. This tumor has also been noted in the vagina, retroperitoneum, mediastinum, and pineal gland.[13] It can metastasize to lymph nodes, lung, liver, and bone. *Dysgerminoma* or *seminoma* is unusual in childhood except when it occurs in the ovary, mediastinum, or central nervous system or is related to gonadal dysgenesis and undescended testes.

Teratomas represent the most common histologic type of pediatric germ-cell tumors. Virchow[14] originally recognized the gross anatomic structures within these tumors and labeled them as "teratoma" from the Greek terms *teratos* ("monster") and *onkoma* ("swelling"). The origin of teratomas from primordial germ cells is generally accepted, and they are defined by the presence of all three embryonic layers: ectoderm, endoderm, and mesoderm. Teratomas contain tissue foreign to the anatomic site, which cannot be the result of metaplasia of cells normally

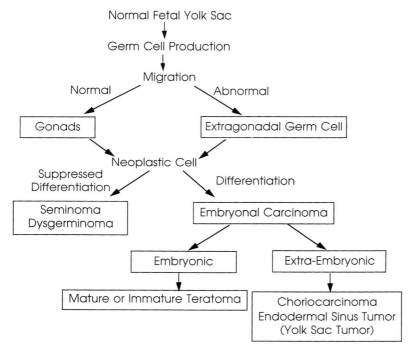

Figure 13–1 • Classification system for development of germ-cell tumors.

found there. Although technically these tumors have all three embryonic tissues, at the time of clinical presentation one layer may be the predominant, and occasionally the only recognizable, tissue type (*monodermal teratoma*). A large single-institution review of 245 teratomas noted the following anatomic and age distributions: sacrococcygeal 42% (newborns), ovary 35% (median age of 13 years), head and neck 6% (newborns), retroperitoneum 5% (median age of 5 months), mediastinum 4% (median age of 8 months median), brain and spinal cord 4% (median age of 2½ years) and testes 3% (median age of 3½ years).[15] In general, the treatment of any mature teratoma in childhood is excision alone.

Immature teratomas contain various amounts of immature tissue consisting most frequently of neuroectodermal tissue.[16–19] They are generally graded according to the system of Norris and coworkers:[20] Grade I tumors have immaturity with primitive neuroepithelium limited to one lower magnification (40×) field per slide; Grade II, less than four fields per slide; and Grade III, greater than four per slide. The risk of recurrence for gonadal immature teratomas is thought to be higher for high-grade tumors. This hypothesis is based on work by Norris[20] and coworkers evaluating ovarian immature teratomas treated with surgery alone. The relationship between histologic grade and recurrence for immature teratomas at other sites, such as the sacrococcygeal region, is not clear.[21, 22] A study involving 262 mature and immature teratomas in children reported a 13% overall relapse rate with surgery alone; 10% for children with mature teratomas and 20% for those with immature teratomas.[23] Of the relapses, 46% experienced relapse with malignant components. The relationship of relapse to grade was as follows: 10% for Grade 0 (mature teratoma), 14% for Grade I, 23% for Grade II, and 33% for Grade III. Risk of relapse by site was 19% for the coccyx, 7% for the ovary, and 6% for other sites. Of interest, the strongest predictor of relapse was the extent of resection; there was 4% recurrence with complete resection versus 41% with incomplete resection.

GENETICS AND RISK FACTORS

A study from the Children's Cancer Group correlated several parental factors with risk of malignant germ-cell tumors occurring in offspring.[24] Adverse factors (primarily maternal) included exposure to chemicals or solvents and plastic or resin fumes and maternal urinary tract infection, the latter being associated with a 3.1-fold increased risk. This study suggests maternal influence through disease states, hormonal influence, and environmental exposure may contribute to subsequent development of germ-cell tumors.

Studies of adult germ-cell tumors have identified isochromosome 12p [i(12p)] as an abnormality seen exclusively in germ-cell tumors, occurring in 80% to 100% of adult testicular tumors.[25] The presence of more than three copies of i(12p) has been associated with an increased risk of treatment failure.[26] The prevalence of this abnormality in pediatric germ-cell tumors is not known, but it is being investigated in the intergroup study of germ-cell tumors involving the Pediatric Oncology Group (POG) and the Children's Cancer Group (CCG). Several studies have noted that infantile endodermal sinus tumors lack the i(12p).[27, 28]

Studies of DNA content of tumors in adults (primarily testicular) have demonstrated aneuploid stemlines in most. The prognostic significance of this finding in adults is unclear.[29–31] One study in children indicated that childhood tumors are distinct.[32] Infantile testicular endodermal sinus tumors were tetraploid or diploid, and all sacrococcygeal teratomas regardless of grade were diploid. Ovarian immature teratomas of Grades I and II were diploid, whereas Grade III teratomas were aneuploid. This study, as well as the lack of i(12p), suggests a different pathogenesis for pediatric germ-cell tumors than for those in adults and may explain differences in their clinical behavior.

Although familial germ-cell cancers have been noted in cases of gonadal dysgenesis, the occurrence in normal siblings and offspring is rare. A study[33] including first- and second-degree relatives of 78, 46 XX patients with malignant ovarian germ-cell tumors (in newborns and patients up to 20 years old) identified no increased risk of similar tumors. There is, however, one report of two sisters (both with normal karyotype) presenting malignant ovarian germ-cell tumors (one dysgerminoma and one mixed tumor)[34] and another of three siblings with ovarian tumors (two germ-cell and one sarcoma) whose mother had a tumor excised as a teenager.[35]

Intersex Disorders and Risk of Malignancy

Patients with intersex disorders may have a 30% chance of development of a *gonadoblastoma*,[36] an in situ form of germ-cell tumor with the ability to transform most commonly into dysgerminoma (50% of cases) but also yolk-sac tumor, immature teratoma, or choriocarcinoma. Gonadoblastomas consist of germ-cell and sex-cord elements. Children so affected are typically male pseudohermaphrodites (under-androgenized males) with testosterone deficiency, androgen insensitivity syndromes (complete = testicular feminization, incomplete = Reifenstein), or 5α-reductase deficiency. They also may have pure or mixed gonadal dysgenesis.

The risk of tumor development in cases of gonadal dysgenesis is approximately 10% at age 20 and 19% at age 30.[37] Most such patients are phenotypic females with 46, XY karyotypes or mosaics such as 45, XO/46, XY. Most investigators recommend gonadectomy for these patients if there is any portion of a Y chromosome present, this being the presumed risk factor.[37–40] In addition, patients with Turner's syndrome (45, X) may be at risk if they have any portion of a Y fragment and thus should have chromosomal evaluation.[38]

In a review of 102 children with intersex disorders Ramani[41] and coworkers noted a 6% incidence of *intratubular germ-cell neoplasia*, a known precursor of invasive germ-cell cancer, in the testes of children and adolescents, with a higher incidence after puberty. Intratubular germ-cell neoplasia progresses to invasive germ-cell cancer in 50% of patients within 5 years if the gonad is not removed.[42]

Androgen insensitivity (formerly known as *testicular feminization syndrome*) is one of the male pseudohermaphrodite syndromes characterized by 46, XY karyotype with complete or partial resistance of the end organs to the peripheral effect of androgens. In the complete form, the external genitalia appear normal; in the incomplete form they vary from that of a virilized female to that of an undervirilized male with severe hypospadias. Patients with the complete form frequently present with an inguinal hernia with a testis noted in the inguinal region. These gonads have a risk for development of malignancy, so gonadectomy is required. The risk of malignancy is low in childhood, 3.6% at age 20, but rises to 22% at age 30 and 33% at age 50.[37, 43] Carcinoma in situ, however, has been diagnosed at 2 months of age[44] and invasive seminoma at puberty.[45] In addition, a yolk-sac tumor has been reported in a 17-month-old child 4 months after the diagnosis of complete androgen insensitivity was established at herniorrhaphy.[46] Delayed gonadectomy is recommended by some to allow time for the effect of testicular estrogens on secondary sex characteristics[46]; however, most contend that early gonadectomy with estrogen replacement is safer.[47, 48]

The Undescended Testes and Cancer

Several large series of adult patients with testicular cancer have demonstrated a 3.5% to 12% incidence of undescended testes.[49, 50] As the incidence of undescended testes in the general population is approximately 0.4%, patients with undescended testes are thought to have a 30- to 50-times normal incidence of testicular cancer.[51] For intra-abdominal testes there may be a 200-fold increase in the incidence of testicular cancer. In a collective review, Campbell[52] noted that although intra-abdominal testes account for only 14.3% of undescended testes, they account for 48.5% of all tumors in undescended testes. The risk also appears to increase with age at orchiopexy.[51] Of interest is that 20% of tumors in patients with an undescended testis occur in the scrotal testis.[53, 54]

Seminomas account for 60% of cancers in patients with undescended testes compared with a 30% to 40% incidence of seminoma in adolescent and adult patients with descended testes.[55, 56] In one study of 34 patients with cryptorchid testes cancer, 9 had had prior orchiopexy.[57] Of these, only 22% had seminomas whereas 64% of those without prior orchiopexy had seminomas. In this study orchiopexy did not lead to a lower stage at presentation because of the advanced stage of the nonseminomas, but it did appear to decrease the risk of a seminoma developing. The actual effect of orchiopexy on the rate of testicular cancer is presently unknown. It does, however, facilitate examination for screening purposes.

TUMOR MARKERS

Human chorionic gonadotropin (hCG) and alpha-fetoprotein (AFP) are two useful markers of germ-cell tumors. In general, their failure to return to normal levels indicates residual, recurrent, or progressive disease. AFP is a major serum protein in the human fetus produced by the embryonic liver, yolk sac, and gastrointestinal tract. It is normally elevated in fetal life. AFP synthesis does not cease completely at birth, and some hepatocytes still produce AFP in early postnatal life.[58] Wu[59] and coworkers have noted the half-life of AFP to be 5 1/2 days from birth to 2 weeks of age, 11 days from 2 weeks to 2 months of age, and 33 days from 2 to 4 months of age. After 8 months of life the AFP half-life is 5 days. Tsuchida[60] and coworkers, in a report on 55 normal newborns, infants, and children, noted markedly elevated levels of AFP in newborns that dropped to normal levels by 9 months of age.

AFP is a sensitive marker when endodermal sinus tumor forms a portion of a malignant germ-cell tumor. It can also be elevated in association with benign or malignant hepatic conditions. In nonmalignant cases, elevations have been attributed to liver damage secondary to drugs (chemotherapy, anesthetic, or antiseizure medication), viral conditions, or alcoholism.[61] Tsuchida[62] and coworkers have reported the ability to differentiate between yolk-sac and hepatic AFPs by means of immunoelectrophoresis.

The beta subunit of hCG can serve as another marker when syncytiotrophoblasts are present in the tumor, typically in a choriocarcinoma. The half-life of hCG is 16 hours. Lactate dehydrogenase (LDH) is also elevated in many germ-cell tumors but is not a specific marker. Lactate dehydrogenase isoenzyme 1 (LDH-1) is frequently elevated in dysgerminomas.[63]

OVARIAN TUMORS

Clinical Presentation

The ovary is the second most common location for germ-cell tumors that develop in childhood behind the sacrococcygeal region. Although up to one half of them are benign, malignancy is more common in the younger child.[64] Tumors can arise from the epithelium, germ cells, or sex-cord/stromal tissues. A large review of 1002 primary ovarian tumors in children noted that approximately 71% were germ-cell, 17% epithelial, and 12% sex-cord/stromal tumors.[65] Most series reporting on both benign and malignant ovarian lesions in children note a predominance of benign conditions, with cysts and mature teratomas the most common.[66, 67]

Among ovarian germ-cell tumors, teratomas are the most common, the majority being mature teratomas. Immature teratoma, dysgerminoma, and endodermal sinus tumors are the most common ovarian malignancies, followed by embryonal carcinoma, choriocarcinoma, polyembryoma, and mixed tumors. A large review of 148 children with ovarian tumors noted the following histologic incidences: 47% mature teratomas, 12% immature teratomas, 10% yolk-sac tumors, 5% dysgerminomas, less than 1% choriocarcinomas, 14% epithelial tumors, and 13% sex-cord tumors.[68] Although the exact percentage of distribution may vary from study to study, this is a fairly representative histologic distribution.

Most patients with ovarian tumors present with an abdominal pain or mass.[69] The mass can lead to gastrointestinal symptoms produced by compression or can occasionally undergo torsion leading to acute pain. In addition, ovarian cystic lesions may be noted in newborns on routine physical examination or prenatal ultrasounds and are commonly present in older girls.

In addition to a thorough physical examination, ultrasound examination should be done to allow evaluation of the location and nature of the lesion. If a cyst is identified, a repeat study in 1 to 2 weeks may be a reasonable approach. Computed tomography allows further definition of the lesion and evaluation of the retroperitoneal lymph nodes (Fig. 13–2). Serum hCG and AFP levels are measured prior to surgery.

Non-Germ-Cell Ovarian Cysts

Cystic lesions in newborns are usually benign and can generally be managed with observation. Many are diagnosed in the fetus. Although routine removal of palpable cysts or those greater than 4 cm to 5 cm by ultrasound has been recommended,[64, 70] others have argued for the conserva-

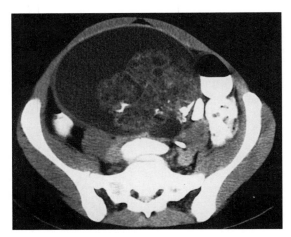

Figure 13–2 • Computed tomography scan demonstrates a large (2.5 kg) immature ovarian teratoma (Grade III).

tive management of large cysts.[71] In a review of patients with fetal ovarian cysts followed after birth, Calisti[71] and coworkers noted that cysts greater than 5 cm were more likely to be removed surgically and had produced a slightly higher incidence of ultrasound or operative signs of torsion than their smaller counterparts (46% versus 33%). Nonoperative management by observation was successful in some of the patients with larger cysts and no symptoms or signs of torsion. The same results were obtained in other studies.[72, 73]

Complex ovarian cysts are those with a fluid-debris level, cystic or retracting clot, septation, or echogenic wall. Most recommend removal of these lesions in neonates and infants less than 1 year of age[72, 74] owing to the high incidence of torsion. Some, however, recommend that if the complex nature was noted prenatally, observation is appropriate, as spontaneous asymptomatic involution may occur.[71] The laparoscopic approach to neonatal ovarian cysts has been described and may be useful in selected cases.[75]

Ovarian cysts are also common in older children, and most are benign.[76, 77] Warner[76] and coworkers noted resolution in 46 of 51 (90%) large cysts both simple and complex. They recommended operative intervention in cases of persistent symptoms, complications resulting from the size of the mass, suspicion of neoplasm, or failure to decrease in size on follow-up ultrasound over a period of 1 to 2 weeks.

Non-Germ-Cell Ovarian Tumors

Epithelial tumors account for approximately 15% of all ovarian tumors.[64, 68] Cystadenoma is the most common of these tumors and may be serous or mucinous. *Nonpapillary serous cystadenomas* are large benign lesions, and *papillary serous cystadenomas* are also usually benign except when ruptured. *Mucinous cystadenomas* are often very large lesions[15] in which pseudomyxoma peritonei may occasionally be noted with implantation of tumor on the peritoneal surface. Some of these tumors with cellular atypia and proliferation of surface epithelium are termed *borderline malignancies*.[69] Cystadenocarcinomas are very rare in children and may be either serous or mucinous.

Sex-cord/stromal tumors account for 10% to 13% of ovarian tumors.[64, 68] Small benign sex-cord tumors have been noted in 5% to 12% of patients with Peutz-Jeghers syndrome.[78] Most sex-cord/stromal tumors are juvenile *granulosa-cell tumors*, usually associated with precocious pseudopuberty in prepubertal girls[79] as a result of estrogen production from the tumor. There may be breast or labial enlargement, vaginal bleeding, or advanced development of pubic or axillary hair. Most cases have a benign course and can be treated with unilateral oophorectomy if they are Stage I. Müllerian inhibiting substance has been reported as a marker in these tumors.[80]

Thecoma-fibroma tumors are less common than granulosa-cell tumors. They are usually unilateral and benign and can be treated by excision only. *Sertoli-Leydig cell tumors* are also rare, usually occurring in postmenarchal girls, although a 7-year-old girl has been treated at Indiana University School of Medicine. These tumors are frequently androgenic and have been referred to in the past as "androblastoma" and "arrhenoblastoma."

Burkitt's lymphoma is a common cause of malignant ovarian tumors in some countries.[81, 82] Cases have also been reported in the United States.[15] Non-Hodgkin's lymphoma has been noted in the ovary as well.[83] Plus, there is a report of 25 primary neuroectodermal tumors of the ovary in girls as young as 6 years of age (the average age being 23 years).[84]

Operative Management and Staging

The goal of surgical management in children is complete tumor removal, accurate staging, and preservation of reproductive capability whenever possible. The use of reproduction-sparing techniques has been supported in the literature. Slayton[55] and coworkers noted that the survival rate in patients with Stage I ovarian tumors was the same with unilateral salpingo-oophorectomy or total abdominal hysterectomy. There are many reports of successful pregnancy after chemotherapy, so the contralateral ovary should be preserved whenever possible.[56-91] The details of the operative approach are listed in Table 13–1. An adequate incision is required for thorough inspection of all surfaces of the peritoneum including the diaphragm. Most surgeons recommend a midline incision for adults; however, in children the operation can frequently be performed with an infra-umbilical transverse incision.

If the presence of a malignancy in the involved ovary is uncertain, a wedge biopsy and frozen section analysis may be helpful. The contralateral ovary should be closely examined and a biopsy taken if tumor involvement is suspected. Some recommend bivalving a normal-appearing contralateral ovary for internal inspection. This procedure may be more appropriate in cases of dysgerminoma, in which a 10% to 15% bilateral rate is reported.

The staging system of POG and CCG is presented in Table 13–2. It is somewhat different from the International Federation of Gynecologists and Obstetritians (FIGO) staging system presented in Table 13–3, a system that was devised for epithelial neoplasms.[92] The value of peritoneal washings is well established for epithelial tumors but is less so for germ-cell tumors.[93] Patients with evidence of recurrent disease or persistently elevated markers after induction che-

Table 13–1 • Operative Procedure for Malignant Ovarian Germ-Cell Tumors

Collect ascites; if absent, peritoneal washings should be used for cytology.
Examine entire peritoneal surface and liver—excise suspicious lesions.
Perform unilateral oophorectomy.
Perform wedge biopsy of contralateral ovary if it looks suspicious.
Perform omentectomy.
Perform bilateral retroperitoneal lymph node sampling of internal iliac, common iliac, low para-aortic, and perirenal areas.

Table 13–2 • CCG-POG Staging System for Pediatric Ovarian Germ-Cell Tumors

Stage I	Limited to ovary or ovaries; peritoneal washings normal; tumor markers normal after appropriate half-life decline (AFP 5 days, hcG 16 hours).
Stage II	Microscopic residual disease or disease in lymph nodes (<2 cm); peritoneal washings normal; tumor markers either normal or showing evidence of malignancy.
Stage III	Lymph node involvement (>2 cm); gross residual disease or biopsy only; contiguous visceral involvement (omentum, intestine, bladder); peritoneal washings positive for malignant cells; tumor markers either normal showing evidence of malignancy.
Stage IV	Distant metastases, including to the liver.

motherapy require surgical exploration and excision of residual disease if possible.

PostSurgical Therapy and Pathology

Modern-day chemotherapy has dramatically influenced the survival rate of patients with ovarian germ-cell tumors. Therapy with vincristine, actinomycin D, and cyclophosphamide (VAC) in the 1960s and 1970s improved the survivorship of adults with malignant germ-cell tumors; however, relapse rates were still as high as 46%, even with complete resection.[55] The efficacy of VAC in children was substantiated in a report by Cangir and coworkers[94] (from M.D. Anderson) in which all Stage I and II patients, 86% of Stage III, and 20% of Stage IV children survived with VAC chemotherapy. FIGO staging was used. The introduction of Einhorn-type chemotherapy for initial treatment of malignant testicular germ-cell tumors has been the major factor in improved survival rates in the 1980s and 1990s.[95] Initial reports[96, 97] on treatment with cisplatin, vinblastine, and bleomycin (PVB) for ovarian germ-cell tumors noted improved survival rates, too. One of the initial major trials comparing VAC to Einhorn-type therapy (BEP: bleomycin, etoposide, cisplatin [platinol]) was a Gynecologic Oncology Group (GOG) study of adults with a 24% relapse rate with VAC compared with only 4% for BEP.[98]

The current treatment of unilateral germ-cell

Table 13–3 • FIGO Staging System for Primary Carcinoma of the Ovary

Stage I: Growth limited to the ovaries:
    IA. Growth limited to one ovary; no ascites; no tumor on the external surface; capsule intact.
    IB. Growth limited to both ovaries; no ascites; no tumor on the external surface; capsule intact.
    IC. Tumor either Stage IA or IB, but with ascites or peritoneal washings containing malignant cells; tumor on surface or capsule ruptured.
Stage II: Growth involving one or both ovaries with pelvic extension:
    IIA. Extension or metastases to the uterus or the tubes.
    IIB. Extension to other pelvic tissues.
    IIC. Tumor either Stage IIA or IIB, but with ascites or peritoneal washings containing malignant cells; tumor on surface or capsule ruptured.
Stage III: Tumor involving one or both ovaries with peritoneal implants outside the pelvis or positive retroperitoneal or inguinal nodes; superficial liver metastasis equals Stage III; tumor is limited to the true pelvis but with histologically proved malignant extension to small bowel or omentum.
    IIIA. Tumor grossly limited to the true pelvis with negative nodes but with histologically confirmed microscopic seeding of abdominal peritoneal surfaces.
    IIIB. Tumor of one or both ovaries with histologically confirmed implants of abdominal peritoneal surfaces, none exceeding 2 cm in diameter; nodes are negative.
    IIIC. Abdominal implants greater than 2 cm in diameter or positive retroperitoneal or inguinal nodes
Stage IV: Growth involving one or both ovaries with distant metastases; if pleural effusion is present, there must be positive cytology to allot a case to Stage IV; parenchymal liver metastasis equals Stage IV.

tumors is unilateral salpingo-oophorectomy followed by cisplatin, etoposide, and bleomycin, allowing high cure rates along with maintenance of fertility,[99] even in the case of dysgerminoma, a disease treated in the past with radiation therapy and resulting in loss of fertility.

The current intergroup protocol of POG and CCG is listed in Figure 13–3. Patients in all stages receive chemotherapy except those with immature teratomas, who are treated with surgery and observation. The POG/CCG intergroup study (POG 9048/CCG 8891) of immature teratomas and Stage I and II ovarian and testes germ-cell tumors closed in 1995, and results were unavailable at the time of this writing. One major concern of the high-dose cisplatin etoposide-bleomycin (HDPEB) arm for advanced tumors is the possible increased toxicity.

Malignant germ-cell tumors of the ovary are dysgerminomas (the female homologues of seminomas) or nondysgerminomas, including endodermal sinus tumor, embryonal carcinoma, choriocarcinoma, immature teratoma, and mixed tumor. Malignant elements rarely arise within a mature teratoma.

Teratomas are the most common ovarian tumor of childhood, accounting for approximately one half of all germ-cell ovarian tumors. Benign mature teratomas are frequently cystic. Patients may present with a very large abdominal mass,

pain, or torsion. Calcifications may be noted on plain radiographs. Pathologic evaluation demonstrates all three primordial germ layers; however, ectodermal elements usually predominate. Malignant transformation is very rare (<1%) in childhood; it occurs mainly in older patients and can include malignant germ-cell elements (endodermal sinus, choriocarcinoma, dysgerminoma) or non-germ-cell lesions, such as squamous cell carcinoma, melanoma, and carcinoid.[100] Some are classified as monodermal when one cell type predominates. Rarely, thyroid tissue forms a mass within a teratoma referred to as *struma ovarii*, but these are rare in children.[101] Another group of monodermal teratomas consists almost exclusively of neuroectodermal elements. Rarely a mature or an immature ovarian teratoma may be associated with implantation of mature glial tissue on the peritoneum and omentum referred to as *gliomatosis peritonei*.[102, 103] This is a benign disorder; nevertheless, sampling of the lesions should be performed to exclude the possibility of immature tissue. Bilateral involvement occurs in 10% of cases. Treatment of mature teratomas is excision with the ovary preserved if possible. Solid lesions usually require a unilateral oophorectomy. Observation after surgery is the current standard of care.

Immature teratomas demonstrate various degrees of immature elements and, as noted pre-

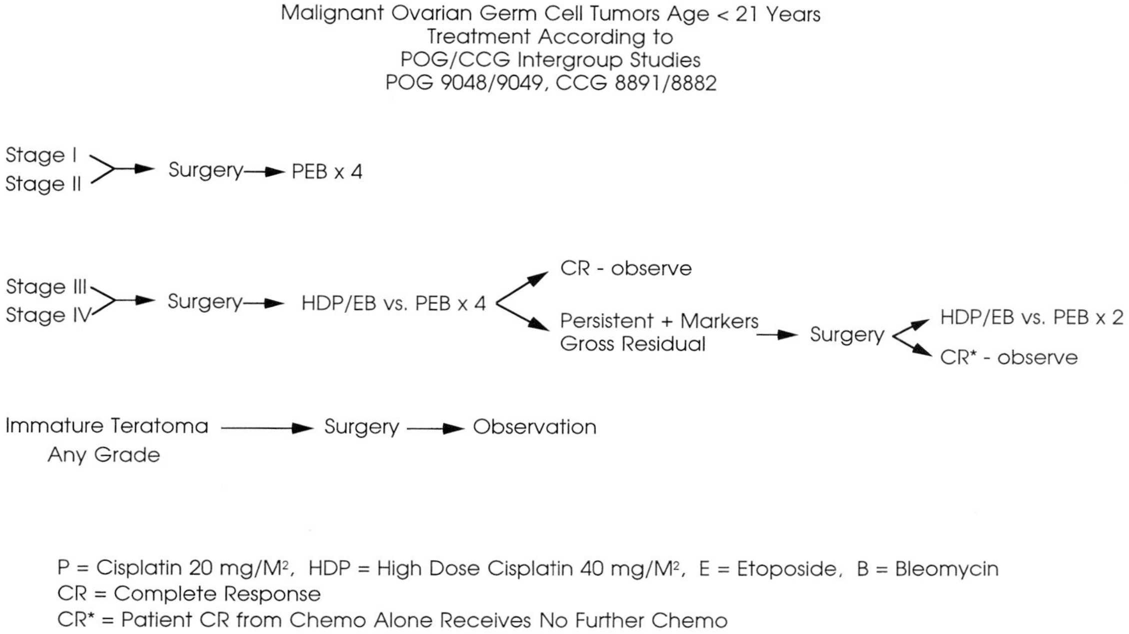

Malignant Ovarian Germ Cell Tumors Age < 21 Years
Treatment According to
POG/CCG Intergroup Studies
POG 9048/9049, CCG 8891/8882

Stage I
Stage II ⟩⟶ Surgery ⟶ PEB x 4

Stage III
Stage IV ⟩⟶ Surgery ⟶ HDP/EB vs. PEB x 4 ⟨
    CR - observe
    Persistent + Markers / Gross Residual ⟶ Surgery ⟨ HDP/EB vs. PEB x 2 / CR* - observe

Immature Teratoma ⟶ Surgery ⟶ Observation
    Any Grade

P = Cisplatin 20 mg/M², HDP = High Dose Cisplatin 40 mg/M², E = Etoposide, B = Bleomycin
CR = Complete Response
CR* = Patient CR from Chemo Alone Receives No Further Chemo

Figure 13–3 • Schema of treatment for malignant ovarian tumors. All stages receive chemotherapy.

viously, are graded as I, II, or III. Malignant elements may be present, so thorough pathologic evaluation is required. The post-surgical treatment of these lesions is controversial. Norris and coworkers[20] reviewed a total of 58 cases of immature teratomas in which 40 Stage I patients were treated initially with only surgery. Disease-free survival and overall survival were directly related to tumor grade. Thirteen of 14 patients (93%) with Grade I lesions survived, compared with 11 of 20 (55%) Grade II patients and 2 of 6 (33%) Grade III patients. It is noteworthy that several of the patients were children, and four of them suffered recurrent disease: two who had Grade II disease (ages 5 and 10) and two who had Grade III disease (ages 10 and 13). It is conceivable that some of these lesions had malignant elements missed at initial pathologic evaluation.

Gershenson and coworkers[104] from M.D. Anderson subsequently demonstrated improved survival rates with VAC therapy for immature teratomas, with only 1 of 11 Stage I patients disease-free after surgery alone compared with 10 of 11 disease-free after surgery plus VAC therapy. Similar results were obtained by others,[105] including Slayton[85] and colleagues in a Gynecologic Oncology Group (GOG) study in

which only 1 of 20 patients with immature teratomas of Grade II or III developed recurrent disease after being treated with VAC. Subsequent studies from GOG have demonstrated improved survival rates with BEP compared with VAC, and this is the current protocol of choice. Most adult centers recommend observation after surgery for Stage I, grade I immature teratomas and PEB for Grade II and III lesions.

In the CCG/POG intergroup study, all ovarian immature teratomas regardless of grade were treated by surgery alone. Preliminary evaluation of 31 patients with pure immature teratomas treated by surgery alone noted that all were free of recurrent malignant disease.[106] Long-term follow-up is needed to determine if observation is adequate therapy for children with higher grades of disease and to evaluate the salvage rate when there is recurrent disease.

Dysgerminomas occur at an average patient age of 16 years and are usually large tumors. Although most occur in otherwise normal females, dysgerminomas can also occur in those with dysgenic gonads. Lactic dehydrogenase (LDH), and specifically LDH-1, are frequently elevated in patients with dysgerminomas.[63, 107] The tumors are bilateral in 10% to 15% of cases, and thus the contralateral ovary should be examined at the time of surgery. Treatment of Stage I lesions by surgery only is associated with a 17% recurrence rate.[108] The tumors are radiosensitive, as are seminomas, and so radiation has been the cornerstone of therapy for years. As data from adult groups indicate that this tumor is chemosensitive to cisplatin, etoposide, and bleomycin. (PEB)[109–110] treatment with surgery to preserve reproductive function and avoid radiation is now accepted. Some recommend observation for Stage IA.[111]

The ovary is the second most common location for *endodermal sinus tumors* behind the sacrococcygeal region. As with tumors in other locations, AFP elevation is nearly always associated with ovarian tumors. Bilateral involvement occurs only 1% of the time. This is a friable tumor with rupture noted before or during surgery in about one third of cases.[112] Most are Stage IA lesions (FIGO classification). The inadequacy of surgery alone for Stage I lesions of this type was demonstrated by Kurman and Norris,[113] who reported only 5 survivors out of 27 patients (19%) treated with surgery alone. Although some improvement was noted with the addition of VAC[105, 113] therapy, the greatest response has been obtained with the addition of PEB.[110]

Although AFP is an excellent tumor marker in most patients, there is no correlation between the initial level of AFP and the stage of disease or the ultimate prognosis.[86, 114] Early studies[115] reported that patients with tumors less than 10 cm in size did better than those with larger tumors, but at least one study[86] does not substantiate this finding. Survival does correlate with stage and residual disease. Stage I patients do better than higher-stage patients, and those with no residual disease after surgery do better than those with some residual disease, and those with less than 2 cm residual disease do better than those with more than 2 cm residual disease.[86]

Embryonal carcinoma is the least differentiated of the germ-cell tumors. These tumors have been confused previously with endodermal sinus tumors.[69] They frequently have syncytiotrophoblasts and therefore usually secrete hCG. Hormonal manifestations, including precocious puberty, abnormal vaginal bleeding, and positive results on pregnancy tests, occur in approximately 60% of cases.[15]

Choriocarcinoma is a very rare pediatric germcell tumor[15] that can be gestational, arising from a pregnancy, or can be from an abnormal germcell differentiation. It is characterized by an elevated hCG level that may lead to isosexual pseudoprecocious puberty in the prepubertal female.[112] The hCG marker provides a means to follow results of treatment according to extent of surgical resection, response to therapy, and recurrence, although in a poorly sampled initial tumor, a nonchoriocarcinoma germ-cell element may recur without an elevated hCG.

Polyembryoma is an extremely rare lesion with very few reported cases; one series included one case of a 9-year-old girl.[116] Most other series have not included any patients with this lesion.[15]

Mixed tumors represent approximately 8% of malignant germ-cell tumors.[115, 117] The most common combinations are yolk sac–endodermal sinus with dysgerminoma or immature teratoma, but any combination is possible. Patients with immature teratomas that have components of endodermal sinus tumor may have an elevated AFP level. Current recommendations are to treat these lesions based on the endodermal sinus tumor component.

TESTICULAR GERM-CELL TUMORS

Clinical Presentation

Testicular cancer is rare in prepubertal children. Tumors are usually divided into those of germcell origin, which in prepubertal children are usually endodermal sinus tumor or teratomas, and those of non-germ-cell origin, including tumors of Sertoli and Leydig cells as well as sarcomas of the paratesticular tissues. Prepubertal children are much more likely to have non-germcell tumors than pubertal or adult male patients, in whom nearly all testicular tumors are germcell tumors.

The clinical presentation and histology of pediatric testicular germ-cell tumors are significantly different than those of tumors in adults. Approximately 35% of adults present with Stage I disease, compared with 80% to 85% of prepubertal children.[118–119] In addition, children usually have endodermal sinus tumor, which is less common in adults. Adults usually have seminomas or nonseminomatous lesions, including embryonal carcinoma, teratocarcinoma, or choriocarcinoma, which are rare in childhood.[120] A review of the Danish Cancer Registry also lends support to the idea of a different origin for germ-cell tumors in adolescents than in infants.[121] According to that registry, usually infants with tumors presented prior to 3 years of age and were either yolk-sac tumors or teratomas. The tumors of puberty were morphologically and immunohistochemically similar to those of adulthood.

Other differences involve the relationship of intratubular germ-cell neoplasia, a precursor of testicular germ-cell cancer, to pediatric versus adult cases of testicular cancer. These lesions have been identified in the seminiferous tubules adjacent to testicular germ-cell tumors in 85% to 100% of adult cases.[122] They have also been noted in biopsies of (1) an undescended testis of a child who later developed a germ-cell tumor as an adult[123] and (2) the testes of infertile men who later developed cancer.[124] Although this lesion has been identified in children with dysgenic gonads and androgen insensitivity, it has not been noted in infants with endodermal sinus tumors.[125–128] In a study comparing infantile with adolescent cases of germ-cell tumors, Jorgensen and coworkers[129] noted that the adolescent cases were associated with both normal germ cells and carcinoma in situ cells (intratubular germ-cell neoplasia), just as the adult cases were. In contrast, the infantile cases were generally not associated with carcinoma in situ cells, again suggesting that the etiology of germ-cell tumors in infants may be fundamentally different from that in adolescents and adults.

Since testicular tumors in infants appear to differ from those in adolescents, and those in adolescents appear identical to those in adults this section covers only the infantile type. The recommendation of CCG and POG is to treat adolescent boys with gonadal germ-cell tumors according to adult protocols.

Testicular tumors usually appear as a painless scrotal mass. The mass is solid and does not transilluminate, although one third of patients may have an associated hydrocele. Testicular ultrasound may be helpful in some cases. Workup includes physical examination of the abdomen and contralateral testes, computed tomography of the abdomen and chest to detect metastatic spread, and determination of serum markers (AFP, hCG). As noted earlier, endodermal sinus tumors represent the most common histologic type in children. AFP is elevated in approxi-

mately 85% of cases, and hCG is rarely elevated.[130–131]

Testicular teratomas are the second most common germ-cell tumor of the testes in children, accounting for 10% to 40% of cases.[64, 118, 130, 132, 133] Approximately 80% are mature teratomas and the remainder immature.[132] They are benign lesions, and there have been no reported cases of metastases from testicular teratomas in prepubertal boys.[134–136]

Operative Management and Staging

After an inguinal surgical approach with initial occlusion of the cord structures with a vessel loop, the testicle is mobilized into the field. If a mass is present, a radical orchiectomy is performed, with resection of the testes, epididymis, and cord structures and high ligation at the level of the internal ring. Transcrotal biopsy or excision is not utilized because of the risk of local recurrence and, as noted in the staging and treatment discussion in this chapter, such transcrotal procedures have an adverse effect on staging and mandate chemotherapy. The staging of testicular cancer for CCG and POG purposes is presented in Table 13–4. Patients with higher-stage disease, III–IV, undergo retroperitoneal lymph node sampling and debulking. No attempt is made to perform a standard retroperitoneal lymph node dissection in order to avoid complications associated with this procedure. Levels of lymph node sampling include high infrarenal (renal vein to infe-

Table 13–4 • CCG-POG Staging System for Pediatric Testicular Germ-Cell Tumors

Stage I	Limited to testis; tumor markers normal after appropriate half-life decline (AFP 5 days, hCG 16 hours).
Stage II	Transscrotal orchiectomy; microscopic disease in scrotum or high in spermatic cord (<5 cm from proximal end); retroperitoneal lymph node involvement (<2 cm) and/or increased tumor markers after appropriate half-life decline.
Stage III	Retroperitoneal lymph node involvement (>2 cm) but no visceral or extra-abdominal involvement.
Stage IV	Distant metastases, including to the liver.

rior mesenteric artery), low infrarenal (inferior mesenteric artery to aortic bifurcation), and iliacs.

Although the management of teratomas has generally been orchiectomy, in view of the benign course in prepubertal boys, testicular-sparing surgery may be a reasonable alternative. Rushton and coworkers[137] reported five patients successfully treated with enucleation. They note that teratoma can be suspected if the AFP level is normal, there are no endocrine manifestations of a Leydig cell tumor, and ultrasound demonstrates a circumscribed, partly cystic mass. The operative approach is the same except that the tumor suspected of being a teratoma is enucleated. If frozen section confirms the diagnosis of teratoma, the testicular blood supply is restored and the testis placed back in the scrotum. Although extremely rare, intratubular germ-cell neoplasia adjacent to a teratoma has been reported in two cases, one being an 8-month-old boy with an immature teratoma of the testis[138] and another being a 3-year-old boy with a mature teratoma.[139]

Treatment

Survival rates for patients with pediatric germ-cell tumors have improved with modern-day chemotherapy. As described, current protocols utilized by CCG and POG include cisplatin, etoposide, and bleomycin (PEB). These current protocols are attempting to confirm the 85% to 100% reported survival rate of patients with Stage I testicular germ-cell tumors treated with only surgery[140–142] and to evaluate the value of dissecting retroperitoneal lymph nodes. The current scheme for treatment of prepubertal testes cancer is shown in Figure 13–4. All patients with evidence of disease outside the scrotum receive chemotherapy.

Although the results of the current studies are pending as of this writing, several reports have substantiated the effectiveness of management of Stage I tumors with post-surgical observation. A report of 24 patients with Stage I endodermal sinus testes tumors noted the same 3-year survival rate (96%) for those treated with chemotherapy as for those treated by post-surgical observation.[143] Several other relatively small series have also noted excellent results in the management of Stage I patients by orchiectomy followed by observation without chemotherapy.

The report of the Testicular Tumor Registry on 181 yolk-sac tumors noted that orchiectomy without retroperitoneal lymph node dissection or chemotherapy was adequate for Stage I patients.[130] The United Kingdom Children's Cancer Study Group also supports the adequacy of observation after surgery for disease limited to the testes in patients whose AFP levels return to normal.[131] A large study of 76 yolk-sac tumors (73 of them Stage I) reported a disease-free survival rate of 98%.[145] Of the patients with Stage I lesions, 56 were treated with observation after retroperitoneal lymphadenectomy to confirm Stage I; and of these, nine (16%) required delayed chemotherapy, and all but one were salvaged.

The value of hemiscrotectomy in clinical Stage I tumor is controversial.[146–150] In the current staging system scrotal contamination mandates Stage II classification and therefore chemotherapy. The current POG-CCG protocol calls for hemiscrotectomy in this situation. The literature on adult patients has supported this procedure in cases of scrotal violation in order to lower the local recurrence rate.[147–149] Yet, one series of adults with Stage I tumors and scrotal contamination demonstrated no increase in the relapse or recurrence rate among those treated by observation alone after removal of tumor.[150] Some believe that children with clinical Stage I tumors and scrotal violation should not undergo hemiscrotectomy because of the low yield and overall favorable outcome in these patients.[146] Notwithstanding, reports of metastatic seeding resulting from needle biopsy contamination suggest that hemiscrotectomy may indeed be appropriate.[146, 151]

The role of retroperitoneal lymphadenectomy or sampling is also somewhat controversial. Early studies recommended ipsilateral retroperitoneal lymphadenectomy. In a review of 11 cases, Hopkins[118] and coworkers noted improved survival rates with lymphadenectomy and chemotherapy compared with orchiectomy alone, although none who underwent lymphadenectomy had any identifiable retroperitoneal tumor. The improved survival rate may have been related to chemotherapy not lymphadenectomy. Some reports have noted the incidence of lymphatic spread to be 12% to 33%.[152, 153] Others have noted a 0% yield of retroperitoneal lymphadenectomy in

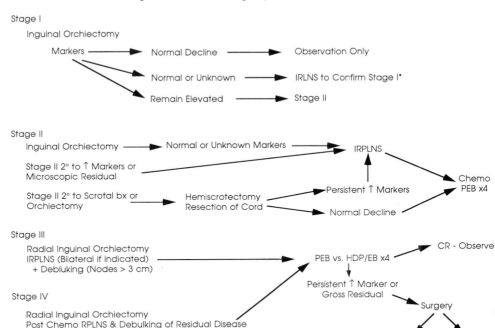

Testicular Germ Cell Malignancies - Age < 10 Years
Treatment Accordingto POG/CCG Intergroup Studies (POG 9048/9049, CCG 8891/8882)

P = Cisplatin 20 mg/M², HDP = High Dose Cisplatin 40 mg/M², E = Etoposide, B = Bleomycin
CR = Complete Response
CR* = Patient CR from Chemo Alone Receives No Further Chemo
IRPLNS = Ipsilateral Retroperitoneal Lymph Node Sampling

Figure 13–4 • Schema of treatment for malignant prepubertal testicular germ cell tumors.

those with clinical Stage I disease.[154] A collective review of 39 clinical Stage IA cases noted only 2 (5%) with retroperitoneal disease.[132]

The current POG-CCG protocol recommends lymph node sampling in order to avoid when possible the complications related to retroperitoneal lymph node dissection. One point of controversy concerns the evaluation of patients with Stage I or II disease and tumor markers that are normal or present inconclusive evidence: is retroperitoneal lymph node sampling needed or not? Some would contend that CT imaging and observation are sufficient. In a review of 12 patients with clinical Stage I disease subjected to lymphadenectomy, Bracken and coworkers[154] noted that all had negative results on biopsy. Those with retroperitoneal disease had presented with clinical evidence of nodes.

After chemotherapy, residual retroperitoneal disease must be excised or a biopsy taken, as it is not possible to differentiate malignancy from benign teratoma.[155] Those patients who have a complete response from chemotherapy alone (benign retroperitoneal disease) receive no further therapy. Those with viable tumor receive additional courses of chemotherapy.

Teratomas of the testes in prepubertal children are treated with surgery followed by observation, even if immature elements are present. Immature testicular teratomas in young children act as benign tumors; in adults they have a more aggressive course and are treated as a malignancy.[156] If these teratomas are present in the pubertal male, they are treated as adult malignancies with chemotherapy.

EXTRAGONADAL GERM-CELL TUMORS
Etiology and Incidence

Extragonadal germ-cell tumors were initially thought to represent metastases from an unrecognized gonadal primary. Autopsy studies of patients with anterior mediastinal germ-cell tumors, however, failed to support this idea.[157] Moreover, autopsy studies of patients with testicular germ-cell cancer identified fewer than 1% of patients with isolated mediastinal metastases.[158, 159] In addition, many patients with extragonadal germ-cell tumors have been successfully treated with only surgery or radiation, experiencing no progression of gonadal disease.[160]

Most currently accept that extragonadal germ-cell tumors of the pineal, mediastinum, and sacrococcygeal regions arise from germ cells distributed aberrantly to these locations. Retroperitoneal extragonadal tumors may arise from aberrant germ cells or may be related to gonadal disease. One study of 39 retroperitoneal, presumed extragonadal tumors in which testicular biopsies were performed identified 42% with carcinoma in situ,[161] or, more accurately, *intratubular germ-cell neoplasia,* a known precursor of invasive germ-cell tumors. In contrast, none of the patients with mediastinal or pineal disease had testicular lesions.

Extragonadal germ cell tumors account for 5% to 10% of germ-cell tumors in adults[162] but are more common in children, accounting for approximately two thirds of all pediatric germ-cell tumor cases.[160] The most common sites in children are the sacrococcygeal, anterior mediastinal, and pineal regions. Rare sites include the retroperitoneum, neck, stomach, and vagina. The staging system used by POG and CCG is presented in Table 13–5. Thus far, patients with malignant extragonadal tumors have had a less favorable prognosis (particularly when the site is the mediastinum) than those with gonadal disease. Their prognosis may improve with the advent of platinum-based chemotherapy,[163] but it has been poor enough to prompt a high-risk CCG-POG protocol of etoposide and bleomycin plus either standard or high-dose cisplatin for all extragonadal patients.

Sacrococcygeal Tumors

Clinical Presentation

Sacrococcygeal tumors in childhood generally appear in two clinical patterns—as large, predominantly benign masses noted in the neonatal period or as primarily pelvic lesions, predominantly

Table 13–5 • CCG-POG Staging System for Malignant Extragonadal Germ-Cell Tumors

Stage I	Complete resection at any site; coccygectomy for sacrococcygeal site; normal tumor margins; tumor markers either normal or showing evidence of malignancy.
Stage II	Microscopic residual disease; lymph nodes normal; tumor markers either normal or showing evidence of malignancy.
Stage III	Gross residual disease or biopsy only; retroperitoneal nodes either normal or showing evidence of malignancy; tumor markers either normal or showing evidence of malignancy.
Stage IV	Distant metastases, including to the liver.

malignant, noted at some point between birth and 4 years.

In neonates the *sacrococcygeal teratoma (SCT)* is the most common type of teratoma, accounting for 40% to 70% of teratomas in most series. SCT has a reported incidence of 1 in 35,000 live births.[164] There is a strong female preponderance, with a 3–4:1 female-to-male ratio in most series.[16, 165, 166] Most SCTs are noted at delivery when the characteristic mass is seen protruding from the space between the anus and the coccyx (Fig. 13–5).

The diagnosis of SCT is occasionally made by prenatal ultrasound. Because of the size of the mass, fetal dystocia may occur, requiring cesarean section. Abdominal delivery should be considered in cases of tumors larger than 5 cm to avoid dystocia and tumor rupture.[167, 168] In addition to dystocia, other fetal problems can include polyhydramnios, preterm delivery with lung immaturity, and tumor hemorrhage with anemia and hydrops. Hydrops can also develop if the tumor behaves as an arteriovenous fistula, resulting in high-output cardiac failure and placentomegaly.[169]

In a collective review of fetal SCTs, Flake and coworkers[168] noted that most were presented at 22 to 34 weeks of gestation and were associated with a large uterus or polyhydramnios symptoms. Late presentation means a better prognosis: six of eight fetuses in whom the condition was diagnosed after 30 weeks of gestation survived versus only one of 14 in whom diagnosis was made

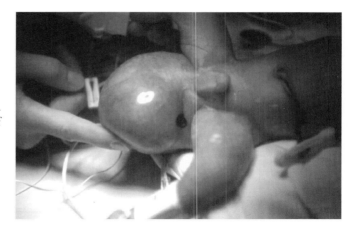

Figure 13–5 • A large sacrococcygeal teratoma in a newborn. Note the deviation of the rectum to the left of the midline.

earlier. If hydrops is diagnosed after 30 weeks of gestation, delivery should be delayed until the fetus's lungs are mature. Some fetuses of less than 30 weeks of gestation with hydrops may benefit from in utero fetal surgery. Two fetal SCT resections have been reported. Unfortunately, one newborn died after a premature delivery 12 days after fetal repair, and the other was delivered prematurely 8 days after surgery and

died during resection of the residual tumor on the 13th day of life.[170]

Although many SCTs are apparent at delivery, some are quite small and may have a minimal external abnormality (Fig. 13–6). Still others may be entirely within the pelvis. Altman and coworkers,[166] in a survey of the Surgical Section of the American Academy of Pediatrics (AAP) involving 405 patients, classified SCTs according to the

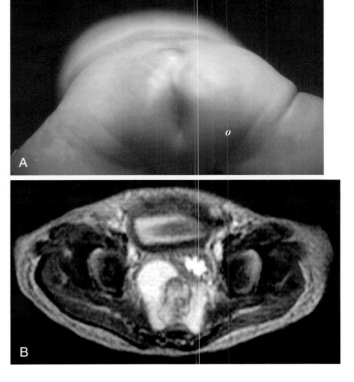

Figure 13–6 • *A*, A 4-week-old boy with a small external component of a sacrococcygeal teratoma. *B*, An MRI scan identified the larger pelvic portion of the tumor as AAP Type III.

degree of intrapelvic extension (Fig. 13–7): Type I, predominantly external (46.7%); Type II, external with significant intrapelvic extension (34.7%); Type III, visible externally but with predominant pelvic and abdominal extension (8.8%); and Type IV, entirely presacral (9.8%).

The occurrence of malignancy in SCTs appears related to the age of the child at resection, and it has been postulated that a delay in diagnosis leads to an increased incidence of malignancy. Altman's[166] AAP survey evaluated the incidence

of malignancy based on location and size of tumor and age of patient. As regards location and size of tumor, 8% of Type I, 21% of Type II, 34% of Type III, and 38% of Type IV lesions were malignant. Altman suggested this finding may have been due to delayed diagnosis in the less apparent lesions. As regards age of patient, there was a much higher rate of malignancy in cases in which diagnosis was made after 2 months of age. There was a higher malignant rate in boys: in children younger than 2 months, the

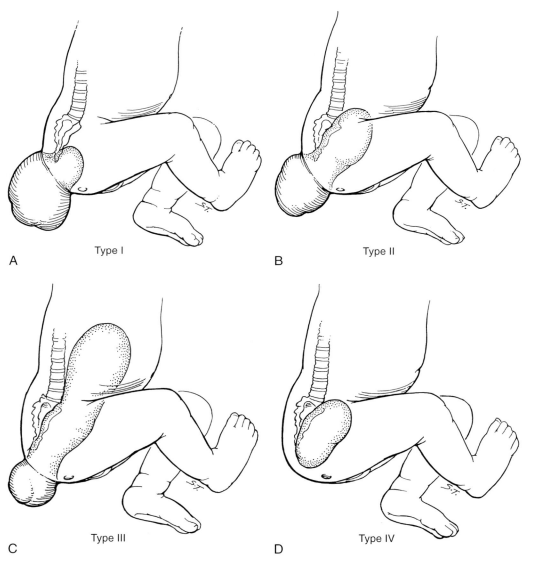

Type I

A

Type II

B

Type III

C

Type IV

D

Figure 13–7 • Classification of sacrococcygeal teratomas based on Altman's AAP series.[166] Type I is predominantly external; Type II is external with intrapelvic extension; Type III is visible externally but predominantly pelvic and abdominal; and Type IV is entirely presacral.

rate of malignancy was 10% for boys versus 7% for girls, and in children older than 2 months, it was 67% for boys versus 48% for girls. Most of these older patients had no apparent mass at birth.

Delays in diagnosis of SCT may be due to earlier misdiagnosis. In Altman's series there were 24 cases in which SCT was not diagnosed until 1 year of age, and 5 (21%) of these were malignant. These tumors were present at birth, and the delay presumably allowed malignant degeneration or allowed a small focus of malignant cells to grow. In a preliminary review of data from CCG surgeons involving 114 neonates, 6 with a mass noted at birth underwent delayed surgery (at 1.5 to 24 months of age). Malignant germ-cell tumors were noted in two cases (33%), metastases being discovered in one at the time of surgery.[171]

The second clinical scenario involves infants and children with SCTs presenting at some time after birth, in patients up to 4 years of age.[16] These children generally have no external portion noted at birth. The tumors are usually located in the pelvis, and symptoms are related to compression of the rectum or bladder. The rate of malignancy is considerably higher. Altman's AAP survey, as noted earlier, had a much higher rate of malignancy in this older group of patients, and others have also noted 50% to 90% malignancy rates in these older children.[166, 172–174] The germ cells presumably either undergo malignant transformation, or a small focus of malignancy intitially present becomes the major tissue type.[175] Most malignancies in these cases are yolk-sac tumors (endodermal sinus). In some cases of large malignant tumors, initial biopsy followed by chemotherapy and delayed resection may be appropriate.

In 1965 Ashcraft and Holder[176] described two patients with presacral teratomas and anal stenosis. Subsequent to this diagnosis, several other family members of these two patients had presacral tumors. In 1979 Ashcraft and Holder[177] reported 17 cases of presacral tumors and sacral defects in kindreds of 6 of those in the earlier series. Twelve of these patients had anorectal stenosis. These 17 cases suggest the autosomal dominant nature of this trait, which has been substantiated by others as well.[178–180] Currarino and coworkers[181] added three cases to the literature in 1981 in support of the theory that the etiology might be related to either persistent adhesions between the endoderm and neural ectoderm causing a split notochord or a primary split notochord. All reports emphasize the close attachment of the sacral mass to the rectum and dura, and several cases of meningitis have been reported as developing after resection. In addition, two cases of intradural extension of primary sacrococcygeal teratomas have been reported.[182, 183]

Operative Management

Prior to surgical resection, the degree of pelvic or abdominal extension of an SCT should be assessed by either ultrasound, computed tomography, or magnetic resonance imaging. These procedures also allow evaluation for a myelomeningocele, which can occasionally be difficult to find on physical examination.

Complete surgical excision of the SCT with resection of the coccyx is the initial procedure of choice (Fig. 13–8). The importance of resecting the coccyx was emphasized by Gross and others,[184–186] who noted SCT recurrence rates of up to 37% when the coccyx was not removed. If the tumor extends cephalad to the bony pelvis, an initial abdominal incision may be required to mobilize the upper portion of the tumor and divide the blood supply to the tumor from the middle sacral artery. Resection of the external portion is performed with the patient in the prone position. An inverted V-type incision allows excellent exposure and maximal preservation of the levator ani muscles and the muscle complex around the rectum. Placement of sutures between the anal sphincter and presacral fascia allows formation of the gluteal crease.[187]

Nearly all large series of patients with SCT report deaths as a result of operative complications.[16, 188] In a collective review of CCG surgeons involving 114 patients, there were 7 perioperative deaths.[171] Neonatal factors in such deaths include hydrops, anemia and intratumor hemorrhage, or tumor rupture due to delivery trauma. In addition, some neonates have abnormal coagulation parameters preoperatively.[189] SCTs can be difficult to resect and thus result in significant intraoperative blood loss and death. Hypothermia and coagulopathy related to blood loss are other serious problems.

Some neonates may benefit from a staged ap-

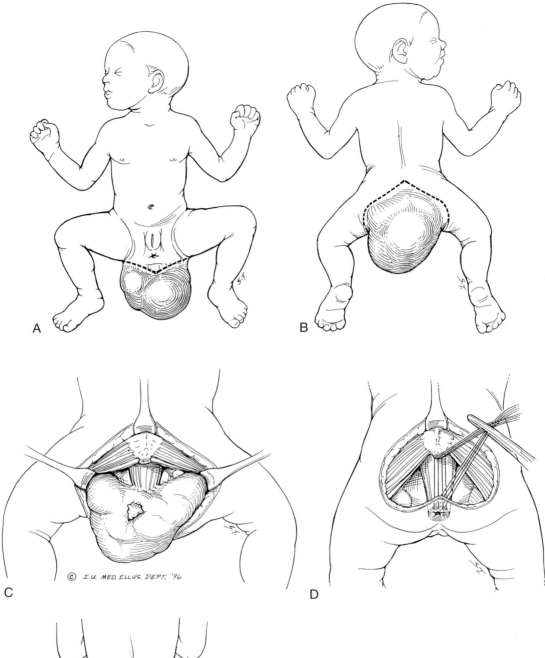

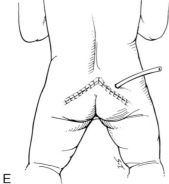

Figure 13–8 • Operative excision of sacrococcygeal teratoma. *A* and *B*, An inverted **V** incision. *C*, The tumor along with the coccyx is excised, taking care to avoid injury to the rectum. *D*, Placement of sutures between anal sphincter and presacral fascia. *E*, Wound closure with drainage.

proach with initial ligation of the vascular supply. Robertson and coworkers[190] described a premature infant (26 weeks old) with a large SCT treated by initial ligation of the middle sacral artery and both internal iliac arteries as well as a diverting colostomy. The external portion was excised 36 hours later and the pelvic portion on the 111th day of life. Lindahl[191] and Teitelbaum and coworkers[192] have described placement of an elastic vessel loop around the aorta just above the bifurcation in order to totally occlude blood flow during the resection if necessary. Lund and colleagues[193] reported extracorporeal membrane oxygenation and hypothermic hypoperfusion to allow safe resection of a giant SCT in a premature child. Older infants and children with large pelvic and abdominal masses at presentation may benefit from initial biopsy followed by chemotherapy and a delayed resection. If a laparotomy is required in a child past the neonatal period, retroperitoneal lymph node sampling should be performed. The CCG-POG protocol also recommends sampling of ascitic fluid or performing peritoneal washings.

Postoperative Management

In general, mature and immature SCTs are treated with initial surgery only, and malignant lesions are treated with surgery and chemotherapy. Postoperatively all infants should be closely followed, with periodic rectal examinations every 3 months until 3 years of age and then every 6 months until 4 or 5 years of age. The recommendation to follow cases this way is based on the CCG-POG report of Hawkins and coworkers[194] that noted a recurrence as late as 33 months. AFP levels should be followed after surgery to ascertain that they decline according to the normal graphs reported by Tsuchida.[60] Any elevation should prompt evaluation for recurrent disease.

Close follow-up is essential because a small focus of malignancy could be missed during pathologic examination of the specimen or overlooked at the time of surgery. In a combined CCG-POG study, four of six children with malignant recurrence after neonatal resection of mature or immature SCTs were noted on review to have microscopic foci of yolk-sac tumor in the original specimen.[194] The recurrences were 7 to 33 months after the initial procedure (a mean of 17 months). Gilcrease and coworkers[156] reported

a case involving a premature child who underwent resection of a Grade I immature SCT with no evidence of malignancy in the specimen but who died intraoperatively. At autopsy a small focus of residual tumor that contained yolk-sac tumor was identified.

Recurrent SCTs, either benign or malignant, have been reported after excision of mature and immature teratomas. In the CCG experience, 6 of 72 patients with mature teratoma experienced recurrence 6 to 33 months after the initial procedure; 1 had a benign teratoma, and 5 had malignant recurrences.[171] All with malignancy survived after treatment by surgery and chemotherapy. One of 22 patients with immature teratoma experienced recurrence of a mature teratoma at 6 months of age. In a review of 28 patients with initial benign tumors, Bilik[195] noted 6 (22%) recurrences; 3 were benign, and 3 were malignant endodermal sinus tumors. Two patients with malignancy survived after surgery and chemotherapy (one with disease), and one died. All with benign disease survived after surgery alone. Most recurrences are local, managed with surgery followed by chemotherapy only if malignant elements are identified.

A long-term follow-up study of 45 patients for 4 to 43 years after resection of SCT demonstrated 2 benign recurrences and 1 malignant.[196] The malignancy, occurring 43 years after treatment, was a mucinous adenocarcinoma, probably originating from a benign epithelial residual component of the original teratoma.

As noted previously, the significance of immature SCT is not clear.[197, 198] The current recommendation of both CCG and POG is to treat this initially by surgery alone. Although the exact survival rate for malignant SCTs treated in the modern era of chemotherapy is not precisely known, the combined CCG-POG study ongoing at the time of this writing should answer this question. This study utilizes cisplatin, etoposide, and bleomycin for four cycles. The doses are modified for infants younger than 12 months. Most reports of malignant tumors primarily involve older children, with only 6% to 18% of the cases being neonates. A large series by Schropp and coworkers[16] involving 16 malignant SCTs noted improved survival rates with the advent of Einhorn type chemotherapy; 11% survived prior to 1978, and 86% survived after 1978. Results from POG also noted improved survival rates with cisplatin, bleomycin, and vinblastine.[163]

Long-term sequelae are rarely reported apart from recurrent disease. In a long-term study of adults who had undergone surgery for SCTs as infants, Rintala and coworkers[199] noted good fecal continence in 88%; however, only 27% had normal bowel habits, and 27% had minor soiling. In a report on 27 patients, Malone and colleagues[200] noted that 8 (30%) had chronic constipation and soiling, and 6 (22%) had urinary incontinence. The voiding dysfunction is usually neurogenic in origin.[201] Havranek and coworkers[202] noted fecal soiling in 40% of patients and urinary incontinence in 16% in their series. Anorectal manometry in 14 such patients demonstrated normal anal resting tone and squeezing pressures in 10 but below normal levels in 4. These 4 also had soiling problems. Reinberg and coworkers,[203] in a follow-up series of 29 patients, noted neurogenic bladder in 12%, uretheral obstruction in 10%, and vesicoureteral reflux in 7%. The highest incidence of urologic complication (81%) was seen in patients who had had Type IV (presacral) tumors.

Long-term orthopedic follow-up in one series has demonstrated an 80% incidence of vertebral anomalies by the mean age of 21 years.[204] Spondylolysis of the lumbosacral spine was associated with extrapelvic tumors, and intrapelvic tumors were associated with spina bifida occulta lesions and other abnormalities. In addition, congenital dislocation of the hip was noted in 7% of cases.

Mediastinal Tumors

Clinical Presentation

Anterior mediastinal tumors may be noted incidentally on chest radiographs or may be manifested by signs and symptoms such as cough, dyspnea, and orthopnea due to mechanical airway obstruction or superior vena cava syndrome (Fig. 13–9). They commonly occur in the teenage years and account for approximately 7% of all germ-cell tumors in children.[205] They also account for 20% of mediastinal masses in children.[206] Klinefelter's syndrome has been noted in approximately 20% of these patients.[160]

The most common type of abnormal histology in children is that associated with teratoma. In a series of 15 patients with mediastinal teratomas,

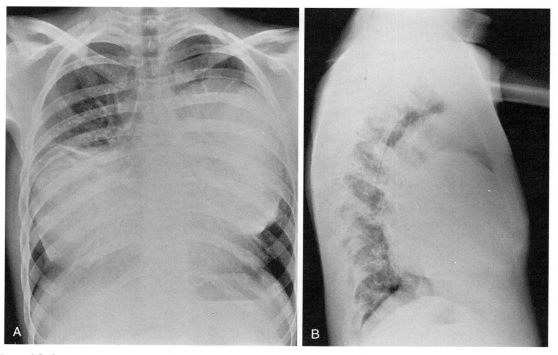

Figure 13–9 • Radiographs of a 15-year-old boy with a large anterior mediastinal teratoma: A, Anterior-posterior view; B, lateral view. The tumor was totally excised through a median sternotomy.

2 had mature tumors, 10 had immature tumors, and 3 had malignant tumors.[206] All the patients with malignancies were older than 12 years of age. Mediastinal primary tumors have been noted to have a high incidence of non-germ-cell elements, including neuroblastoma, embryonal rhabdomyosarcoma, small-cell carcinoma, and adenocarcinoma.[207, 208] Hematologic malignancies in association with mediastinal germ-cell tumors have also been reported.[209]

Treatment

Standard evaluation for mediastinal tumors includes determination of tumor markers as well as a careful examination of the testes, perhaps including ultrasound. A chest CT scan identifies the extent of the lesions. A fine-needle aspiration with cytologic examination may be useful to evaluate other anterior mediastinal tumors as well as to assist in differentiating a germ-cell tumor from lymphoma.

Surgical removal is the treatment of choice. A median sternotomy usually provides excellent exposure. Care should be taken to avoid injury to the phrenic nerves. In addition, the anesthetic management is of critical importance as the loss of spontaneous respiratory effort with pharmacologic paralysis may allow the mass to further compress the airway. Treatment is as with other germ-cell tumors; mature and immature teratomas are treated with surgery and observation and malignant lesions with surgery and chemotherapy.

Cervicofacial Teratomas

Cervicofacial teratomas are rare lesions, accounting for approximately 5% to 6% of all teratomas.[15, 210] Nearly all are discovered in the neonatal period, and one third are associated with polyhydramnios.[211] Azizkhan and coworkers[212] reported a CCG study of 20 neonates, 14 with cervical and 6 with orofacial lesions. Life-threatening airway obstruction occurred in 7; 2 died in the delivery room, and 2 required immediate tracheostomies. Of the 18 patients who survived past the delivery room, 17 survived surgical resection. Most of the lesions were mature or immature teratomas; however, 4 patients had malignant lesions, 2 of them with pulmonary metastases. One of these patients died. The sur-

viving child, interestingly, had neuroblastoma-like cells in the primary tumor as well as in metastases to the liver, lung, subcutaneous tissue, and buttock.[212, 213] This child was successfully treated with excision of the primary lesion and all metastatic lesions, without chemotherapy.

Prenatal diagnosis of these lesions allows preparation for delivery. The airway should be secured, preferably orally. Personnel experienced in tracheostomy should be in attendance just in case they are needed. Operative management consists of early excision of the primary lesion and all metastatic lesions. Chemotherapy is reserved for infants with disseminated disease that has not differentiated and those with residual disease.[212]

Rare Sites

Teratomas

Gastric. Teratomas of the stomach are unusual lesions, accounting for less than 1% of all teratomas in most series.[214, 215] Most of the approximately 50 reported gastric teratomas have occurred in male patients, in contrast to the teratomas of other sites that predominate in female patients. The female patient with a gastric teratoma reported in 1995 was only the sixth such case.[216]

Patients with gastric teratomas usually present within the first few months of life as an abdominal mass or symptoms of gastric distention or, rarely, gastrointestinal bleeding.[217] The treatment is complete excision. There have been no reported malignant teratomas at this location.

Pancreas. There have been ten reported cases of pancreatic teratoma, five of them in children.[218] The most common symptoms have been nausea, vomiting, and abdominal or lumbar pain. Most have been benign cystic lesions. Resection is the treatment of choice as marsupialization can result in a fistula.[219]

Vaginal-Endodermal Sinus Tumor

Endodermal sinus tumor of the vagina is a rare tumor occurring exclusively in children younger than 3 years of age.[13, 220, 221] These girls usually present with vaginal bleeding, and the mass may be confused with a sarcoma botyroides. The initial reports of radical surgery had survival rates of less than 50%.[222] In 1985 Copeland and co-workers[220] reported four of six (66%) survivors of radical surgery with VAC therapy. Hwang and coworkers[221] reported two patients treated with excision and vaginal preservation and VAC chemotherapy. It is noteworthy that a recurrence in one was successfully treated with PEB. Current treatment attempts vaginal-preserving surgery and includes PEB chemotherapy with close observation of AFP levels.

References

1. Dehner LP: Gonadal and extragonadal germ-cell neoplasia of childhood. *Hum Pathol* 14:493, 1983.
2. Brown NJ: Teratomas and yolk-sac tumours. *J Clin Pathol* 29:1021, 1976.
3. Gillman J: The development of the gonads in man with consideration of the role of fetal endocrines and the histogenesis of ovarian tumors. *Contrib Embryol* 32:83, 1948.
4. Witschi E: Migration of the germ cells of human embryos from the yolk sac to the primitive gonadal fold. *Contrib Embryol* 32:69, 1948.
5. Teilum G: Classification of endodermal sinus tumor (mesoblastoma vitellinum) and so-called "embryonal carcinoma" of the ovary. *Acta Pathol Microbiol Scand* 64:407, 1965.
6. Willis RA: *Pathology of tumours*, 4th ed. London: Butterworths, 1967.
7. Collins DH, Pugh RCB: Pathology of testicular tumours. *Br J Urol* 36(suppl):1–112, 1964.
8. Stevens LC: Embryonic potency of embryoid bodies derived from transplantable testicular teratoma of the mouse. *Dev Biol* 2:285, 1960.
9. Pierce BG, Dixon FJ: Testicular teratomas 1. Demonstration of teratogenesis by metamorphosis of multipotential cells. *Cancer* 12:573, 1959.
10. Pierce GB, Midgley AR Jr: The origin and function of human syncytiotrophoblastic giant cells. *Am J Pathol* 43:153, 1963.
11. Inoue M, Fujita M, Azuma C, et al: Histogenetic analysis of ovarian germ cell tumors by DNA fingerprinting. *Cancer Res* 52(24):6823, 1992.
12. Teilum G: Endodermal sinus tumors of ovary and testis: Comparative morphogenesis of the so-called mesonephroma ovarii (Schiller) and extra-embryonic (yolk sac-allantoic) structures of the rat's placenta. *Cancer* 23:1092–1105, 1959.
13. Graivier L, Bronsther B: Endodermal sinus tumors in infants and children. In Brooks BF(ed): *Malignant Tumors of Childhood*. Austin, TX: University of Texas Press, 1986, p. 131.
14. Virchow R: *Ueber die Sakralgeschwulst des Schliewener Kindes. Klin Wschr* 46:132, 1869.
15. Lack EE, Young RH, Scully RE: Pathology of ovarian neoplasms in childhood and adolescence. *Pathol Annu* 27:281, 1992.
16. Schropp KP, Lobe TE, Rao B, et al: Sacrococcygeal teratoma: The experience of four decades. *J Pediatr Surg* 27(8):1075, 1992.
17. Dehner LP: Gonadal and extragonadal germ cell neoplasms-teratomas in childhood. In Finegold MJ (ed): *Pathology of Neoplasia in Children and Adolescents*. Philadelphia: W.B. Saunders Co., 1986, p. 291.
18. Bale PM: Sacrococcygeal developmental abnormalities and tumors in children. *Perspect Pediatr Pathol* 1:9, 1984.
19. Damjanov I: Pathology of human teratomas. In Damjanov I, Knowles B, Solter D (eds): *The Human Teratomas. Experimental and Clinical Biology*. Clifton, NJ: The Humana Press, 1983, p. 23.
20. Norris HJ, Zirkin HJ, Benson WL: Immature (malignant) teratoma of the ovary: A clinical and pathological study of 58 cases. *Cancer* 37:2359, 1976.
21. Gonzalez-Crussi F, Winkler RF, Mirkin DL: Sacrococcygeal teratomas in infants and children. Relationship of histology and prognosis in 40 cases. *Arch Pathol Lab Med* 102:420, 1978.
22. Valdiserri RO, Yunis EJ: Sacrococcygeal teratomas: A review of 68 cases. *Cancer* 48:217, 1981.
23. Gobel G, Calaminus G, Harms D: SIOP teratoma 95, a randomized cooperative protocol for chemotherapy. *Med Pediatr Oncol* 25:319, 1995.
24. Shu XO, Nesbit ME, Buckley JD, et al: An exploratory analysis of risk factors for childhood malignant germ-cell tumors: Report from the Children's Cancer Group (Canada, United States). *Cancer Causes Control* 6:187, 1995.
25. Samaniego F, Rodriguez E, Houldsworth J, et al: Cytogenetic and molecular analysis of human male germ cell tumors: Chromosome 12 abnormalities and gene amplification. *Genes, Chromosomes and Cancer* 1:289, 1990.
26. Bosl GJ, Dmitrovsky E, Reuter VE, et al: Isochromosome of chromosome 12: Clinically useful marker for male germ-cell tumors. *J Natl Cancer Inst* 81:1874, 1989.
27. Oosterhuis JW, Castedo SMMJ, de Jong B, et al: Karyotyping and DNA flow cytometry of an orchidoblastoma. *Cancer Genet Cytogenet* 36:7, 1988.
28. Perlman EJ, Henneberry J, Hawkins E, et al: Cytogenetic and ploidy analysis of endodermal sinus tumors in infants. *Mod Pathol* 6:7, (abstract) 1993.
29. Fossa SD, Nesland JM, Waehre H, et al: DNA ploidy in the primary tumor from patients with nonseminomatous testicular germ-cell tumors clinical stage I. *Cancer* 67:1874, 1991.

30. Fossa SD, Pettersen EO, Thorud E, et al: DNA flow cytometry in human testicular cancer. *Cancer Lett* 28:55, 1985.

31. Sledge GW Jr, Eble JN, Roth BJ, et al: Flow cytometry derived DNA content of the primary lesions of advanced germ-cell tumours. *Intl J Androl* 10:115, 1987.

32. Silver SA, Wiley JM, Perlman EJ: DNA ploidy analysis of pediatric germ-cell tumors. *Mod Pathol* 7(9):951, 1994.

33. Shulman LP, Muram D, Marina N, et al: Lack of heritability in ovarian germ-cell malignancies. *Am J Obstet Gynecol* 170(6):1803, 1994.

34. Blake KI, Gerrard MP: Malignant germ-cell tumours in two siblings. *Med Pediatr Oncol* 21(4):299, 1993.

35. Weinblatt M, Kochen J: An unusual family cancer syndrome manifested in young siblings. *Cancer* 68(5):1068, 1991.

36. Rutgers JL, Scully RE: Pathology of the testis in intersex syndromes. *Semin Diagn Pathol* 4:275, 1987.

37. Manuel M, Katayama KP, Jones HW: The age of occurrence of gonadal tumours in intersex patients with a Y chromosome. *Am J Obstet Gynecol* 124:293, 1976.

38. Krasna IH, Lee ML, Smillow P, et al: Risk of malignancy in bilateral streak gonads. The role of the Y chromosome. *Pediatr Surg* 27(1):1376, 1992.

39. Shellhas HF: Malignant potential of the dysgenetic gonad. *Obstet Gynecol* 44:298, 1974.

40. Donahoe PK, Schnitzer JJ: Evaluation of the infant who has ambiguous genitalia, and principles of operative management. *Semin Pediatr Surg* 5(1) 30, 1996.

41. Ramani P, Yeung CK, Habeebu SS: Testicular intratubular germ-cell neoplasia in children and adolescents with intersex. *Am J Surg Pathol* 17(11):1124, 1993.

42. Skakkebaek NE, Berthelsen JG, Visfeldt J: Clinical aspects of testicular carcinoma-in-situ. *Int J Androl* 4:153, 1981.

43. Morris JM, Mahesh VB: Further observations on the syndrome, "testicular feminization." *Am J Obstet Gynecol* 87(6):731, 1963.

44. Muller J, Skakkebaek NE: Testicular carcinoma in situ in children with the androgen insensitivity (testicular feminization) syndrome. *Br Med J* 288:1419, 1984.

45. Hurt WG, Bodurtha JN, McCall JB, et al: Seminoma in pubertal patients with androgen insensitivity syndrome. *Am J Obstet Gynecol* 161:530, 1989.

46. Handa N, Nagasaki A, Tsunoda M, et al: Yolk sac tumor in a case of testicular feminization syndrome. *J Pediatr Surg* 30(9):1366, 1995.

47. Duckett JW: Yolk sac tumor in a case of testicular feminization syndrome. *J Pediatr Surg* 30(6) 1367 (editorial), 1995.

48. Shah R, Woolley MM, Costin G: Testicular feminization: The androgen insensitivity syndrome. *J Pediatr Surg* 27(6):757, 1992.

49. Fonkalsrud EW: The undescended testis. *Curr Probl Surg* 15:5, 1978.

50. Gilbert JB, Hamilton JB: Incidence and nature of tumors in ectopic testes. *Surgery* 71:731, 1940.

51. Fonkalsrud EW: Current management of the undescended testis. *J Pediatr Surg* 5(1):2, 1996.

52. Campbell HE: Incidence of malignant growth of the undescended testicle. *Arch Surg* 44:353, 1942.

53. Johnson DE, Woodhead DM, Pohl DR, et al: Cryptorchidism and testicular tumorigenesis. *Surgery* 63:919, 1968.

54. Altman BL, Malament M: Carcinoma of the testis following orchiopexy. *J Urol* 97:498, 1967.

55. Sohval AR: Testicular dysgenesis as an etiologic factor in cryptorchidism. *J Urol* 72:693, 1954.

56. Einhorn LH, Williams SD, Donohue JP, et al: Cancer of the testes. In DeVita VT Jr, Hellman S, Rosenberg SA (eds): *Cancer, Principles and Practice of Oncology*, 2nd ed. Philadelphia: J.B. Lippincott, 1985, p. 979.

57. Jones BJ, Thornhill JA, O'Donnell B, et al: Influence of prior orchiopexy on stage and prognosis of testicular cancer. *Eur Urol* 19(3):201, 1991.

58. Gitlin D: Normal biology of alpha-fetoprotein. *Ann N Y Acad Sci* 259:7, 1975.

59. Wu JT, Book L, Sudar K: Serum alpha-fetoprotein levels in normal infants. *Pediatr Res* 15:50, 1981.

60. Tsuchida Y, Endo Y, Saito S, et al: Evaluation of alpha-fetoprotein in early infancy. *J Pediatr Surg* 13(2):155, 1978.

61. Germa JR, Llanos M, Tabernero JM, et al: False elevations of alpha-fetoprotein associated with liver dysfunction in germ-cell tumors. *Cancer* 72(8):2491, 1993.

62. Tsuchida Y, Kaneko M, Fukui M, et al: Three different types of alpha-fetoprotein in the diagnosis of malignant solid tumors: Use of a sensitive lectin-affinity immunoelectrophoresis. *J Pediatr Surg* 24(4):350, 1989.

63. Zondag HA: Enzyme activity in dysgerminoma and seminoma. A study of lactic dehydrogenase isoenzymes in malignant disease (the 1963 Fiske essay). *Rhode Island Med J* 47:273, 1964.

64. Snyder CL, Holder TM: Miscellaneous tumors. In Ashcraft KW, Holder TM (eds): *Pediatric Surgery*, 2nd ed. Philadelphia: W.B. Saunders, Co., 1993, p. 898.

65. Breen JL, Maxson WS: Ovarian tumors in children and adolescents. *Clin Obstet Gynecol* 20:607, 1977.

66. Brown MF, Hebra A, McGeehin K, et al: Ovarian masses in children: A review of 91 cases of malignant and benign masses. *J Pediatr Surg* 28(7):930, 1993.

67. Ehren IM, Mahour GH, Isaacs H Jr: Benign and malignant ovarian tumors in children and adolescents: A review of 63 cases. *Am J Surg* 147:339, 1984.

68. Lack EE, Goldstein DP: Primary ovarian tumors in childhood and adolescence. In Leventhal JM (ed): *Current Problems in Obstetrics and Gynecology* Chicago: Year Book, 1984, p. 1.

69. Gribbon M, Ein SH, Mancer K: Pediatric malignant ovarian tumors: A 43-year review. *J Pediatr Surg* 27(4):480, 1992.

70. Brandt ML, Luks FI, Filiatrault D, et al: Surgical indications in antenatally diagnosed ovarian cysts. *J Pediatr Surg* 26(3):276, 1991.

71. Calisti A, Pintus C, Celli S, et al: Fetal ovarian cysts: Postnatal evolution and indications for surgical treatment. *Pediatr Surg Int* 4:341, 1989.

72. Bagolan P, Rivosecchi M, Giorlandino C, et al: Prenatal diagnosis and clinical outcome of ovarian cysts. *J Pediatr Surg* 27(7):879, 1992.

73. Campbell BA, Garg RS, Garg K, et al: Perinatal ovarian cyst: A nonsurgical approach. *J Pediatr Surg* 27(12):1618, 1992.

74. Croitoru DP, Aaron LE, Laberge JM, et al: Management of complex ovarian cysts presenting in the first year of life. *J Pediatr Surg* 26(12):1366, 1991.

75. Van der Zee DC, van Seumeren IGC, Bax KMA, et al: Laparoscopic approach to surgical management of ovarian cysts in the newborn. *J Pediatr Surg* 30(1):42, 1995.

76. Warner BW, Kuhn JC, Barr LL: Conservative management of large ovarian cysts in children: The value of serial pelvic ultrasonography. *Surgery* 112(4):749, 1992.

77. Thind CR, Carty HML, Pilling DW: The role of ultrasound in the management of ovarian masses in children. *Clin Radiol* 40:180, 1989.

78. Scully RE: Sex cord tumor with annular tubules. A distinctive ovarian tumor of the Peutz-Jeghers syndrome. *Cancer* 25:1107, 1970.

79. Lemerle J: Juvenile granulosa cell tumor of the ovary in children: A clinical study of 15 cases. *J Clin Oncol* 6:990, 1988.

80. Gustafson ML, Lee MM, Asmundson L, et al: Müllerian inhibiting substance in the diagnosis and management of intersex and gonadal abnormalities. *J Pediatr Surg* 28(3); 439, 1993.

81. Junaid JA: Ovarian neoplasms in children and adolescents in Ibadan, Nigeria. *Cancer* 47:610, 1981.

82. Ferry JA, Young RH: Malignant lymphoma, pseudolymphoma, and hematopoietic disorders of the female genital tract. In Rosen PP, Fechner RE (eds): *Pathology Annual*, 26th ed. Norwalk, CT: Appleton & Lange, 1991, p. 227.

83. Skinner MA, Schlatter MG, Heifetz SA, et al: Ovarian neoplasms in Children. *Arch Surg* 128:849, 1993.

84. Kleinman GM, Young RH, Scully RE: Primary neuroectodermal tumors of the ovary: A report of 25 cases. *Am J Surg Path* 17(8):764, 1993.

85. Slayton RE, Park RC, Silvergerg SG, et al: Vincristine, dactinomycin, and cyclophosphamide in the treatment of malignant germ-cell tumors of the ovary: A gynecologic oncology group study (a final report). *Cancer* 56:243, 1985.

86. Kawai M, Kano T, Furuhasi Y, et al: Prognostic factors in yolk sac tumors of the ovary: A clinicopathologic analysis of 29 cases. *Cancer* 67(1):184, 1991.

87. Davis TE, Loprinzi CL, Buchler DA: Combination chemotherapy with cisplatin, vinblastine, and bleomycin for endodermal sinus tumor of the ovary. *Gynecol Oncol* 19:46, 1984.

88. Sessa C, Bonazzi C, Landoni F, et al: Cisplatin, vinblastine, and bleomycin combination chemotherapy in endodermal sinus tumor of the ovary. *Obstet Gynecol* 70:220, 1987.

89. Forney JP: Pregnancy following removal and chemotherapy of ovarian endodermal sinus tumor. *Obstet Gynecol* 52:360, 1978.

90. Karlen JR, Kastelic JE: Endodermal sinus tumor of the ovary: An improving prognosis. *Gynecol Oncol* 10:206, 1980.

91. Wu PC, Huang RL, Lang JH, et al: Treatment of malignant ovarian germ-cell tumors with preservation of fertility: A report of 28 cases. *Gynecol Oncol* 40(1):2, 1991.

92. FIGO Cancer Committee. Staging announcement. *Gynecol Oncol* 25:303, 1986.

93. Valente PT, Schantz HD. Edmonds PR, et al: Peritoneal cytology of uncommon ovarian tumors. *Diagn Cytopathol* 8(2):98, 1992.

94. Cangir A, Smith J, van Eys J, et al: Improved prognosis in children with ovarian cancers following modified VAC (vincristine sulfate, dactinomycin, and cyclophosphamide) chemotherapy. *Cancer* 42(3):1234, 1978.

95. Einhorn LH, Donohue J: *Cis*-diamminedichloroplatinum, vinblastine, and bleomycin combination chemotherapy in disseminated testicular cancer. *Ann Intern Med* 87:293, 1977.

96. Carlson RW, Sikic BI, Turbow MM, et al: Combination cisplatin, vinblastine, and bleomycin chemotherapy (PVB) for malignant germ-cell tumors of the ovary. *J Clin Oncol* 1(10):645, 1983.

97. Jacob AJ, Harris M, Deppe G, et al: Treatment of recurrent and persistent germ-cell tumors with cisplatin, vinblastine, and bleomycin. *Obstet Gynecol* 59:129, 1982.

98. Williams SD, Blessing JA, Slayton R, et al: Ovarian germ-cell tumors: Adjuvant trials of the gynecologic oncology group. In Salmon S (ed): *Proceedings of the Sixth International Conference on the Adjuvant Therapy of Cancer*, 1990, p. 501.

99. Hicks ML, Piver MS: Conservative surgery plus adjuvant therapy for vulvo-vaginal rhabdomyosarcoma, diethylstilbestrol clear-cell adenocarcinoma of the vagina, and unilateral germ-cell tumors of the ovary. *Obstet Gynecol Clin North Am* 19(1):219, 1992.

100. Peterson WF: Malignant degeneration of benign cystic teratomas of the ovary: A collective review of the literature. *Obstet Gynecol Surv* 12:793, 1957.

101. Kempers RD, Dockerty MD, Hoffman DL, et al: Struma ovarii—ascitic, hyperthyroid and asymptomatic syndromes. *Ann Intern Med* 72:883, 1970.

102. Robboy SJ, Scully RE: Ovarian teratoma with glial implants on the peritoneum: An analysis of 12 cases. *Hum Pathol* 1:643, 1970.

103. Truong LD, Jurco S III, McGavran MH: Gliomatosis peritonei: Report of two cases and review of literature. *Am J Surg Pathol* 6:443, 1982.

104. Gershenson DM, Del Junco G, Silva EG, et al: Immature teratoma of the ovary. *Obstet Gynecol* 68:624, 1986.

105. Curry SL, Smith JP, Gallaher HS: Malignant teratoma of the ovary: Prognostic factors and treatment. *Am J Obstet Gynecol* 131:845, 1978.

106. Cushing B, Biller R, Cohen L, et al: Surgery alone is effective treatment of resected ovarian immature teratoma (OIT) in children: A pediatric intergroup report (POG 9048/CCG 8891). ASCO Annual Meeting (abstract), May 1996.

107. Friedman M, White RG, Nissenbaum MM, et al: Serum lactic dehydrogenase—A possible tumor marker for an ovarian dysgerminoma: A literature review and report of a case. *Obstet Gynecol Surv* 39:247, 1984.

108. Gordon A, Lipton D, Woodruff D: Dysgerminoma: A review of 158 cases from the Emil Novak ovarian tumor registry. *Obstet Gynecol* 58:497, 1981.

109. Gershenson DM, Morris M, Cangir A, et al: Treatment of malignant germ-cell tumors of the ovary with bleomycin, etoposide and cisplatin. *J Clin Oncol* 8:715, 1990.

110. Williams SD, Blessing J, Hatch K, et al: Chemotherapy of advanced ovarian dysgerminomas: Trials of the Gynecologic Oncology Group. *Proc Am Soc Clin Oncol* 9:155(abstract), 1990.

111. Williams SD: Chemotherapy of ovarian germ-cell tumors. *Hematol Oncol Clin of North Am* 5(6):1261, 1991.

112. Copeland LJ: Malignant gynecologic tumors. In Sutow WW, Fernbach GJ, Vietti TJ (eds): *Clinical Pediatric Oncology*, 3rd ed. St. Louis: C.V. Mosby Co., 1984, p. 744.

113. Kurman RJ, Norris HJ: Endodermal sinus tumor of the ovary. *Cancer* 38:2404, 1976.

114. Ohta M, Kano T, Nishida Y, et al: Embryonal carcinoma (Higuchi Kato) of the ovary: Clinical analysis and recent improvement using AFP as a tumor marker. *Acta Obstet Gynecol Jpn* 38:887, 1986.

115. Kurman RJ, Norris HJ: Malignant mixed germ-cell tumors of the ovary: A clinical and pathological analysis of 30 cases. *Obstet Gynecol* 48:579, 1976.

116. Nakashima N, Murakami S, Fukatsu T, et al: Characteristics of "embryoid bodies" in human gonadal germ-cell tumors. *Hum Pathol* 19:1144, 1988.

117. Kurman RJ, Norris HJ: Malignant germ-cell tumors of the ovary. *Hum Pathol* 8:551, 1977.

118. Hopkins TB, Jaffe N, Colodny A, et al: The management of testicular tumors in children. *J Urol* 12:96, 1978.

119. Einhorn LH, Donohue JP: Combination chemotherapy in disseminated testicular cancer: The Indiana University Experience. *Semin Oncol* 6:87, 1979.

120. Brosman S, Gondos B: Testicular tumors in children. In Johnston JH, Goodwin WE (eds): *Review in Pediatric Urology*, New York: American Elsevier Publishing Co., 1974, p. 162.

121. Visfeldt J, Jorgensen N, Muller J, et al: Testicular germ-cell tumours of childhood in Denmark, 1943–1989: Incidence and evaluation of histology using immunohistochemical techniques. *J Pathol* 174:39, 1994.

122. Jacobsen GK, Pedersen BN: Placental alkaline phosphatase in testicular germ-cell tumours and carcinoma in situ of the testis: An immunohistochemical study. *Acta Pathol Microbiol Immunol Scand* 92:323, 1984.

123. Muller J, Skakkebaek NE Nielsen OH, et al: Cryptorchidism and testis cancer: Atypical infantile germ cells followed by carcinoma in situ and invasive carcinoma in adulthood. *Cancer* 54:629, 1984.

124. Skakkebaek NE: Carcinoma in situ of the testis: Frequency and relationship to invasive germ-cell tumours in infertile men. *Histopathology* 2:157, 1978.

125. Guinand S, Hedinger C: Cellules germinales atypiques intratubulaires et tumeurs germinales testiculaires del'enfant. *Ann Pathol* 1:251, 1981.

126. Manivel JC, Cimonton JS, Lester E, et al: Absence of intratubular germ-cell neoplasia in testicular yolk sac tumours in children. *Arch Pathol Lab Med* 112:641, 1988.

127. Manivel JC, Reinberg Y, Niehans GA, et al: Intratubular germ-cell neoplasia in testicular teratomas and epidermoid cysts. *Cancer* 64:715, 1989.

128. Soosay GN, Bobrow L, Happerfield L, et al: Morphology and immunohistochemistry of carcinoma in situ adjacent to testicular germ-cell tumours in adults and children: Implications for histogenesis. *Histopathology* 19:537, 1991.

129. Jorgensen N, Muller J, Giwercman A, et al: DNA content and expression of tumour markers in germ cells adjacent to germ-cell tumours in childhood: Probably a different origin for infantile and adolescent germ cell tumours. *J Pathol* 176(3):269, 1995.

130. Kaplan GW, Gromie WC, Kelalis PP, et al: Prepubertal yolk sac tumors—Report of the Testicular Tumor Registry. *J Urol* 140:1109, 1988.

131. Huddart SN, Mann JR, Gornall P, et al: The UK Children's Cancer Study Group: Testicular Malignant Germ Cell Tumours 1979–1988. *J Pediatr Surg* 25(4):406, 1990.

132. Filler RM, Hardy BE: Testicular tumors in children. *World J Surg* 4:63, 1980.

133. Karamehmedovic O, Woodti W, Pluss HJ: Testicular tumors in childhood. *J Pediatr Surg* 10:109, 1975.

134. Brosman SA: Male genital tract. In Kelalis PP, King LR, Belman AB (eds): *Clinical Pediatric Urology*, 2nd ed. Philadelphia: W.B. Saunders Co., 1985, p. 1202.

135. Weissbach L, Altwein JE, Steins R: Germinal testicular tumors in childhood. Report of observations and literature review. *Eur Urol* 10:73, 1984.

136. Brown NJ: Teratomas and yolk sac tumours. *J Clin Path* 29:1021, 1976.

137. Rushton HG, Belman AB, Sesterhenn I, et al: Testicular-sparing surgery for prepubertal teratoma of the testis: A clinical and pathological study. *J Urol* 144:726, 1990.

138. Stamp IM, Barlebo H, Rix M, et al: Intratubular germ-cell neoplasia in an infantile testis with immature teratoma. *Histopathology* 22:69, 1993.

139. Renedo DE, Trainer TD: Intratubular germ-cell neoplasia (ITGCN) with p53 and PCNA expression and adjacent mature teratoma in an infant testis: An immunohistochemical and morphologic study with a review of the literature. *Am J Surg Pathol* 18(9):947, 1994.

140. Exelby PR: Testis cancer in children. *Semin Oncol* 6:116, 1976.

141. Peckham MJ, Barrett A, Husband JE, et al: Orchiectomy alone in testicular Stage I non-seminomatous germ cell tumors. *Lancet* 11:678, 1982.

142. Carroll WL, Kempson RL, Govan DE, et al: Conservative management of testicular endodermal sinus tumor in childhood. *J Urol* 133:1011, 1985.

143. Flamant F, Nihoul-Fekete C, Palte C, et al: Optimal treatment of stage I yolk sac tumor of the testes in children. *J Pediatr Surg* 21:108, 1986.

144. Griffin GC, Raney Jr RB, Snyder HM, et al: Yolk sac carcinoma of the testis in children. *J Urol* 137:954, 1987.

145. Haas RJ, Schmidt P, Gobel U, et al: Testicular germ-cell tumors: Results of the GPO MAHO studies −82, −88, −92. *Klin Padiatr* 207(4):145, 1995.

146. Rogers DA, Rao BN, Meyer WH, et al: Indications for hemiscrotectomy in the management of genitourinary tumors in children. *J Pediatr Surg* 30(10):1437, 1995.

147. Giguere JF, Stablein DM, Spaulding JT, et al: The clinical significance of unconventional orchiectomy approaches in testicular cancer: A report from the Testicular Cancer Intergroup study. *J Urol* 139:1225, 1988.

148. Bredael JJ, Vugrin D, Whitmore WF: Recurrences in surgical stage I nonseminomatous germ-cell tumors of the testis. *J Urol* 130:476, 1983.

149. Boileau MA, Steers WD: Testis tumors: The clinical significance of the tumor-contaminated scrotum. *J Urol* 132:51, 1984.

150. Kennedy CL, Hendry WF, Peckham MJ: The significance of scrotal interference in Stage I testicular cancer managed by orchiectomy and surveillance. *Br J Urol* 58:705, 1986.

151. Denton KJ, Cotton DWK, Nakielnyu RA, et al: Secondary tumor deposits in needle biopsy tracks: An underestimated risk. *J Clin Pathol* 43:83, 1990.

152. Kaplan WE, Filit CF: Treatment of testicular yolk sac carcinoma in the young child. *J Urol* 126:663, 1981.

153. Homsy Y, Arroja-Vila F, Khoriaty N, et al: Yolk sac tumor of the testicle: Is retroperitoneal lymph node dissection necessary? *J Urol* 132:532, 1984.

154. Bracken RB, Johnson DE, Cangir A, et al: Regional lymph nodes in infants with embryonal carcinoma of testis. *Urology* 11:376, 1978.

155. Stomper PC, Kalish LA, Barnick MB, et al: CT and pathologic predictive features of residual mass histologic findings after chemotherapy for nonseminomatous germ-cell tumors: Can residual malignancy or teratoma be excluded? *Radiology* 180(3):711, 1991.

156. Gilcrease MZ, Brandt ML, Hawkins EP: Yolk sac tumor identified at autopsy after surgical excision of immature sacrococcygeal teratoma. *J Pediatr Surg* 30(6):875, 1995.

157. Luna M, Valenzuela-Tamariz J: Germ-cell tumors of the mediastinum: Postmortem findings. *Am J Clin Pathol* 65:450, 1976.

158. Luna M, Johnson P: Postmortem findings in testicular tumors. In Johnson DE (ed): *Testicular Tumors*, New York: New York Medical Examination Publishing, 1976.

159. Lynch M, Blewett G: Choriocarcinoma arising in the male mediastinum. *Thorax* 8:157, 1953.

160. Nichols CR, Fox EP: Extragonadal and pediatric germ-cell tumors. *Hematol Oncol Clin North Am* 5(6):1189, 1991.

161. Daugaard G, Rorth M, von der Maase H, et al: Management of extragonadal germ-cell tumors and the significance of bilateral testicular biopsies. *Ann Oncol* 3(4):283, 1992.

162. Collins D, Pugh R: Classification and frequency of testicular tumours. *Br J Urol* 36(1):11, 1964.

163. Hawkins EP, Finegold MJ, Hawkins HK, et al: Nongerminomatous malignant germ-cell tumors in children: A review of 89 cases from the Pediatric Oncology Group, 1974–1984. *Cancer* 58:2579, 1986.

164. Pantoja E, Llobet R, Gonzales-Flores B: Retroperitoneal teratoma: Historical review. *J Urol* 115:520, 1976.

165. Grosfeld JL, Billmire DF: Teratomas in infancy and childhood. *Curr Probl Cancer* 9(9):1, 1985.

166. Altman RP, Randolph JG, Lilly JR: Sacrococcygeal teratoma: American Academy of Pediatrics Surgical Section Survey—1973. *J Pediatr Surg* 9(3):389, 1974.

167. Harrison MR, Adzick NS: The fetus as a patient: Surgical considerations. *Ann Surg* 213(4):279, 1991.

168. Flake AW, Harrison MR, Adzick NS, et al: Fetal sacrococcygeal teratoma. *J Pediatr Surg* 21(7):563, 1986.

169. Bond SJ, Harrison MR, Schmidt KG, et al: Death due to high-output cardiac failure in fetal sacrococcygeal teratoma. *J Pediatr Surg* 25(2):1287, 1990.

170. Flake AW: Fetal sacrococcygeal teratoma. *J Pediatr Surg* 2(2):113, 1993.

171. Rescorla FJ: Preliminary report of the CCG surgery survey of neonatal sacrococcygeal teratomas. Presented November 1994, Dallas, TX.

172. Grosfeld JL, Ballantine TVN, Lowe D, et al: Benign and malignant teratomas in children: Analysis of 85 patients. *Surgery* 80:297, 1976.

173. Donnellan WA, Swenson O: Benign and malignant sacrococcygeal teratoma. *Surgery* 64:834, 1968.

174. Hickey RC, Layton JM: Sacrococcygeal teratoma. *Cancer* 7:1031, 1954.

175. Ein SH, Mancer K, Adeyemi SD: Malignant sacrococcygeal teratoma-endodermal sinus, yolk sac tumor—in infants and children: A 32-year review. *J Pediatr Surg* 20(5):473, 1985.

176. Ashcraft KW, Holder TM: Congenital anal stenosis with presacral teratoma. *Ann Surg* 162:1091, 1965.

177. Ashcraft KW, Holder TM: Hereditary presacral teratoma. *J Pediatr Surg* 9(5):691, 1974.

178. Yates VD, Wilroy RS, Whitington GL, et al: Anterior sacral defects: An autosomal dominantly inherited condition. *Pediatrics* 102(2):239, 1983.

179. Cohn J, Bay-Nielsen E: Hereditary defect of the sacrum and coccyx with anterior sacral meningocele. *Acta Paediatr Scand* 58:28, 1969.

180. O'Riordain, DS, O'Connell PR, Kirwan WO: Hereditary sacral agenesis with presacral mass and anorectal stenosis: The Currarino triad. *Br J Surg* 78:536, 1991.

181. Currarino G, Coln D, Votteler T: Triad of anorectal, sacral, and presacral anomalies. *AJR* 137:395, 1981.

182. Powell RW, Weber ED, Manci EA: Intradural extension of a sacrococcygeal teratoma. *J Pediatr Surg* 28(6):770, 1993.

183. Teal LN, Angtuaco TL, Jimenez JF, et al: Fetal teratomas: Antenatal diagnosis and clinical management. *J Clin Ultrasound* 16:329, 1988.

184. Gross RE, Clatworthy HWJ, Meeker IAJ: Sacrococcygeal teratoma in infants and children. *Surg Gynecol Obstet* 92:341, 1951.

185. Waldhausen JA, Kolman JW, Vellios F, et al: Sacrococcygeal teratoma. *Surgery* 54:933, 1963.

186. Mahour HG, Woolley MM, Trivedi SN, et al: Sacrococcygeal teratoma: A 33-year experience. *J Pediatr Surg* 10:183, 1975.

187. Wooley MM: Teratomas. In Ashcraft KW, Holder TM (eds): *Pediatric Surgery*, 2nd ed. Philadelphia: W.B. Saunders, 1993, p. 847.

188. Billmire DF, Grosfeld JL: Teratomas in childhood: Analysis of 142 cases. *J Pediatr Surg* 21:548, 1986.

189. Murphy JJ, Blair GK, Fraser GC: Coagulopathy associated with large sacrococcygeal teratomas. *J Pediatr Surg* 27(10):1308, 1992.

190. Robertson FM, Crombleholme TM, Frantz III ID, et al: Devascularization and staged resection of giant sacrococcygeal teratoma in the premature infant. *J Pediatr Surg* 30(2):309, 1995.

191. Lindahl H: Giant sacrococcygeal teratoma: A method of simple intraoperative control of hemorrhage. *J Pediatr Surg* 23(11):1068, 1988.

192. Teitelbaum D, Teich S, Cassidy S, et al: Highly vascularized sacrococcygeal teratoma: Description of this atypical variant and its operative management. *J Pediatr Surg* 29(1):98, 1994.

193. Lund DP, Soriano SG, Fauza D, et al: Resection of a massive sacrococcygeal teratoma using hypothermic hypoperfusion: A novel use of extracorporeal membrane oxygenation. *J Pediatr Surg* 30(11): 1557, 1995.

194. Hawkins E, Issacs H, Cushing B, et al: Occult malignancy in neonatal sacrococcygeal teratomas. *Am J Pediatr Hematol Oncol* 15(4):406, 1993.

195. Bilik R, Shandling B, Pope M, et al: Malignant benign neonatal sacrococcygeal teratoma. *J Pediatr Surg* 28(9):1158, 1993.

196. Lahdenne P, Heikinheimo M, Nikkanen V, et al: Neonatal benign sacrococcygeal teratoma may recur in adulthood and give rise to malignancy. *Cancer* 72(12):3727, 1993.

197. Gonzalez-Crussi F, Winkler RF, Mirkin DL: Sacrococcygeal teratomas in infants and children: Relationship of histology and prognosis in 40 cases. *Arch Pathol Lab Med* 102:420, 1978.

198. Valdiserri RO, Yunis EJ: Sacrococcygeal teratomas: A review of 68 cases. *Cancer* 48:217, 1981.

199. Rintala R, Lahdenne P, Lindahl H, et al: Anorectal function in adults operated for a benign sacrococcygeal teratoma. *J Pediatr Surg* 28(9):1165, 1993.

200. Malone PS, Spitz L, Kiely EM, et al: The functional sequelae of sacrococcygeal teratoma. *J Pediatr Surg* 25(6):679, 1990.

201. Boemers TMl, van Gool JD, de Jong TPVM, et al: Lower urinary tract dysfunction in children with benign sacrococcygeal teratoma. *J Urol* 151:174, 1994.

202. Havranek P, Hedlund H, Rubenson A, et al: Sacrococcygeal teratoma in Sweden between 1978 and 1989: Long-term functional results. *J Pediatr Surg* 27(7):916, 1992.

203. Reinberg Y, Long R, Manivel JC, et al: Urological aspects of sacrococcygeal teratoma in children. *J Urol* 150:948, 1993.

204. Lahdenne P, Heikinheimo M, Jaaskelainen J, et al: Vertebral abnormalities associated with congenital sacrococcygeal teratomas. *J Pediatr Orthop* 11:603, 1991.

205. Dehner L: Gonadal and extragonadal germ-cell neoplasms in childhood. *Hum Pathol* 14:493, 1983.

206. Lakhoo K, Boyle M, Drake DP: Mediastinal teratomas: Review of 15 pediatric cases. *J Pediatr Surg* 28(7):1161, 1993.

207. Loehrer P, Mandelbaum I, Hui S, et al: Resection of thoracic and abdominal teratoma in patients after cisplatin-based chemotherapy for germ-cell tumor. *J Thorac Cardiovasc* 92:676, 1986.

208. Ulbright T, Loehrer P, Roth L, et al: The development of non-germ-cell malignancies within germ-cell tumor: A clinicopathologic study in 11 cases. *Cancer* 54:1824, 1984.

209. Nichols C, Roth B, Heerema N, et al: Hematologic neoplasia associated with primary mediastinal germ-cell tumors: An update. *N Engl J Med* 322:1425, 1990.

210. Teal LN, Angtuaco TL, Jimenez JF, et al: Fetal teratomas: Antenatal diagnosis and clinical management. *J Clin Ultrasound* 16:329, 1988.

211. Rosenfeld CR, Coln CD, Duenhoelter JH: Fetal cervical teratomas as a cause of polyhydramnios. *Pediatrics* 64:176, 1979.

212. Azizkhan RG, Haase GM, Applebaum H, et al: Diagnosis, management and outcome of cervicofacial teratomas in neonates: A Children's Cancer Group study. *J Pediatr Surg* 30(2):312, 1995.

213. Touran T, Applebaum H, Frost DB, et al: Congenital metastatic cervical teratoma: Diagnostic and management considerations. *J Pediatr Surg* 24:21, 1989.

214. Mahour GH, Landing BH, Woolley MM: Teratomas in children: Clinicopathologic studies in 133 patients. *Z Kinderchir* 23:365, 1978.

215. Srikanth MS, Ford EWG, Mahour GH: Gastric teratoma: Report of two cases. *Contemp Surg* 44:166, 1994.

216. Gengler JS, Ashcraft KW, Slattery P: Gastric teratoma: The sixth reported case in a female infant. *J Pediatr Surg* 30(6):889, 1995.

217. Cairo MS, Grosfeld JL, Wheetman RM: Gastric teratoma: Unusual case for bleeding of the upper gastrointestinal tract in the newborn. *Pediatrics* 67:721, 1981.

218. Mester M, Trajber HJ, Compton CC, et al: Cystic teratomas of the pancreas. *Arch Surg* 125:1215, 1990.

219. Dennis WA: Dermoid cysts of the pancreas. *Surg Clin North Am* 3:1319, 1923.

220. Copeland LJ, Sneige N, Ordonez NG, et al: Endodermal sinus tumor of the vagina and cervix. *Cancer* 55:2558, 1985.

221. Hwang EH, Han SJ, Lee MK, et al: Clinical experience with conservative surgery for vaginal endodermal sinus tumor. *J Pediatr Surg* 31(2):219, 1996.

222. Young RH, Scully RE: Endodermal sinus tumor of the vagina: A report of nine cases and review of literature. *Gynecol Oncol* 18:380, 1984.

Hodgkin's and Non-Hodgkin's Lymphoma

• *Thomas Whalen, M.D.*

Lymphoma is the second most common malignancy of childhood. Although similar histologically, Hodgkin's disease (HD) and Non-Hodgkin's lymphoma (NHL) are vastly different in biology, treatment, and prognosis.

The role of the pediatric surgeon in treatment of these diseases is in evolution now, with a trend toward minimal involvement. For HD staging, laparotomy remains undisputedly the most accurate method to delineate extent of disease precisely. Yet, for therapy of all HD patients, young and old, chemotherapy has taken a predominant role. Oncologists thus believe that the precise staging afforded by laparotomy has come to have academic value and no clinical import. Second malignancies are, however, increasingly reported and need to be prominently considered in risk-benefit calculations when recommending treatment options.

BACKGROUND

Hodgkin's Disease

The incidence of Hodgkin's disease is increasing. This is especially so in the pediatric population and is led by an increase in the incidence of the nodular-sclerosis histologic subtype.[1] When comparing the 5-year intervals of 1973–1977 versus 1983–1987, one sees a dramatic increase in this subtype, rising from 1.1 per 100,000 to 1.6 per 100,000. The overall incidence of HD is reviewed in Figure 14–1. One can see in that

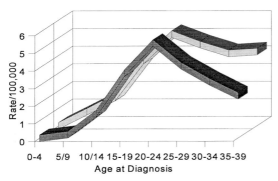

Figure 14–1 • Patients' ages at diagnosis of Hodgkin's disease in first four decades of life. (From SEER Data (Surveillance, Epidemiology, and End Results): 1983–1987. In Medeiros LJ, Greiner TC: Hodgkin's disease. *Cancer* 75(suppl. 1):357–359, 1995, with permission.)

same figure that HD is not a disease of the very young. In the experience at Stanford University, from 1961 through 1991 there were 2238 patients seen with HD, of whom only 91, or 4%, were below the age of 10 years at the time of original diagnosis.[2] Outcome in this age group is highly favorable; the 5-year survival rate is 94%, and the 10-year survival rate is 92%, either when comparing all patients and/or when stratifying them by stage. There may be an advantage in this age group for those with Stage III and IV disease over adolescents and adults, although the incidence decreases; 25-year actuarial survival rate is 89% for those younger than 10 at time of diagnosis compared with 28% for adolescents and 41% for adults.

More than 85% of patients with HD will prove to have disease within the chest. Computerized tomography is superior to plain chest radiographs in detecting disease within the chest.[3]

Non-Hodgkin's Lymphoma

Non-Hodgkin's lymphoma (NHL) is far less common than HD. It may occur throughout the body. Biopsy is the primary role for the pediatric surgeon, although occasional intra-abdominal disease may be encountered that needs to be surgically removed as a primary therapy.

Approximately 10% of NHL cases in the pediatric population involve the nasal-paranasal oropharyngeal area. Sites of primary occurrence include the maxillary sinus, tonsil, posterior

pharynx, orbit, and mandible.[4] Such malignancies are curable in three quarters of patients when treated with aggressive chemotherapy and radiation therapy.

One classification of NHL allows for *indolent lymphomas,* low-grade lymphomas accounting for about 25% of patients with NHL that are usually quite sensitive to chemotherapy, even with a single agent, or are radiosensitive. Unfortunately, such sensitivity relates to remission, not cure, and even more aggressive treatment regimens have failed to prevent the near-uniform frequent relapses that occur. The only patients likely to be cured are younger patients with early-stage disease responding to radiation.[5] For the rare pediatric patient presenting with a low-grade or indolent lymphoma, the typical approach to the patient in the fifth or sixth decades of life, namely a conservative, no initial therapy approach, is clearly unacceptable. It will lead to a median survival of only 10 years. Yet there are few established effective treatments for such patients. One technique involves high-dose therapy with BCNU, etoposide, cytosine arabinoside, and melphalan, followed by marrow purging and autologous bone marrow transplantation. Preliminary results are favorable, but longer follow-up will be necessary for evaluation of efficacy.[6]

BIOLOGY

Hodgkin's Disease

The classic differentiation of HD has been and continues to be histologic classification. There are four major histologic types recognized:

Lymphocyte predominant	3%
Lymphocyte depleted	5%
Mixed cellularity	25%
Nodular sclerosis	67%

Lymphocyte-depleted histology is extremely rare in children and adolescents. Nodular-sclerosis histology is not only the most common type overall but also accounts for the continuing increase in the incidence of this disease in the young.

Long-term analysis has called into question the value of simple histologic differentiation.[7] Figure 14–2 shows graphically by long-term survival rates of the 1770 patients in the Stanford series that histology does not differentiate survival rates at all. Rosenberg[7] states in the just

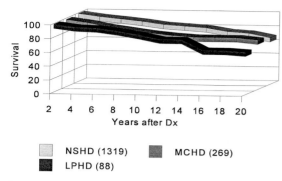

NSHD (1319)   MCHD (269)
LPHD (88)

Figure 14–2 • Overall survival of patients with Hodgkin's disease according to histology. (From Rosenberg SA: The treatment of Hodgkin's disease. *Ann Oncol* 5(suppl. 2):17–21, 1994, adapted with permission from Kluwer Academic Publishers.)

cited article, "The classic prognostic factors of histologic subtype, stage, and extent of disease are no longer relevant in predicting cure and survival of patients with Hodgkin's disease."

Whether derived by imaging (clinical staging) or histology (staging laparotomy with pathologic staging), there is a recognized staging system that uses the results of that process to set prognosis and to some extent therapy. This time-honored system is that of the Ann Arbor staging system (Table 14–1). The Cotswold modification has also been proposed (Table 14–2). Either system can help in making a prognosis.

In more than 80% of cases, HD begins above the diaphragm and proceeds stepwise from one nodal group to another. The essential biologic behavior and natural history of the disease are no different in adults than in children.[8] Disease that exists beneath the diaphragm will determine if the patient is Stage III or IV, and most often such disease will not exist at a sufficiently gross level to allow imaging by any available modality. The most common locus of this microscopic disease remains the spleen. In 26% of patients who have been clinically staged as I or II, disease is found within the spleen at a microscopic level. Of those patients with unimaged infradiaphragmatic disease, 50% will have only splenic disease within all submitted tissues.[9]

New frontiers in the biology of HD exist in several areas. Much literature exists on the association of HD and the Epstein-Barr virus.[10, 11] Geographic variations in the prevalence of the virus in association with HD are quite marked.

Table 14–1 • Ann Arbor Staging Classification for Hodgkin's Disease

Stage	Definition
I	Involvement or a single lymph node region (I) or of a single extra lymphatic organ or site (I_E)
II	Involvement of two or more lymph node regions on the same side of the diaphragm (II) or localized involvement of an extra lymphatic organ or site and one or more lymph node lesions on the same side of the diaphragm (II_E)
III	Involvement of lymph node regions on both sides of the diaphragm (III), which may be accompanied by involvement of the spleen (III_S) or by localized involvement of an extra lymphatic organ or site (III_E) or both (III_{ES})
IV	Diffuse or disseminated involvement of one or more extra lymphatic organs or tissues with or without associated lymph node involvement

From Hoekstra HJ, Tamminga RYJ, Timens W: Partial splenectomy in children: An alternative for splenectomy in the pathological staging of Hodgkin's disease. *Ann Surg Oncol* 1:480–486, 1994.

Patients in the Western World will have the virus as little as 30% of the time compared with 100% for those in Third World countries. Since the virus is associated with at least three other

Table 14–2 • Cotswold's Staging Classification

Stage	Definition
I	Involvement of single lymphoid region or structure
II	Involvement of two or more lymphoid regions on same side of diaphragm
III	Involvement of lymphoid structures on both sides of diaphragm
III_1	Involvement limited to upper abdomen or spleen
III_2	Involvement in lower abdomen or pelvis
IV	Diffuse involvement
A	No symptoms
B	Fever, night sweats, weight loss
X	Nodal mass greater than 10 cm, or mediastinum widened greater than one third
E	Extranodal involvement
CS	Clinical stage
PS	Pathologic stage (staging laparotomy)

From Lister TA, Crowther D, Sutcliffe SB: Report of a committee convened to discuss the evaluation and staging of patients with Hodgkin's disease: Cotswold's meeting. *J Clin Oncol* 7:1630–1636, 1989.

malignancies—Burkitt's lymphoma, nasopharyngeal carcinoma, and post-transplant lymphoma—the demonstrated ability to induce tumors and immortalize lymphoid cells in the laboratory may be part of the oncogenesis of HD as well.

Non-Hodgkin's Lymphoma

Molecular biology is investigating NHL tumors with vigor. The *MIC2* gene has been known to geneticists for more than 15 years. It was first shown to be expressed highly in acute lymphocytic leukemias of the T-cell type. Subsequently, many small-, round-cell tumors of childhood have been found to express the *MIC2* gene, including Ewing's sarcoma and primitive neuroectodermal tumors, but the gene is not seen in small-cell osteosarcomas, neuroblastomas, or most rhabdomyosarcomas. The *MIC2* gene has been shown to be expressed in lymphoblastic lymphomas.[12]

There has been a well-known link between Epstein-Barr virus (EBV) and Burkitt's lymphoma for some time. The virus is also associated with other large-cell lymphomas in immunosuppressed patients. The apparent pathophysiology is that EBV infection of B-lymphocytes leads to activation of cellular growth-related pathways, and at least one study has posited that EBV latent protein serves to activate the *bcl*-2 oncogene. This has the effect of prolonged cell survival by protecting the cell from apoptosis.[13]

MEDICAL THERAPY

Once the central component of treatment for HD, radiation therapy (RT) has been receiving less and less emphasis. Children in the early 1970s would receive 35–40 Gy of RT. This treatment would lead to skeletal and soft-tissue hypoplasia in most prepubertal children. Consequently, reduced doses of RT were designed to avert this complication: 20–25 Gy in more limited fields, along with chemotherapy.[14] Such a change in approach has led to essentially equivalent outcomes as measured by event-free survival rates and 10-year survival rates. The design of multimodal therapy in children in the hope of averting the severe complications of high-dose radiation is attributed to Donaldson and Kaplan.[15]

Chemotherapy is thus at the core of all protocols of treatment for HD. Formerly the mainstay of therapy was MOPP, which is the acronym for mechlorethamine, vincristine (Oncovin), procarbazine, and prednisone. In the 1970s, however, the newer multiagent therapy of ABVD was designed: doxorubicin (Adriamycin), bleomycin, vinblastine, and dacarbazine (DTIC).[16] This therapy was shown as early as 1975 to be superior to MOPP and was moreover effective in MOPP crossover treatment failures. ABVD also has the long-term advantage of fewer delayed second malignancies at least as far as the most prominent histologic variant of acute nonlymphoblastic leukemia (ANLL) (Fig. 14–3).

If a reliable diagnosis of limited Hodgkin's disease is made in a child, then radiation may become an optional component of therapy or may even be omitted.[17] Patients with this localized disease at Stanford were randomized to receive either combination chemotherapy with RT or chemotherapy alone. Follow-up at the time of report averaged 38 months, and no difference was found in event-free survival rates. Patients who received RT had a greater amount of toxic side effects.

A newer, less well-known therapy that has also been employed in an attempt to reduce treatment morbidity is termed the *Vancouver hybrid*.[18] This therapy incorporates seven drugs: mechlorethamine, vincristine (Oncovin), procar-

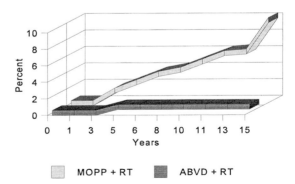

Figure 14–3 • Risk of acute nonlymphoblastic leukemia (ANLL) in patients treated with MOPP (mechlorethamine, vincristine [Oncovin], procarbazine, prednisone) plus RT (radiation therapy) versus ABVD (doxorubicin [Adriamycin], bleomycin, vinblastine, dacarbazine) plus RT. (From Bonadonna G: Modern treatment of malignant lymphomas: A multidisciplinary approach? The Kaplan Memorial Lecture. *Ann Oncol* 5(suppl. 2):5–16, 1994, adapted with permission from Kluwer Academic Publishers.)

bazine, prednisone, doxorubicin (Adriamycin), bleomycin, and vinblastine (MOPP/ABV). It allows the number of courses of treatment to be reduced by half. Long-term analyses of late complications of second malignancies and fertility problems are not yet available, and these issues remain of high concern. But in at least one series, the need for RT has been markedly reduced and has even been eliminated in patients without any evidence of involvement of the mediastinum.[19]

For treatment failures with MOPP or ABVD, or either one combined with RT, there exist advanced protocols based upon high-dose cyclophosphamide, carmustine, and etoposide sequenced to dose-limited radiation followed by bone marrow transplantation.[20] These advanced protocols have been employed for patients with either HD or NHL as well as acute lymphoblastic leukemia. Such patients who have already maximized their RT options have a dismal prognosis, and this advanced protocol, too, remains less than ideal, with disease-free survival rates being less than 20%.

Non-Hodgkin's Lymphoma

Most NHL that seems to be localized at time of diagnosis is in fact disseminated, as has now become apparent. The treatment of choice for most patients remains chemotherapy with a regimen containing doxorubicin, usually accompanied by RT to the involved field. Such treatment leads to an impressive 95% survival rate in Stage I patients and 75% rate in Stage II patients.

High-grade NHL occurs primarily in the pediatric age range. If a child with a small-, noncleaved-cell lymphoma presents with limited disease, the prognosis is generally excellent. Even patients with more advanced disease have an encouraging outlook with newer therapies. Small-, noncleaved-cell lymphomas in children are found mostly in the abdomen (more than 50%). At St. Jude's Hospital, a series of 24 children with unresectable tumors were treated with high-dose, fractionated cyclophosphamide, vincristine, doxorubicin, high-dose methotrexate, and cytarabine.[21] Most of them (20 of 24) were alive and event-free after a median follow-up period of 4 years. Of the 4 who relapsed, 3 were seen to have a pleural effusion, whereas only 1 of 17 patients without pleural effusion relapsed.

MORBIDITY OF THERAPY

With refinement of therapy over the past four decades, the improvement in survival rates for patients with HD in particular and lymphomas in general has been remarkable. Indeed, this is one of the most dramatic examples of success in the treatment of cancer. Yet the many survivors of treatment have lived only to experience numerous long-term complications of therapy. Foremost among these have been second malignancies, both solid tumors and acute non-lymphoblastic leukemia. Debilitating myocardial damage and lung fibrosis have also been seen, as well as growth abnormalities. Late iatrogenic complications of RT in patients with HD include lung fibrosis, myocardial damage, growth disturbance, and secondary malignancies, including acute nonlymphocytic leukemia, and a variety of solid tumors.[5]

Both RT and chemotherapy have been incriminated in significant damage to the heart and the lungs. In the lungs, the entity of *radiation pneumonitis* has long been recognized; it is minimized, although not prevented, by modern, more precise techniques. Also, the pulmonary toxicity of bleomycin has been recognized since the time of the initial use of the drug. The toxicity of doxorubicin is also well known, and cases are followed fastidiously by oncologists who employ the agent. Nevertheless, the incidence of doxorubicin-induced cardiomyopathy in patients with HD is low considering the dosages employed.

The question of whether RT causes damage to the heart is more controversial. Reports surfaced in the 1960s and 1970s of seemingly early myocardial infarctions in patients thus treated. The apparent isolated atherosclerosis in the mediastinal vessels but minimal or no such changes in the arteries in the rest of the body lent credence to the theory that something in the high-dose mediastinal radiation then employed led to this phenomenon. Yet subsequent nonanecdotal reviews have cast doubt upon the theory. Most of the literature supports the idea that the overall risk of myocardial infarction is not increased among patients who have received mediastinal irradiation but that there may be some contribution to the development of atherosclerosis.

An objective analysis of the effect of radiation upon the height of the former pediatric oncology patient has been provided by Willman and colleagues.[22] In a series of 124 children who had undergone radiation before the age of 16 for boys and 14 for girls, baseline height measurements were taken at time of diagnosis of HD and again at least 2 years after therapy was completed. On average, when compared with U.S. population means there was a highly statistically significant decrease of 7.7%, which translated to a loss of 13 cm of height for these patients. The most severely affected children were those who had had prepubertal radiation to the entire spine. Nevertheless, even when growth was impaired overall, it was seen to be proportionate.

Mantle radiation, with its invariable inclusion of the thyroid gland, will produce hypothyroidism as a frequent complication.[23] When hypothyroidism was rigorously searched for using hormone levels, it was found in as many as two thirds of these patients, although overt clinical hypothyroidism occurs much less frequently. The highest incidence of the problem occurs in patients who receive lymphangiography as part of their evaluation for extent of disease. The postulated mechanism here is that the iodine load greatly stimulates the thyroid gland and makes it much more susceptible to radiation-induced damage. Children may be at higher risk than adolescents or adults for radiation-induced damage to the thyroid.[24] At least one fifth of the children treated with conventional RT will develop overt thyroid problems. Levels of thyroid-stimulating hormone show that nearly 100% have abnormalities of thyroid function.

Chemotherapy has also led to significant long-term complications, notably those of second malignancies and of infertility. The latter is most noted in patients who underwent the effects of alkylating agents with MOPP. This finding was first drawn to attention by a report upon testis biopsies in 15 men who had had cyclophosphamide as a part of their therapy.[25] Ten of these patients were found to have germinal aplasia. Other evaluations have shown that those males who receive MOPP therapy have an overwhelming subsequent incidence of azoospermia, or at least oligospermia sufficient to cause functional infertility.[26] Damage to the testis is not limited to the germinal centers. Leydig-cell damage has been seen as well.

Although testosterone levels may be decreased from normal in these patients, hormonal replacement is rarely necessary. In Table 14–3 one can

Table 14–3 • Testicular Dysfunction after MOPP and ABVD in Patients <40 Years of Age

	Azoospermia		
	Cases	(%)	Recovery
MOPP plus RT	28	97	3/21 (14%)
ABVD plus RT	24	33	13/13 (100%)
MOPP/ABVD	77	87	17/42 (40%)

Data from Bonadonna G: Modern treatment of malignant lymphomas: A multidisciplinary approach? The Kaplan Memorial Lecture. Ann Oncol 5(suppl. 2):5–16, 1994.

easily see that in the significant minority of patients who had azoospermia after ABVD, the reversal rate was 100%, whereas such reversal after MOPP is quite rare. If there is a compelling reason why alkylating agents should be used for more than three cycles of therapy, then certainly the young man who envisions any chance of wishing to be a parent should be offered the opportunity to preserve his sperm in a long-term sperm bank.

The ability to do semen analysis provides an easy assay of fertility in the male patient. Nevertheless, there have been extensive investigations into the effect of therapy on female fertility as well. Primary ovarian failure is seen in over half the women treated with MOPP chemotherapy.[27] And chemotherapy is not the only treatment agent that has affected women treated for HD. Radiation may also, of course, provide significant gonadal dysfunction, and as little as 625 rads to the ovary can induce amenorrhea that is permanent.[28] The practice of oopheropexy during staging laparotomy may minimize this complication. If iliac RT is still considered, then perhaps oopheropexy as an isolated laparoscopic procedure should be considered as well.

Second malignancies in survivors of treated HD have been increasingly reported, and efforts have been extensive to design treatment protocols that will reduce or avoid totally this troubling complication. Among 499 patients treated for HD at St. Jude's Hospital between 1962 and 1993, a second malignancy developed in 25.[29] The median duration to occurrence of the second process was 9 years with a range of 0.1 to 27.4 years. The majority (19) were solid tumors. Acute nonlymphoblastic leukemia, NHL, and chronic myeloid leukemia were also seen. These second malignancies were more common among patients who were adolescent females at the time of original diagnosis and therapy. In the experience at Stanford University with 2037 patients treated for HD from 1968 through 1992 (all ages), actuarial projections for second malignancies were 26% for NHL, 19% for leukemia, and 4% for other cancers.[7]

SURGICAL THERAPY

There are few reports in the literature on the use of operative resection as a primary therapy in lymphoma. One such report applies to isolated mediastinal lymphoma.[30] The instances in which such a technique would be applicable are rare and the efficacy in wide trials has never been tested. In the cited series, there were just over 100 preoperative patients who were thought to have isolated mediastinal disease. Fourteen (11 with HD and 3 with NHL) were candidates at the time of operation for a local radical resection. Another 5 underwent debulking subtotal resections. All 14 patients who underwent a total gross resection of disease were alive and well 1 to 14 years after surgery. Adjuvant therapy varied from low-dose local RT to conventional RT combined with chemotherapy. Among the 5 patients who underwent a debulking resection, the 3 with HD were alive and well 5 to 11 years postoperatively. The 2 with NHL both died 3 years after surgery.

STAGING LAPAROTOMY

Laparotomy with multiple tissue sampling was first used for staging at Stanford University in the late 1960s.[31] The classic staging laparotomy should produce 13 separate specimens (Table 14–4). Despite the widespread knowledge of these tissue requirements, many national cooperative studies fail to fulfill all of them. The most common omissions are among the lymph node requirements.

Staging laparotomy has been repeatedly shown to enable the highest accuracy in diagnosis of disease stage. Despite advances in the technology of imaging, approximately one third of the patients clinically staged this way and determined to have only supradiaphragmatic disease are found to have infradiaphragmatic disease after a complete staging laparotomy. An equivalent number of those determined by imaging to have Stage III disease are found on staging laparotomy to have no histologic evidence of disease.

Table 14–4 • Tissues Sampled in a Complete Staging Laparotomy

The complete spleen
Liver biopsies
  Right and left lobe
  Needle and wedge biopsies
  Biopsy any gross disease
Lymph node areas
  Superior periaortic
  Inferior periaortic
  Perisplenic
  Porta hepatis
  Mesenteric
  Right iliac
  Left iliac
Bone marrow biopsy

In some centers up to 80% of adult patients undergo staging laparotomy to help clinicians plan therapy for HD.[32] In children, an analysis of CT scanning at Stanford University revealed that its sensitivity in detecting splenic involvement as compared with histology from laparotomy was only 19%.[33] Even when CT was combined with lymphography, staging laparotomy in children altered the stage in 37% of the cases.

Benefits may accrue from the surgical removal of the spleen and hence avoidance of radiation to that field. Enlarged portals of treatment for patients with an intact spleen may lead to damage to the left kidney and lung base.[34] In centers where patients with Stage I or II disease undergo radiation as the primary treatment, the complications of extended field radiation, especially long term, can be avoided. One opinion states that the induction of high platelet counts and white blood cell counts after splenectomy allows for more aggressive immediate chemotherapy when necessary.[35]

At Children's Hospital in Boston there remains a decided partiality toward performance of staging laparotomy.[36] Through the early 1990s staging laparotomy remains "part of the routine diagnostic evaluation." Over the 22 years ending in December of 1991, 247 patients underwent this procedure. Overall, 25% of the patients had altered staging as a result, with 25% of the Clinical Stage (CS) I or II patients re-evaluated to Stage III or IV, and 27% of CS III or IV patients re-evaluated to I or II. An analysis was done of risk factors for altered staging. Three subgroups had less than a 10% chance of restaging: (1) CS I and II patients with lymphocyte predominant histology, (2) CS I female patients, and (3) CS III and IV female patients with nonlymphocyte predominant histology. Yet even in these cases, patients under age 15 were deemed most likely to benefit from combined modality therapy, in which case staging laparotomy would be marginally useful.

Overall, the severe morbidity that radiation can produce on the growing skeleton has prevented this therapy from being used in the growing child in most pediatric oncology centers. On a practical level, patients diagnosed with HD are nearly always first referred to the pediatric oncologist, and the sentiment is strong within that discipline to avoid staging laparotomy in these patients. It is, however, worthwhile to keep in mind the words of Jesse Ternberg:[37] "There are risks and complications associated with chemotherapy and radiotherapy, but the fact that many of these occur later in the course of treatment or follow-up has served to minimize the impression that the therapy can be a problem."

COMPLICATIONS OF STAGING LAPAROTOMY

In the literature on adult patients, few complications are reported for the staging operation in HD. Those major complications that are listed include wound infection or dehiscence, subphrenic abscess, cardiopulmonary arrest, sepsis, pancreatitis, and adhesive small bowel obstruction. Overall, these standard complications for open intra-abdominal procedures have an incidence of 5% to 13%.[38] Furthermore, many if not most series report no operative mortality.

One retrospective review[39] of 133 patients of all ages who underwent staging laparotomy demonstrated after a median 15-year follow-up that overwhelming post-splenectomy infection was seen 7% of the time, but in none of the patients who had received pneumococcal vaccination preoperatively. The obvious recommendation—standard practice today in every elective splenectomy—is to administer pneumococcal vaccination in advance of splenectomy.

Long-term risks also exist for the procedures done at staging, centrally that of splenectomy. Evaluating such risks can, however, be confounded by the fact that radiation to an intact spleen may also eradicate any effective splenic function. Nevertheless, it is undeniable that splenectomy will predispose a patient to the markedly lethal complication of overwhelming post-splenectomy sepsis, which occurs at a rate of 0.5%.[40] Moreover, there is a known risk of delayed second malignancy, as acute nonlymphoblastic leukemia has been found to double in those patients who have had their spleens removed.[41]

It seems that children undergoing staging laparotomy experience a high incidence of subsequent adhesive bowel obstruction. From the Children's Cancer Group an experience has been reported with 49 patients who underwent staging laparotomy, of whom 3 were rehospitalized for adhesive bowel obstruction.[42] In another series small bowel obstruction occurred in 10% of the patients, two thirds of them requiring operation for correction of the obstruction.[39]

MINIMALLY INVASIVE SURGERY

The wave of enthusiasm for minimally invasive surgery in the abdomen has not yet embraced the lymphomas. A few reports exist of the use of laparoscopy for formal staging, but no widespread study protocol currently exists. Both Lefor[43] and Childers[44] reported on staging laparoscopy in 1993. As the latter points out, each of the component portions of the staging laparotomy had been reported before, and so information on the technical details of the procedure was not lacking. What was then, and still is, missing is outcome analysis that delineates whether or not the minimally invasive technique holds any concrete advantage over classic open laparotomy for staging. Childers[44] also states that based upon experience with para-aortic lymphadenectomy for other diseases, there is reason to extrapolate that obesity and adhesions will limit the utility of the laparoscopic procedure. This researcher writes an addendum to the referenced article on three further cases in which a laparoscopic splenectomy was attempted but needed to be abandoned and an open procedure done instead because of bleeding complications. It is perhaps unlikely that a rigorous study of minimally invasive surgery to stage HD will ever come about in view of the pervasive opinion among oncologists to treat primarily with chemotherapy.

Table 14–5 • Annual Death Rates (per 1,000,000 Persons) for Hodgkin's Disease According to Sex, Race, Age Group, and Region in United States: 1979, 1983, 1988

	Year			Risk Ratio for 1988/1979 (95% CI)	% Decreased (1988/1979)
	1979 (n = 2563)	*1983* (n = 2431)	*1988* (n = 2205)		
Total	11.4	10.4	9.0	0.8 (0.7, 0.8)	21.1
Sex					
Male	14.2	12.5	11.0	0.8 (0.7, 0.8)	22.5
Female	8.8	8.4	7.0	0.8 (0.7, 0.9)	20.5
Race					
White	12.2	11.2	9.7	0.8 (0.8, 0.8)	20.5
Black	7.4	6.7	6.2	0.8 (0.7, 1.0)	16.2
Other	1.9	2.0	1.6	0.9 (0.4, 2.0)	15.8
Age group (yr)°					
0–14	0.5	0.3	0.3	0.7 (0.4, 1.2)	40.0
15–34	7.8	7.1	6.1	0.8 (0.7, 0.9)	21.8
35–54	11.9	10.8	9.5	0.8 (0.7, 0.9)	20.2
55+	29.1	25.9	21.6	0.7 (0.7, 0.8)	25.8
Region					
Northeast	14.1	12.1	12.0	0.9 (0.8, 1.0)	14.9
North central	11.8	11.3	9.6	0.8 (0.7, 0.9)	18.6
South	10.5	9.2	7.9	0.8 (0.7, 0.8)	24.8
West	9.5	9.5	7.1	0.8 (0.7, 0.9)	25.3

CI = confidence interval.
°Age not included for one death in 1983.
From Hooper WC, Holman RC, Strine TW, et al: Hodgkin's disease mortality in the United States: 1979–1988. *Cancer* 70:1166–1171, 1992.

OUTCOME

Among children up to the age of 14 diagnosed with HD, the outlook continues to improve. Data from the National Center for Health Statistics reveal an overall mortality reduction of 21% from the 1970s to the 1980s for all patients with HD.[45] The youngest age group had a 40% reduction in mortality (Table 14–5).

References

1. Medeiros LJ, Greiner TC: Hodgkin's disease. *Cancer* 75(suppl. 1):357–359, 1995.
2. Cleary SF, Link MP, Donaldson SS: Hodgkin's disease in the very young. *Int J Rad Oncol Biol Phys* 28:77–83, 1994.
3. Castellino RA, Blank N, Hoppe RT: Hodgkin's disease: Contribution of chest CT in the initial staging evaluation. *Radiology* 160:603–605, 1986.
4. Wollner N, Mandell L, Filippa D, et al: Primary nasal-paranasal oropharyngeal lymphoma in the pediatric age group. *Cancer* 65:1438–1444, 1990.
5. Kwak LW, DeVita VT, Longo DL: Lymphomas. In Pinedo HM, Longo DL, Chabner BA (eds): *Cancer Chemotherapy and Biological Response Modifiers Annual 14.* New York: Elsevier Science Publishers, 1993, pp 383–426.
6. Fouillard L, Gorin NC, Laporte JPH, et al: Feasibility of autologous bone marrow transplantation for early consolidation of follicular non-Hodgkin's lymphoma. *Eur J Haematol* 46:279–284, 1990.
7. Rosenberg SA: The treatment of Hodgkin's disease. *Ann Oncol* 5 (Suppl. 2):17–21, 1994.
8. Bonadonna G: Modern treatment of malignant lymphomas: A multidisciplinary approach? The Kaplan Memorial Lecture. *Ann Oncol* 5(suppl. 2):5–16, 1994.
9. Leibenhaut MH, Hoppe RT, Efron B, et al: Prognostic indicators of laparotomy findings in clinical stage I-II supradiaphragmatic Hodgkin's disease. *J Clin Oncol* 7:89–91, 1989.
10. Chan JKC, Yip TTC, Tsang WYM, et al: Detection of Epstein-Barr virus in Hodgkin's disease occurring in an Oriental population. *Hum Pathol* 26:314–318, 1995.
11. Khan G, Coates PJ: The role of Epstein-Barr virus in the pathogenesis of Hodgkin's disease. *J Pathol* 174:141–149, 1994.
12. Riopel M, Dickman PS, Link MP, et Al: *MIC2* analysis in pediatric lymphomas and leukemias. *Hum Pathol* 25:396–399, 1994.
13. Henderson S, Rowe M, Gregory C, et al: Induction of bcl-2 expression by Epstein-Barr virus latent membrane protein 1 protects infected B-cells from programmed cell death. *Cell* 65:1107–1115, 1991.

14. Maity A, Goldwein JW, Lange B, et al: Comparison of high-dose and low-dose radiation with and without chemotherapy for children with Hodgkin's disease: An analysis of the experience at the Children's Hospital of Philadelphia and the Hospital of the University of Pennsylvania. *J Clin Oncol* 10:929–936, 1992.

15. Kaplan HS: *Hodgkin's Disease*, 2nd ed. Cambridge: Harvard University Press, 1980.

16. Bonadonna G: Chemotherapy strategies to improve the control of Hodgkin's disease: The Richard and Hinda Rosenthal Foundation Award Lecture. *Cancer Res* 42:4309–4320, 1982.

17. Link MP, Donaldson SS, Berard CW, et al: Results of treatment of childhood localized non-Hodgkin's lymphoma with combination chemotherapy with or without radiotherapy. *N Engl J Med* 322:1169–1174, 1990.

18. Klimo P, Connors JM: MOPP/ABV hybrid program: Combination chemotherapy based on early introduction of seven effective drugs for advanced Hodgkin's disease. *J Clin Oncol* 3:1174–1182, 1985.

19. Khan SP, Gilchrist GS, Arndt CAS, et al: Vancouver hybrid: Preliminary experience in the treatment of Hodgkin's disease in childhood and adolescence. *Mayo Clin Proc* 69:949–954, 1994.

20. Demirer T, Weaver CH, Buckner CD, et al: High-dose cyclophosphamide, carmustine, and etoposide followed by allogenic bone marrow transplantation in patients with lymphoid malignancies who had received prior dose-limiting radiation therapy. *J Clin Oncol* 13:596–602, 1995.

21. Sandlund JT, Crist WM, Abromowitch M, et al: Pleural effusions associated with a poor treatment outcome in Stage III small noncleaved cell lymphoma. *Leukemia* 5:71–74, 1991.

22. Willman KY, Cox RS, Donaldson SS: Radiation-induced height impairment in pediatric Hodgkin's disease. *Int J Rad Oncol Biol Phys* 28:85–92, 1994.

23. Adler RA, Corrigan DF, Wartofsky L: Hypothyroidism after X irradiation to the neck: Three case reports and a brief review of the literature. *Johns Hopkins Med J* 138:180–184, 1976.

24. Constine LS, Donaldson SS, McDougall IR, et al: Thyroid dysfunction after radiotherapy in children with Hodgkin's disease. *Cancer* 53:878–883, 1984.

25. Sherins RJ, DeVita VT: Effect of drug treatment for lymphoma on male reproductive capacity: Studies of men in remission after therapy. *Ann Intern Med* 79:216–220, 1973.

26. Whitehead E, Shalet Sm, Blackledge G, et al: The effects of Hodgkin's disease and combination chemotherapy on gonadal function in the adult male. *Cancer* 49:418–422, 1982.

27. Chapman RM, Sutcliffe SB, Malpas JS: Cytotoxic-induced ovarian failure in women with Hodgkin's disease: I. Hormone function. *JAMA* 242:1877–1881, 1979.

28. Rubin P, Casarett GW: *Clinical Radiation Pathology*, Philadelphia: W.B. Saunders, 1968, p. 396.

29. Beaty O, Hudson MM, Greenwald C, et al: Subsequent malignancies in children and adolescents after treatment for Hodgkin's disease. *J Clin Oncol* 13:603–609, 1995.

30. Ricci C, Rendina EA, Venuta F, et al: Surgical approach to isolated mediastinal lymphoma. *J Thorac Cardiovasc Surg* 99:691–695, 1990.

31. Leibenhaut MH: The changing role of staging laparotomy in the management of Hodgkin's disease. In Dana B (ed): *Malignant Lymphomas, Including Hodgkin's Disease: Diagnosis, Management and Special Problems*, Boston: Kluwer Academic Publishers, 1993, pp. 1–19.

32. Mauch P, Larson D, Osteen R, et al: Prognostic factors for positive surgical staging in patients with Hodgkin's disease. *J Clin Oncol* 8:257–265, 1990.

33. Baker LL, Parker BR, Donaldson SS, et al: Staging of Hodgkin's disease in children: Comparison of CT and lymphography with laparotomy. *AJR* 154:1251–1255, 1990.

34. Le Bourgeois JP, Meignan M, Parmentier C, et al: Renal consequences of irradiation of spleen in lymphomas. *Br J Radiol* 52:55–60, 1979.

35. Schreiber DP, Jacobs C, Rosenberg SA, et al: The potential benefits of therapeutic splenectomy for patients with Hodgkin's disease and non-Hodgkin's lymphoma. *Int J Radiat Oncol Biol Phys* 11:31–36, 1985.

36. Breurer CK, Tarbell NJ, Mauch PM: The importance of staging laparotomy in pediatric Hodgkin's disease. *J Pediatr Surg* 29:1085–1089, 1994.

37. Ternberg JL: Changing role of surgery in childhood lymphomas. *Semin Surg Oncol* 9:541–544, 1993.

38. Taylor MA, Kaplan HS, Nelson TS: Staging laparotomy with splenectomy for Hodgkin's disease: The Stanford experience. *World J Surg* 9:449–460, 1980.

39. Jockovich M, Mendenhall NP, Sombeck MD, et al: Long-term complications of laparotomy in Hodgkin's disease. *Ann Surg* 219:615–624, 1994.

40. Abrahamsen AF, Borge L, Holte H: Infection after splenectomy for Hodgkin's disease. *Acta Oncol* 29:167–170, 1990.

41. Kaldor JM, Day NE, Clarke EA, et al: Leukemia following Hodgkin's disease. *N Engl J Med* 322:7–13, 1990.

42. Hays DM, Fryer CJ, Pringle KC, et al: An evaluation of abdominal staging procedures performed in pediatric patients with advanced Hodgkin's disease: A report from the Children's Cancer Study Group. *J Pediatr Surg* 27:1175–1180, 1992.

43. Lefor AT, Flowers JL, Heyman MR: Laparoscopic staging of Hodgkin's disease. *Surg Oncol* 2:217–220, 1993.

44. Childers JM, Balserak JC, Kent T, et al: Laparoscopic staging of Hodgkin's lymphoma. *J Lapar Surg* 5:495–499, 1993.
45. Hooper WC, Holman RC, Strine TW, et al: Hodgkin's disease mortality in the United States: 1979–1988. *Cancer* 70:1166–1171, 1992.
46. Hoekstra HJ, Tamminga RYJ, Timens W: Partial splenectomy in children: An alternative for splenectomy in the pathological staging of Hodgkin's disease. *Ann Surg Oncol* 1:480–486, 1994.
47. Lister TA, Crowther D, Sutcliffe SB: Report of a committee convened to discuss the evaluation and staging of patients with Hodgkin's disease: Cotswold's meeting. *J Clin Oncol* 7:1630–1636, 1989.
48. Medeiros LJ, Greiner TC: Hodgkin's disease. *Cancer* 75:(suppl. 1):357–359, 1995.

Thyroid Malignancy

• *David M. Powell, M.D.* • *Kurt D. Newman, M.D.*

Several issues contribute to the continuing controversy regarding the optimal management of thyroid malignancy in children. The low incidence of childhood thyroid cancer, combined with the indolent nature of the disease even in the presence of metastases, makes it difficult to determine the effects of various surgical and medical treatment strategies on long-term outcome. Individual patient-care decisions are, therefore, based upon personal experience and the comparison of results published in retrospective reports of various aggressive and conservative surgical approaches. No published randomized trials currently exist to guide the clinician in determining the strategy most likely to yield optimal long-term results.

Pediatric thyroid cancer was exceedingly rare until the 1950s, when it was common to use external-beam irradiation for benign childhood medical conditions such as thymic enlargement[1,2] and acne.[3] With a latent period extending from 5 to 35 years,[4-8] the incidence of pediatric thyroid cancer increased gradually through the 1960s. Perhaps owing to the abandoning of this irradiation approach over the past two decades, the incidence has decreased from 5 to less than 1 new case per 1 million.[9,10] Primary thyroid carcinoma represents 10% to 15% of all pediatric head and neck cancers,[11] and 10% of all cases of thyroid carcinoma are diagnosed in children.[9]

The biology of thyroid cancer in children is different from that in adults. When compared with their counterparts in adults, thyroid masses in children are more than twice as likely to be malignant,[12] and pediatric thyroid tumors are frequently larger and more often multicentric than those in adults. Children are likely to have a higher rate of lymphatic and pulmonary metastases[13] and a higher rate of recurrences.[14] Despite the seemingly aggressive nature of pediatric thyroid malignancies at the time of presentation, only 14% of children with distant metastases die from the disease compared with 68% of adults.[15]

PATHOLOGY

Based upon histologic appearance, malignant primary tumors of the thyroid gland are classified as papillary, follicular, medullary, or anaplastic.

Approximately 80% are *papillary carcinomas* originating from the epithelial elements of the gland. These tumors are more common in females, and their incidence increases with patient age. For this reason most pediatric studies note a peak incidence in adolescence. Grossly, surgical specimens are grayish white, solid lesions. Histologically, papillary carcinomas display nuclear changes of enlargement, grooving, and clearing ("Orphan Annie" nuclei).[16] Concentric rings of calcification known as psammoma bodies are present in almost half of all papillary cancers (Fig. 15–1). The diffuse sclerosing variant of papillary cancer may exhibit an involvement of the thyroid gland and a more aggressive clinical course.[17,18]

True *follicular tumors* are rare in children. Grossly they have thick, fibrous capsules and microscopically display a follicular histology. Distinguishing between a follicular adenoma and carcinoma requires identification of either vascular invasion or capsular involvement. Therefore, if the surrounding architecture is unknown, fine-

needle aspiration cytology can often be inconclusive when follicular cells are identified. Vascular invasion in particular is related to a poorer prognosis.[19] Although follicular thyroid cancer is more likely to be associated with vascular metastases than papillary, the question of whether or not it is more aggressive in the pediatric age group remains unanswered.[18] The presence of follicular components within a predominantly papillary tumor does not alter the prognosis, and mixed papillary-follicular variant lesions are treated as if they were pure papillary tumors.

Medullary carcinoma constitutes 2% to 3% of thyroid cancer in children and arises from the calcitonin-secreting parafollicular, or C-cells, of the thyroid. C-cell hyperplasia may be a precursor.[20] The gene predisposing children to this syndrome has been located on chromosome 10. Although medullary carcinoma is most often present in children with the autosomal dominant familial *multiple endocrine neoplasia, type 2* (MEN2) syndromes, other sporadic cases do exist. Grossly these lesions characteristically occur in the upper two thirds of the thyroid and are fleshy, gray, well-circumscribed masses. Bilateral disease is the rule (Fig. 15–2). In view of the multicentricity, total thyroidectomy in indicated. Histologically, amyloid is usually present and confirms the diagnosis of medullary carcinoma when found in a thyroid nodule (Fig. 15–3). Results of immunohistochemical staining for calcitonin are positive.

Medullary carcinomas associated with the MEN2B syndrome are characterized by the aforementioned multicentricity and by frequent metastases and local invasiveness.[21] Children at

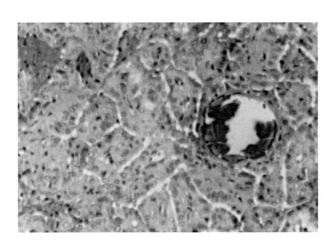

Figure 15–1 • Histologic appearance of papillary carcinoma of the thyroid with prominent psammoma body. (From Newman KD: The current management of thyroid tumors in children. *Semin Pediatr Surg* 2:69–74, 1993, with permission.)

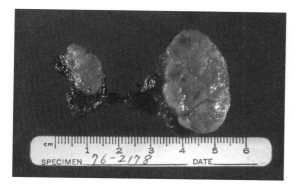

Figure 15–2 • Gross appearance of bissected total thyroidectomy specimen of child with MEN 2B syndrome displaying medullary carcinoma in both lobes.

risk are screened by serial monitoring of stimulated serum calcitonin levels to allow for early surgical treatment.[22] Unfortunately, even when medullary carcinoma is detected solely by biochemical evaluation and treated by total thyroidectomy, a significant number of patients suffer recurrence. Now that molecular biologic techniques exist, children identified as *ret* proto-oncogene mutation carriers by DNA screening have been offered prophylactic thyroidectomy before the development of either clinical or biochemical evidence of disease.[23–26] Children in whom medullary carcinoma of the thyroid is diagnosed, and their relatives, should be evaluated for the other components of the syndrome.

Rarer still in children is *anaplastic thyroid cancer*. Unfortunately, when present, these tumors are extremely aggressive and often metastatic. Because of their associated high mortality,

an aggressive surgical posture in the form of total thyroidectomy is warranted.

On a molecular level, several oncogenes (*c-myc*, *c-fos*,[27] *erb* B-2[28]) have been implicated in the development of thyroid cancer. Rearrangement of the tyrosine kinase proto-oncogenes *ret* and *trk* have been identified in papillary carcinomas,[29] the *ras* proto-oncogene may be involved in follicular carcinoma,[30] and a p53 mutation may lead to the transition from differentiated to anaplastic carcinoma.[31] The absence of p53 expression in childhood thyroid carcinoma may explain the better prognosis associated with the disease in children.[32] Further advances in determining the role of genetic defects in thyroid disease may permit early identification of children at risk for thyroid cancer.

PRESENTATION

The typical patient with thyroid malignancy is an adolescent who presents with an asymptomatic cervical mass (Fig. 15–4). The mass may represent a thyroid nodule or a metastatic lymph node.[33] The incidence of malignancy in pediatric thyroid nodules is as high as 50%.[34] Benign causes of thyroid masses in children are simple cyst, adenoma, goiter, and thyroiditis. Rarely, a thyroid nodule will be a manifestation of lymphoma.[35] Since extracapsular invasion is unusual in children, symptoms related to direct tumor extension such as nerve or airway compression are likewise rare.

Children exposed to (1) radiation for the treat-

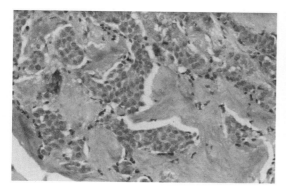

Figure 15–3 • Histologic appearance of medullary carcinoma of the thyroid with abundant amyloid.

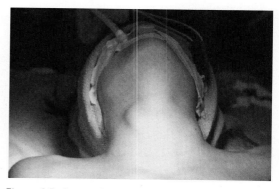

Figure 15–4 • Visible neck mass, representing a nodal metastasis, in an adolescent with thyroid cancer. (From Newman KD: The current management of thyroid tumors in children. *Semin Pediatr Surg* 2:69–74, 1993, with permission.)

ment of malignant disease or (2) environmental contaminants constitute a special population at increased risk. Patients treated with head and neck irradiation for pediatric Hodgkin's disease are at a 3- to 15-fold risk for the development of thyroid cancer.[36] In more than 2% of children receiving head and neck radiation for benign conditions, thyroid cancer developed during a follow-up period with a median of 20 years. Interestingly, the subsequent outcomes for these patients mirrored those for patients with childhood thyroid cancer without an antecedent radiation exposure.[37]

An 80-fold increase above the predicted rate of thyroid cancer in children was noted in Belarus following the 1986 Chernobyl nuclear accident.[38–40] The tumors began to be identified following a shorter latent period than had existed for other patients with radiation exposure. The tumors displayed an extremely aggressive histologic appearance and clinical behavior.[41]

The sensitivity of the pediatric thyroid gland to radiation is most likely inversely related to age, with the earliest cases of neoplasia identified in children exposed in utero.[42] Children who receive either therapeutic or environmental thyroid radiation should be followed closely and have lifelong annual neck examinations in the attempt at early detection.[43]

Thyroid carcinoma may be associated with preexisting benign thyroid disease. Although pathologic specimens excised for malignancy may have thyroiditis occasionally identified on preoperative fine-needle aspiration or in tissue adjacent to the malignant nodule, a causal relationship has been difficult to establish.[9,44]

DIAGNOSTIC EVALUATION

Classically, the evaluation of a neck mass that may represent thyroid cancer begins with an ultrasound examination to confirm the proximity of the mass to the thyroid gland and to determine whether it is solid or cystic (Fig. 15–5).[45–47] A thyroid scan is then used to differentiate functioning from nonfunctioning (cold) nodules (Fig. 15–6). Although most surgeons rely upon these studies to complete the diagnostic evaluation, some investigators question their usefulness as they may have no bearing on treatment or prognosis.[48]

Although fine-needle aspiration (FNA) cytology is used frequently and accurately in adults to assist in diagnosing thyroid malignancy preoperatively,[49] its role in treating patients with large masses[50,51] and in children, who are more likely to have large masses, is less clear. The requirement for sedation in small children and reliance on the experience of the pathologists in interpreting cytologic specimens may limit its usefulness.

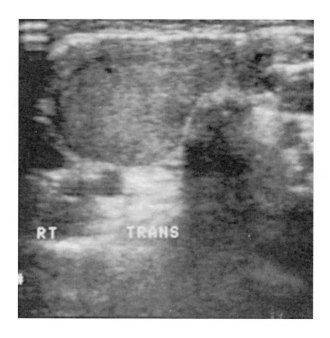

Figure 15–5 • Ultrasound of an anterior neck mass revealing a solid, homogeneous mass in the thyroid gland. (From Newman KD: The current management of thyroid tumors in children. *Semin Pediatr Surg* 2:69–74, 1993, with permission.)

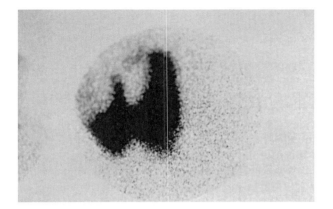

Figure 15–6 • Thyroid radionuclide scan demonstrating a nonfunctioning "cold" nodule in the right upper lobe. (From Newman KD: The current management of thyroid tumors in children. *Semin Pediatr Surg* 2:69–74, 1993, with permission.)

Positive FNA results can be helpful in discussing an operative strategy with parents, but negative or nondiagnostic FNA results cannot be used to rule out the presence of a malignancy because of sampling error. Nevertheless, an effort to avoid the one third of thyroid operations that are performed for benign disease, some investigators rely on FNA to determine surgical management. Patients with persistently suspect nodules are thus subjected to annual FNA examinations as well as a potential delay in diagnosis.[52] Perhaps the safest approach in children is to resect all nonfunctioning thyroid masses.

A chest radiograph should be included in the evaluation of all children thought to have thyroid cancer because of the high incidence of pulmonary metastases.[53] Since the likelihood of malignancy is higher in childhood, the practice of attempting to shrink a nodule with exogenous thyroid hormone suppression, usual in adults, is discouraged in children.

SURGICAL APPROACH

Potential options for thyroid resection include nodulectomy, lobectomy with or without isthmusectomy, ipsilateral lobectomy with contralateral subtotal or near total lobectomy, and total thyroidectomy. In choosing the most appropriate procedure, one must consider this single issue: does the long-term patient survival benefit of additional extensive thyroid resection outweigh the increased surgical risk of a more aggressive procedure? Nodulectomy is associated with unacceptably high recurrence rates and should be avoided in malignant disease.[54] Intraoperative

frozen section diagnosis may assist in surgical decision making.[55]

Advocates of an aggressive surgical approach suggest that total thyroidectomy is most likely to achieve local disease control given the high frequency of multifocal, multicentric, and contralateral disease found when totally resected glands are examined pathologically.[56] For children in high-risk groups (i.e., those with a history of radiation exposure, medullary carcinoma, or anaplastic carcinoma), total thyroidectomy removes all such affected thyroid tissue (Fig. 15–7). Removal of all functioning thyroid tissue also simplifies subsequent radioablative therapy and radionuclide scans.

Total thyroidectomy carries with it a higher rate of operative complications. A multicenter review of 329 patients followed for a mean of 11 years failed to identify any significant survival benefit for children who underwent more than lobectomy and isthmusectomy.[57] Given the increase in risk without a documented increase in benefit, many surgeons prefer the more conservative approach. Data do not currently exist on the significance of the potential for cancer developing in the unresected lobe and its effect on prognosis.

Regardless of the extent of thyroid resection, dissection of palpable regional lymph nodes is recommended because of the high rate of nodal spread. Areas of local (i.e., jugular) lymph node drainage should be directly inspected and clinically involved nodes removed. Formal neck dissection may be indicated in some patients depending on the histologic findings.

The reported rates of hypoparathyroidism and recurrent laryngeal nerve injury following thyroid

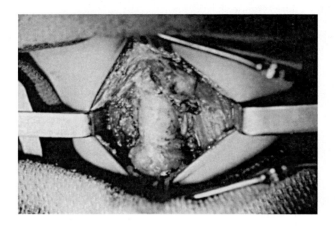

Figure 15–7 • Operative field after total thyroidectomy performed for multifocal papillary carcinoma in a patient who received neck radiation for Hodgkin's disease. (From Newman KD: The current management of thyroid tumors in children. *Semin Pediatr Surg* 2:69–74, 1993, with permission.)

surgery for malignancy are highly variable.[58] In children the risk of surgical complications is related to the extent of surgery and inversely related to the age of the patient. The incidence of complications in children is greater than that in adults, with rates of permanent hypocalcemia and recurrent nerve paralysis being 15% and 14%, respectively. The major complication rate for total or subtotal thyroidectomy is 20% to 40% higher than that for lobectomy or biopsy, depending upon the age of the patient.[59] The most important variable in the frequency of complications may be the surgeon's experience.

ADJUVANT THERAPY

All patients undergoing total thyroidectomy receive postoperative thyroid hormone replacement. Exogenous thyroid suppression is usually administered to children who have undergone lobectomy, but specific data regarding the effectiveness of this approach in preventing recurrence are lacking. Presumably, thyroid hormone administration decreases the thyroid-stimulating hormone effect on tumor cells. Replacement therapy is discontinued and the patient allowed to become hypothyroid for 2 to 6 weeks prior to the administration of iodine[131] scans used to identify metastases.

Radioiodine has been found effective in the treatment of local recurrences as well as lymph node and pulmonary metastases.[60–62] Although the treatment is usually well tolerated, pulmonary fibrosis has been seen in patients receiving large doses of the isotope. The value of radioiodine in the initial treatment of disease in children remains unproven.[57]

PROGNOSIS AND FOLLOW-UP

Even though children frequently present with advanced disease, the prognosis for children with thyroid cancer is excellent.[63] In one study with a mean follow-up of 13 years, despite the fact that 40% of patients had persistent or recurrent disease, the overall survival rate at 10 and 25 years was 98% and 78%, respectively.[64] For papillary carcinoma, the overall recurrence rate in one large series was approximately 2% per year. When followed for 30 years, the survival curves of children with papillary carcinoma of the thyroid were very similar to those of the general population, and the death rate in the presence of pulmonary metastases was only 3.4%.[15]

The search for clinically useful markers that might identify patients with a worse prognosis has been disappointing. The only clinical factors that correlate with disease progression are a young age at diagnosis and the presence of positive margins after surgical resection.[57] Higher mortality is associated with tumors greater than 2 cm in size, nondiploid DNA, and identification of psammoma bodies or anaplastic type on histology. Overexpression of the p21 *ras* protein[65] or focal adhesion kinase (FAK)[66] and *ret* proto-oncogene activation[67] may some day serve as markers for more aggressive tumors.

Because of the indolent nature of the disease, frequent and meticulous follow-up is required for all patients treated for thyroid cancer. Physical examination remains the most useful tool for detecting local and regional recurrence. Serum thyroglobulin levels can be monitored in those patients who have undergone total thyroidectomy, and an increase in thyroglobulin may be the most sensitive indicator of recurrence.[68] Although they require cessation of thyroid supplementation for optimal sensitivity, radioisotope scans can be employed to detect and localize recurrence and metastases. Not all metastases may concentrate isotope, making the thyroid scan less than completely sensitive.

SUMMARY

Clearly, the most important factor in the outcome for children with thyroid cancer is the choice of a surgical strategy that completely removes the tumor with a minimum of morbidity. In the absence of multicentric disease, medullary carcinoma, or anaplastic carcinoma, lobectomy and isthmusectomy are appropriate. Clinically involved lymph nodes should be excised at the time of presentation or recurrence. Distant metastases respond well to radioiodine. The most significant variable seems to be not the type of procedure performed but the biologic behavior of a given tumor. Perhaps as the molecular basis of thyroid cancer becomes more clearly elucidated, surgical strategies can become more individualized.

The optimal long-term management of thyroid cancer in children requires input from the patient, family, pediatrician, endocrinologist, radiotherapist, pathologist, and pediatric surgeon. The striking differences between the outcomes in adult versus pediatric patients combined with the rarity of the disease dictate a specific surgical approach tailored to the particular case. Although the foundation of any effective approach must include complete resection, clear data regarding more aggressive operative or adjuvant strategies do not exist at this time. The goal of continued investigation should be centered on identification of those patients in whom the benefit of a more aggressive surgical or medical treatment outweighs the risk.

References

1. Simpson CL, Hempelmann LH, Fuller LM: Neoplasia in children treated with x-rays in infancy for thymic enlargement. *Cancer* 10:42–56, 1955.
2. Hempelmann LH, et al: Neoplasms in persons treated with x-rays in infancy for thymic enlargement. A report of the fourth follow-up in twenty years. *J Natl Cancer Inst* 55:519–530, 1975.
3. Albright EC, Allday RW: Thyroid carcinoma after radiation therapy for adolescent acne vulgaris. *JAMA* 199:280–281, 1967.
4. Duffy BJ, Fitzgerald PJ: Cancer of the thyroid in children: A report of 28 cases. *J Clin Endocrinol* 10:1296–1308, 1950.
5. Clark DE: Association of irradiation with cancer of the thyroid in children and adolescents. *JAMA* 149:1007–1009, 1955.
6. Rooney DR, Powell RW: Carcinoma of the thyroid in children after x-ray therapy in early childhood. *JAMA* 169:1–4, 1959.
7. Silverman C, Hoffman DA: Thyroid tumor risk from radiation during childhood. *Prev Med* 4:100–105, 1975.
8. Favus MJ, Scheider AB, Stachur ME, et al: Thyroid cancer occurring as late consequence of head and neck irradiation: Evaluation of 1056 patients. *N Engl J Med* 294:1019–1025, 1976.
9. Gorlin JB, Sallan SE: Thyroid cancer in childhood. *Endocrinol Metab Clin North Am* 19:649–662, 1990.
10. Young J, Percy C, Asire A: Surveillance, epidemiology and end results: Incidence and mortality data, 1973-1977. *NCI Monog* 57:1981.
11. Clark RM, Rosen IB, Laperreire NJ: Malignant tumors of the head and neck in a young population. *Am J Surg* 144:459–462, 1982.
12. Belfiore A, Giuffrida D, La Rosa GL, et al: High frequency of cancer in cold thyroid nodules occurring at young age. *Acta Endocrinol* 121:197–202, 1989.
13. Winship T, Rosvoll R: Childhood thyroid carcinoma. *Cancer* 14:734–743, 1961.
14. Samaan NA, Schultz PN, Hickey RC, et al: The results of various modalities of treatment of well differentiated thyroid carcinoma: A retrospective review of 1599 patients. *J Clin Endocrinol Metab* 75:714–720, 1992.
15. Zimmerman D, Hay ID, Gough IR, et al: Papillary thyroid carcinoma in children and adults: Long-term follow-up of 1039 patients conservatively treated at one institution during three decades. *Surgery* 104:1157–1166, 1988.
16. Ferreiro JA, Weiland LH: Pediatric surgical pathology of the head and neck. *Semin Pediatr Surg* 3:169–181, 1994.
17. Carcangui ML, Bianchi S: Diffuse sclerosing variant of papillary carcinoma of the thyroid: Clinicopathologic study of 15 cases. *Am J Surg Pathol* 13:1041–1049, 1989.
18. Fujimoto Y, Obara T, Ito Y, et al: Diffuse sclerosing variant of papillary carcinoma of the thyroid: Clinical importance, surgical treatment, and follow-up study. *Cancer* 66:2306–3212, 1990.
19. Van Heeden JA, Hay ID, Goellner JR, et al: Follicular thyroid carcinoma with capsular invasion alone: A non-threatening malignancy. *Surgery* 112:1130–1136, 1992.
20. Vribe M, Grimes M, Fenoglio-Preiser CM, et al: Medullary carcinoma of the thyroid gland: Clinical, pathological, and immunohistochemical

features with review of the literature. *Am J Surg Pathol* 9:577–594, 1985.

21. Norton JA, Froome LC, Farrell RE, et al: Multiple endocrine neoplasia type IIb—The most aggressive form of medullary thyroid carcinoma. *Surg Clin North Am* 59:109–118, 1979.

22. Wells SA Jr, Baylin SB, Leight GS, et al: The importance of early diagnosis in patients with hereditary medullary thyroid carcinoma. *Ann Surg* 195:595–599, 1982.

23. Shimotake T, Inwa N, Yangigara J: Prediction of affected MEN2A gene carriers by DNA linkage analysis for early total thyroidectomy: Progress in clinical screening program for children with hereditary cancer syndrome. *J Pediatr Surg* 27:444–446, 1992.

24. Pacini F, Romei C, Miccoli P, et al: Early treatment of hereditary medullary thyroid carcinoma after attribution of multiple endocrine neoplasia type 2 gene carrier status by screening for *ret* gene mutations. *Surgery* 118:1031–1035, 1995.

25. Frilling A, Dralle H, Eng C, et al: Presymptomatic DNA screening in families with multiple endocrine neoplasia type 2 and familial medullary thyroid carcinoma. *Surgery* 118:1099–1104, 1995.

26. Skinner MA, DeBenedetti MK, Moley JF, et al: Medullary thyroid carcinoma in children with multiple endocrine neoplasia types 2A and 2B. *J Pediatr Surg* 31:177–182, 1996.

27. Terrier P, Sheng ZM, Schlumberger M, et al: Structure and expression of c-*myc* and c-*fos* proto-oncogenes in thyroid carcinomas. *Br J Cancer* 57:43–47, 1988.

28. Mincione G, Cirafici AM, Lazzareschi D, et al: Loss of thyrotropin regulation and transforming growth factor β-induced growth arrest in *erb* B-2 overexpressing rat thyroid cells. *Cancer Res* 53:5548–5553, 1993.

29. Bongarzone I, Pierotti MA, Monzini N, et al: High frequency of activation of tyrosine kinase oncogenes in human papillary carcinomas and their lymph-nodal metastases. *Nature* 328:170–172, 1987.

30. Lemoine NR, Mayall ES, Wyllie FS, et al: Activated *ras* oncogenes in human thyroid cancers. *Cancer Res* 48:4459–4463, 1988.

31. Fagin JA, Matsuo K, Karmakar A, et al: High prevalence of mutations of the p53 gene in poorly differentiated human thyroid carcinomas. *J Clin Invest* 91:179–184, 1993.

32. Kobayashi T, Nakanishi H, Yana I, et al: Clinicopathological findings and p53 expression of thyroid cancer in children. *Surg Today* 25:217–221, 1995.

33. Hayles AB, Johnson LM, Beahrs OH, et al: Carcinoma of the thyroid gland in children. *Am J Surg* 106:g735–743, 1963.

34. Hung W, August GP, Randolph JG, et al: Solitary thyroid nodules in children and adolescents. *J Pediatr Surg* 3:225–229, 1982.

35. Compagno J, Oertel JE: Malignant lymphoma and other lymphoproliferative disorders of the thyroid gland: A clinicopathologic study of 245 cases. *Am J Clin Pathol* 74:1–11, 1980.

36. Flemming ID, Black TL, Thompson EI, et al: Thyroid dysfunction and neoplasia in children receiving neck radiation for cancer. *Cancer* 55:1190–1194, 1985.

37. Viswanathan K, Gierlowski TC, Schneider AB: Childhood thyroid cancer: Characteristics and long-term outcome in children irradiated for benign conditions of the head and neck. *Arch Pediatr Adolesc Med* 148:260–265, 1994.

38. Kazakov VS, Demidchik EP, Astokhovl LN: Thyroid cancer after Chernobyl. *Nature* 359:21, 1992.

39. Baverstock K, Egloff B, Pinchera A: Thyroid cancer after Chernobyl. *Nature* 359:21–22, 1992.

40. Baverstock KF: Thyroid cancer in children in Belarus after Chernobyl. *World Health Stat Q* 46:204–208, 1993.

41. Nikiforov Y, Gnepp DR: Pediatric thyroid cancer after the Chernobyl disaster: Pathomorphologic study of 84 cases. *Cancer* 74:748–66, 1994.

42. Korff JM, Degroot LJ: The management of radiation-induced tumors of the thyroid. *Endocrinol Metabol Clin North Am* 10:299–315, 1981.

43. Kaplan MM, Garnick MB, Gelber R, et al: Risk factors for thyroid abnormalities after neck irradiation for childhood cancer. *Am J Med* 74:272–280, 1983.

44. Dailey ME, Lindsay S, Skahen R: Relation of thyroid neoplasms in Hashimoto's disease of the thyroid gland. *Arch Surg* 70:291–297, 1955.

45. Bachrach LK, Daneman D, et al: Use of ultrasound in childhood thyroid disorders. *J Pediatr* 103:547–552, 1983.

46. Brander A, Viikinoski P, Nickels J, et al: Thyroid gland: US screening in a random adult population. *Radiology* 181:683–687, 1991.

47. Garcia CJ, Daneman A, McHugh K, et al: Sonography in thyroid carcinoma in children. *Br J Radiol* 65:977–982, 1992.

48. Moir CR, Telander RL: Papillary carcinoma of the thyroid in children. *Semin Pediatr Surg* 3:182–187, 1994.

49. Gharib H, Goellner JR: Fine-needle aspiration biopsy of the thyroid: An appraisal. *Ann Intern Med* 118:282–289, 1993.

50. Gharib H: Fine-needle aspiration biopsy of thyroid nodules: Advantages, limitations, and effect. *Mayo Clin Proc* 69:44–49, 1994.

51. Meko JB, Norton JA: Large cystic/solid thyroid nodules: A potential false-negative fine-needle aspiration. *Surgery* 118:996–1004, 1995.

52. Telander RL, Zimmerman D, Kaufman BH, et al: Pediatric endocrine surgery. *Surg Clin North Am* 65:1551–1557, 1985.

53. Vassilopoulou-Sellin R, Klein MJ, Smith TH, et al: Pulmonary metastases in children and young adults with differentiated thyroid cancer. *Cancer* 71:1348–1352, 1993.

54. Cohn KH, Backdahl M, Forsslund G, et al: Biologic considerations in operative strategy in papillary thyroid carcinoma: Arguments against the routine performance of total thyroidectomy. *Surgery* 96:957–968, 1984.
55. Gibb GK, Pasieka JL: Assessing the need for frozen sections: Still a valuable tool in thyroid surgery. *Surgery* 118:1005–1010, 1995.
56. Ceccaralli C, Pacini F, Lippie F, et al: Thyroid cancer in children and adolescents. *Surgery* 104:1143–1148.
57. Newman KD, Black T, Heller G, et al: Differentiated thyroid cancer: Determinants of disease progression in patients <21 years of age at diagnosis. *Children's Cancer Group*, unpublished data.
58. Foster RF: Morbidity and mortality after thyroidectomy. *Surg Gynecol Obstet* 146:423–429, 1978.
59. LaQuaglia MP, Corbally MT, Heller G, et al: Recurrence and morbidity in differentiated thyroid carcinoma in children. *Surgery* 104:1149–1156, 1988.
60. Turner JE, Weir GJ: Pulmonary metastasis from thyroid carcinoma detectable only by I131 scan: Treatment and response. *J Nucl Med* 13:852–855, 1972.
61. Beierwaltes WH: The treatment of thyroid carcinoma with radioactive iodine. *Semin Nucl Med* 8:79–94, 1978.
62. Vassilopoulou-Sellin R, Libshitz HI, Haynie TP: Papillary thyroid cancer with pulmonary metastases beginning in childhood: Clinical course over three decades. *Med Pediatr Oncol* 24:119–122, 1995.
63. Buckwalter JA, Nelson JG, Thomas CG: Cancer of the thyroid in youth. *World J Surg* 5:15–25, 1981.
64. Schlumberger M, Vathaire F, Travagli JP, et al: Differentiated thyroid carcinoma in childhood: Long-term follow-up of 72 patients. *J Clin Endo Metab* 65:1088–1094, 1987.
65. Basolo F, Pinchera A, Fugazzola L, et al: Expression of p21 *ras* protein as a prognostic factor in papillary thyroid cancer. *Eur J Cancer* 30:171–174, 1994.
66. Owens LV, Xu L, Dent GA, et al: Focal adhesion kinase as a marker of invasive potential in differentiated human thyroid cancer. *Ann Surg Oncol* 3:100–105, 1996.
67. Jossart GH, Greulich KM, Siperstein AE, et al: Molecular and cytogenetic characterization of a t(1;10;21) translocation in the human papillary thyroid cancer cell line TPC-1 expressing the *ret/*H4 chimeric transcript. *Surgery* 118:1018–1023, 1995.
68. Kirk JM, Mort C, Grant D, et al: The usefulness of serum thyroglobulin in the follow-up of differentiated thyroid carcinoma in children. *Med Pediatr Oncol* 20:201–208, 1992.

Gastrointestinal Tumors

• *Edward G. Ford, M.D.*

Malignant lesions of the gastrointestinal (GI) tract in children occur at rates far below those of the central nervous system, neuroblastoma, nephroblastoma, lymphoma, and leukemia. When tumors of the liver are excluded (Chapter 11), the remaining solid tumors of the intestine are extremely rare. Most GI tumors in adults are of epithelial tissues, whereas tumors in children are usually lymphatic or stromal. Of 39 childrenwith GI tumors at James Whitcomb Riley Hospital for Children, Indianapolis, 30% had benign lesions. The mean age of presentation was 9 years. About one third of children complained of abdominal pain, one third had a palpable mass, and about one fourth had rectal bleeding. Of those children with malignant lesions, 81% had non-Hodgkin's lymphoma and 14% had adenocarcinoma of the colon. One child had a leiomyosarcoma of the stomach.[1] This relatively small number of patients, which was collected over 20 years at a major children's hospital, speaks to the rarity of GI tumors in children.

Children with acquired immune deficiency syndrome (AIDS) have a number of GI manifestations that are caused by opportunistic infections, lymphoproliferative diseases, and cancers. GI tumors are becoming more common in this patient population, especially lymphomas, Kaposi's sarcomas, and smooth-muscle tumors.[2,3]

A convenient method of discussing intestinal tumors is to use the World Health Organization (WHO) histologic typing of intestinal tumors.[4] In this system, tumors are identified by site (small intestine, appendix, large intestine, and rectum) and then classified as epithelial tumors, carcinoid tumors, nonepithelial tumors, hematopoietic/

lymphoid neoplasms (Chapter 14), unclassified tumors, secondary tumors, or tumor-like lesions. This chapter uses the WHO outline where practical. GI tumors in children are so rare that each histologic subtype may not be represented for each anatomic site listed. The primary anatomic sites to be discussed are the esophagus, stomach, small intestine, appendix, and large intestine.

THE ESOPHAGUS

Apparent "tumors" of the esophagus in children are usually the result of external compression (vascular ring,[5] mediastinal masses) or benign lesions (leiomyoma, enterogenous cysts, bronchogenic foregut malformations).[6] True malignant lesions of the esophagus in children are rare.

Epithelial Tumors

Gastroesophageal reflux (GER) is a normal finding in newborns; persistence of reflux is a common problem in the pediatric population. Symptomatic or persistent reflux is treated with medication or antireflux surgery. Children with both untreated and treated (medically and surgically) GER may be at risk for the development of dysplasia and the subsequent adenocarcinoma of the esophagus.[7]

Patients with long-standing GER may develop glandular metaplasia (Barrett's esophagus) of the distal esophagus (Fig. 16–1).[8] Whereas over 250 reports have been published in the past 5 years alone concerning identification and treatment of Barrett's esophagus in adults, fewer than 200 pediatric patients have been presented in all the literature. Up to 10% of adults with Barrett's syndrome may be expected to develop adenocarcinoma, but only two children with adenocarcinoma have been reported to date.[9] The disparity may be the result of a surveillance and reporting error. Routine biopsy of the distal esophagus of those children with GER is unusual, unless clinical changes are noted, so the true incidence of metaplasia in children is unknown. According to statistical observations from the Riley Children's Hospital experience, an estimated 33 of 100 children with Barrett's esophagus will eventually (over a 50-year follow-up) develop adenocarcinoma.[4] These investigators conclude the following:

1. Barrett's esophagus in children is more common than previously suspected, and its prevalence will increase owing to an increasing number of children with GER. As the cohort of children at high risk matures, an increased number of cases of Barrett's esophagus may be expected.
2. Because the epithelium of Barrett's syndrome is often not visually evident in children, accurate diagnosis will require screening endoscopic biopsies of children with GER before and after treatment.
3. As in adults, metaplasia of Barrett's syndrome in children rarely reverts to normal squamous epithelium despite a successful antireflux procedure.
4. Children with small-intestinal metaplasia are at higher risk for developing malignant transformation than those with fundic or junctional epithelium only.
5. In order to achieve successful resection and improved cure rates, long-term surveillance is needed to detect cases of dysplasia or esophageal carcinoma before transmural infiltration occurs.
6. Children demonstrating severe dysplasia should be considered for early esophageal resection.

These recommendations are reasonable, considering that esophagectomy for adenocarcinoma in the esophagus of a patient with Barrett's syndrome is curative—if the resection is undertaken while the carcinoma is still intramucosal or intramural.[10]

Nonepithelial Tumors

Smooth muscle makes up the predominant tissue of the esophagus. Benign and malignant smooth-muscle tumors (leiomyoma and leiomyosarcoma) are common in adults, but less than 5% are found in children. Smooth-muscle tumors in children are strangely opposite those of adults. Adult tumors are isolated, more common in men, and sporadic. Pediatric tumors are multiple or diffuse, more common in girls, and frequent in syndromic patients (i.e., those with multiple congenital anomalies). The presenting symptoms are those of esophageal obstruction, that is, dysphagia, retained foodstuffs, emesis of undigested food, and chest pain. Contrast esophagrams may

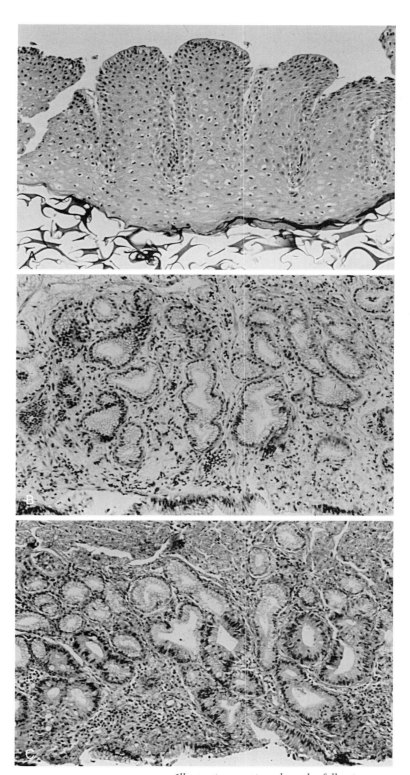

Figure 16–1 • Histologic changes in the development of adenocarcinoma of the esophagus from gastroesophageal reflux. *A*, Histologic changes consistent with reflux esophagitis. The papillae of the lamina propria extend farther into the epithelium than normal, occupying about two thirds of its thickness. There is mild hyperplasia of the basal zone, and increased numbers of lymphocytes are present. *B*, Columnar epithelial-lined (Barrett's) esophagus. The epithelium present in this biopsy closely resembles that normally found in the gastric cardia and can be diagnosed as Barrett's esophagus only in light of the knowledge that it came from above the lower esophageal sphincter. *C*, Barrett's esophagus with mild epithelial dysplasia. The epithelium is similar to that seen in Figure 16-1*B* except that the nuclei are hyperchromatic, crowded, and stratified. The epithelium in the deeper parts of the mucosa remains normal.

Illustration continued on the following page

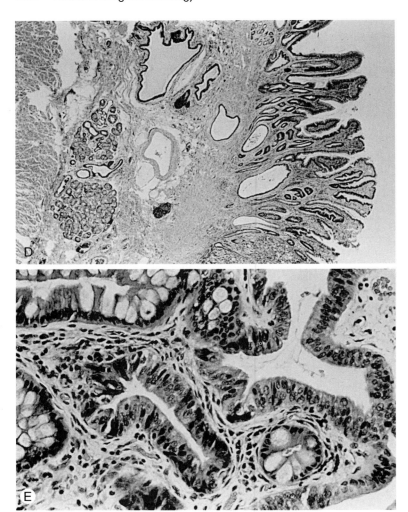

Figure 16–1 • *Continued D*, Barrett's esophagus with epithelial dysplasia and adenocarcinoma. The submucosal glands seen here confirm its esophageal origin. The columnar epithelium has given rise to an early adenocarcinoma (far right). *E*, High-power examination of the previous plate reveals small intestine–appearing epithelium as well as the presence of marked epithelial dysplasia. (From Roger C. Haggitt, M.D., Department of Pathology, The University of Washington, Seattle, WA, with permission. Used earlier in American Society of Clinical Pathologists Educational Courses.)

show a dilated proximal esophagus interpreted as achalasia rather than an intramural tumor. Esophagoscopy will reveal a mucosa-covered constriction suggestive of stricture. Symptoms will not resolve without surgical resection. Because of the usual diffuse nature of the tumor, the required resections may be extensive and must be tailored for each patient. Large resections may require esophageal substitution.

Leiomyosarcomas may occur in any portion of the GI tract. Only three reports of these lesions have appeared in the literature on pediatric patients. None involved tumors of the esophagus. The first case was that of a 12-year-old who was included in a cohort of 191 patients studied from 1957 to 1987 at M.D. Anderson Cancer Center.[11] The report detailed general patterns of failure in

GI leiomyosarcomas and did not specify details of the pediatric patient.

The second case was that of a 4-year-old girl with disseminated leiomyosarcoma associated with AIDS.[12] She presented with abdominal pain, anorexia, and epigastric tenderness. Initial barium upper GI series (UGI), abdominal sonogram (U/S), and esophagogastroduodenoscopy (EGD) were not helpful in diagnosis. Complaints persisted, and follow-up EGD showed numerous raised nodules in the stomach, duodenum, and small intestine. Biopsy was unrevealing. Persistence and worsening of the abdominal pain eventually prompted laparotomy and appendectomy. The appendix showed nodules consistent with leiomyosarcoma. The patient died 5 months later. Postmortem examination showed over 40 intestinal tumors with metastases in the lungs and brain.

The third case was that of a 12-year-old with leiomyosarcoma of the stomach included in the review of GI tumors from Riley Children's Hospital. She presented with GI bleeding and abdominal pain. She underwent partial gastrectomy and received adjuvant chemotherapy. Two years later she returned with widespread metastasis to the liver and died 6 years after diagnosis.

THE STOMACH

Nonepithelial Tumors

Most neoplasms are composed of cells derived from a single cell line and histologically resemble one another. Teratomas are tumors of multiple germ layers composed of distinct well-differentiated tissues such as skin, teeth, brain, respiratory epithelium, fat, and muscle.[13] Uncertainty regarding the etiopathology of teratomas is reflected by the large number of theories presented. The three most common etiologic theories suggest (1) an abortive attempt at twinning, (2) a pathogenetic development of a single unfertilized gamete (parthenogenetic tumors), and (3) a development of pluripotent cells lost during the tissue-differentiation stage of embryogenesis.[14,15] Teratomas occur as benign, well-differentiated cystic lesions or as solid malignant tumors. Most benign teratomas occur in younger infants (<4 months of age), with malignancy rates directly related to the patient's age.

A large study from Children's Hospital of Los Angeles showed that teratomas are seen, in order of frequency, in the sacrococcygeal region (42.9%), ovary (38.3%), testes (4.5%), retroperitoneum (3.8%), mediastinum (3%), intracranial loci (3%), and other sites (4.5%).[16] Gastric tumors comprise less than 1% of all childhood teratomas, usually present in the first 3 months of life, and are located along the greater curvature.[17] Common clinical presentations include abdominal mass (75%), abdominal distention (56%), emesis (18%), hematemesis or melena (15%), respiratory distress (15%), and anemia (15%). Gastric teratomas differ from other teratomas in that most occur in males (96%), they originate from the visceral wall, and no reported case exists of malignant gastric teratoma (although there are three reports of immature gastric teratomas in

children.[18]) Gastric teratomas are large tumors, usually exceeding 10 cm in diameter. Of 40 cases reviewed by Moriuchi[18a], 20 arose from the posterior gastric wall, eight from the anterior wall, five from the lesser curvature, three from the greater curvature, two from the entire stomach, and one from the fundus.

Plain films and UGI series usually show a large soft-tissue mass limited to one quadrant of the abdomen, which deforms the stomach; displaces the intestine; and usually contains coarse, globular calcifications resembling bone and teeth.[19,20] Ultrasonography and computed tomography (CT) scans may identify characteristic cystic and solid areas within the tumor (Fig. 16–2). Cysts are homogeneously anechoic and sharply marginated. Solid areas are homogeneous with focal high intensity echoes characteristic of calcification. A CT scan is specific in the detection of fat in the periphery of the tumor or within the septations dividing cystic areas.

Needle aspiration for diagnosis is unnecessary and may be misleading. In one report, an aspiration biopsy from an area of brain tissue within a teratoma led to an erroneous diagnosis of neuroblastoma and subsequent radiotherapy.[21] Simple excision and reconstruction of the stomach are the treatment of choice. In a review of 46 patients with gastric teratomas, 32 underwent simple excision, 10 partial gastrectomy, and 1 total gastrectomy.[22,23] Patients undergoing partial or total gastrectomy must be carefully followed as they may develop iron deficiency anemia, B_{12} and folate deficiency, steatorrhea, gastroesophageal reflux, or growth retardation.

THE SMALL INTESTINE

Hematopoietic/Lymphoid Neoplasms

The predominant GI malignant tumors in children are non-Hodgkin's lymphomas of the distal small bowel, cecum, and appendix.[1] As children become older, the pattern of presentation in them approaches that of adults, with the typical location being the stomach.[24] More male patients are seen with intestinal lymphoma than with gastric lymphoma. About one half of the children have a palpable mass, and about one half have an initial complaint of intermittent/crampy abdominal pain. No patient presents with Stage I disease. Of those patients with Stage II disease

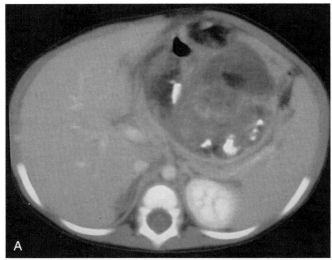

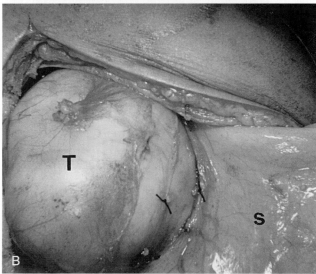

Figure 16–2 • *A*, Computed tomogram of the abdomen of a child with a gastric teratoma. The mass is lateral to the liver and medial to the spleen, contains multiple coarse calcifications, and is multiseptate. *B*, Intra-operative photograph of the teratoma: S = stomach; T = tumor.

(73%), 81% survive for a mean follow-up period of 4.5 years. There are no survivors among Stage III or IV patients. Treatment modalities available for GI lymphoma include chemotherapy, radiation, and surgical resection.

Some controversy exists as to the role of surgical resection. In large reviews, patients with *gastric lymphoma* had the same 5-year survival rate irrespective of whether the primary tumor was resected.[25] Patients with *intestinal lymphoma* who did not experience perforation or hemorrhage did well with surgical resection.[26] In one report patients undergoing complete resection did well even if they were not treated with adjuvant chemotherapy.[27] The patients who did

poorly were those with intestinal tumors who underwent tumor debulking or partial resection followed by chemotherapy.

As many as one half of patients reported as "nonresected" were those who presented with perforations. This group has a mortality of >90%. The relationship of the high mortality to the perforation, the degree of tumor resection, or whether the patient's course was complicated by profound malnutrition (because of advanced tumor burden, unresectable tumor mass, or leukopenia following an intensive chemotherapy regimen for unfavorable histology) is yet undefined. Those patients who present with intestinal lymphoma with obstruction, perforation, or hemorrhage are probably best treated by attempted resection of the tumor and primary anastomosis.

Some also suggest that surgical intervention may not even significantly improve staging accuracy, provided there is a thorough nonoperative staging protocol including multiple endoscopies, CT scan, and lymphangiography.

THE PANCREAS

Pancreatic cancers in children are rare. The children will present with a palpable mass, and a typical history may include abdominal pain, weight loss, intestinal obstruction, diarrhea, or lower leg edema. Jaundice is an infrequent finding.[28] The types of tumors (adenocarcinomas) encountered in children are similar to those in adults, and treatment includes standard surgical resection. Infants and children tolerate pancreatoduodenectomy well, with a reported 9% mortality.[29,30] Occasionally (30% of cases), children may have functioning or nonfunctioning islet-cell tumors. There is an association of islet tumors and the Type I *multiple endocrine neoplasia* (MEN) syndrome, so that children in families with this syndrome must be carefully evaluated and followed. These tumors are usually non-beta islet tumors, and patients may present as the Zollinger-Ellison syndrome.

THE APPENDIX
Carcinoid Tumors

Carcinoid tumors are derived from enterochromaffin cells within the crypts of Lieberkühn, located throughout the GI tract. Most carcinoids are clinically silent and are discovered incidentally at surgery or autopsy. All carcinoid tumors are potentially malignant; however, their tendency toward metastasis depends upon the site of origin. Carcinoids are most commonly found in the ileum (30%) and appendix (30%); less frequently in the cecum, duodenum, and jejunum; and very rarely in the rectum or pylorus. Most reports detail patient presentations made from 5 years of age and older (mean 50 years); those patients with carcinoid of the appendix average 32 years of age at time of diagnosis. Patients in whom tumors occur before age 5 are extremely rare and reportable. Enterochromaffin cells are usually not apparent within the intestinal tract until approximately 4 years of age, and it is thought that this probably contributes to the extreme rarity of carcinoid tumors in very young children.

The age-standardized incidence of carcinoid tumor in the United States is 1.3 per 100,000 per year in men and 1.6 per 100,000 per year in women. The incidence in children between 10 and 15 years of age is 0.4 per 100,000 per year in boys and 0.8 per 100,000 per year in girls. Some have suggested that the higher incidence in females may represent a tendency toward a higher laparotomy rate in women with abdominal pain. Approximately 50% of patients with appendiceal tumors present with acute abdominal symptoms suggestive of appendicitis.[31]

Approximately 60% of carcinoid tumors are confined to the bowel at the time of diagnosis; metastatic disease may be present in the remaining 40% of cases. Appendiceal carcinoids are almost never metastatic, whereas 70% of ileal and all cecal carcinoids are metastatic. Classifying carcinoid tumors as benign or malignant is usually not possible based simply on histology. The tumors show very little in the way of pleomorphism, nuclear hyperchromasia, or increased mitotic activity, and local intramural invasion does not indicate advanced or metastatic disease. The distinction between a benign and malignant carcinoid is based on the presence or absence of metastases.

The carcinoid syndrome occurs in 15% to 25% of patients and consists of various clinical manifestations. Flushing and diarrhea occur in about three fourths of patients; less frequently, patients may have telangiectasias, cyanosis, bronchial constriction suggestive of asthma, cardiac valvular anomalies, pellagra, or carcinoid crisis. The syndrome occurs when tumors secrete vasoactive substances such as serotonin, histamine, bradykinin, or prostaglandins. The diagnosis of carcinoid in symptomatic patients may be confirmed by identifying elevated urinary levels of 5-hydroxyindoleacetic acid (5-HIAA), the metabolic product of serotonin. The disease progresses slowly, and patients should be treated symptomatically. Octreotide is a long-acting parenteral somatostatin analog that is effective in alleviating the clinical symptoms. Conventional chemotherapy has little place in treating metastatic carcinoid.

Appendectomy is the treatment for appendiceal carcinoid. Carcinoids found in the small intestine and stomach are frequently multicentric, and the intestine must be thoroughly examined for other tumors. Ileal tumors should undergo wide resection, including removal of the regional lymph nodes.[32]

THE LARGE INTESTINE

Epithelial Tumors

In the Riley Children's Hospital experience, adenocarcinoma of the large intestine was the second most common GI tumor. One half of the tumors were of the right colon, and the remainder were equally distributed between the left colon and rectum. All of the children had advanced disease at presentation, three fourths with Duke's Stage C and one fourth with Duke's Stage D with metastasis to the liver. Three fourths of the patients died from disease, and one fourth are living with residual disease. Surgical treatment involves tumor resection en bloc with regional lymph nodes. Results of adjuvant therapy are variable but consistently disappointing. Resection of large, fixed rectal tumors may be facilitated by preoperative radiation therapy.

Tumor-like Lesions

Polyps, by far, outnumber actual tumors of the GI tract in children. Polyps may occur either spontaneously or in association with inherited (familial) polypoid diseases.[33] The majority of polypoid lesions and diseases are benign. The spectrum of diseases associated with intestinal polyps in children is presented in Table 16–1.

Table 16–1. • Inherited and Spontaneous Polypoid Lesions Found in Children

Juvenile polyps
Juvenile polyposis
Lymphoid polyps
Inflammatory polyps
Inherited polyps
Cronkhite-Canada syndrome
Peutz-Jeghers syndrome
Familial adenomatous polyposis
Turcot's syndrome
Gardner's syndrome

Juvenile Polyps

Approximately 1% of children have benign, asymptomatic intestinal juvenile polyps. The peak instance of clinical presentation occurs at 4 years of age, with boys twice as likely to come to medical attention as girls. The most common clinical presentation is painless rectal bleeding. Next most commonly, patients will have intestinal prolapse with the polyp as a lead point or protrusion of the polyp itself through the anus. Approximately 10% of patients will undergo auto-amputation and pass the polyp with stool.

Most polyps (60%) are located within 10 cm of the anus, greater than 1 cm in diameter, and easily identifiable with a standard proctoscope. Fewer than 10% are located more than 20 cm from the anus.[34]

Juvenile polyps are smooth, round, beefy-red tumor-like growths with a stalk. The cut surface shows numerous mucous cysts. Microscopically, the bulk of the tumor is connective tissue with normal-appearing epithelial structures.[35] These polyps are hamartomas and have no malignant potential.

Diagnosis of polyp in the patient with rectal bleeding can usually be made using proctosigmoidoscopy. The lesion can be removed transanally. In patients presenting with prolapse of the intestine or transanal tumor, control of the polypoid stalk must be achieved prior to resection. If the tumor is amputated prior to control of the stalk, it is common for the intestine to quickly retract and thereby return to its normal location at a distance far enough from the anal verge to make hemostatic control difficult. Barium enema or colonoscopy may be used to identify lesions in patients in whom the polyps are suspected but are apparently located beyond the reach of a standard proctosigmoidoscope. Colonoscopy provides the advantage of allowing polyp resection (polypectomy) during the diagnostic endeavor.

Juvenile polyps are usually solitary, but as many as one half of children may have between 2 and 10 polyps. Since these lesions are hamartomas, if they are otherwise asymptomatic and located in areas not amenable to endoscopy (i.e., small intestine), the patient may be followed clinically. Patients who have polyps greater than 1 cm in diameter with an irregular surface, or who have a family history of polyps, may have an adenomatous polyp and should have the polyp removed.

Juvenile Polyposis

A few children with multiple juvenile polyps may have *juvenile polyposis syndrome*.[36] In about one third of patients, other family members are affected, suggesting an autosomal dominant mode of inheritance. Polyps are distributed throughout the GI tract, including the stomach and small intestine. Patients with juvenile polyposis have a clinical course clearly distinct from the relatively benign presentation of juvenile polyps. Large numbers of polyps increase the chances of chronic bleeding, which subsequently leads to iron deficiency anemia, hypoproteinemia, and failure to thrive.[37] Disease in infants and younger children may be devastating. In these small patients, the secondary effects of hemorrhage and protein loss contribute to a high mortality. Juvenile polyposis is considered a potentially premalignant condition by some because children with polyposis may have a family history of adenomatous polyposis and carcinoma of colon. Approximately 6% of these patients develop malignancy.[38] Multiple polyps may be removed by polypectomy during repeated gastroscopy and colonoscopy. Alternatively, children with polyps too numerous to remove endoscopically may undergo surgical resection by laparotomy and multiple enterotomy. Microscopically, these polyps are mucous-retention polyps.

Cronkhite-Canada Syndrome

The *Cronkhite-Canada syndrome* is a variant of juvenile polyposis in which the GI polyposis is associated with skin hyperpigmentation, alopecia, and nail changes.[39] Hair loss and skin and nail changes may be evident long before the GI symptoms. Polyps are found in the stomach and large intestine in almost every patient. Microscopically the polyps are hamartomas. Patients with this syndrome characteristically have a great deal of diarrhea and malabsorption, which leads to vitamin deficiency, hypoproteinemia, and fluid/electrolyte abnormalities. Such patients may also develop malignant neoplasms of the colon, so close follow-up is advised. Polyps may be identified during follow-up and removed endoscopically. Surgical resections may be appropriate when a large number of polyps appear in a small segment of intestine.

Peutz-Jeghers Polyps

Peutz-Jeghers syndrome is a familial autosomal dominant association of GI polyps with altered pigmentation of the mouth and skin.[40] The skin changes include clusters of black or dark brown spots 1 mm to 2 mm in diameter about the lips and buccal mucosa, fingers, and toes, which may be obvious at birth and disappear by puberty. Mucosal pigment changes tend to persist throughout life. Most polyps are found in the small intestine (particularly the jejunum), but may also occur in the stomach, colon, and rectum. Patients may present with abdominal pain from intestinal obstruction by a large polypoid mass or an intussusception. They may also present with rectal bleeding, prolapse of a polyp, passage of spontaneously amputated polyps, hematemesis, or anemia. Many patients will undergo multiple abdominal operations for small bowel obstruction or bleeding.

The polyps are large and pedunculated and microscopically may represent hamartomas or adenomatous polyps. Several reviews have suggested a spectrum of hamartomas proceeding to carcinomatous changes.

Malignancy in this syndrome approaches 50%, with patients having approximately a 50% chance of dying from cancers by age 60 years.[41] Cancers may develop in both GI and non-GI tissues.

Treatment is tailored to the individual. For asymptomatic patients with polyps limited to the small bowel, a course of watchful observation may be undertaken. Gastric or colon polyps may be removed by endoscopic polypectomy. Those patients with significant bleeding, bowel obstruction, or intussusception require laparotomy and polypectomy.

Familial Adenomatous Polyposis Coli

Familial adenomatous polyposis coli is a rare, autosomal dominant polyposis syndrome in which hundreds of adenomatous polyps are found throughout the colon (Fig. 16–3). The disease is further subdivided into Gardner's syndrome and Turcot's syndrome.

The median patient age for presentation of polyposis is 16 years. Intestinal symptoms appear at a median age of 29 years, colorectal cancer a median of 36 years, and death from malignancy a median of 40 years. Patients develop extracolonic

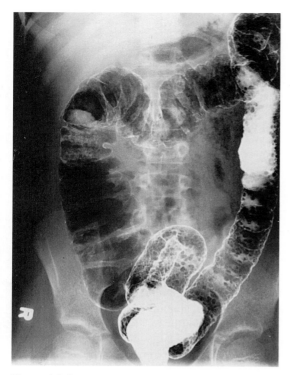

Figure 16–3 • Air contrast barium enema in patient with familiar adenomatous polyposis. Hundreds of polyps are evident throughout the colon.

manifestations that define the characteristic syndromes.

Gardner's syndrome combines colonic polyps with benign extra colonic soft- and hard-tissue tumors. Bone tumors are the most common (80%), followed by inclusion cysts (35%), and desmoid tumors (18%). Epidermal inclusion cysts appear during the first decade of life at a time when there are few, if any, colonic polyps. Lipomas, fibromas, desmoid tumors, and benign bone and cartilage tumors occur during the second decade. Periampullary malignancies may develop during the third or fourth decade at rates much more common than in the general population.

Turcot's syndrome combines GI polyposis with malignant brain tumors. All patients with this syndrome develop carcinoma of the colon as young adults. Colonic adenocarcinomas, which may be multicentric, occur both in the colonic polyps and in mucosa between the polyps.

Familial adenomatous polyposis coli syndromes are usually suspected early in life be-

cause of their strong family history. Diagnostic investigation should begin during the second decade and be continued annually. Clinical symptoms may be similar to those of the polypoid lesions listed earlier—that is, chronic bloody diarrhea, hypoproteinemia, weight loss, anemia, malnutrition, bowel obstruction, and intussusception. Polyps begin as small lesions and gradually increase in both number and size. They are finely lobulated and said to have a raspberry-like appearance. Histologically, the polyps are adenomatous; cellular dysplasia heralds malignant transformation. Dysplasia may occur simultaneously in more than one polyp or in other (nonpolypoid) areas of the colon.

Surgical Management

The surgical options for patients with adenomatous polypoid disease of the colon are several, but each requires colectomy. If the rectum is relatively spared, the patient may undergo total abdominal colectomy with ileoproctostomy. This approach assumes that the patient is willing to undergo frequent endoscopic evaluations of the remaining rectum and polypectomy as lesions arise. If the lesions become dysplasic, the patient may require a completion proctectomy.

Alternatively, the patient may undergo a total abdominal colectomy and abdominal perineal resection of the rectum. These are the only surgical procedures that absolutely guarantee removal of the tissue at risk for development of carcinoma. The disadvantage is that the patient is then subjected to lifelong ileostomy.

An alternative to complete proctocolectomy is total abdominal colectomy with rectal mucosectomy and ileoanal anastomosis. This operative approach removes the entire colon and the mucosa of the rectum. Since the mucosa is the tissue in which dysplasia develops, its removal avoids the risk of malignancy. Yet normal continence is maintained and permanent diverting ostomy unnecessary. The operative procedure may be undertaken in a one-stage procedure, but it is usually combined with a temporary diverting ileostomy to protect the operative field. Reconstruction may be accomplished with a straight ileoanal pull-through, or the distal ileum may be fashioned into a reservoir with a J- or S-type ileal pouch. The long-term results are similar either way.

Lymphoid Polyps

Lymphatic tissues are normally located just below the submucosa of the entire intestine. Children are subjected to a variety of bacterial and viral illnesses that cause hypertrophy of intestinal lymphoid tissue. These lymphoid nodules may enlarge and assume a polypoid shape by the normal traction of intestinal propulsion. Lymphoid polyps are actually pseudopolyps. They are extremely common and may be identified in a majority of pediatric barium air contract enemas. The polyps may occur with some bleeding, as erosion of the overlying mucosa is common. These polyps spontaneously resolve with the inciting clinical event. There is no specific surgical treatment recommended. On occasion, surgeons will be asked to remove these lesions when the patient is suspected to have a true polyp.

Inflammatory Polyps

Inflammatory polyps include several different processes. The most characteristic inflammatory polyp is that associated with chronic ulcerative colitis (discussed later). A second type of inflammatory polyp is termed the *inflammatory fibroid polyp*. These polyps are solitary polypoid or sessile lesions that develop from local inflammation. They are not restricted to any age group, although lesions are most commonly found in the sixth decade. Polyps may be located throughout the GI tract, most commonly the gastric antrum (70%) and small bowel (20%), and they may cause obstruction. The radiographic appearance is that of a smooth, spheric intraluminal mass.

Microscopically, the polyps are similar to granulation tissue, with loose fascicles of proliferating fibroblasts surrounded by capillaries. Very little resemblance is seen to any other soft-tissue tumor, and there is no evidence that these lesions are true vascular tumors. The polyp is thought to simply represent an inflammatory overgrowth of granulation tissue that is confined to the GI tract.[42, 43]

A disease often confused with inflammatory polyps is eosinophilic gastroenteritis. The age distribution is comparable to that of inflammatory polyps, and symptoms suggest upper GI obstruction. Often there is a history of recurrent attacks. Many patients (70%) have a personal or family history of allergies. A barium GI series shows mucosal irregularities and pseudopolyposis that may simulate Crohn's disease or gastric malignancy. Microscopically there is intense edema of the submucosa and diffuse eosinophilic infiltration. The causes of this disease are unknown, although allergies seem most likely. The disease has been found in association with roundworm larvae, various parasites, and gluten and dermatitis herpetiformis. The treatment for eosinophilic gastroenteritis involves identification and removal of the allergen from the diet.

Table 16–2. • Factors Predisposing Colon Cancer in Patients with Ulcerative Colitis

Ulcerative colitis of the entire colon
Prolonged duration of illness
Continuous disease (as compared with intermittent disease)
Severity of disease

ULCERATIVE COLITIS

Patients with inflammatory bowel disease are at risk for developing dysplastic mucosal changes and subsequent adenocarcinomas. Carcinomas of the colon arising in patients with ulcerative colitis (UC) have been evident since the original report in 1925.[44] A number of factors are significant in identifying patients at risk for developing carcinomas (Table 16–2); however, the age of UC onset is not one of these factors.

The earliest that patients develop carcinoma is approximately 7 years from the onset of the inflammatory disease. There is an increased risk of carcinoma with increased duration of the disease (Table 16–3). The overall incidence of carcinoma in UC patients is reported as between 2% and 5% for boys and girls, respectively. Patients

Table 16–3. • Cumulative Risk of Cancer in Ulcerative Colitis

Age (years)	Risk (%)
25	25
30	35
35	45
40	65

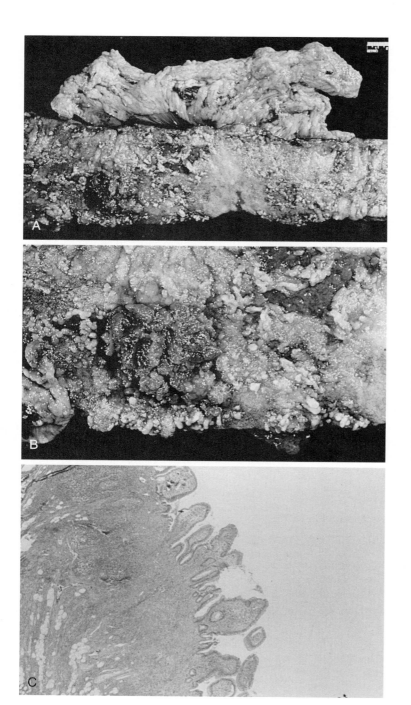

Figure 16–4 • *A*, Gross changes evident in colectomy specimen from a 15-year-old patient with ulcerative colitis. The specimen is not uniform, and multiple areas of hemorrhage are evident. *B*, Mucosa of the colon shows an irregular pattern with multiple true polyps and pseudopolyps. *C*, Representative microscopic section of the colon showing thickened basement tissues infiltrated with large numbers of inflammatory cells and loss of the normal mucosal barrier.

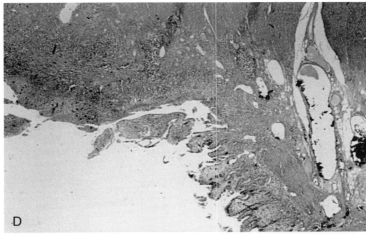

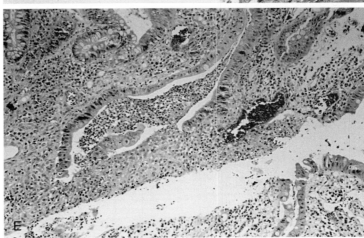

Figure 16–4 • *Continued D,* Ulceration of the colonic mucosa with loss of mucosa, erosion of basement tissues, and dense inflammatory infiltrate. *E,* Crypt abscess in the same patient.

Illustration continued on the following page

with left-sided disease tend to develop cancers about a decade earlier than those with total colon disease. Patients with cancer may be asymptomatic.

The adenocarcinoma in patients with UC is somewhat different from standard adenocarcinoma of the colon in that it tends to be infiltrative, dysplastic, and aggressive. Half the patients will have colloid cancers with mucous-secreting tumors of the signet-ring cell type.[44] Patients who develop colonic strictures should be considered to have carcinomas until proved otherwise. Stricture is an indication for surgical intervention. In one report, 11 of 15 patients with strictures were found to have carcinomas on biopsy.[45]

Among patients with chronic symptomatic UC who present with cancers, 40% have Duke's A or B as compared with 63% if the cancers arise in the absence of active disease. Conversely, 60%

of patients with cancer and colitis will have Duke's C and D tumors, whereas 37% will have carcinomas alone (i.e., asymptomatic patients have advanced tumors). Among those with cancer, 23% have multicentric tumors. Survival is 72% at 5 years in those patients who undergo prophylactic colectomy.[46]

Colonoscopy and proctosigmoidoscopy may not be consistently accurate in the identification of patients with carcinoma. This is particularly true when the patients are examined only when symptomatic. Based upon a great deal of collective experience, the current recommendation is that patients who have had disease for a minimum of 7 years should undergo surveillance endoscopy at least every other year. During these endoscopic interventions, the patient should undergo multiple biopsies of any demonstrated lesion, and multiple random biopsies should be

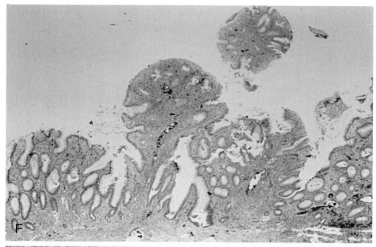

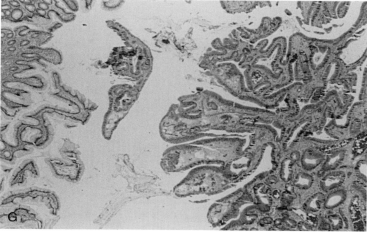

Figure 16–4 • *Continued F*, Inflammatory pseudopolyp in the same patient. *G*, Villous adenoma in the same patient.

taken throughout the colon (a minimum of 10 biopsies). If the biopsies demonstrate severe dysplasia or frank adenocarcinoma, the patient should undergo proctocolectomy.

The surgical options for treatment of patients with chronic ulcerative colitis are similar to those listed earlier for polypoid disease. The risk of cancer is deleted if the entire colon is removed along with the mucosa of the rectum. If the rectal mucosa is left in place, there is a higher risk (3% to 5%) than in the general population for the development of rectal cancer.[47,48] More than one half of these patients have disseminated disease at the time of rectal removal. The estimated cumulative probability of developing cancer in the rectum following colectomy alone is approximately 17% at 27 years.[47] The large number of possible histologic changes in patients with long-standing possible UC are shown in Figure

16–4. This patient had failed to improve despite multiple immunosuppressive medications; colectomy and mucosal proctectomy were prompted by the identification of severe dysplasia on annual colon biopsy.

CONCLUSION

Numerous other lesions may occur within the GI tract as "tumors." For example, the *blue rubber bleb nevus syndrome* is present in children with cutaneous and intestinal hemangiomatoses.[49] The cavernous hemangiomas may occur within the GI tract and appear as bleeding or chronic anemia. Contrast studies of the patient population show "tumors" of the GI tract that may be suggestive of any one of a number of different syndromes. The cutaneous hemangiomas help delineate this particular syndrome. Surgical intervention is confined to regional intestinal segmentectomy for the treatment of bleeding or delayed diagnosis.

Another unusual childhood disease is the *Carney triad*,[50] involving gastric epithelioid tumors, pulmonary chondromas, and extra-adrenal paragangliomas. The gastric tumors have been classified as epithelioid leiomyosarcomas, which also have ultrastructural evidence of being autonomic nervous tumors. Surgical interventions are limited to biopsy and resection of tumors identified by endoscopy or contrast studies.

There are many reports of isolated tumors of the GI tract or tumors associated with other diseases that may be metastatic. These are not discussed here.

Lesions of the GI tract should be histologically explained when identified by either endoscopy or contrast studies. Endoscopic biopsy and resection or enterotomy with biopsy or segmental intestinal resection by formal laparotomy may be required. The more common diseases are outlined in this chapter.

References

1. Skinner MA, Plumley DA, Grosfeld JL, et al: Gastrointestinal tumors in children: An analysis of 39 cases. *Ann Surg Oncol* 1(4):283–289, 1994.
2. Haller JO, Cohen HL: Gastrointestinal manifestations of AIDS in children. *Am J Radiol* 162:387–393, 1994.
3. DiCarlo FJ Jr, Joshi VV, Oleske JM, et al: Neoplastic diseases in children with acquired immunodeficiency syndrome. *Prog AIDS Pathol* 2:163–185, 1990.
4. Morson BC, Sobin LH: Histological Typing of Intestinal Tumours. International Histological Classification of Tumours. Paper No. 15, presented at the World Health Organization, Geneva, 1976.
5. Backer CL, Ilbawi MN, Idriss FS, et al: Vascular anomalies causing tracheoesophageal compression. Review of experience in children. *J Thorac Cardiovasc Surg* 97(5):725–731, 1989.
6. Srikanth MS, Ford EG, Stanley P, et al: Communicating bronchopulmonary foregut malformations. Classification and embryogenesis. *J Pediatr Surg* 27(6):732–736, 1992.
7. Cheu HW, Grosfeld JL, Heifetz SA, et al: Persistence of Barrett's esophagus in children after antireflux surgery: Influence on follow-up care. *J Pediatr Surg* 27(2):260–266, 1992.
8. Chow W-H, Finkle WD, McLaughlin JK, et al: The relation of gastroesophageal reflux disease and its treatment to adenocarcinomas of the esophagus and gastric cardia. *JAMA* 274(6):474–477, 1995.
9. Hoeffel JC, Nihoul-Fekete C, Schmitt M: Esophageal adenocarcinoma after gastroesophageal reflux in children. *J Pediatr* 115(2):259–261, 1989.
10. DeMeester TR, Attwood SE, Smyrk TC, et al: Surgical therapy in Barrett's esophagus. *Ann Surg* 212(4):528–542, 1990.
11. Ng E-H, Pollock RE, Romsdahl MM: Prognostic implications of patterns of failure for gastrointestinal leiomyosarcomas. *Cancer* 69(6):1334–1341, 1992.
12. McLoughlin LC, Nord KS, Joshi VV, et al: Disseminated leiomyosarcoma in a child with acquired immune deficiency syndrome. *Cancer* 67(10):2618–2621, 1991.
13. Cotran RS, Kumar V, Stanley RL: Diseases of infancy and childhood. In *Pathologic Basis of Disease*, 4th ed. Philadelphia: W.B. Saunders Co., 1989, pp. 241, 538.
14. Haley T, Dimler M, Hollier P: Gastric teratoma with gastrointestinal bleeding. *J Pediatr Surg* 21(11):949–950, 1986.
15. Gerald PS: Origin of teratomas. *New Engl J Med* 292(2):103–104, 1975.
16. Mahour GH, Landing BH, Woolley MM: Teratomas in children: Clinicopathologic studies in 133 Patients. *Z Kinderchir* 23(4):365–80, 1978.
17. Cairo MS, Grosfeld JL, Weetman RM: Gastric teratoma: Unusual cause for bleeding of the upper gastrointestinal tract in the newborn. *Pediatrics* 67(5):721–724, 1981.
18. Sharma AK, Sarin YK, Agarwal LD: Immature gastric teratoma in a neonate. *Indian Pediatr* 31(3):357–360, 1994.
18a. Moriuchi A, Nakayama I, Muta H, et al: Gastric teratoma of children—a case report with review of the literature. *Acta Pathologica Japonica* 27:749–758, 1977.
19. Esposito G, Cigliano B, Paludetto R: Abdominothoracic gastric teratoma in a female newborn infant. *J Pediatr Surg* 18(3):304–305, 1983.
20. Azpiroz JC, Valle EM, Herberth AF, et al: Gastric teratoma in infants. *Am J Surg* 128(3):429–432, 1974.
21. Handelsman JC, Reinhoff WF III, Ward GE: Benign teratoma of the stomach in an infant. *Am J Dis Child* 90:196–198, 1955.
22. De Angelis VR: Gastric teratoma in a newborn infant: Total gastrectomy with survival. *Surgery* 66(4):794–797, 1969.
23. Purvis JM, Miller RC, Blumenthal BI: Gastric teratoma: First reported case in a female. *J Pediatr Surg* 14(1):86–87, 1979.
24. Libson E, Mapp E, Dachman AH: Hodgkin's disease of the gastrointestinal tract. *Clin Radiol* 49(3):166–169, 1994.
25. d'Amore F, Brincker H, Grønbæk K, et al: Non-Hodgkin's lymphoma of the gastrointestinal tract: A population-based analysis of incidence, geographic distribution, clinical pathologic presentation features, and prognosis. *J Clin Oncol* 12(8):1673–1684, 1994.

26. Rivera-Luna R, Guerra GM: Abdominal lymphoma and intestinal perforation. *J Clin Oncol* 7(2):285–286 (letter), 1989.

27. Morton JE, Leyland MJ, Hudson GV, et al: Primary gastrointestinal non-Hodgkin's lymphoma: A review of 175 British National Lymphoma Investigation cases. *Br J Cancer* 67:776–782, 1993.

28. Sty JR, Wells RG: Other abdominal and pelvic masses in children. *Semin Roentgenol* 23(3):216–231, 1988.

29. Smith JH 3d, Baugh C, Reppun T: Obstructive jaundice secondary to pancreatic adenocarcinoma in a seven-year-old male. *J Pediatr Surg* 20(2):184–185, 1985.

30. Rich RH, Weber JL, Shandling B: Adenocarcinoma of the pancreas in a neonate managed by pancreatoduodenectomy. *J Pediatr Surg* 21(9):806–808, 1986.

31. Newton JN, Swerdlow AJ, dos Santos Silva IM, et al: The epidemiology of carcinoid tumours in England and Scotland. *Br J Cancer* 70(5):939–942, 1994.

32. Marshall JB, Bodnarchuk G: Carcinoid tumors of the gut: Our experience over three decades and review of the literature. *J Clin Gastroenterol* 16(2):123–129, 1993.

33. Watne AL: Syndromes of polyposis coli and cancer. *Curr Probl Cancer* 7(1):1–31, 1982.

34. Mazier WP, MacKeigan JM, Billingham RP, et al: Juvenile polyps of the colon and rectum. *Surg Gynecol Obstet* 154(6):829–832, 1982.

35. Morson BC: Some peculiarities in the histology of intestinal polyps. *Dis Colon Rectum* 5:337–344, 1962.

36. McColl I, Bussey HJ, Veale AMO, et al: Juvenile polyposis coli. *Proc R Soc Med* 57:896–897, 1964.

37. Grosfeld JL, West KW: Generalized juvenile polyposis coli: Clinical management based on long-term observations. *Arch Surg* 121:530–534, 1986.

38. Desai DC, Neale KF, Talbot IC, et al: Juvenile polyposis (review). *Br J Surg* 82(1):14–17, 1995.

39. Cronkhite LW, Canada WJ: Generalized gastrointestinal polyposis: Unusual syndrome of polyposis syndrome, pigmentation, alopecia and onychatrophia. *N Engl J Med* 252:1011, 1955.

40. Peutz JLA: Very remarkable case of familial polyposis of mucous membrane of the intestinal tract and nasal pharynx accompanied by peculiar pigmentations of skin and mucous membrane. *Nederal Maandschr V Geneesk* 10:134, 1921.

41. Spigelman AD, Murday V, Phillips RK: Cancer and the Peutz-Jeghers syndrome. *Gut* 30(11):1588–1590, 1989.

42. Santos G da C, Zucoloto S: Inflammatory fibroid polyp: Review of the literature. *Arq Gastroenterol* 30(4):107–111, 1993.

43. Blackshaw AJ, Levison DA: Eosinophilic infiltrates of the gastrointestinal tract. *J Clin Pathol* 39:1–7, 1986.

44. Stahl D, Tyler G, Fischer JE: Inflammatory bowel disease—Relationship to carcinoma. In *Current Problems in Cancer.* Chicago: Year Book Medical Publishers, 1981, p. 5.

45. Lashner BA, Turner BC, Bostwick DG, et al: Dysplasia and cancer complicating strictures in ulcerative colitis. *Dig Dis Sci* 35:349–352, 1990.

46. Van Heerdeen JA, Beart RW Jr: Carcinoma of the colon and rectum complicating chronic ulcerative colitis. *Dis Colon Rectum* 23(3):155–159, 1980.

47. Johnson WR, McDermott FT, Hughes ES, et al: The risk of rectal carcinoma following colectomy in ulcerative colitis. *Dis Colon Rectum* 26(1):44–46, 1983.

48. Grundfest SF, Fasio V, Weiss RA, et al: The risk of cancer following colectomy and ileorectal anastomosis for extensive mucosal ulcerative colitis. *Ann Surg* 193(1):9–14, 1981.

49. Sumi Y, Taguchi N, Kaneda T: Blue rubber bleb nevus syndrome with oral hemangiomas. *Oral Surg Oral Med Oral Pathol* 71(1):84–86, 1991.

50. Perez-Atayde AR, Shamberger RC, Kozakewich HW: Neuroectodermal differentiation of the gastrointestinal tumors in the Carney triad: An ultrastructural and immunohistochemical study. *Am J Surg Pathol* 17(7):706–714, 1993.

Primary Bronchopulmonary Tumors

• C. Thomas Black, M.D.

Cancer of the lung is one of the most common forms of malignancy in adults but is quite uncommon in children. A variety of tumors of the lungs and airways, both benign and malignant, has been reported in children, but the scarcity of each tumor type makes it difficult to assess accurately the natural histories and optimal methods of treatment of each type.

In a large series of 230 cases of actual primary lung tumors in children reported by Hartman and Shochat,[1] 151, or 66%, were classified as malignant and 34% as benign (Table 17–1). Distinctions between malignant and benign forms of pediatric primary lung tumors are often subtle. Another review found that the majority of such tumors were benign.[2] Generally, small differences in a chest radiograph or CT scan are all one has upon which to base a diagnosis. Even when tissue is available for the pathologist, many histologic types have been identified, and classification may be difficult.

BENIGN TUMORS

Benign bronchopulmonary masses include the inflammatory pseudotumors, chondromas, leiomyomas, hemangiomas, and granular-cell myoblastomas, and an assortment of radiographic conditions grouped together as pulmonary *coin lesions*.

Inflammatory Pseudotumor

More than half of the benign tumors in the large series just mentioned were postinflammatory

Table 17–1 • Primary Bronchopulmonary Tumors in 230 Children: Classification by Type of Tumor

Type of Tumor	No. Patients (230 total)	
Benign	**64**	
Inflammatory pseudotumor		45
Neurogenic tumor		9
Leiomyoma		6
Mucous gland adenoma		2
Myoblastoma		2
Possibly malignant	**80**	
Pulmonary hamartoma		15
Bronchial adenoma		65
Malignant	**86**	
Bronchogenic carcinoma		47
Pulmonary blastoma		14
Leiomyosarcoma		9
Rhabdomyosarcoma		6
Hemangiopericytoma		3
Lymphoma		3
Teratoma		2
Plasmacytoma		1
Myxosarcoma		1

Adapted from Hartman GE, Shochat SJ: Primary pulmonary neoplasms of childhood: A review. *Ann Thorac Surg* 36:108–119, 1983, with permission of the publisher.

pseudotumors. The term *postinflammatory pseudotumor* or simply *inflammatory pseudotumor* denotes a benign and non-neoplastic lesion comprised of proliferating spindle cells (fibroblasts and myoblasts) with mitotic figures and inflammatory cells, particularly plasma cells. This entity has been variously termed plasma-cell granuloma, xanthofibroma, fibrous xanthoma, sclerosing hemangioma,[3, 4] benign fibrous histiocytoma, and xanthogranuloma; the multiplicity of terms for similar if not identical lesions has contributed to the confusion surrounding this lesion.

Prior to development of the mass there is generally a characteristic mild respiratory infection with symptoms of cough, dyspnea, fever, and hemoptysis lasting several months, although nearly half of affected patients are asymptomatic. Females are disproportionately affected compared with males, at a ratio of between 4 to 1 and 10 to 1. The radiographic pattern shows a single, sharply circumscribed mass in any lobe of the lungs, although the right lower lobe is the most common site. Calcification may be present. The mass frequently occludes totally a mainstem

bronchus. Because of the tumor's benign nature, its excision along with unsalvagable lung tissue is curative.[5] The cause is unknown. There is experimental evidence suggesting a viral etiology; however, one case was preceded by a *Mycoplasma pneumoniae* infection.[6]

Plasma-cell granulomas are sometimes classified as a subset of the inflammatory pseudotumors. They have been associated with high levels of interleukin-1 beta and interleukin-6 as well as hypergammaglobulinemia and may result from a dysregulation of cytokine production.[7] The lesions may be as large as 12 cm in diameter, although they are usually between 2 cm and 5 cm. Their size generally prompts a diagnostic surgical procedure. Treatment consists of thoracotomy with wedge or segmental resection and frozen section or permanent histopathologic correlation. The histologic picture is chiefly one of chronic inflammation with fibrosis.

The plasma-cell granuloma and the *fibrous histiocytoma* share several features.[8] Pulmonary fibrohistiocytic lesions range from the benign fibrous histiocytoma (a form of inflammatory pseudotumor[9]) to fibrohistiocytic lesions of borderline malignant appearance, to frankly malignant fibrous histiocytoma.

Fibrous Tumors

Although not truly malignant, invasive *fibrous tumors* of the trachea and major bronchi may recur unless completely resected.[10] Proliferating fibroblasts and moderate nuclear pleomorphism are seen, but mitotic activity is low. It is important to differentiate these invasive tumors from less invasive inflammatory pseudotumors and to differentiate them from more malignant mesenchymal tumors, such as the fibrous histiocytoma, in order to achieve adequate but not unnecessary resection.

Coin Lesions

Overlapping to some extent with the inflammatory pseudotumors are the *coin lesions*, so-called because of their radiographic appearance as spherical intrapulmonary masses. These may be localized inflammatory lesions, particularly if they appear during or following an upper respiratory infection. Twenty-one such coin lesions occurred during a 10-year period at the Children's Medical Center in Seattle.[11] These lesions were acute inflammatory processes that generally resolved with antibiotic therapy, although some small ones persisted for several months.

Coin lesions have been associated with an atypical measles infection.[12] In this reported case, the patient had a history of partial immunization to measles with the development of an atypical skin rash beginning on the extremities and spreading toward the trunk with a febrile illness. In such a situation, the lesion should be observed. When no previous history suggests measles or upper respiratory infection, any coin lesion persisting over 4–6 weeks should be biopsied by wedge resection.

Leiomyomas

Leiomyomas are benign tumors of smooth muscle.[13] About half are found within the pulmonary parenchyma, where they are usually asymptomatic, and only serendipitously found on chest radiography. About one third are found within the bronchi, where they produce symptoms of partial or complete obstruction with wheezing and distal hyperinflation or atelectasis resulting in chronic infection and tissue destruction. Tracheal lesions may mimic bronchial asthma.[14] One young HIV-positive child developed two bronchial leiomyomas,[15] but no association has been established as yet between the two conditions.

Hemangiomas

Several patients with capillary or other forms of *hemangiomas* of the bronchi are reported in the medical literature.[16,17] Presenting symptoms of bronchial irritation or obstruction are similar to those of many other benign tumors that occur within the trachea or mainstem bronchus (Fig. 17–1). When such symptoms are present, a cutaneous hemangioma may portend intrabronchial hemangioma. Bronchial resection and reanastomosis are ideal treatment; attempted bronchoscopic biopsy or excision, or attempted use of the laser for fulguration, may result in profuse hemorrhage.

Granular-Cell Tumors (Myoblastomas)

Granular-cell tumors are of neurogenic origin and are rarely found in the lower respiratory tract.[18, 19] One granular-cell tumor in the trachea of a 12-year-old boy was successfully resected by tracheal resection and end-to-end anastomosis.[20] Most frequently, hoarseness is the presenting symptom of such a tumor on the true vocal cords or in the subglottic area.

Chondroma

Although pulmonary *chondromas* themselves are recognized as benign lesions, a fascinating association of gastric leiomyosarcoma, extra-adrenal paragangliomas, and pulmonary chondroma (Carney's triad) has been reported in more than 20 patients, the overwhelming majority of them young girls.[21–24]

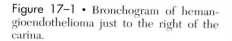

Figure 17–1 • Bronchogram of hemangioendothelioma just to the right of the carina.

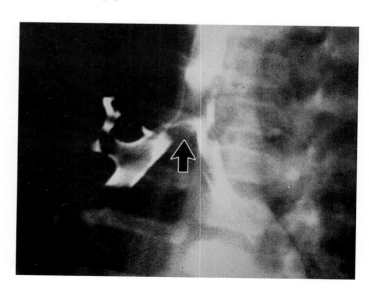

POSSIBLY MALIGNANT TUMORS

A subset of tumors that are variably benign but have a low-grade malignant potential includes some of the more common types of bronchopulmonary tumors, including the pulmonary hamartoma, various forms of bronchial adenoma, and papillomatosis.

Hamartoma

The *hamartoma* is a benign tumor consisting of tissue normally occurring in a particular organ but arranged in an abnormal fashion.[25] This is a rare occurrence in the lung but may be suspected when there is a persistent, smooth, round density, possibly containing calcium, on a chest X ray or computed tomography (CT) scan (Fig. 17–2). Skin tests should be performed to rule out tuberculosis and fungal infections, but diagnosis is frequently not made until after thoracotomy and surgical resection have been performed.

Although hamartomas elsewhere are considered to be benign, complications of pulmonary hamartomas include sudden hemorrhage into a cyst from adjacent pulmonary vessels or hemopneumothorax from the rupture of a subpleural cyst.

One report described an 11-year-old boy with a pulmonary hamartoma known to have been present over an 8-year period in whom poorly differentiated adenocarcinoma of the lung developed.[26] Several other children have developed mesenchymal sarcomas in cystic hamartomas.[27, 28] Our group resected a left upper lobe mass from a newborn child that was found to be a congenital pulmonary hamartoma with fibrosarcoma arising from within. Although pulmonary hamartomas are classified as benign masses, the current recommendation is to resect them.

Bronchial Adenoma

Bronchial adenomas as a group include carcinoids, adenoid cystic carcinomas or cylindromas, and mucoepidermoid carcinomas. They constitute about 35% of all primary pulmonary neoplasms in children. They are not, as their name erroneously implies, always benign tumors.[29]

Bronchial Carcinoids

Bronchial carcinoid tumors are the most common of the bronchial adenomas and account for approximately 60% of all reported cases. The most frequent presenting signs are hemoptysis, cough, and pneumonia. The duration of symptoms ranges from 1 month to 12 years, with a mean of just over 1 year. These tumors generally involve major bronchi, which explains the fact that the symptoms and physical signs are those of bronchial obstruction. The right lung is affected approximately twice as often as the left. Bronchoscopic biopsy is diagnostic in the majority of

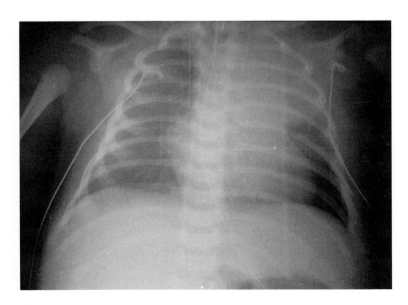

Figure 17–2 • Operative photo of hemangioma within the bronchus intermedius.

cases; however, these tumors are quite vascular and may hemorrhage if biopsied.

Carcinoid tumors generally occur in one of two patterns: (1) as endobronchial polypoid masses that produce segmental bronchial obstruction followed by atelectasis and infection and (2) as iceberg lesions with predominantly extrabronchial growth—the small intrabronchial extent of which gives rise to mucosal ulceration and hemoptysis. In routine histologic preparations, bronchial and intestinal carcinoids usually are indistinguishable from each other but may be distinguishable when levels of enzymes such as monoamine oxidase are assayed.[30]

Carcinoid tumors of the lung consist histologically of "festoons" and "ribbons" of small polyhedral cells with central nuclei and eosinophilic cytoplasm, arranged in a plexiform or an organoid pattern that resembles the pattern of carcinoid tumors (argentaffinomas) of the gastrointestinal tract (Fig. 17–3). Distant metastases are extremely rare, and no documented cases of carcinoid syndrome have been reported, although one symptomatic patient was found to have an elevated serum 5-hydroxyindolacetic acid level.

Adenoid Cystic Carcinomas

Adenoid cystic carcinomas (cylindromas) represent the second group of bronchial adenomas, accounting for about 10% of the total. These are most commonly found in the trachea and are made up of cuboidal or flattened epithelial cells arranged in two layers. Histologically, they resemble mixed tumors of the salivary glands and basal cell carcinomas of the skin. Clinical presentation, physical signs, and diagnostic approach are all similar to those in patients with carcinoids. There is an approximately 40% chance of malignancy with this tumor.

Mucoepidermoid Carcinomas

Approximately 30% of bronchial adenomas are mucoepidermoid carcinomas.[31] These are pedunculated endobronchial tumors that generally arise from the trachea or major bronchi. The epithelial component has somewhat of an epidermoid appearance, and the glandular lumen shows abundant mucus. The incidence of malignancy reported for children with this tumor appears to be extremely low, and survival should be at least 90%.

Papillomatosis

Papillomatosis is a common laryngeal tumor of infancy and childhood associated with the human papilloma virus Type II. The lesions occasionally spread distally into the trachea and occasionally into the bronchi and even the pulmonary parenchyma. Treatment has generally consisted of serial laser fulgeration of the lesions. The development of squamous cell carcinoma, with fatal results, within areas of papilloma has been reported several times.[32] When irradiation has also been administered, the risk of developing squamous cell carcinoma rises an estimated 16-fold.[33]

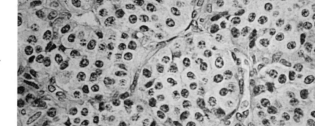

Figure 17–3 • Chest radiograph of pulmonary hamartoma.

Interferon alfa-n1 has been used to induce remission of the lesions of papillomatosis with a success rate of over 50%.[34] Unfortunately, squamous cell carcinoma of the bronchus developed in a child whose papillomas had regressed following treatment with interferon alfa-n1. This finding seems to indicate that the interferon has an antiviral effect but not an antitumoral effect.[35]

Another report outlined the complete regression of juvenile laryngobronchial papillomatosis following the systemic administration of bleomycin. A total of 240 units/m^2 was given over the 6 months of treatment with minimal clinical toxicity.[36]

MALIGNANT TUMORS

Malignant bronchopulmonary tumors of the lung are rare in childhood; there are fewer than 50 cases reported in the literature. These include bronchogenic squamous cell carcinoma, pulmonary blastoma, teratoma, a variety of sarcomas, and lymphoma.

Squamous Cell Carcinoma

In adults squamous cell carcinoma is associated with a prolonged history of cigarette smoking; in children papillomatosis is a common antecedent. A 1995 review of bronchogenic squamous cell carcinoma in children found five cases in the medical literature and added a sixth—an 11-year-old patient who was treated by surgical resection and external irradiation.[37] Although this boy was well and free of disease 4 years later, the average life expectancy for a child with squamous cell carcinoma is approximately 6 months after the onset of symptoms.

Other histologic cell types that have been reported include oat-cell carcinomas, small-cell carcinomas, and anaplastic carcinomas. As might be imagined, owing to less suspicion of malignancy in pediatric cases, diagnosis of malignant disease is usually delayed and metastases are frequently present by the time of diagnosis.

Pulmonary Blastoma

Pulmonary blastomas are malignant neoplasms that histologically resemble fetal lung tissue.[38] Because abnormalities of chromosome 2q have been noted in both this and other embryonal tumors, a common genetic mechanism has been postulated.[39] There have been about 60 reported cases in children and about three times that many in adults.[40, 41] Pulmonary blastomas generally arise in the peripheral portion of the lung but may arise in extrapulmonary tissue and resemble extralobar sequestrations. Like most pulmonary tumors, pulmonary blastomas are present with cough, fever, and occasionally lobar atelectasis or even abdominal pain. Despite variable clinical behavior, patients with these tumors have uniformly poor survival rates. Identification of the tumor is frequently first made either at thoracotomy or at autopsy. Operable lesions should be treated by lobectomy or pneumonectomy, as effective chemotherapy has not yet been determined.[40, 41]

Teratoma

Primary teratomas of the lung are both quite malignant and rare.[42]

Pulmonary Sarcomas

Fibrosarcoma

Primary bronchopulmonary fibrosarcoma (PBPF) occurs as intrabronchial or intraparenchymal masses of fibrous tissue, often pedunculated. These tumors consist of sheets and bundles of spindle cells displaying varying degrees of mitotic activity. About 30 cases of PBPF have been reported in the literature.[43] Fever is the most common presenting symptom and is accompanied by signs of distal infection secondary to obstruction. The diagnosis is most appropriately established by bronchoscopy. Resection is possible through the bronchoscope, but a high incidence of local recurrence accompanies PBPF, so that a more complete resection is the treatment of choice. PBPF is primarily invasive locally and should be resected even when extensive, as survival is likely.

Leiomyosarcoma

Jimenez and coworkers[44] collected 10 cases of primary pulmonary leiomyosarcoma in patients younger than 8 years of age but found no cases in the literature of patients 8–19 years of age. Since then, one 14-year-old patient has been reported.[45] The tumor obviously affects predominantly the younger age group. Since 1990 four children 8 years of age and younger with profound immunosuppression due to AIDS were found to have pulmonary and gastrointestinal leiomyosarcomas,[46, 47] raising the question of a possible association or even a direct or an indirect viral etiology. Such patients have presented with the usual signs and symptoms of cough, dyspnea, and obstructive pneumonitis. Complete surgical resection has usually resulted in a good outcome, with respect to the tumor at least, and the data seem to indicate that the prognosis is better in children.

Rhabdomyosarcoma

Numerous cases of primary rhabdomyosarcoma of the lung in children have been reported.[48–50] Although the radiographic appearance varies, a history of a rapidly enlarging mass compressing surrounding structures is consistent. The prognosis seems worse than for rhabdomyosarcoma at most other sites, and there may be a disposition for developing intracerebral metastases.[51] Of particular concern are numerous descriptions of rhabdomyosarcoma developing within or adjacent to a congenital pulmonary cyst.[52] Both bronchogenic cysts and cystic adenomatoid malformations have been implicated, although the risk for developing rhabdomyosarcoma within malformed pulmonary tissue has not been quantified. Most pediatric surgeons have deliberated how best to manage a prenatally or perinatally diagnosed congenital pulmonary cyst that resolves spontaneously within a few days of birth. Some surgeons advocate the prophylactic resection of all cystic malformations, whereas others advocate regular radiographic studies of the area, unconvinced that a major operation is justified.

Lymphomas

Although both primary Hodgkin's and non-Hodgkin's lymphomas may arise in the lung,[53,54] the lung is most commonly involved secondarily by direct spread from the mediastinal lymph nodes or thymus, or by disseminated lymphoma. The differential diagnosis must include pseudolymphoma[55] and lymphocytic interstitial pneumonitis. One case was reported of a non-Hodgkin's lymphoma arising within the bronchus of a 10-year-old boy.[56] Several cases have been reported of primary pulmonary lymphomas arising in immunosuppressed children. One HIV-positive child developed a low-grade B-cell pulmonary lymphoma.[57] Three others who had been undergoing chemotherapy for acute lymphoblastic leukemia also developed various forms of primary pulmonary lymphomas.[58] Since the lung is a highly unusual site for the development of lymphoma, these cases suggest that a compromise of the host's immune system may contribute to the development of pulmonary lymphoma in children. Although the mass is occasionally resected or biopsied, nonsurgical treatment is the rule.

CLINICAL FEATURES

Signs and Symptoms

Children with pulmonary parenchymal masses are frequently asymptomatic. In those with symptoms, a persistent cough refractory to the usual antitussive agents and expectorants is most frequent and generally indicates the presence of an endobronchial mass. Other symptoms include fever, recurrent pneumonia, respiratory distress that may resemble asthma, weight loss, pain, and hemoptysis.

Evaluation

Chest radiographs are extremely helpful in the majority of cases; these will show either hyperlucencies of a lung field due to air trapping (Fig. 17–4) or pulmonary infiltrates due to bronchial

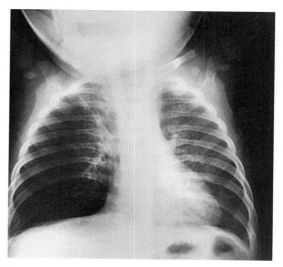

Figure 17–4 • Photomicrograph of bronchial carcinoid.

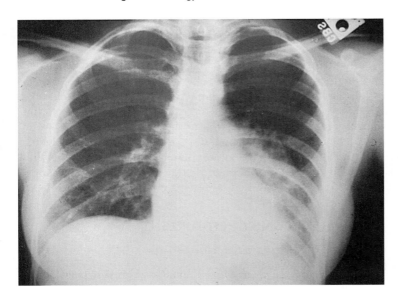

Figure 17–5 • Chest radiographs. *A*, hyperinflation due to a capillary hemangioma within the bronchus intermedius; *B*, left lower lobe infiltrate due to a bronchial carcinoid obstructing the left lower lobe bronchus.

obstruction (Fig. 17–5). The symptomatic infant or toddler is frequently suspected of having aspirated a foreign body and undergoes early diagnostic bronchoscopy. Diagnostic procedures are more likely to be delayed in the older child or adolescent with similar complaints. Sputum collection and diagnostic cytology are rarely of benefit in the pediatric age group. Since the majority of lung tumors in the pediatric age group occur in the trachea or in the main bronchi, biopsy of lesions detected during diagnostic bronchoscopy facilitates early diagnosis and treatment. If biopsy is unsuccessful or contraindicated, diagnostic thoracotomy will be necessary.

TREATMENT

Early intervention may prevent the destruction of pulmonary parenchyma due to the effects of chronic obstruction and recurrent infection. The treatment of both benign and malignant primary tumors consists of a thorough bronchoscopic examination and biopsy, followed by a thoracotomy or possibly thoracoscopy, although there are few bronchopulmonary tumors that can be adequately managed using current thoracoscopic techniques. Limited bronchial and pulmonary resection may salvage normal lung tissue when the tumor is benign. As with other endobronchial tumors, sleeve resection or resection of a damaged lobe with limited bronchial excision may prevent unnecessary resection of normal lung.

Many techniques of bronchoplastic reconstruction have been described[16] and should be employed to preserve lung tissue. Awareness of the possibility of both benign and malignant bronchopulmonary lesions occurring in infants, children, and adolescents is vital to early recognition and treatment.

References

1. Hartman GE, Shochat SJ: Primary pulmonary neoplasms of childhood: A review. *Ann Thorac Surg* 36:108–119, 1983.
2. Eggli KD, Newman B: Nodules, masses, and pseudomasses in the pediatric lung. *Radiol Clin North Am* 31:651–666, 1993.
3. Guibaud L, Pracos JP, Rode V, Dijoud F, Foray P, Chapelon C, Tran-Minh VA: Sclerosing hemangioma of the lung: Radiological findings and pathological diagnosis. *Pediatr Radiol* 25:S207–S208, 1995.
4. Hsu NY, Chen CY, Kwan PC, Chen CL, Hsu CP, Lin CT, Wang JH, Wang PY: Sclerosing hemangioma of the lung: A clinicopathologic study. *Chung Hua I Hsueh Tsa Chih* 52:149–154, 1993.
5. Daudi FA, Less GM, Higa TE: Inflammatory pseudotumours of the lung: Two cases and a review. *Can J Surg* 34:461–464, 1991.
6. Kim I, Kim WS, Yeon KM, Chi JG: Inflammatory pseudotumor of the lung manifesting as a posterior mediastinal mass. *Pediatr Radiol* 22:467–468, 1992.
7. Rohrlich P, Peuchmaur M, Cocci SN, Gasselin ID, Garel C, Aigrain Y, Galanaud P, Vilmer E, Emilie D: Interleukin-6 and interleukin-1 beta

production in a pediatric plasma cell granuloma of the lung. *Am J Surg Pathol* 19:590–595, 1995.

8. Spencer H: The pulmonary plasma cell/histiocytoma complex. *Histopathology* 8:903–916, 1984.

9. Schwartz EE, Katz SM, Mandell GA: Postinflammatory pseudotumors of the lung: Fibrous histiocytoma and related lesions. *Radiology* 136:609–613, 1980.

10. Tan-Liu NS, Matsubara O, Grillo HC, Mark EJ: Invasive fibrous tumor of the tracheobronchial tree: Clinical and pathologic study of seven cases. *Hum Pathol* 20:180–184, 1989.

11. Rose RW, Ward BH: Spherical pneumonias in children simulating pulmonary and mediastinal masses. *Radiology* 106:179–182, 1973.

12. Laptook A, Wind E, Nussbaum M, Shenker IR: Pulmonary lesions in atypical measles. *Pediatrics* 62:42–46, 1978.

13. Ozcelik U, Kotiloglu E, Gocmen A, Senocak ME, Kiper N: Endobronchial leiomyoma: A case report. *Thorax* 50:101–102, 1995.

14. Olgun N, Ozaksoy D, Ucan ES, Turkmen MA, Canda T, Oto O, Akkoclu A, Cevik N: Paediatric endobronchial leiomyoma mimicking asthma. *Respir Med* 89:581–582, 1995.

15. Balsam D, Segal S: Two smooth-muscle tumors in the airway of an HIV-infected child. *Pediatr Radiol* 22:552–553, 1992.

16. Black CT, Luck SR, Raffensperger JG: Bronchoplastic techniques for pediatric lung salvage. *J Pediatr Surg* 23:653–656, 1988.

17. Paul KP, Borner C, Muller KM, Vogt-Moykopf I: Capillary hemangioma of the right main bronchus treated by sleeve resection in infancy. *Am Rev Resp Dis* 143:876–879, 1991.

18. Conley SF, Milbrath MM, Beste DJ: Pediatric laryngeal granular cell tumor. *J Otolaryngol* 21:450–453, 1992.

19. Lazar RH, Younis RT, Kluka EA, Joyner RE, Storgion S: Granular-cell tumor of the larynx: Report of two pediatric cases. *Ear Nose Throat J* 71:440–443, 1992.

20. Spandow O, Lindholm CE: Granular-cell tumour in a child's trachea—A diagnostic and therapeutic challenge. *Int J Pediatr Otorhinolaryngol* 30:159–166, 1994.

21. Carney JA: The triad of gastric epitheliod leiomyosarcoma, pulmonary chondroma, and functioning extra-adrenal paraganglioma: A five-year review. *Medicine* 62:159–169, 1983.

22. Dajee A, Hinrichs S, Lillington G: Pulmonary chondroma, extra-adrenal paraganglioma, and gastric leiomyosarcoma: Carney's triad. *J Thorac Cardiovasc Surg* 84:377–381, 1982.

23. Raafat F, Salman WD, Roberts K, Ingram L, Rees R, Mann JR: Carney's triad: Pulmonary chondroma and extra-adrenal paraganglioma in young females. *Histopathology* 10:1325–1333, 1986.

24. Acha T, Picazo B, Garcia-Martin FJ, Urda A, Campos J: Carney's triad: Apropos of a new case. *Med Pediatr Oncol* 22:216–220, 1994.

25. Fudge TL, Ochsner JL, Mills NL: Clinical spectrum of pulmonary hamartomas. *Ann Thorac Surg* 30:36–39, 1980.

26. Kojima R, Mizuguchi M, Bessho F, Oka T, Watanabe H, Yonezawa M, Asano N, Iwanaka T: Pulmonary carcinoma associated with hamartoma in an 11-year-old boy. *Am J Pediatr Hematol Oncol* 15:439–442, 1993.

27. Bove KE: Sarcoma arising in pulmonary mesenchymal cystic hamartoma. *Pediatr Pathol* 9:785–792, 1989.

28. Hedlund GL, Bisset GS, Bove KE: Malignant neoplasms arising in cystic hamartomas of the lung in childhood. *Radiology* 173:77–79, 1989.

29. Wang LT, Wilkins EW Jr, Bode HH: Bronchial carcinoid tumors in pediatric patients. *Chest* 103:1426–1428, 1993.

30. Feldman JM, Benning TL, Saltzman H: Biochemical and ultrastructural differences between muco-epidermoid and carcinoid tumors of the bronchus. *J Surg Oncol* 37:227–231, 1988.

31. Patel RG, Norman JR: Unilateral hyperlucency with left lower lobe mass in a patient with bronchial asthma. *Chest* 107:569–570, 1995.

32. Parichartikanond P, Parichartikanond P, Ratanarapee S, Sinrachtanand C: Carcinomatous transformation of juvenile squamous cell papillomas of the larynx and tracheobronchial tree. *J Med Assoc Thai* 65:499–504, 1982.

33. Lindeberg H, Elbrønd O: Malignant tumours in patients with a history of multiple laryngeal papillomas: The significance of irradiation. *Clin Otolaryngol* 16:149–151, 1991.

34. Leventhal BG, Kashima HK, Mounts P, Thurmond L, Chapman S, Buckley S, Wold D: Long-term response of recurrent respiratory papillomatosis to treatment with lymphoblastic interferon alfa-n1. *N Eng J Med* 325:613–617, 1991.

35. Schouten TJ, van den Broek P, Cremers CW, Jongerius CM, Meyer JW, Vooys GP: Interferons and bronchogenic carcinoma in juvenile laryngeal papillomatosis. *Arch Otolaryngol* 109:289–291, 1983.

36. Mehta P, Herold N: Regression of juvenile laryngobronchial papillomatosis with systemic bleomycin therapy. *J Pediatr* 97:479–480, 1980.

37. Keita O, Lagrange JL, Michiels JF, Soler C, Garcia J, Valla JS, Thyss A: Primary bronchogenic squamous cell carcinoma in children: Report of a case and review of the literature. *Med Pediatr Oncol* 24:50–52, 1995.

38. Ashworth TG: Pulmonary blastoma, a true congenital neoplasm. *Histopathology* 7:585–594, 1983.

39. Sciot R, Dal Cin P, Brock P, Moerman P, Van Damme B, De Wever I, Casteels-Van Daele M, Van den Berghe H, Desmet V: Pleuropulmonary blastoma (pulmonary blastoma of childhood): Genetic link with other embryonal malignancies? *Histopathology* 24:559–563, 1994.

40. Lobo-Sanahuja F, Garcia I, Santamaria S,

Barrantes JC: Case report: Pulmonary blastoma in children—Response to chemotherapy. *Med Pediatr Oncol* 26:196–200, 1996.

41. Schmaltz C, Sauter S, Opitz O, Harms D, Kremens B, Lohner M, Metz K, Brandis M, Niemeyer C: Pleuro-pulmonary blastoma: A case report and review of the literature. *Med Pediatr Oncol* 25:479–484, 1995.

42. Walrond ER, Prussia PR: Pulmonary teratoma. *West Indian Med J* 36:39–42, 1987.

43. Pettinato G, Manivel JC, Saldana MJ, Peyser J, Dehner LP: Primary bronchopulmonary fibrosarcoma of childhood and adolescence: Reassessment of a low-grade malignancy. Clinicopathologic study of five cases and review of the literature. *Hum Pathol* 20:463–471, 1989.

44. Jimenez JF, Uthman EO, Townsend JW, Gloster ES, Seibert JJ: Primary pulmonary leiomyosarcoma in childhood. *Arch Pathol Lab Med* 110:348–351, 1986.

45. Beluffi G, Bertolotti P, Mietta A, Manara G, Luisetti M: Primary leiomyosarcoma of the lung in a girl. *Pediatr Radiol* 16:240–244, 1986.

46. Sabatino D, Martinez S, Young R, Balbi H, Ciminera P, Frieri M: Simultaneous pulmonary leiomyosarcoma and leiomyoma in pediatric HIV infection. *Pediatr Hematol Oncol* 8:355–359, 1991.

47. Chadwick EG, Conner EJ, Hanson IC, Joshi VV, Abu-Farsakh H, Yogev R, McSherry G, McClain K, Murphy SB: Tumors of smooth-muscle origin in HIV-infected children. *JAMA* 263:3182–3184, 1990.

48. Allan BT, Day DL, Dehner LP: Primary pulmonary rhabdomyosarcoma of the lung in children: Report of two cases presenting with spontaneous pneumothorax. *Cancer* 59:1005–1011, 1987.

49. Shariff S, Thomas JA, Shetty N, D'Cunha S: Primary pulmonary rhabdomyosarcoma in a child, with a review of literature. *J Surg Oncol* 38:261–264, 1988.

50. Schiavetti A, Dominici C, Matrunola M, Capocaccia P, Ceccamea A, Catello MA: Primary pulmonary rhabdomyosarcoma in childhood: Clinico-biologic features in two cases with review of the literature. *Med Pediatr Oncol* 26:201–207, 1996.

51. Micallef-Eynaud PD, Goulden NT, Langdale-Brown B, Eden TB, Steers JW: Intracerebral recurrence of primary intrathoracic rhabdomyosarcoma. *Med Pediatr Oncol* 21:132–136, 1993.

52. Murphy JJ, Bair GK, Fraser GC, Ashmore PG, LeBlanc JG, Sett SS, Rogers P, Magee JF, Taylor GP, Dimmick J: Rhabdomyosarcoma arising within congenital pulmonary cysts: Report of three cases. *J Pediatr Surg* 27:1364–1367, 1992.

53. Suzuki L, Funari M, Rocha M de S, Cristofani LM, Odone Filho V, Vieira GS: Calcification in primary lung non-Hodgkin's lymphoma. *Rev Hosp Clin Fac Med Sao Paulo* 50:227–229, 1995.

54. Tamura A, Komatsu H, Yanai N, Homma J, Nagase A, Memoto E, Hirai T, Hashizume T, Kawata K, Ishikawa S, et al: Primary pulmonary lymphoma: Relationship between clinical features and pathologic findings in 24 cases. *Jpn J Clin Oncol* 25:140–152, 1995.

55. Koss MN, Hochholzer L, Nichols PW, Wehunt WD, Lazarus AA: Primary non-Hodgkin's lymphoma and pseudolymphoma of lung: A study of 161 patients. *Hum Pathol* 14:1024–38, 1983.

56. Carr T, Stevens RF, Marsden HB, Morris-Jones P, Kumar S: An unusual presentation of non-Hodgkin's lymphoma (NHL) in a child. *Eur J Oncol* 12:193–195, 1986.

57. Teruya-Feldstein J, Temeck BK, Sloas MM, Kingma DW, Raffeld M, Pass HI, Mueller B, Jaffe ES: Pulmonary malignant lymphoma of mucosa-associated lymphoid tissue (MALT) arising in a pediatric HIV-positive patient. *Am J Surg Pathol* 19:357–363, 1995.

58. Drut R, Angiocentric B-cell lymphoma of the lung in an immunocompromised boy. *Pediatr Pathol* 8:395–400, 1988.

Nonrhabdo-myosarcoma Soft-Tissue Sarcomas

• *Deborah Belchis, M.D.* • *Peter Dillon, M.D.*

Nonrhabdomyosarcoma soft-tissue tumors in children comprise a diverse group of neoplasms. Some overlap exists between childhood and adult tumors, but many of these sarcomas are either unique to childhood or possess special characteristics that distinguish them from their adult counterparts. Our knowledge of these tumors is rapidly evolving as the fields of immunohistochemistry and molecular biology bring new insights into their underlying histogenesis and genetic makeup. Advances in therapy have also spurred greater recognition of the different subtypes and emphasized the need for correct classification of these tumors.

Tumors arising from soft tissues are very uncommon in children. They account for approximately 6% of all childhood malignancies and are the fourth most common type of solid tumor seen in the pediatric population.[1-3] Just over one half of all soft-tissue tumors originate from striated muscle as *rhabdomyosarcomas* (RMS). The other group consists of a heterogeneous collection of subtypes referred to as *nonrhabdomyosarcoma soft-tissue sarcomas* (NRSTSs).[4]

These NRSTS tumors have been well studied in adults, and in the past this information has dictated management strategies for children. A number of clinical studies of children with these lesions have been reported. These have begun to improve our understanding. This chapter reviews the current data available on the pathologic features, treatments, and current outcomes of childhood NRSTS.

EPIDEMIOLOGY

NRSTS has been reported in children of all ages ranging from newborn infants to young adults. The median age of patients in most studies has ranged from 11 to 13 years, with a slight male predominance.[1, 5–7] The majority of patients have been white, but children of all ethnic groups have been represented.

A number of preexisting conditions have been reported, of which the most widely recognized is neurofibromatosis. In studies of malignant peripheral nerve-sheath tumors, neurofibromatosis has been noted in 39% to 70% of the patients.[8–11] Other preexisting conditions have included Down's syndrome, spina bifida, giant pigmented nevus, and prior radiation exposure.[6]

CLINICAL PRESENTATION

The most common complaint at the time of presentation of NRSTS is usually that of a slow-growing mass, often noted for a long period of time. Pain localized to the lesion occurs in up to one third of the patients. Quite often the mass is first detected in relation to a traumatic event, with the result that long delays in evaluation and treatment have resulted from the unfortunate assumption that the mass is simply a temporary swelling. Other signs that have been reported include weakness and muscular atrophy.

On physical examination the mass is usually well demarcated, although deep-seated lesions may be difficult to palpate. Local skin involvement or breakdown is very unlikely except in the case of epithelioid sarcomas. Rarely, regional lymph nodes are enlarged. Since dissemination of tumor occurs via hematogenous pathways, the most common site of metastatic disease is the lung. Liver metastases can occur from sarcomas arising in the gastrointestinal tract, and brain lesions have been reported in patients with diffuse metastatic disease.[6, 12]

In a prospective analysis of pediatric patients with these tumors, the extent of disease at presentation was found to be localized in 70%, regionalized in 9%, and metastatic in 21% of the cases.[5]

SITE AND PATHOLOGY

NRSTS can be found anywhere in the body, but the most common anatomic site has been the extremities, followed by the trunk and abdominal region, the thorax, and the head and neck area. In the extremities, tumors have been found most often in the lower limbs.[5]

One of the major difficulties in studying NRSTS has been the fact that these tumors comprise a heterogeneous collection of different subtypes with histologic features that are occasionally difficult to differentiate and classify. The development of new molecular markers and immunohistochemical techniques (discussed shortly) has improved the pathologist's ability to accurately identify and classify these tumors. As a result, the most common NRSTSs reported in children have been synovial cell sarcomas.[1, 4, 5] Other common sarcomas have included malignant fibrous histiocytomas, fibrosarcomas, and malignant peripheral nerve-sheath tumors.[6, 7] Additional histologic subtypes include leiomyosarcoma, alveolar soft-part sarcoma, angiosarcoma, liposarcoma, epithelioid sarcoma, and extraskeletal chondrosarcoma (Table 18–1). Even with current techniques a number of lesions are too primitive or undifferentiated to be classified.

For each anatomic site a broad spectrum of tumor types has been reported. The most common lesions of the extremities are synovial cell sarcomas, followed by malignant fibrous histiocy-

---

Table 18–1 • Nonrhabdomyosarcoma Soft-Tissue Tumors in Children: Listed in Order of Commonness

Synovial cell sarcoma
Fibrosarcoma
Primitive neuroectodermal tumor (PNET)
Malignant fibrous histiocytoma (MFH)
Neurogenic sarcomas
   Malignant schwannoma
   Neurofibrosarcoma
   Malignant peripheral nerve-sheath tumor
Leiomyosarcoma
Angiosarcoma
Alveolar soft-part sarcoma
Hemangiopericytoma
Clear-cell sarcoma
Epithelioid sarcoma
Malignant mesenchymoma
Intra-abdominal desmoplastic small round cell tumor (DSRCT)
Extraskeletal chondrosarcoma

tomas, malignant neurogenic tumors, and fibrosarcomas. Tumors of the trunk are predominantly malignant fibrous histiocytomas or neurogenic in origin.[1, 5]

A universally applicable and reproducible grading system is of paramount importance in studying these lesions. A great deal of variation exists in the grading systems employed in most major studies. The important points of a grading system proposed by Coindre[13] included the degree of differentiation of the tumor, the extent of necrosis, and the mitotic index. Table 18–2 shows a grading system based on the analysis of pediatric NRSTS that has refined these histologic determinants into a structured formula with excellent clinical correlation.[14–16] Factors important in this analysis include an evaluation for mitotic activity, cytologic pleomorphism and cellularity, necrosis degree, and patient age. Incorporation of patient age into the grading system is important for childhood tumors, as certain infantile sarcomatous lesions may be histologically aggressive but clinically benign. Most NRSTSs in children, except for malignant fibrous histiocytoma and fibrosarcoma, tend to be immature and poorly differentiated, approximately half have a histologic grade of G3.[1, 5] No correlation between anatomic site and histologic grade has been reported.

EVALUATION

For all patients the clinical evaluation should include routine hemograms, renal and liver function studies, and occasionally bone scans. Diagnostic imaging studies should include plain radiographs of the lesion as well as of the chest to evaluate for extent of disease. In the past, special tests have included intravenous pyelograms, lymphangiograms, and angiograms. These have been supplanted by the routine use of CT scans with contrast and magnetic resonance imaging (MRI). MRI is considered the imaging modality of choice for the evaluation of local and regional disease, particularly in the extremities, the pelvis, and head and neck regions, and should be obtained after initial plain radiographic evaluation.[17] Pulmonary metastatic disease and some abdominal tumors may be best evaluated with contrast-enhanced CT scans.

Advantages of MRI include superior soft-tissue resolution, multiplanar image acquisition, no requirement for iodinated contrast agents or ionizing radiation, and less of the streak artifact that may appear on CT scans.[18] Whether one can differentiate a benign from a malignant soft-tissue tumor on MRI is debated.[19] Image characteristics used to predict benign tumors include small size, homogenous signal intensity, and smooth, well-defined margins. Because they tend to outgrow their blood supply and develop areas of necrosis, malignant lesions are usually larger and display an inhomogenous signal intensity on T2-weighted images.[18] Gadolinium-enhanced imaging strengthens the signal intensity on T1-weighted images and helps to distinguish cystic and necrotic areas from cellular regions and to allow assessment of overall tumor vascularity.

STAGING

Several systems are utilized for staging based in part upon either pre- or postoperative informa-

---

Table 18–2 • NRSTS Tumor Grading System Correlating Histology and Patient Age with Cytologic Characteristics of Degree of Necrosis, Mitotic Index, and Cellularity

Grade 1 (G1): Myxoid, well-differentiated liposarcoma; deep-seated dermatofibrosarcoma protuberans; extraskeletal chondrosarcoma; well-differentiated leiomyosarcoma; malignant hemangiopericytoma; peripheral nerve-sheath tumor; infantile fibrosarcoma

Grade 2 (G2): Sarcomas not included in G1 or G3 with <15% necrosis, a mitotic index of <5 to 10 per high-power field, and absence of marked nuclear atypia or cellularity; fibrosarcoma and malignant hemangiopericytomas in children younger than 4 years are G1 or G2 despite high cellularity or mitotic index

Grade 3 (G3): Pleomorphic liposarcoma; mesenchymal chondrosarcoma; extraskeletal osteosarcoma; Triton tumor; alveolar soft-part sarcoma; all other sarcomas not in G1 or G2 with >15% necrosis or mitotic index of >5 to 10 per high-power field

From Parham D, Webber BL, Jenkins JJ, et al: Nonrhabdomyosarcomatous soft tissue sarcomas of childhood: Formulation of a simplified system for grading. *Mod Pathol* 8:705–710, 1995, with permission.

tion. The most widely used is the postsurgical scheme derived from the Intergroup Rhabdomyosarcoma Study (IRS):

Stage I	Complete resection of localized disease
Stage II	Gross resection with microscopic residual disease
Stage III	Incomplete resection with macroscopic residual disease, or biopsy only
Stage IV	Metastatic disease

This system does not take into account the size of the tumor or the degree of the tumor infiltration at the primary site. Therefore, an alternative system involving the TNM classification has been proposed:[15, 20, 21]

T1N0M0	Tumor limited to tissue or organ of origin
T2N0M0	Tumor invasion of contiguous organs or tissues
T1/2N1M0	T1 or T2 with lymph node involvement
T1/2N0/1M1	T1 or T2, N0 or N1 with distant metastasis

With this system, T1 lesions are confined to the tissue of origin and are subgrouped into lesions that are smaller than 5 cm (a) or larger than 5 cm (b). Lesions with the T2 classification are those that have invaded local structures outside the margin of the tissue of origin. They also are subgrouped by size into lesions smaller than 5 cm (a) or 5 cm or larger (b). Tumor size as reflected in the "a" or "b" classification is an essential prognostic factor for all stages. Clinical studies have shown that the TNM staging system is more relevant than the IRS system in analyzing treatment results.

DIAGNOSIS

In the evaluation of a soft-tissue lesion, the procurement of an adequate tissue specimen for histologic classification and grade determination without compromising subsequent treatment options is one of the first challenges facing the surgeon. The optimal method for obtaining tissue—fine-needle aspiration (FNA) cytology, needle-core biopsy (NCB), incisional biopsy, or excisional biopsy—is open to debate. FNA cytology and NCB are useful in the diagnosis of soft-

tissue lesions.[22] Both techniques have been shown to have high sensitivity and specificity for benign and malignant neoplasms in adults.[23–25] Yet, 37% of FNAs were unsatisfactory in one study and required NCB evaluation.[26] FNA is a useful diagnostic tool in the initial evaluation of soft-tissue tumors or possible metastatic lesions, but NCB is better at providing enough tissue to permit accurate histologic subtyping of a sarcoma.

Excisional biopsy is an inadequate procedure for diagnosing a soft-tissue sarcoma and should never be used. A pseudocapsule containing malignant cells builds up around the tumor as it enlarges. Simple excision of the tumor violates this tissue plane and results in the dissemination of tumor cells throughout the operative field. Subsequent surgery in the region is thereby compromised, since the margins of tumor involvement become indistinct. Proper surgical treatment may be further hindered by an improperly placed incision at the time of the initial biopsy.

The initial procedure of choice for obtaining a tissue diagnosis of a suspected soft-tissue sarcoma is an incisional biopsy. For tumors of the extremities, head and neck, or truncal regions, such a biopsy requires a properly planned approach so that definitive surgical therapy can be pursued once the diagnosis is confirmed. For tumors in the thoracic or abdominal cavities, CT-guided NCBs can be considered, but often a thoracotomy or laparotomy may be required. The techniques of minimally invasive surgery with video-assisted thoracoscopy and laparoscopy have been successfully employed in children with malignancies and may prove to be quite effective for tissue procurement.[27]

Once tissue has been obtained, proper handling is essential. The specimen should be delivered sterile and fresh to the pathologist on gauze moistened with normal saline. The pathologist must then carefully apportion tissue for electron microscopy, microbial culture, DNA/RNA analysis, cytogenetics, and routine processing—each test with its own special handling requirements. Additionally, touch preparations for use in fluorescence in situ hybridization can be invaluable.

TREATMENT

For children with NRSTSs surgical resection is the treatment of choice. The surgical management of soft-tissue sarcomas in general has undergone a considerable evolution with the realization that multimodal therapy provides the best chance for survival. The success of such therapy in adults is quite evident for extremity tumors with various limb-salvage protocols.[28–30]

Soft-tissue sarcomas were thought to be radioresistant, and so radical surgery offered the only chance for a cure. With extremity tumors in particular, recurrence rates depended directly on the extent of the initial surgical procedure. An excisional biopsy or a simple enucleation of the tumor resulted in local recurrence rates of 60% to 90%. If a 2 cm to 3 cm margin of tissue around the tumor was taken, the recurrence rates fell to 25% to 60%. Radical surgery including amputation produced the lowest rates of recurrence at 7% to 18%.[28, 31] Advances in radiotherapy have subsequently demonstrated that these tumors are responsive to such an approach and have allowed the development of less radical limb-sparing surgical procedures in combination with the radiotherapy. Local control rates as high as 95% have been reported with such multimodal therapy in adults.[30]

Wide local excision or en bloc resection should be the primary form of treatment in children with NRSTSs. The main goal of such surgical therapy is the complete eradication of local disease to minimize the risk of recurrence. All attempts should be made to obtain margins negative for tumor cells on microscopic examination. Skene and coworkers[4] reported that radical or wide local excisions were possible in 22 of 28 patients (78%), whereas McCoy and coworkers[32] and Rao and coworkers[2] were able to perform such operations on 85% and 58% of their patients, respectively. What constitutes an adequate margin of tissue is still debated. In certain sites, such as the head and neck region, mediastinum, and retroperitoneum, wide local excision with clean margins may be impossible to achieve because of the proximity of important structures. Such anatomic limitations are the reason for high rates of local recurrence in these areas.[33]

For most extremity tumors such resections are technically feasible as part of a limb-salvage procedure. Skene and coworkers[4] reported that limb salvage was possible in all 11 of their patients. In one of the largest studies of pediatric NRSTSs, Rao and colleagues[16] were able to perform a limb-sparing procedure on 46 of 64 patients

(72%). Adjuvant therapy was utilized in selected patients. In terms of surgical techniques the efficacy of a compartmental resection over a wide excision in achieving local tumor control has not been demonstrated.

The rate of amputation as a primary form of surgical intervention is variable in the few pediatric studies reported but appears to be higher than in most adult series—5% to 15%.[33, 34] In the study by Rao,[1] 19 of 69 (27%) patients underwent primary amputation. In a limited study of sarcomas in the antecubital or popliteal fossae, 3 of 14 (21%) patients were treated with amputation.[35] The investigators concluded that preservation of a functional limb was possible for the majority of soft-tissue sarcomas in an extremity and that postoperative radiation therapy was an essential component of treatment. Amputation is warranted if invasion of a major neurovascular bundle is identified. In adult series, results of amputation have been compared with results of limb-sparing procedures. It has been proposed, as a result of these comparative studies, that amputation be recommended when a limb-sparing procedure cannot achieve a gross resection of the tumor and still preserve a useful extremity.[34] Although amputation has been found to be superior to limb-sparing surgery in preventing local disease recurrence, survival rates have not been different for the two procedures, probably because neither procedure addresses the problem of systemic disease.[36] One reason for the higher amputation rate in children may be a reluctance to administer radiation therapy to the extremity. Concerns regarding the functional outcome and long-term effects of such therapy, including the risk of developing secondary malignancies, are significant.

In adults, local disease control is of crucial importance because the development of a local recurrence reportedly affects survival adversely.[37, 38] This fact has tremendous implications for surgical treatment strategies. Following an attempted surgical resection, the finding of microscopic involvement of the surgical margins has been highly predictive for local disease recurrence, distant disease recurrence, and diminished overall survival.[38] Zornig and coworkers[39] reported that 67 of 189 (35%) patients did not have safe margins at the time of the initial operation and required reexcision of the primary site. Repeat en bloc resection was accomplished in 59 of the patients, and residual tumor was found in 45% of the specimens. The researchers concluded that primary reexcision should have priority over any adjuvant treatment.[39] Rao[1] reported that 88 of 154 pediatric patients (57%) underwent reexcision of the primary site. Upon reexploration, residual tumor was found in 36% of these patients. Thus, there should be no hesitation to reexplore a tumor site if residual disease is suspected after the initial procedure.

The role of regional lymph node dissection is less clear. Lymph node metastases from soft-tissue sarcomas are quite rare except in the case of a clear-cell sarcoma.[40] In an extensive study in adults, Mazeron and Suit[41] found an incidence of lymph node metastases of 3.9%. In children, positive lymph nodes have been demonstrated in 9% and 6% of patients, and the majority of tumors involved are high-grade G3 lesions.[5, 15] Lawrence and Neifeld[33] have proposed that there is no indication for lymph node dissection unless lymphadenopathy is present or the primary lesion is in the lymph node region.

Adjuvant Therapy

Radiotherapy

Adjuvant radiotherapy in the management of soft-tissue sarcomas, particularly of the extremities, has become standard practice for adult patients. Radiation therapy is currently utilized in conjunction with limb-sparing surgery for local tumor control with excellent clinical results.[28, 30, 42] There are no clear guidelines as to the optimal dose of radiotherapy, although Fein and colleagues[42] noted a local control rate of better than 95% in patients who received greater than 62.5 Gy. Unfortunately, improved local control in some studies does not translate into either decreased distant metastasis or improved survival in adults.[43]

Radiation therapy has been used sparingly in children because of concerns about its long-term effects.[44] Nevertheless, results indicate that it is as effective in local control of extremity tumors in children as it is in adults. Philippe and coworkers[35] administered radiation therapy to 5 patients with flexor fossa tumors and reported complete local control in all. Rao and coworkers[16] treated a total of 16 patients with radiation therapy and had no local failures. In a later study by Rao,[1]

radiation therapy appeared to contribute to an improved overall survival in those patients who had microscopic residual disease. In contrast, in a retrospective study of synovial sarcoma in children, Fontanesi and coworkers[45] examined the results of radiotherapy to the primary tumor site in 16 patients, and they found improved local control in those who had incomplete resections or biopsies only; there was no advantage in overall survival resulting from such treatment.[45] These observations were supported by Maurer and colleagues'[46] prospective, randomized study of NRSTSs in children receiving radiotherapy and chemotherapy. When results were analyzed by tumor grade, they concluded that patients with completely resected Grade I and II sarcomas did not need postoperative radiotherapy. Children with incompletely resected tumors however, required such therapy for local tumor control and were entered into multimodal trials that included postoperative radiotherapy if amputation was not chosen.

A number of new techniques in radiotherapy administration are evolving that may be applicable to children. In adults preoperative radiotherapy with or without chemotherapy has proved effective in reducing tumor size and yet has higher morbidity in regard to wound healing than postoperative radiotherapy.[29] Unfortunately, preoperative radiotherapy may change the tumor margins, making the extent of surgical resection more difficult to determine. No reports exist on the use of preoperative radiotherapy in children.

The technique of brachytherapy has been described in both adults and children. The theoretic advantage of brachytherapy is that it is designed to treat only the tumor bed with no more than a 2 cm margin, thus sparing surrounding normal tissue. In adults the effect of brachytherapy on local tumor control is most significant with high-grade lesions.[43] In children brachytherapy has been utilized in a pilot project involving 13 patients, 6 of whom had various NRSTSs.[47] Local control was reported to be equivalent to standard external-beam therapy. No significant complications were noted. As further clinical experience is gained with this technique, it may be particularly suitable for pediatric patients. Another radiotherapy modality that is being employed in trials for soft-tissue sarcomas—particularly for retroperitoneal sarcomas—is *intraoperative electron-beam radiotherapy (IORT)*[48, 49]

Initial results in adults have demonstrated an improvement in local control with IORT.[50] Such therapy has been attempted in children with intra-abdominal solid tumors, but no long-term results are known.[51] Future studies will determine its therapeutic role.

Chemotherapy

The role of chemotherapy in the treatment of patients with NRSTSs remains unclear and under intense investigation. In adults few trials have demonstrated any benefit other than a prolongation in disease-free survival but not in long-term outcome.[52] The major chemotherapeutic agents that have demonstrated activity in both adults and children have been doxorubicin and ifosfamide. Maurer and coworkers[46] reported a prospective analysis of chemotherapy in children utilizing a protocol of alternating cycles of vincristine, doxorubicin, and cyclophosphamide with VAC over a period of 1 year.[46] They found that disease-free survival was 74% in the chemotherapy group and 76% in the observed group, with overall survival rates of 95% and 97%, respectively. Patients with G3 tumors fared poorly despite chemotherapy. These investigators concluded that children with completely or grossly resected G1 and G2 NRSTSs do not benefit from adjuvant chemotherapy but that chemotherapy trials should be developed for patients with G3 tumors and inoperable or metastatic lesions (IRS groups III and IV). Trials being evaluated at the time of this writing include high-dose ifosfamide as well as combination therapy of ifosfamide, etoposide, and doxorubicin.[53–56]

In Europe a treatment strategy for patients with NRSTSs has been devised involving surgery, chemotherapy, and radiotherapy based on histology and grade of tumor.[56] This plan breaks the tumors into three groups:

Group A: Extraosseous Ewing's sarcoma, peripheral neuroectodermal tumor, synovial sarcoma, undifferentiated sarcoma, and unclassified sarcoma. This group should be treated with protocols from the rhabdomyosarcoma studies.

Group B: Malignant fibrous histiocytoma, leiomyosarcoma, vascular sarcoma, alveolar soft-part sarcoma, liposarcoma, and rhabdoid tumor. The main therapy is surgical resection with chemotherapy utilized depending upon the grade of the tumor. Radiotherapy is administered for marginal or incomplete resections.

Group C: Malignant peripheral nerve-sheath tumor, fibrosarcoma, and neurofibrosarcoma. Surgery is the main treatment employed as there is no evidence that chemotherapy or radiotherapy is curative. Chemotherapy may be used preoperatively to reduce tumor size, and radiotherapy may be used postoperatively for incomplete resections.

Only time will tell how this protocol will compare with those that emphasize surgical control of the primary tumor, radiotherapy for incomplete resection, and chemotherapy for all G3 lesions and metastatic diseases.

OUTCOME

Overall survival rates in children with NRSTSs have been quite variable and may be affected by institutional bias and retrospective analysis. Rao and coworkers[16] originally reported an overall survival rate of 65% in children with extremity tumors, whereas Hayani and coworkers[6] reported an overall survival rate of 64% and a disease-free rate of only 51%. McCoy and colleagues[32] reported a 5-year survival rate of 92% and a disease-free rate of 61%. Maurer and coworkers[46] had almost similar results in a 3-year prospective study. In both studies there was little difference between overall and disease-free survival rates for Grade I and Grade II tumors, but, the survival rates for Grade III tumors were significantly lower. McCoy[32] noted a 5-year survival rate of only 39% for such tumors.

In the largest pediatric review to date, Rao[1] studied 154 children and reported a survival rate of 58%. The large number of cases allowed for an in-depth analysis of factors related to survival. The best survival rates were noted in those patients who had either complete resection (IRS group I) or microscopic residual with adjuvant therapy (IRS group II) (Table 18–3). Again, histologic grade had a bearing on survival with 82% of patients with Grade I and II tumors surviving but only 27% of those with Grade III tumors.

When clinical outcomes in Rao's[1] study were analyzed in relationship to tumor invasiveness,

Table 18–3 · Survival in Children with NRSTS Based on Intergroup Rhabdomyosarcoma Staging System

IRS Grade	Survival (%)
I	82
II	67
III	12
IV	5

Adapted from Rao BN: Nonrhabdomyosarcomas in children: Prognostic factors influencing survival. *Semin Surg Oncol* 9:524–531, 1993, with permission of Wiley-Liss, Inc., a division of John Wiley & Sons, Inc.

just under half of the patients had T1 lesions, and survival in this group was 90%. Children with Grade I or II tumors in this group had survival rates of 93%; those with Grade III tumors had an 80% survival rate. The clinical results were not as good for patients with T2 lesions; overall survival was only 30%, and although patients with Grade I and II tumors had a higher survival rate, it was only 65%. Just over two thirds of the T2 lesions were Grade III, and the survival rate for these patients was dramatically

reduced to 12% (Fig. 18–1). All studies have found that most local recurrences involve invasive T2 primary lesions. In the case of extremity lesions, the presence of involved lymph nodes is associated with a mortality rate of 66%.

Rao's[1, 16] data suggest that the two most important prognostic factors in children with NRSTSs are tumor invasiveness and histologic grade. Patients with T2 and Grade III tumors have the poorest survival rates despite current adjuvant treatment protocols. Tumor size, although related to degree of invasion, was not a factor in multivariate analysis.

PATHOLOGY OF NONRHABDOMYOSARCOMA SOFT-TISSUE TUMORS

Immunohistochemistry and Molecular Pathology

Once a diagnosis of a sarcoma is made, accurate histopathologic subtyping is required for proper grading and prognosis. For certain tumors, such

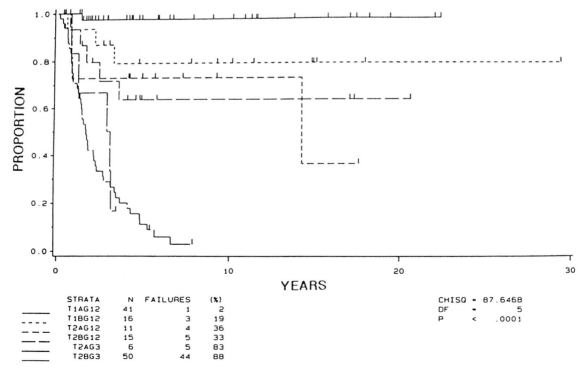

STRATA	N	FAILURES	(%)
T1AG12	41	1	2
T1BG12	16	3	19
T2AG12	11	4	36
T2BG12	15	5	33
T2AG3	6	5	83
T2BG3	50	44	88

CHISQ = 87.6468
DF = 5
P < .0001

Figure 18–1 · Survival curves by stage for children with nonrhabdomyosarcoma soft-tissue sarcomas. (From Rao BN: Nonrhabdomyosarcomas in children: Prognostic factors influencing survival. *Semin Surg Oncol* 9:524–531, 1993, with permission.)

as alveolar soft-part sarcoma, biphasic synovial sarcoma, and malignant fibrous histiocytoma, light microscopy in conjunction with clinical information is sufficient for diagnosis. For other tumors a differential diagnosis must be developed, in which case immunohistochemistry can be of great assistance.[57, 58] The evaluation of immunohistochemical markers will help to confirm a diagnosis in 30% to 40% of cases, will select the correct diagnosis from several different possibilities in 50% to 60% of the cases, and will be indeterminate in 10% of the cases.[57]

As a general rule, immunoperoxidase stains reflect the degree of differentiation of tumors and can help classify them as epithelial, neural, myoid, histiocytic, lymphoid, endothelial, or melanocytic in origin. As most markers are not specific, and tumors can demonstrate variable expression of these markers, a panel of several antibodies is the recommended approach to correctly categorize a neoplasm.[57] The importance of using a panel of antibodies is well illustrated by studies describing the many and varied tumors that stain with an antibody to the MIC2 gene product, a glycoprotein located in the pseudoautosomal region of both the X and Y chromosomes.[59, 60] Originally thought to be specific for extraosseous Ewing's sarcoma and peripheral neuroectodermal tumor, this glycoprotein has been found to stain a number of different tumors, including synovial cell sarcoma, malignant peripheral nerve-sheath tumor, alveolar rhabdomyosarcoma, and lymphoblastic lymphoma.[61]

A number of technical factors must be considered in evaluating the immunohistochemical staining pattern of any tumor or tissue. These factors include the type of fixative, length of fixation, use of antigen retrieval or other special techniques to enhance staining, and specificity of the marker.

Specific Markers

Vimentin

Vimentin was originally used as a marker of mesenchymally derived neoplasms. It is expressed by virtually all types of sarcomas, many adenocarcinomas, and some squamous cell carcinomas. Vimentin also serves as an important internal immunohistochemical control, as a negative vimentin result calls into question the retention of antigenicity of the specimen block.

Epithelial Markers

Cytokeratins

Cytokeratins are expressed on soft-tissue tumors with evidence of epithelial differentiation, that is, epithelial sarcoma and synovial sarcoma. Coexpression of vimentin with cytokeratin can be very helpful in differentiating epithelioid sarcoma from granulomatous reactions. Yet, aberrant cytokeratin reactivity can also be found in several nonepithelial neoplasms including liposarcomas and hemangiopericytomas.[57, 58]

Epithelial membrane antigen (EMA)

Epithelial membrane antigen (EMA) is a collective term given to a group of carbohydrate-rich, protein-poor, high-molecular-weight substances found on the surface of epithelial cells. EMA is widely expressed on epithelial tumors. Coexpression of EMA and cytokeratin is supportive of true epithelial differentiation.

Endothelial markers

The most specific and sensitive endothelial marker is CD31, a transmembrane glycoprotein and member of the immunoglobulin supergene family. The antigen is present on the surface of endothelial cells and some hematopoietic cells. Virtually all benign vascular tumors and 80% to 100% of angiosarcomas express this antigen. Other markers in this category include Factor VIII–related antigen and *Ulex lectin*. CD34, a human progenitor cell antigen, was thought initially to be somewhat specific for vascular endothelium, but it is now known to have a much broader spectrum of reactivity and is particularly helpful in diagnosing certain adult soft-tissue tumors, such as solitary fibrous tumors and Kaposi's sarcoma.[62, 57]

Myoid markers

The most common myoid markers include desmin, muscle-specific actin (HHF35), smooth-muscle actin, and myoglobin, and the newest muscle marker, MyoD1. Tumors with muscle differentiation as well as myofibroblastic differentiation react with these markers.

Desmin, an intermediate filament, forms an integral part of the cytoskeleton of cardiac, skeletal, and smooth-muscle fibers. This antibody is most useful in the diagnosis of small-, round-cell tumors. Depending upon the method of fixation, it is expressed in 80% to 100% of rhabdomyosarcomas, even those that appear undifferentiated by light microscopy. Desmin's expression is interpreted as indicative of myofibroblastic differentiation. HHF35 and smooth-muscle actin must be interpreted with caution owing to nonspecific reactions, whereas myoglobin staining is very specific but not very sensitive.[58]

Histiocytic markers

Histiocytic markers are notorious for their lack of specificity, and their interpretation must be made cautiously with careful attention to the morphologic appearance of the tumor. CD68/KP1, a macrophage antigen, reacts with tissue histiocytes but also with any cells containing lysosomes, including granular-cell tumors. Other histiocytic markers include MAC387 and Factor XIIa.[58]

Neural markers

Neural filament, an intermediate filament, is specific for neuronal cells. Additional neuronal markers include neuron-specific enolase (NSE), synaptophysin, and chromogranin. S-100, Leu-7/HNK-1, GFAP, and HMB45 are all nerve-sheath markers. S-100 is an acidic protein widely distributed in the central and peripheral nervous systems. It is most useful in the diagnosis of benign nerve-sheath tumors and melanoma.[58]

Molecular Biology of Soft-Tissue Tumors

Current advances in our understanding of the molecular pathology of malignant tumors are having a profound effect upon the categorization of various tumors. The most remarkable example of this change is the Ewing's family of tumors, which has been found to share a common translocation t(11;22)(q24;q12).[63] Prior to this discovery, peripheral neuroectodermal tumor, extraosseous Ewing's sarcoma, and thoracopulmonary tumor of childhood (Askin's tumor)[64] were thought of as distinct entities. The discovery of a common molecular link raises the possibility that these tumors are either the same or represent a spectrum of neuroectodermal tumors that are related neoplasms.

Specific and consistent translocations have been identified in a number of childhood and some adult soft-tissue tumors (Table 18–4). The translocation of the Ewing's tumor family results in a chimeric mRNA involving a gene on chromosome 22 known as the *ews* gene and a human homologue of the *fli*-1, a member of the *ets*-1 transcription factor family on chromosome 11. Biochemical studies have demonstrated that the fusion product is a potent transcriptional activator. The production of unique chimeric fusion proteins that result from these specific translocations has been a consistent finding. The role of these proteins in the behavior and development of these tumors remains to be discovered. The fact that most of these proteins appear to be tumor-specific has suggested the possibility that the identification of these products may help to confirm histologic diagnosis or delineate prognostic or therapeutic significance.[65–68]

Table 18–4 • Molecular Translocations of Pediatric Sarcomas

Tumor	Translocation	Chimeric Product
Alveolar rhabdomyosarcoma	t(2;13)(q35;q14)	PAX3/FKHR
	t(1;13)(p36;q14)	PAX7/FKHR
Ewing's sarcoma/PNET	t(11;22)(q24;q12)	EWS/FLI1
	t(21;22)(q22;q12)	EWS/ERG
Synovial sarcoma	t(X;18)(p11;q11)	SYT/SSX
	t(X;18)(p11.2;q11.2)	
Clear cell sarcoma	t(12;22)(q13;q12)	ATF-1/EWS
Mesenchymal chondrosarcoma	t(11;22)(q24;q12)	
Desmoplastic small round cell tumor (DSRCT)	t(11;22)(p13;q12)	EWS-WT1

SPECIFIC PATHOLOGY

Extraosseous Ewing's Sarcoma (EOE)/ Peripheral Neuroectodermal Tumor (PNET)

Extraosseous Ewing's sarcoma (EOE) and peripheral neuroectodermal tumor (PNET) are closely related sarcomas of presumed neuroectodermal origin. As discussed earlier, the common molecular translocation indicates that these sarcomas may represent a spectrum of tumors, with EOE being the more primitive, histologically less differentiated lesion and PNET being more differentiated.[69, 70] PNET and EOE accounted for 22% of the soft-tissue sarcomas reported in the Kiel Tumor Registry.[7]

Clinically, there is a great deal of overlap between the two tumors. The median age of presentation is 18 to 20 years, and both show a predisposition for the paravertebral region, chest wall, and lower extremities. EOEs tend to afflict adolescents and young adults age 15 to 30, whereas PNETs have been described in all ages.[69, 71, 72]

Grossly, both tumors are soft, friable, and often show large areas of necrosis and hemorrhage. Histologically, EOE is identical to its intraosseous counterpart (Fig. 18–2). The tumor is composed of sheets of uniform, round cells with an even distribution of nuclear chromatin and clear to amphophilic cytoplasm. Cytoplasmic glycogen is a characteristic and diagnostically useful feature of the tumor. Four histologic patterns have

been described.[73] Of these, the filigree pattern resulting from extensive tumor necrosis has been associated with the worse prognosis.[73, 74] Mitoses are rare.

In contrast, the cells of PNETs are arranged in lobules separated by fibrous septa (Fig. 18–3). Rosette formation can be focal, or it may be widespread. PNETs show frequent mitoses, nuclear pleomorphism, and indistinct cell borders.

Reported survival rates for patients with these two tumors have been variable. Schmidt[75] reported that patients with EOE had a 60% disease-free survival rate compared with 45% for those with PNET. Other studies have not supported this result.[76, 77] One analysis indicated that with current therapy, the survival rate for both tumors is the same.[78]

Intra-abdominal Desmoplastic Small Round Cell Tumor (DRSCT)

Intra-abdominal desmoplastic small round cell tumor (DRSCT) is a highly aggressive tumor that has a predilection for children and adolescent males. It usually is associated with widespread intra-abdominal growth without any obvious connection to an organ system. The patient usually presents with a palpable, painful mass that may cause abdominal distension, bowel or ureteral obstruction, or constipation.[71, 79]

Histologically, the small round tumor cells are arranged in nests surrounded by an abundant desmoplastic stroma (Fig. 18–4). Immunohisto-

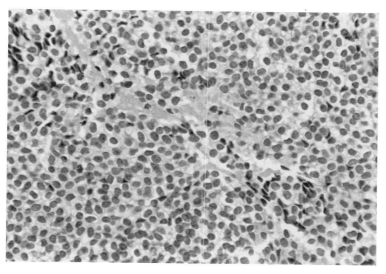

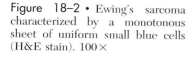

Figure 18–2 • Ewing's sarcoma characterized by a monotonous sheet of uniform small blue cells (H&E stain). 100×

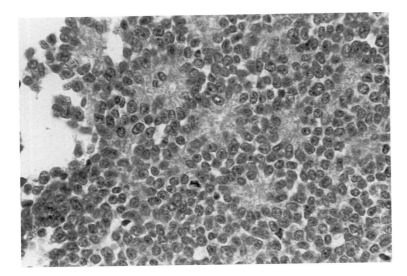

Figure 18–3 • Peripheral neuroectodermal tumor with prominent rosette formation (H&E stain). 100×

chemical analysis of the tumor cells shows evidence of divergent differentiation, with positive staining for epithelial, neural, and muscle markers. These tumors are often mistaken for rhabdomyosarcomas as they contain cells that have rhabdoid features. Molecular analysis has demonstrated a unique translocation t(11;22) (p13;q12) involving the fusion of the Ewing's sarcoma and *WT1* genes with expression of a chimeric *EWS/WT1* product[63, 65–67, 80] The prognoses for patients with these tumors are quite poor. Despite intensive multimodal therapy most patients succumb to widespread metastatic disease a few years after diagnosis. The inability to completely excise these tumors because of their

diffuse infiltrative nature combined with the presence of multiple peritoneal implants impedes therapy.

Synovial Sarcoma

Synovial sarcomas are malignant soft-tissue neoplasms that usually arise in close association with tendon sheaths, bursae, and joint cavities, but despite their name, it is rare for these tumors to involve the synovial membrane. The cell of origin is believed to be a primitive mesenchymal precursor cell. Eighty percent (80%) of these tumors occur in the extremities, primarily in the para-

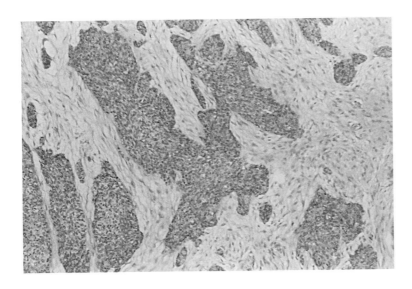

Figure 18–4 • Intra-abdominal desmoplastic small round-cell tumor demonstrating classic irregular tumor nests within a desmoplastic stroma (H&E stain). 100×

articular regions, with 60% noted in the lower extremities.[81] Tumors have been reported in the head and neck (9%) and trunk areas (8%) as well as in the tongue, parapharyngeal region, and abdominal wall.[81, 82]

Grossly, the tumors are multilobular, sharply circumscribed, yellow to gray-white colored lesions that can compress surrounding structures. A pseudocapsule may be present, and cyst formation can be a prominent feature of the tumor. Histologically, this sarcoma can demonstrate three patterns: biphasic, monophasic, or a poorly differentiated variant. The biphasic pattern is the most differentiated and contains columnar or cuboidal epithelial cells surrounded by a fibrosarcomatous stroma that may show hyalinization or myxoid change (Fig. 18–5). The monophasic variant lacks the epithelial component and shows only the sarcomatous stroma. The poorly differentiated tumor is characterized by solidly packed oval or spindle-shaped cells that can have prominent branching vasculature and clinically is associated with the worst prognosis of the three. Calcification is found in 20% of the tumors.

A number of immunohistochemical markers are expressed in the analysis of this tumor. Important markers include vimentin, low-molecular-weight cytokeratins, epithelial membrane antigen (EMA), neuron-specific enolase (NSE), protein S-100, Leu-7, and collagen type IV.[81] Molecular analysis of this tumor has revealed a characteristic balanced translocation between chromosome X and 18 t(X;18)(p11.2;q11.2) in greater than 90% of cases.[83–85] A second translocation has been reported in less than 1% of synovial sarcoma cases as t(X;18)(p11;q11).

Current treatment strategies involve multimodal protocols with surgery and radiation therapy; the role of chemotherapy remains to be defined. Survival rates ranging from 53% to 89% have been reported.[81, 86] Poor prognostic features include age (>20 years), tumor size (>5 cm), high mitotic count (>15/10 HPF), few mast cells (<20 cells/10 HPF), the presence of rhabdoid cells, high-stage, vascular invasion, and high nuclear grade.[87, 88]

Alveolar Soft-Part Sarcoma

Alveolar soft-part sarcomas account for 5% of pediatric nonrhabdomyosarcoma soft-tissue tumors. These are indolent tumors of uncertain histogenesis.[1] The tumor is usually associated with the muscles or fascial planes of the lower extremities, thighs, and buttocks and has been reported in children in the head and neck region, including the orbit and tongue.[89] Metastatic disease at the time of initial diagnosis is rare, but the tumor has a propensity for the development of pulmonary, bone, or brain metastases many years later. In one study 38% of the metastases developed 10 years or later after the original diagnosis.[90, 91]

On gross examination the tumors are firm and variegated in color. Areas of necrosis and hemorrhage are frequent. Histologically, the tumor is

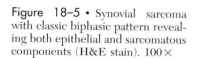

Figure 18–5 • Synovial sarcoma with classic biphasic pattern revealing both epithelial and sarcomatous components (H&E stain). 100×

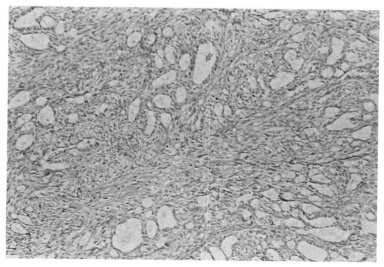

characterized by an alveolar or a pseudoalveolar arrangement of cells separated by thin vascular septa. The tumor cells are polygonal and possess abundant granular eosinophilic cytoplasm. A distinguishing feature of the tumor is the presence of intracytoplasmic glycogen and diastase-resistant crystals noted with PAS staining. The immunohistochemical profile of this tumor has yielded conflicting results, with both neural and muscle cell markers reported.[85, 92, 93] Neuron-specific enolase, S-100, and desmin have been observed in up to 40% of the cases and support a possible neural-cell origin of the tumor.[94] Evidence of MyoD1 expression, which is one of a small set of regulatory genes that control the development and differentiation of myoblasts, has been reported.[95]

Surgery remains the only effective form of therapy, since no study has demonstrated a response to chemotherapy. In adults, radiotherapy has proved to be a useful adjunct for local tumor control in incomplete resections. These tumors are highly vascular, and massive hemorrhage may be a serious complication at the time of surgery. Long-term survival rates vary from 59% to 89%.[94]

Epithelioid Sarcoma

Epithelioid sarcoma is a high-grade tumor that is histologically innocuous and easily mistaken for an inflammatory condition. Predominantly affecting young adults, these tumors most commonly occur in the fingers, hands, and forearms. They are reportedly the most common malignant soft-tissue tumor of the hand. They tend to occur as solitary nodules, but multiple masses have been reported. The nodules in the dermis frequently ulcerate and create the impression of an indurated ulcer or inflammatory lesion. Deep-seated lesions may be attached to tendons, tendon sheaths, or fascial structures.[89]

Grossly, epithelioid sarcomas are gray with a glistening outline. By light microscopy, these tumors consist of nodular arrangements of epithelioid cells with a tendency to undergo central necrosis—mimicking a granulomatous reaction. Calcification and bone formation occur in 10% to 20% of cases.[89]

Multiple recurrences are an important feature of this tumor. An aggressive initial surgical resection appears to be crucial in preventing recurrent growth.[89, 96]

Malignant Fibrous Histiocytoma (MFH)

Malignant fibrous histiocytoma (MFH) is one of the most frequently diagnosed soft-tissue tumors in adults but accounts for less than 5% of such tumors in children.[97, 98] Childhood MFH appears to affect both sexes equally and, unlike the adult version, occurs most often in the head and neck region (30% to 45% of pediatric cases).[98] Of interest, MFH is a frequent postirradiation sarcoma and has also been found following surgery and chronic inflammatory reactions.[97]

The histologic appearance of MFHs is quite variable. Four subtypes have been described: storiform-plexiform, myxoid (myxofibrosarcoma), giant-cell, and inflammatory. The prognosis and clinical behavior have been related in part to the subtype. Storiform-plexiform MFH is the most aggressive. The histogenesis of these tumors remains unclear. Although they were originally considered to be of histiocytic origin, immunohistochemistry and other ancillary tools have been unable to prove this theory.[99, 100] A myofibroblastic origin is postulated for at least some subtypes.[101] There is current debate as to whether or not MFH represents a group of pleomorphic sarcomas.[100]

The overall prognosis for patients with MFH is poor with 5-year survival rates under 60%. In 40% of patients, recurrence or metastatic disease develops, and the survival rate with documented metastases is 20% at 4 years. Complete surgical excision is the major form of treatment.

Angiomatoid MFH

Angiomatoid MFH is a low-grade malignancy with a predilection for childhood; 70% of cases occur in the first decade of life. Over 85% arise in the extremities as slowly growing subcutaneous masses. Less than 5% of patients develop metastatic lesions.[99, 100, 102]

Grossly, these tumors are well-circumscribed nodular lesions containing blood-filled spaces. Microscopically, they have a distinctive appearance and consist of cellular sheets of spindled or rounded cells surrounded by a prominent inflammatory infiltrate and a variable fibrous pseudocapsule. The cells lack the nuclear pleomorphism that characterizes other subtypes of MFH. Studies have shown these tumors to be consistently positive for desmin. The precursor cell still remains unknown, but the possibility of a myogenic or myofibroblastic lineage needs to be explored.[100]

Complete surgical excision remains the primary form of treatment. Tumors tend to recur locally in a small number of cases.

Malignant Peripheral Nerve-Sheath Tumors (MPNSTs)

A highly malignant tumor of childhood, malignant peripheral nerve-sheath tumors (MPNSTs) account for less than 5% of all pediatric soft-tissue neoplasms. Predisposing clinical features include neurofibromatosis and irradiation. These tumors arise from a peripheral nerve or differentiate toward peripheral nerve-sheath cells.[97, 103, 104]

The appearance of these tumors on light microscopy is diverse and shows considerable overlap with other soft-tissue sarcomas. Careful gross examination with identification of the tumor's relationship to a nerve or a neurofibroma, if present, is quite helpful in making the correct diagnosis. As these tumors tend to travel along the nerve itself, careful examination of the nerve by the surgeon and the pathologist, with frozen sections if necessary, is required to ensure complete resection.[105]

Histologically, the features suggestive of a MPNST are a fascicular arrangement of the tumor cells, a hypercellular but monomorphic appearance, a well-developed vascular pattern, and a geographic necrosis with palisading at the periphery. Mitoses are usually abundant, and metaplastic tissue is present in up to 15% of the tumors. Tumors with both neural and skeletal muscle differentiation have been termed *Triton tumors* and are the more mature counterpart of the malignant ectomesenchymoma. With immunohistochemical staining, 50% to 70% of these tumors will be S-100 positive; Leu-7 expression has been noted in 45% of the cases.[104] Some of the epithelioid variants may show HMB-45 positivity and be mistaken for malignant melanoma.[86]

In their study of childhood MPNST cases, Meis-Kindblom and Enzinger[106] recognized an unusual histologic variant of the tumor characterized by a plexiform architecture. Analysis of their cases revealed a relatively high rate of local recurrence but an apparently less aggressive course

clinically than for other MPNSTs. They attributed this fact to the absence of adverse prognostic factors; these tumors were small, superficially located, and showed no evidence of necrosis or vascular invasion. The patients were young and had no evidence of neurofibromatosis. Recognition of this entity is important to prevent its misdiagnosis as a cellular schwannoma, plexiform neurofibroma, or hamartoma.

Complete surgical excision to prevent local recurrences and potential metastatic spread is important. Even so, both local recurrence and distant metastates are common with these tumors. In a study of 78 childhood cases, 50% of the tumors recurred by 12 months, and in 50% metastatic disease developed by 24 months.[104] The overall 5- and 10-year survival rates for patients with these tumors was 34% to 39% and 23%, respectively.[107, 108] Meis and coworkers[104] in their study identified the following adverse features: size greater than 5 cm, patient age greater than 7 years, necrosis involving more than 25% of the tumor, and associated neurofibromatosis.

Malignant Ectomesenchymoma

Malignant ectomesenchymoma is a tumor showing neuronal, schwannian, or melanocytic differentiation in combination with one or more malignant mesenchymal components such as rhabdomyosarcoma. The name derives from the theory that these tumors arise from pluripotent ectomesenchyme or migratory neural-crest cells. Others have named these tumors more descriptively as gangliorhabdomyosarcomas.[97] These are extremely rare tumors, with only 7% occurring in infancy.[109] Their behavior is not well described, but it appears to parallel that of embryonal rhabdomyosarcoma.[86]

Hemangiopericytoma

Hemangiopericytomas can be divided into adult and infantile forms. Whereas the appearance of these two entities is similar on light microscopy, the clinical presentation and behavior as well as the presumed histogenesis are different. The adult form of hemangiopericytoma is a malignant tumor of presumed pericyte origin, and 5% to 10% of the adult types of tumors occur in children and adolescents. Microscopically, they consist of a circumscribed, usually solitary mass composed of oval-shaped to spindle-shaped cells surrounding angular or staghorn-like vascular spaces. These tumors are usually deep-seated or retroperitoneal in location. Poor prognosis is indicated by necrosis, high mitotic activity, high cellularity, and hemorrhage. Diagnosis can be quite challenging as many other tumors can show hemangiopericytomatous-like areas, including synovial sarcoma, malignant peripheral nerve-sheath tumors, mesenchymal chondrosarcoma, and MFH.

Immunocytochemistry is of limited use. The tumor cells stain positively for vimentin, factor XIIIa, and CD34. Initial wide local excision is crucial, as local recurrence predicts distant spread.[86]

Infantile Hemangiopericytoma

Infantile hemangiopericytoma is distinct from its adult counterpart. It usually occurs as a dermal or subcutaneous nodule and may be solitary or multifocal. Tumors arising in the oral cavity and upper respiratory tract have also been described.[97, 110, 111] On light microscopy they exhibit a solid, spindle-cell pattern with cleft-like or staghorn-like vascular spaces. Necrosis, calcification, high mitotic rate, and intravascular or perivascular growth are common.[97, 112] Unlike their adult counterparts, however, these tumors behave in a benign fashion and may spontaneously regress. Immunohistochemical analysis has shown that mature spindle-shaped cells stained positively for α-smooth-muscle actin but were negative for desmin, S-100, EMA, and cytokeratin.

The similarities between infantile hemangiopericytoma and infantile myofibromatosis are striking. Both occur either congenitally or within the first year of life. Both types show a predilection for males, and both have the same anatomic distribution, the head and neck region being the most common site, followed by the extremities, then the trunk. Histologically, infantile myofibromatosis often has a central hemangiopericytomatous-like pattern surrounded by bundles of plump spindle-shaped myofibroblasts (Fig. 18–6).

Infantile myofibromatosis has three clinical presentations: a solitary tumor, a multifocal lesion without visceral involvement, and a multifocal lesion with visceral involvement. The prognosis is excellent for the first two types but is poor for the last, which often leads to death resulting from complications of lesions involving the lungs, heart, and gastrointestinal tract.[110, 111] Infantile hemangiopericytoma and infantile myofibromatosis may represent a spectrum of myofibroblastic proliferations, infantile hemangiopericytoma the more immature of the two.[113]

Fibrosarcoma

Another soft-tissue tumor that shows two distinct patterns of behavior, depending upon the age of the patient, is fibrosarcoma. Prior to the recognition of MFH and monophasic synovial sarcoma, fibrosarcoma was a frequently diagnosed tumor.[114] Now that stricter histologic criteria are used, fibrosarcomas account for only about 3% to 7% of pediatric NRSTSs.[97, 103]

Fibrosarcoma typically presents as a slowly growing, painless mass in the extremities. Grossly, these tumors are soft, lobulated, gray-white to yellow lesions. Histologically, fibrosarcomas in infants and adults are similar, characterized by a relatively uniform proliferation of fibroblastic cells arranged in sweeping fascicles with a herringbone pattern. Tumors from both groups may also show nuclear pleomorphism, high mitotic activity, and necrosis, but the similarity ends there. In a study of older children and adults with fibrosarcoma, Scott and coworkers[114] found a strong correlation between the 5-year survival and histologic grade of the tumor. Tumors were evaluated for degree of cellularity, mitotic activity, nuclear pleomorphism and atypia, and necrosis. Survival rates at 5 years were found to be 58% for Grade I and II tumors, 34% for Grade III, and 21% for Grade IV sarcomas. Local recurrence was strongly correlated with the adequacy of the surgical resection and margins.[114]

While histologically appearing quite aggressive, infantile fibrosarcoma behaves in a much more benign fashion than its older counterpart. Five-year survival rates reportedly range between 83% and 94%. The tumor recurs locally in up to 32% of infants following surgical resection, but the incidence of metastatic disease is less than 10%.[111, 115–117]

Molecular analysis of infantile fibrosarcomas by Schofield and coworkers [118] has demonstrated

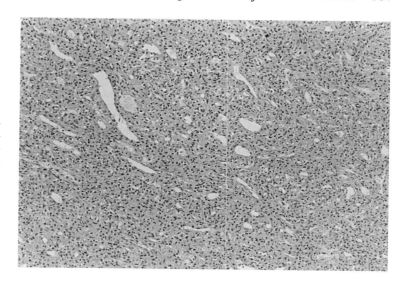

Figure 18–6 • Infantile myofibromatosis demonstrating a hemangiopericytomatous pattern with dilated, stellate vessels (H&E stain). 100×

nonrandom chromosomal gains in genes 8, 11, 17, and 20 in varying combinations in 11 out of 12 fibrosarcomas arising in infants younger than 2 years of age. Additional chromosomal material was not identified in cases of fibrosarcoma from older children or in any of the benign fibromatoses examined.

The therapy of choice for these tumors is wide local excision when possible. Chemotherapy now appears to have some utility, particularly when administered preoperatively to shrink the tumor in order to limit the degree of surgery.[115, 117]

Clear-Cell Sarcoma

Clear-cell sarcoma is a tumor of uncertain histogenesis that accounts for less than 3% of all childhood NRSTSs. Affected individuals usually range from 10 to 64 years of age with a median age of 30. The foot is the most common location in 90% of the reported cases, followed by the knees, hands, and wrists. The tumors tend to be deep-seated.[119, 120]

Histologically, these tumors have the characteristic appearance of clusters of polygonal to spindle-shaped cells arranged in organoid groups separated by fibrous septa. The nuclei are vesicular with prominent nucleoli. Occasional cases show a more diffuse pattern with increased amounts of hyalinized stroma. Abundant intracellular and extracellular iron is present. Cytoplasmic melanin as well as melanosomes can also be seen, suggesting a neural-crest or neuroecto-

dermal origin for these tumors and a link to melanoma. For this reason clear-cell sarcoma has also been referred to as "malignant melanoma of soft parts."[119] The tumor cells stain positively for S-100, HMB-45, Leu-7, NSE, and vimentin. Molecular analysis of clear-cell sarcomas has revealed a characteristic translocation t(12;22)(q13;q12).[86] Of note, the 22q12 gene is the same one involved in the Ewing's/PNET family of tumors.

Clear-cell sarcoma is a highly malignant tumor. The clinical course is characterized by local recurrence and metastatic disease often occurring years after the initial resection. In one review, the 5-year survival rate was 67%, but the 10- and 20-year survival rates were only 33% and 10%, respectively.[120] The propensity for delayed progression is important given the young age of the affected patients.

Current recommendations are for wide local surgical excision. The role of adjuvant therapy is still in question.

Extrarenal Malignant Rhabdoid Tumors

The term *malignant rhabdoid tumors* encompasses a group of tumors that share a specific histologic appearance and aggressive clinical behavior. Originally noted in the kidney, these tumors have now been found in a number of different sites including liver, brain, soft tissues, skin, uterus, and bladder. The lungs, regional lymph

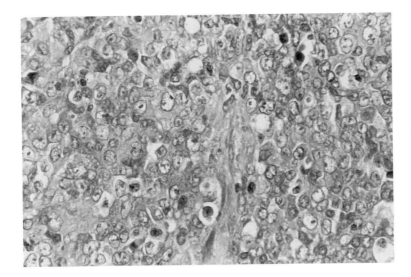

Figure 18–7 • Malignant rhabdoid tumor characterized by large, undifferentiated cells with eccentric nuclei and plump eosinophilic cytoplasm (H&E stain). 400×

nodes, and serosal surfaces are the favored sites of metastases. Rhabdoid or pseudorhabdoid tumors are characterized by an undifferentiated histologic appearance consisting of sheets of cells possessing round to ovoid nuclei, prominent nucleoli, and abundant eccentric eosinophilic cytoplasm (Fig. 18–7). Histologically, the differential diagnosis includes peripheral neuroectodermal tumors, alveolar rhabdomyosarcomas, and hematolymphoid tumors. Immunocytochemical analysis reveals a polyphenotypic profile with expression of cytokeratin, muscle-specific actin, neuron-specific enolase, and epithelial membrane antigen. The tumor cells are negative for MIC2 gene product.[56, 121]

Rhabdoid or pseudorhabdoid cells have also been described in a number of different tumors such as malignant melanoma, poorly differentiated carcinoma, rhabdomyosarcoma, and desmoplastic small round cell tumor.

Other Tumors

Other rare soft-tissue sarcomas in children include myxoid liposarcoma and leiomyosarcoma.[97, 103, 122] The diagnosis of a liposarcoma should be made cautiously as the benign lipoblastomas can closely mimic liposarcomas.

References

1. Rao BN: Nonrhabdomyosarcomas in children: Prognostic factors influencing survival. *Semin Surg Oncol* 9:524–531, 1993.
2. Rao BN, Etcubanas EE, Green AA: Present-day concepts in the management of sarcomas in children. *Cancer Invest* 7:349–356, 1989.
3. Miser JS, Pizzo PA: Soft tissue sarcomas in childhood. *Pediatr Clin North Am* 32:779–800, 1985.
4. Skene AI, Barr L, Robinson M, et al: Adult type (nonembryonal) soft tissue sarcomas in childhood. *Med Pediatr Oncol* 21:645–648, 1993.
5. Dillon PW, Maurer H, Jenkins J, et al: A prospective study of nonrhabdomyosarcoma soft tissue sarcomas in the pediatric age group. *J Pediatr Surg* 27:241–245, 1992.
6. Hayani A, Mahoney DH Jr, Hawkins HK, et al: Soft tissue sarcomas other than rhabdomyosarcomas in children. *Med Pediatr Oncol* 20:114–118, 1992.
7. Harms D: Soft tissue sarcomas in the Kiel Pediatric Tumor Registry. *Curr Top Pathol* 89:31–45, 1995.
8. Decou JM, Rao BN, Parham DM, et al: Malignant peripheral nerve sheath tumors: The St. Jude Children's Research Hospital experience. *Ann Surg Oncol* 2:524–529, 1995.
9. Wanebo JE, Malik JM, VandenBerg SR, et al: Malignant peripheral nerve sheath tumors: A clinicopathologic study of 28 cases. *Cancer* 71:1247–1253, 1993.
10. Storm FK, Eilber FR, Mirra J, et al: Neurofibrosarcoma. *Cancer* 45:126–129, 1980.
11. Ducatman BS, Scheitnauer BW, Peipgras DG, et al: Malignant peripheral nerve sheath tumors: A clinicopathologic study of 120 cases. *Cancer* 57:2006–2021, 1986.
12. Lewis AJ: Sarcoma metastatic to the brain. *Cancer* 61:593–601, 1988.
13. Coindre JM, Trojani M, Contesso G, et al: Reproducibility of a histopathologic grading system for adult soft tissue sarcoma. *Cancer* 58:306–309, 1986.

14. Parham DM: Rhabdomyosarcomas and other soft tissue sarcomas in pediatric patients. *Curr Opin Oncol* 5:672–677, 1993.

15. Parham D, Webber BL, Jenkins JJ, et al: Nonrhabdomyosarcomatous soft tissue sarcomas of childhood: Formulation of a simplified system for grading. *Mod Pathol* 8:705–710, 1995.

16. Rao BN, Santana VM, Parham DM, et al: Pediatric nonrhabdomyosarcomas of the extremities. *Arch Surg* 126:1490–1495, 1991.

17. Lawson JP, Keller MS, Rattner Z: Recent advances in pediatric musculoskeletal imaging. *Radiol Clin North Am* 32:353–375, 1994.

18. Kransdorf MJ, Jelinek JS, Moser RP Jr: Imaging soft tissue tumors. *Radiol Clin North Am* 31:359–371, 1993.

19. Dalinka MK, Zlatkin MB, Chao P, et al: The use of magnetic resonance imaging in the evaluation of bone and soft tissue tumors. *Radiol Clin North Am* 28:461–470, 1990.

20. Jenkin D, Sonley M: Soft tissue sarcomas in the young. *Cancer* 46:621–629, 1980.

21. Horowitz M, Pratt C, Webber B, et al: Childhood malignant soft tissue sarcomas (STS) other than rhabdomyosarcoma: Results of therapy. *Proc Am Soc Clin Oncol* 3:84, 1984.

22. Bennert KW, Abdul-Karim FW: Fine needle aspiration cytology vs. needle core biopsy of soft tissue tumors: A comparison. *Acta Cytol* 38:381–384, 1994.

23. Akerman M, Rydholm A, Persson BM: Aspiration cytology of soft tissue tumors. *Acta Orthop Scand* 56:406–412, 1985.

24. Gonzalez-Campora R, Munoz-Arias G, Otal-Salaverri C, et al: Fine needle aspiration cytology of primary soft tissue tumors: Morphologic analysis of the most frequent types. *Acta Cytol* 36:905–917, 1992.

25. Kissin MW, Fisher C, Carter RL, et al: Value of Tru-Cut biopsy in the diagnosis of soft tissue tumors. *Br J Surg* 73:742–744, 1986.

26. Bennert KW, Abdul-Karim FW: Fine needle aspiration cytology vs. needle core biopsy of soft tissue tumors. *Acta Cytol* 38:381–384, 1994.

27. Holcomb GW, Tomita S, Haase GM, et al: Minimally invasive surgery for pediatric cancer: A Children's Cancer Group experience. *Cancer* 76:121–128, 1995.

28. Dinges S, Budach V, Budach B, et al: Local recurrences of soft tissue sarcomas in adults: A retrospective analysis of prognostic factors in 102 cases after surgery and radiation therapy. *Eur J Cancer* 30A:1636–1642, 1994.

29. Levine EA, Trippon M, Das Gupta TK: Preoperative multimodality treatment for soft tissue sarcomas. *Cancer* 71:3685–3689, 1993.

30. Wilson AN, Davis A, Bell RS, et al: Local control of soft tissue sarcoma of the extremity: The experience of a multidisciplinary sarcoma group with definitive surgery and radiotherapy. *Eur J Cancer* 30A:746–751, 1994.

31. Yang C, Rosenberg SA: Surgery for adult patients with soft tissue sarcoma. *Semin Oncol* 16:289–296, 1989.

32. McCoy DM, Levine EA, Ferrer K, Das Gupta TK: Pediatric soft tissue sarcomas of nonmyogenic origin. *J Surg Oncol* 53:149–153, 1993.

33. Lawrence W, Neifeld JP: Soft tissue sarcomas. In Wells S Jr (ed): *Current Problems in Surgery*, vol. XXVI. Chicago: Year Book Medical Publishers, Inc., 1989.

34. Williard WC, Hajdu SI, Casper ES, et al: Comparison of amputation with limb-sparing operations for adult soft tissue sarcoma of the extremity. *Ann Surg* 215:269–275, 1992.

35. Philippe PG, Rao BN, Rogers DA, et al: Sarcomas of the flexor fossae in children: Is amputation necessary? *J Pediatr Surg* 27:964–967, 1992.

36. Brennan MF, Shiu MH, Collin C, et al: Extremity soft tissue sarcomas. *Cancer Treat Symp* 3:71–81, 1985.

37. Collin C, Godbold J, Hajdu S, Brennan M: Localized extremity soft tissue sarcoma: An analysis of factors affecting survival. *J Clin Oncol* 5:601–605, 1987.

38. Herbert SH, Corn BW, Solin LJ, et al: Limb-preserving treatment for soft tissue sarcomas of the extremities. *Cancer* 72:1230–1238, 1993.

39. Zornig C, Peiper M, Schroder S: Re-excision of soft tissue sarcoma after inadequate initial operation. *Br J Surg* 82:278–279, 1995.

40. Fong Y, Coit DG, Woodruff JM, Brennan MF: Lymph node metastasis from soft tissue sarcoma in adults. *Ann Surg* 217:72–77, 1993.

41. Mazeron JJ, Suit HD: Lymph nodes as sites of metastasis from sarcomas of soft tissue. *Cancer* 60:1800–1808, 1987.

42. Fein DA, Lee WR, Landiano RM, et al: Management of extremity soft tissue sarcomas with limb-sparing surgery and postoperative irradiation: Do total dose, overall treatment time, and the surgery-radiotherapy interval impact on local control? *Int J Radiat Oncol Biol Phys* 32:969–976, 1995.

43. Harrison LB, Franzese F, Gaynor JJ, Brennan MF: Long-term results of a prospective randomized trial of adjuvant brachytherapy in the management of completely resected soft tissue sarcoma of the extremity and superficial trunk. *Int J Radiat Oncol Biol* 27:259–265, 1993.

44. Fromm M, Littman P, Raney RB, et al: Late effects after treatment of twenty children with soft tissue sarcomas of the head and neck. *Cancer* 57:2070–2076, 1986.

45. Fontanesi J, Pappo AS, Parham DM, et al: Role of irradiation in management of synovial sarcoma: St. Jude Children's Research Hospital experience. *Med Pediatr Oncol* 26:264–267, 1996.

46. Maurer HM, Cantor A, Salzberg A, et al:

Adjuvant chemotherapy vs. observation for localized nonrhabdomyosarcoma soft tissue sarcoma in children. *Proc Am Soc Clin Oncol* 11:363, 1992.

47. Nag S, Olson T, Ruymann F, et al: High-dose rate brachytherapy in childhood sarcomas: A local control strategy preserving bone growth and function. *Med Pediatr Oncol* 25:463–469, 1995.

48. Willett CG, Suit HD, Tepper JE, et al: Intraoperative electron beam radiation therapy for retroperitoneal soft tissue sarcoma. *Cancer* 68:278–283, 1991.

49. Thomas L, Delannes M, Stockle E, et al: Intraoperative intersitial iridium brachytherapy in the management of soft tissue sarcomas: Preliminary results of a feasibility phase II study. *Radiother Oncol* 33:99–105, 1994.

50. Dubois JB, Debrigode C, Hay M, et al: Intraoperative radiotherapy in soft tissue sarcomas. *Radiother Oncol* 34:160–163, 1995.

51. Haase GM, Meagher DP, McNeely LK, et al: Electron beam intraoperative radiation therapy for pediatric neoplasms. *Cancer* 73:740–747, 1994.

52. Elias AD: Chemotherapy for soft-tissue sarcomas. *Clin Orthop* 289:94–105, 1993.

53. Santoro A, Tursz T, Mouridsen H, et al: Doxorubicin versus CYVADIC versus doxorubicin plus ifosfamide in first-line treatment of advanced soft tissue sarcomas: a randomized study of the European organization for research and treatment of cancer soft tissue and bone sarcoma group. *J Clin Oncol* 13:1537–1545, 1995.

54. Le Cesne A, Antoine E, Spielmann M, et al: High-dose ifosfamide: Circumvention of resistance to standard-dose ifosfamide in advanced soft tissue sarcomas. *J Clin Oncol* 13:1600–1608, 1995.

55. Saeter G, Talle K, Oyvin PS: Treatment of advanced, high-grade soft tissue sarcoma with ifosfamide and continuous-infusion etoposide. *Cancer Chemother Pharmacol* 36:172–175, 1995.

56. Spicer RD: The management of soft tissue sarcomas in children. *Eur J Surg Oncol* 21:317–320, 1995.

57. Brooks JS: Immunohistochemistry of soft tissue tumors. In Weis SW, Brooks JS (eds): *USCAP Long Course: Soft Tissue Tumors*. Toronto, Ontario: United States and Canadian Academy of Pathology, 1995.

58. Enzinger FM, Weiss SW: Immunohistochemistry of soft tissue lesions. In Enzinger FM, Weiss SW (eds): *Soft Tissue Tumors*. St. Louis: Mosby-Year Book, Inc., 1995, pp. 351–380.

59. Pappo AS, Douglas EC, Meyer WH, et al: Use of HBA 71 and anti-beta 2-microglobulin to distinguish peripheral neuroepithelioma from neuroblastoma. *Hum Pathol* 24:880–885, 1993.

60. Weidner N, Tjoe J: Immunohistochemical profile of monoclonal antibody 013: Antibody that recognizes glycoprotein p30/32^{mic2} and is useful in diagnosing Ewing's sarcoma and peripheral neuroepithelioma. *Am J Surg Pathol* 18:486–494, 1994.

61. Stevenson A, Chatten J, Bertoni F, Miettinen M: CD99 (p30/32^{MIC2}) neuroectodermal/Ewing's sarcoma antigen as an immunohistochemical marker: Review of more than 600 tumors and the literature experience. *Appl Immunohistochemistry* 2:231–240, 1994.

62. Miettinen M, Lindenmayer A, Chaubal A: Endothelial cell markers CD 31, CD 34, and BNH9 antibody to H- and Y-antigens—Evaluation of their specificity and sensitivity in the diagnosis of vascular tumors and comparison with von Willebrand factor. *Mod Pathol* 7:82–90, 1994.

63. Whang-Peng J, Triche TJ, Knutsen T, et al: Chromosome translocation in peripheral neuroepithelioma. *N Engl J Med* 311:584–585, 1984.

64. Askin FB, Rosai J, Sibley JJ, et al: Malignant small cell tumor of the thoracopulmonary region in childhood. *Cancer* 43:2438–2451, 1979.

65. Argatoff LH, O'Connell JX, Mathers JA, et al: Detection of the *EWS/WT1* gene fusion by reverse transcription-polymerase chain reaction in the diagnosis of intra-abdominal desmoplastic small round cell tumor. *Am J Surg Pathol* 20:406–412, 1996.

66. de Alava E, Ladanyi M, Rosai J, et al: Detection of chimeric transcripts in desmoplastic small round cell tumor and related developmental tumors by reverse transcriptase polymerase chain reaction: A specific diagnostic assay. *Am J Pathol* 147:1584–1591, 1995.

67. Gerald WI, Rosai J, Ladanyi M: Characterization of the genomic breakpoint and chimeric transcripts in the *EWS-WT1* gene fusion of desmoplastic small round cell tumor. *Proc Natl Acad Sci USA* 92:1028–1032, 1995.

68. Shivnarain D, Ladanyi M, Zakowski MF: RNA-PCR detection of the t(11;22) as an aid in the cytologic diagnosis of Ewing's sarcoma. *Mod Pathol* 8:44A, 1995.

69. Dehner LP: Primitive neuroectodermal tumor and Ewing's sarcoma. *Am J Surg Pathol* 17:1–13, 1993.

70. Dehner LP: Update on malignant small cell tumors of childhood. In Dehner LP (ed): *17th Annual Conference on Pediatric Disease*. Aspen, Colorado: The Institute for Pediatric Medical Education, 1995.

71. Enzinger FM, Weiss SW: Primitive neuroectodermal tumors and related lesions. In Enzinger FM, Weiss SW (eds): *Soft Tissue Tumors*. St. Louis: Mosby-Year Book, Inc., 1995, pp. 929–964.

72. Kushner BH, Hajdu SI, Gulati SC, et al:

Extracranial primitive neuroectodermal tumors: The Memorial Sloan-Kettering Cancer Center experience. *Cancer* 67:1825–1831, 1991.

73. Triche TJ, Askin FB, Kissane JM: Neuroblastoma, Ewing's sarcoma, and the differential diagnosis of small-, round-, blue-cell tumors. In Finegold M (ed): *Pathology of Neoplasia in Children and Adolescents.* Philadelphia: W.B. Saunders Co., 1986, pp. 145–195.

74. Hartman KR, Triche TJ, Kinsella TJ, Miser JS: Prognostic value of histopathology in Ewing's sarcoma. *Cancer* 67, 163–171, 1991.

75. Schmidt D, Herrmann C, Jurgens H, Harms D: Malignant peripheral neuroectodermal tumor and its necessary definition from Ewing's sarcoma. *Cancer* 68:2251–2259, 1991.

76. Navarro S, Cavazzano AO, Liombart-Bosch A, Triche TJ: Comparison of Ewing's sarcoma of bone and peripheral neuroepithelioma: An immunocytochemical and ultrastructural analysis of two primitive neuroectodermal neoplasms. *Arch Pathol Lab Med* 118:608–615, 1994.

77. Sorenson P, Liu X, Delattre O, et al: Reverse transcriptase PCR amplification of EWS/fil-1 fusion transcripts as a diagnostic test for peripheral primitive neuroectodermal tumors of childhood. *Diag Molec Pathol* 7:147–157, 1993.

78. Hijazi Y, Tsokos M, Steinberg S, et al: Neuroectodermal differentiation does not play a role in the prognosis of Ewing's sarcoma versus primitive neuroectodermal tumor. *Mod Pathol* 9:7A, 1996.

79. Gerald WL, Miler HK, Battifora H, et al: Intra-abdominal desmoplastic small round cell tumor: Report of 19 cases of a distinctive type of high-grade polyphenotypic malignancy affecting young individuals. *Am J Surg Pathol* 15:499–513, 1991.

80. Sawyer JR, Tryka F, Lewis JM: A novel reciprocal chromosome translocation t(11;22)(p13;q12) in an intra-abdominal desmoplastic small round cell tumor. *Am J Surg Pathol* 16:411–416, 1992.

81. Schmidt D, Thum P, Cand M, et al: Synovial sarcoma in children and adolescents: A report from the Kiel Pediatric Tumor Registry. *Cancer* 67:1667–1672, 1991.

82. Enzinger FM, Weiss SW: Synovial sarcoma. In Enzinger FM, Weiss SW (eds): *Soft Tissue Tumors.* St. Louis: Mosby-Year Book, Inc., 1995, pp. 757–786.

83. Fligman I, Lonardo F, Hanwar SC, et al: Molecular diagnosis of synovial sarcoma and characterization of a variant *SYT-SSX2* fusion transcript. *Am J Pathol* 147:1592–1599, 1995.

84. Clark J, Rocques P, Crew A, et al: Identification of novel genes, *SYT* and *SSX*, involved in the t(X;18)(p11.2;q11.2) translocation found in human synovial sarcoma. *Nat Genet* 7:502–508, 1994.

85. De Leeuw B, Suijkerbuijk R, Olde Weghuis D, et al: Distinct Xp11.2 breakpoint regions in synovial sarcoma revealed by metaphase and interphase FISH: Relationship to histologic subtypes. *Cancer Genet Cytogenet* 73:89–94, 1994.

86. Rosai J: Soft tissues. In Rosai J (ed): *Ackerman's Surgical Pathology.* St. Louis: Mosby-Year Book, Inc., 1996, pp. 2021–2134.

87. Kindblom LG, Meis-Kindblom JM, Bertoni F, et al: Synovial sarcoma: Identification of low and high risk groups. *Mod Pathol* 9:8A, 1996.

88. Oda Y, Hashimoto H, Tsuneyoshi M, Takeshita S: Survival in synovial sarcoma: A multivariate study of prognostic factors with special emphasis on the comparison between early death and long-term survival. *Am J Surg Pathol* 17:35–44, 1993.

89. Enzinger FM, Weiss SW: Malignant soft tissue tumors of uncertain type. In Enzinger FM, Weiss SW (eds): *Soft Tissue Tumors.* St. Louis: Mosby-Year Book, Inc., 1995, pp. 1067–1093.

90. Lieberman PH, Brennan MF, Kimmel M, et al: Alveolar soft part sarcoma: A clinico-pathologic study of half a century. *Cancer* 63:1–13, 1989.

91. Auerbach HE, Brooks JJ: Alveolar soft part sarcoma: A clinicopathologic and immunohistochemical study. *Cancer* 60:66–73, 1987.

92. Miettinen M, Ekfors T: Alveolar soft part sarcoma: Immunohistochemical evidence for muscle cell differentiation. *Am J Clin Pathol* 93:32–38, 1990.

93. Cullinane C, Thorner PS, Greenberg ML, et al: Molecular genetic, cytogenetic, and immunohistochemical characterization of alveolar soft part sarcoma: Implications for cell of origin. *Cancer* 70:2444–2450, 1992.

94. Pappo AS, Parham DM, Cain A, et al: Alveolar soft part sarcoma in children and adolescents: Clinical features and outcome of 11 patients. *Med Pediatr Oncol* 26:81–84, 1996.

95. Rosai J, Dias P, Parham DM, et al: MyoD1 protein expression in alveolar soft part sarcoma as confirmatory evidence of its skeletal muscle nature. *Am J Surg Pathol* 15:974–981, 1991.

96. Kodet R, Smelhaus V, Newton WA, et al: Epithelioid sarcoma in childhood: An immunohistochemical, electron microscopic, and clinicopathologic study of 11 cases under 15 years of age and review of the literature. *Pediatr Pathol* 14:431–451, 1994.

97. Coffin CM, Dehner LP: The soft tissues. In Stocker JT, Dehner LP (eds): *Pediatric Pathology.* Philadelphia: J.B. Lippincott Co., 1992, pp. 1091–1132.

98. Zuppan CW, Mierau GW, Wilson HL: Malignant fibrous histiocytoma in childhood: A report of two cases and a review of the literature. *Pediatr Pathol* 7:303–318, 1987.

99. Enzinger FM, Weiss SW: Malignant fibrohistiocytic tumors. In Enzinger FM, Weiss SW (eds): *Soft Tissue Tumors.* St. Louis: Mosby-Year Book, Inc., 1995, pp. 351–380.

100. Hollowood K, Fletcher CD. Malignant fibrous histiocytoma: Morphologic pattern or pathologic entity. *Semin Diag Pathol* 12:210–220, 1995.

101. Mentzel T, Calonje E, Wadden C, et al: Myxofibrosarcoma: Clinicopathologic analysis of 75 cases with emphasis on the low-grade variant. *Am J Surg Path* 20:391–405, 1996.

102. Costa MJ, Weiss SW: Angiomatoid malignant fibrous histiocytoma: A follow-up study of 108 cases with evaluation of possible histologic predictors of outcome. *Am J Surg Pathol* 14:1126–1132, 1990.

103. Coffin CM, Dehner LP: Soft tissue neoplasms in childhood and adolescence: A clinicopathologic review of 944 cases. *Lab Invest* 54:12A, 1986.

104. Meis JM, Enzinger FM, Martz KL, et al: Malignant peripheral nerve sheath tumors (malignant schwannomas) in children. *Am J Surg Pathol* 16:694–707, 1992.

105. Woodruff JM: Pathology of peripheral nerve sheath tumors. In Weiss SW, Brooks, JS (eds): *USCAP Long Course: Soft Tissue Tumors.* Toronto, Ontario: United States and Canadian Academy of Pathology, 1995.

106. Meis-Kindblom JM, Enzinger FM. Plexiform malignant peripheral nerve sheath tumor of infancy and childhood. *Am J Surg Pathol* 18:479–485, 1994.

107. Ducatman BS, Scheithauer BW, Piepgras DG, et al: Malignant peripheral nerve sheath tumors: A clinicopathologic study of 120 cases. *Cancer* 57:2006–2021, 1986.

108. Hruban RH, Shiu MH, Senie RT, et al: Malignant peripheral nerve sheath tumors of the buttock and lower extremity: A study of 43 cases. *Cancer* 66:1253–1265, 1990.

109. Kawanoto EH, Weidner N, Agostini RM, Jaffe R: Malignant ectomesenchymoma of soft tissue: Report of 2 cases and review of the literature. *Cancer* 59:1791–1802, 1987.

110. Coffin CM: Fibroblastic and myofibroblastic proliferations in children and adolescents. In Dehner LP (ed): *17th Annual Aspen Conference on Pediatric Disease.* Aspen, Colorado: The Institute for Pediatric Education, 1995.

111. Coffin CM, Braun JT, Dehner LP: Fibrohistiocytic tumors in children and adolescents: A clinicopathologic study of 107 cases. *Pediatr Pathol* 7:483–484, 1987.

112. Malone M: Soft tissue tumors in childhood. *Histopathology* 23:203–216, 1993.

113. Mentzel T, Calonje E, Nascimento AG, et al: Infantile hemangiopericytoma versus infantile myofibromatosis: Study of a series suggesting a continuous spectrum of infantile myofibroblastic lesions. *Am J Surg Pathol* 18:922–930, 1994.

114. Scott SM, Reiman HM, Pritchard DJ, et al: Soft tissue fibrosarcoma: A clinicopathologic study of 132 cases. *Cancer* 64:925–931, 1989.

115. Coffin CM, Dehner LP: Soft tissue tumors in the first year of life: A report of 190 cases. *Pediatr Pathol* 10:509–526, 1990.

116. Soule EH, Pritchard DJ: Fibrosarcoma in infants and children: A review of 110 cases. *Cancer* 40:1711–1721, 1977.

117. Enzinger FM, Weiss SW: Fibrosarcoma. In Enzinger FM, Weiss SW (eds): *Soft Tissue Tumors.* St. Louis: Mosby-Year Book, Inc., 1995, pp. 269–291.

118. Schofield DE, Fletcher JA, Grier HE, et al: Fibrosarcoma in infants and children: Application of new techniques. *Am J Surg Pathol* 18:14–24, 1994.

119. Enzinger FM, Weiss SW: Malignant tumors of the peripheral nerves. In Enzinger FM, Weiss SW (eds): *Soft Tissue Tumors.* St. Louis: Mosby-Year Book, Inc., 1995, pp. 889–928.

120. Lucas DR, Nascimento A, Sim FH: Clear cell sarcoma of soft tissues: Mayo Clinic experience with 35 cases. *Am J Surg Pathol* 16:1197–1204, 1992.

121. Parham DM, Weeks DA, Beckwith B: The clinicopathologic spectrum of putative extrarenal rhabdoid tumors: An analysis of 42 cases studied with immunohistochemistry or electron microscopy. *Am J Surg Pathol* 18:1010–1029, 1994.

122. Kilpatrick SE, Doyon J, Choong PF, et al: The clinicopathologic spectrum of myxoid and round cell liposarcoma. *Cancer* 77:1450–1458, 1996.

Neonatal Tumors

• *Peter W. Dillon, M.D.* • *Richard G. Azizkhan, M.D.*

A neonate with a malignant neoplasm presents an extremely rare challenge to pediatric surgeon, oncologist, and neonatologist alike. Few specific studies of cancers in the neonatal period exist, with the result being very little experience from which to determine prognostic indicators or treatment strategies. Much of the information regarding specific neoplasms has been gathered from multicenter studies that are dominated by older children or from single-institutional reviews.

The challenge of treating a cancer at this age is further complicated by the physiology and developmental status of the neonate and by the biology of the tumor. Factors such as the age-dependent maturation of various physiologic processes, including renal, gastrointestinal, hematologic, hormonal, and neurodevelopmental systems, make neonates unusually susceptible to the detrimental effects of multimodal approaches, involving radical surgery, chemotherapy, or radiotherapy. The long-term effects of such antineoplastic therapies imposed upon the developing neonate are only now becoming evident. A number of malignant tumors differ markedly in their biologic behavior during this neonatal period as compared with later periods. A proper understanding of such differences is crucial when attempting to institute therapeutic but potentially toxic interventions.

This chapter reviews the current information available on solid malignant tumors in the neonatal period. It is not meant to be an in-depth analysis of each tumor, as such discussions appear in other chapters.

EPIDEMIOLOGY

Most tumors in the newborn period (<30 days of age) are benign lesions. Malignant ones are extremely rare, reportedly constituting only 2% of all childhood cancers, with an incidence of 36.5 per million live births in the United States.[1] This statistic works out to 1 tumor per 27,500 births per year. Overall, no significant differences have been noted according to sex or ethnic group.

The association of cancer with other congenital anomalies has been well documented, but few such cases have been reported in neonatal studies.[2] Parkes and coworkers[3] found associated anomalies in 15% of 170 cases examined. Defects included congenital heart disease, genitourinary abnormalities, CNS abnormalities, and skeletal deformities. Chromosomal abnormalities were documented in three infants with Down's syndrome who had leukemia.[3] Moore and coworkers[4] noted only three patients with chromosomal abnormalities and no other associated conditions in 66 patients studied.[4]

CLINICAL PRESENTATION

Approximately one half of the tumors diagnosed in the neonatal period are evident at the time of birth.[5] The majority of the tumors (59% to 79%) are evident within the first week of life.[4, 5] Physical examination most commonly reveals an anatomic abnormality that must be distinguished from a more common benign lesion. Nonspecific symptoms that may indicate the possibility of an underlying occult malignancy include lethargy, irritability, feeding difficulty, and failure to thrive. Signs of increased intracranial pressure may indicate the presence of a brain tumor. Hematologic abnormalities may indicate possible bone marrow involvement from metastatic spread of a tumor such as neuroblastoma.

PATHOLOGY

The Children's Cancer Group (CCG) has completed the largest multi-institutional retrospective review of solid tumors in infants under 1 month of age ever reported, with a total of 338 patients (Table 19–1). The most common tumor in this study was the teratomatous germ-cell tumor, which accounted for 38% of all tumors reported. Neuroblastomas were the most common malignant lesions, and they were the second most common tumors (27%), followed by soft-tissue sarcomas (9%) and renal tumors (7%).

Table 19–1 • CCG Neonatal Cancer Survey

Type of Cancer	Number of Cases	Percent of Cases
Teratomas	129	38
Neuroblastoma	92	27
Sarcomas	32	9
Renal tumors	25	7
CNS tumors	11	3
Hepatic tumors	10	3
Retinoblastoma	9	2.5
Other		
Histiocytosis	8	
Testicular tumors	4	
Melanoma	3	
Miscellaneous	9	

In a study from the United Kingdom, Parkes and coworkers[3] noted a similar distribution of tumor types: teratomas were most common (46%), followed by neuroblastomas (15%) and soft-tissue tumors (8%). Moore and coworkers[4] reported similar results in a study from South Africa.

Central nervous system (CNS) malignancy, a diagnosis that may be easily overlooked in the newborn period, was reported in 3% to 11% of the tumors studied.

Earlier published reports examining only neonatal solid malignancies noted that neuroblastomas were the most commonly encountered solid cancers in the newborn.[6–9] In contrast, a tertiary referral cancer center reported soft-tissue sarcomas as the most common solid malignancies, followed by neuroblastomas and CNS tumors.[5]

In a study of solid tumors found at the time of perinatal necropsy, teratomas were found to be the most common tumors (57%), followed by benign vascular malformations. Neuroblastomas were identified in 13% of the cases, always as an incidental finding.[10]

EVALUATION

The clinical workup and radiographic evaluation of a solid tumor in the neonatal period should be dictated by the differential diagnosis and suspected pathology. Such evaluations are outlined in the specific chapters concerning each tumor.

The increased use of ultrasound in perinatal

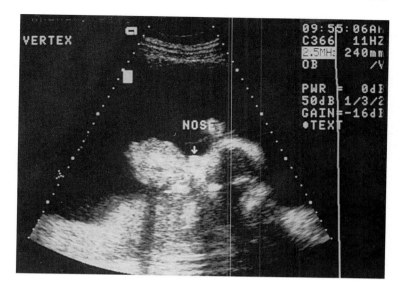

Figure 19–1 • Fetal ultrasound showing soft-tissue mass protruding from the oral pharynx with significant facial distortion. The nose is marked with an arrow.

medicine has aided diagnosis of tumors in the prenatal period. This evaluation has been particularly helpful in the diagnosis of sacrococcygeal and cervical teratomas that might complicate an attempted vaginal delivery or threaten a physiologically compromised fetus or newborn infant (Fig. 19–1).[11, 12] Potential problems with thoracic and abdominal pathology can also be determined on ultrasound, as tumors such as neuroblastoma are frequently detected during fetal development (Fig. 19–2).[13, 14]

TREATMENT

Surgery

At a time when multimodal therapy has proved extremely effective in the treatment of most childhood malignancies, surgery remains the definitive form of treatment of neonatal solid tumors. The timing of surgical intervention and the surgical strategies employed are discussed elsewhere in this book. The principles of neonatal surgery, with strict attention to the special

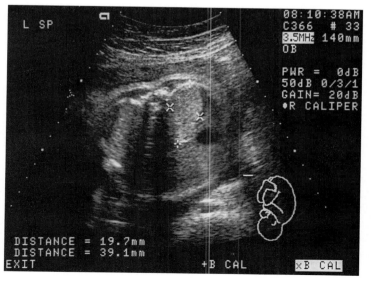

Figure 19–2 • Fetal ultrasound demonstrating intra-abdominal tumor located above the kidney.

physiologic and metabolic processes of the newborn, must be followed.[15] The potential for severe physiologic derangements occurring preoperatively as a direct result of the tumor and intraoperatively as a result of surgical exposure and manipulation is proportionate to the size and location of the tumor. The problems imposed by a giant sacrococcygeal teratoma are a good example. Dependable and adequate venous access must be secured in the event of large third-space fluid losses or significant intraoperative blood loss. Appropriate management plans should be considered to guard against the problems of hypoglycemia, hypocalcemia, and hypothermia, particularly if massive fluid or blood volume replacement is required or prolonged exposure occurs. It is always best to discuss the surgical strategy and potential problems with the pediatric anesthesia team before embarking upon any attempted resection.

Radiation

Most pediatric tumors are radiosensitive, and so radiation therapy has an important role in the management of many of these cases. Although the acute and chronic side effects of radiation exposure in general are well documented, the long-term implications of such therapy in the neonate are essentially still unknown. Treatment parameters such as exposure schedules and maximum doses administered have been empirically derived from studies on older patients and limited neonatal experiences.

Because of ongoing development, it is believed that a number of organs and structures in infants are particularly sensitive to the detrimental effects of radiation therapy and that this sensitivity is inversely related to the age of the child and directly related to the dose.[16] Major organ systems particularly vulnerable to damage include the brain, skeleton, kidney, liver, and lung.[17]

In a study of the late effects of radiotherapy administered to infants less than 2 years of age, Meadows and coworkers[18] found that musculoskeletal abnormalities and growth disturbances were the most common long-term problems. More than 85% of children treated with radiation for selected tumors had later evidence of some degree of bone or soft-tissue abnormality. Following thoracic or spinal irradiation, severe bony abnormalities have been noted, and scoliosis has been reported in as many as 70% of the chil-

dren.[19, 20] Moore and coworkers[4] found that all infants who received radiation therapy had delayed physical development. This problem was also noted by Silber and coworkers.[20] Another major late effect of radiation is on cognitive development in children receiving radiation therapy for leukemia or brain tumors. It is known that young infants treated with cranial radiation for either type of malignancy have a high incidence of learning disabilities and mental retardation, and that this result may be dose-related.[18, 21, 22] Other well-known side effects of radiation therapy include aortic arch dysgenesis, agenesis of the female breast, acute and chronic nephropathy, and hepatic toxicity.[23–25] At least two cases of radiation-induced thyroid carcinoma have been reported in long-term survivors of neonatal cancer.[4, 8]

Chemotherapy

The administration of chemotherapy to the neonate is complicated by the lack of data concerning the pharmacokinetics of such antineoplastic agents in this population. As with radiation therapy, it is generally assumed that newborns are much more sensitive to these agents and have a lower threshold for developing toxic side effects than older children and adults. Increased neurotoxicity has been reported to result from vincristine administration in newborns.[26] Excessive myelosuppression was noted in infants enrolled in the Second National Wilms' Tumor Study, with the resulting recommendation that doses of all agents be reduced by 50% in infants younger than 1 year of age.[27, 28] This approach of reducing doses by 50% has also been followed in the Intergroup Rhabdomyosarcoma Study protocols. Yet, excessive chemotherapy-related toxicities have not been noted in infants with leukemia, and reduced-dosage protocols had an unfavorable impact on clinical response and outcomes in those patients.[29]

Few published studies exist on the disposition of chemotherapeutic agents in infants. McLeod and coworkers[30] examined the pharmacodynamics of a number of such drugs in infants younger than 1 year of age as compared with older children but did not include neonates younger than 2 months of age. They found that methotrexate clearance values tended to be lower in infants younger than 1 year as compared with older

Table 19–2 • Anatomic Location of Germ-Cell Tumors in CCG Neonatal Tumor Survey

Type of Tumor	Percent of Cases
Sacrococcygeal	84
Mature	68
Immature	20
Malignant	12
Cervicofacial	12
Mature	50
Immature	19
Malignant	31
Retroperitoneal	3
Cardiac	1

children and that systemic clearance of doxorubicin was less in children younger than 2 years. No differences were noted in clearance values for teniposide, etoposide, and mercaptopurine.[30] They concluded that empiric dosage protocols based on weight or body surface area alone are inappropriate for young infants and that each agent should be judged instead on its pharmacodynamic characteristics.

SPECIFIC NEOPLASMS

Germ-Cell Tumors

Germ-cell tumors, otherwise known as teratomas, are the most common solid tumors oc-

curring in the neonatal period. Newborn females with these tumors outnumber males by almost a 2:1 ratio.[3] In the CCG study most such tumors occurred in the sacrococcygeal region (84%), followed by the head and neck area (12%) (Table 19–2). Similar anatomic presentations have been noted in other studies.[3, 4, 31]

Sacrococcygeal teratomas most commonly appear as solid or partially cystic masses in the buttock and sacral area. Based on the anatomic location, four types have been described for clinical classification. These four types range from an almost completely external appearance to a localized intra-pelvic presacral lesion.[32] Symptoms are related to the degree of compression of associated structures in the pelvis and may include constipation, urinary frequency, and lower extremity weakness. Cervicofacial teratomas may also appear as solid or partially cystic lesions and frequently cause significant airway and esophageal obstruction in the perinatal period (Fig. 19–3). One third of the cases are associated with maternal polyhydramnios resulting from the inability of the fetus to swallow amniotic fluid.[33]

Pathologically, teratomas are classified into three main types based on the tissue components of the tumor: mature, immature, and malignant. The biologic properties of these neonatal tumors are fascinating, as benign germ-cell tumors have the potential to become malignant.[32] In the CCG Neonatal Cancer Survey, 64% of all teratomas were histologically mature, 21% were immature, and 15% were malignant. When examined by

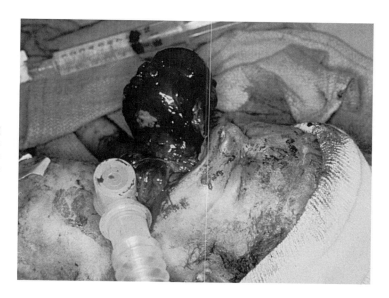

Figure 19–3 • Teratoma originating from the oral pharynx and resulting in complete airway obstruction that required emergency tracheostomy in the delivery room.

site, 12% of the sacrococcygeal teratomas were malignant as were 31% of the cervicofacial tumors. In the literature the reported rate of malignant teratomas varies from 3% to 10%.[32, 34, 35] Malignant germ-cell elements within a teratoma may include germinoma, choriocarcinoma, endodermal sinus tumor, or embryonal carcinoma. Endodermal sinus tumor and embryonal carcinoma are the malignant elements most commonly found in sacrococcygeal tumors.[36] Malignant cervical teratomas are exceedingly rare in the neonate. All cases reported have also had either metastatic disease or extensive local invasion.[12] Neuroectodermal elements and immature neural tissue are the most commonly encountered tissues in metastatic foci and often appear more differentiated than the components of the primary tumor.

Surgical therapy is the treatment of choice for these tumors. Sacrococcygeal teratomas require complete excision including excision of the coccyx to minimize the risk of recurrence. Meticulous attention must be paid to the reconstruction of the gluteal and perineal regions, since severe distortion of structures in these areas can occur from large tumors. Although it is not mandatory immediately following birth, surgical intervention should be carried out as soon as the infant's condition has stabilized and been properly evaluated. Urgent surgery may be required for giant tumors imposing a physiologic stress on the infant such as hyperdynamic congestive heart failure. Tumor rupture with hemorrhage should be immediately controlled with compression or a tourniquet at the base of the tumor and urgent surgical resection.

Early resection of cervicofacial teratomas is also recommended. For these tumors it is most important that a pediatric surgeon be present at the time of delivery, since life-threatening airway obstruction has been reported to occur in 35% of the cases.[12] If respiratory distress is noted at birth and the tumor prevents orotracheal intubation, the surgeon should be prepared to perform fiberoptic or rigid bronchoscopy in the delivery room. If intubation is still impossible, an immediate tracheostomy should be performed. During this time of airway assessment, the maternal-fetal placental circulation must be maintained.[37]

Overall survival rates for neonatal teratomas were 86% in the CCG study and 78% in the study by Parkes and coworkers.[3] For patients with mature sacrococcygeal teratomas the CCG 5-year survival rate was 91%. A number of infants with giant tumors died in the immediate postpartum period. Several cases were obstetric catastrophies in which the tumor was trapped in the birth canal resulting in the asphxiation of the baby. Exsanguinating hemorrhage from the tumor occurred preoperatively as a result of trauma during delivery or intraoperatively as a result of attempted resection in a few cases. Parkes and coworkers[3] reported that 6 of the 11 deaths in their study occurred in patients with benign tumors before surgical excision could be performed. For patients with malignant sacrococcygeal tumors, the long-term survival rate was 54% after 6 years' follow-up in the CCG study. The overall survival rate for patients with cervicofacial teratomas was 85%, with 70% having an excellent functional and cosmetic outcome.[12] Two of the 20 neonates (10%) in the CCG study died in the delivery room without having an airway secured. The long-term survival rates for patients with malignant cervicofacial tumors are not well studied. Among the reported patients that underwent treatment, 73% survived on a very limited follow-up.[12]

Neuroblastomas

Neuroblastomas are the second most common solid tumors appearing in neonates and the most common malignant lesion in neonates. This tumor is diagnosed in the neonatal period in less than 1% of all neuroblastoma cases reported. Most studies have included these neonatal cases in the category of infants younger than 1 year of age for analysis. As a result, a true understanding of these lesions is lacking.

Neonatal neuroblastoma is most often recognized as in situ neuroblastoma.[38, 39] Its unique biologic characteristic is that small neuroblastomas composed of immature neuroblasts can be found during routine neonatal autopsies with a frequency close to 40 times higher than what would be expected for clinically evident disease.[38] Most of these neuroblastomas degenerate and regress spontaneously in a process that may represent normal adrenal development in the fetus. It has been proposed that the appearance of a clinical neuroblastoma may represent a defect in the cellular maturation of these neuroblasts.[40] The tumor usually appears as a solid lesion, but cystic neuroblastomas have been reported.[41] Cystic neuroblastomas may arise from a primary adrenal cyst or may develop as a result of hemorrhage or degeneration within a solid neuroblastoma. It has been found that most tumors diagnosed prenatally have a cystic component to them.[14]

Prenatal ultrasound studies are effective in identifying potential neuroblastoma tumors in the prenatal period.[13, 14, 40, 42, 43] Once an infant is born, it may be difficult to differentiate a neuroblastoma from an adrenal hemorrhage by ultrasound alone. Additional imaging modalities may be required. Other lesions that should also be considered in the differential diagnosis of adrenal tumors found on prenatal ultrasound include congenital mesoblastic nephroma, neonatal Wilms' tumor, hydronephrosis, duplicated renal collecting system, and intra-abdominal extralobar pulmonary sequestration. In older children the diagnosis of neuroblastoma is aided by the fact that urinary catecholamine metabolites are elevated in 85% to 90% of such patients.[44] In younger patients, however, a high percentage of fetal and cystic neuroblastomas are nonfunctioning tumors with negative markers.[41, 45] Nevertheless, catecholamine production by a functioning fetal neuroblastoma can induce maternal symptoms such as hypertension or preeclampsia in the last 2 months of pregnancy.[46, 47] Such symptoms have been associated with Stage 4 and 4s neonatal disease, whereas metastatic neuroblastoma to the placenta can cause similar clinical findings.[40]

Approximately one half of the tumors diagnosed after birth have metastatic spread at that time, usually to the liver. Hepatomegaly or massive abdominal distension may be the initial signs, sometimes associated with significant respiratory distress. Radiographic and biologic marker evaluation in these patients should proceed as for older children (as described elsewhere in this book).

In the CCG Neonatal Cancer Survey 92 newborns with neuroblastoma were reported. Using the Evans classification, a total of 49% were found to be in Stage 1 or 2, and 26% were Stages 3 and 4. The other 25% presented as Stage 4s. In a smaller study group that included infants up to 3 months of age Parkes and coworkers[3] noted a slightly higher proportion of patients presenting in the advanced stages of 3 and 4. Infants in the 4s category were 29% of the group. Patients with tumors diagnosed antenatally seldom present with metastatic disease; 87% of the cases reported by Richards and coworkers[41] had disease confined to the primary tumor site.

Treatment strategies for infants with neuroblastomas are the same as for older children and involve a multimodal approach depending on stage and associated prognostic factors.

Overall, the survival rate of neonates with neuroblastoma appears to be superior to that of older children—a fact that highlights the differing biologic properties of this tumor in the newborn period. But widely varying outcomes have been reported. In the CCG study the survival rate for the entire group was 76% at a mean follow-up period of 6 years. For patients with Stages 1, 2, and 3 disease, the outcomes were excellent; 87% to 95% of the infants survived (Figs. 19–4 and

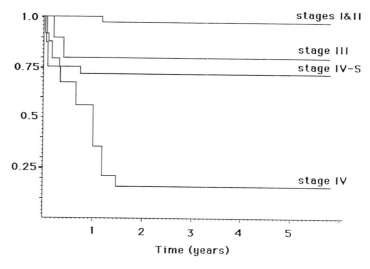

Figure 19–4 • Survival by stage for neonates with neuroblastoma.

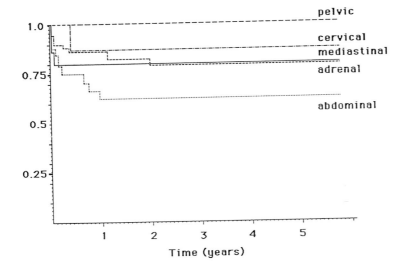

Figure 19–5 • Survival by location of neuroblastoma in neonates at all stages.

19–5). Residual microscopic disease following resection did not adversely affect survival in these newborn infants, confirming the findings of Suita and coworkers,[48] who studied infants younger than 6 months. As in older children, infants with metastatic disease (Stage 4) did poorly. Yet those infants presenting in the special 4s classification of metastatic disease did well, with a long-term survival rate of 74%. The deaths that occurred in Stages 1 and 2 patients were unrelated to the disease process, whereas those occurring in Stages 3, 4, and 4s patients were from disease progression or therapy-related complications. In this study none of the biologic markers (n-*myc*, ferritin, VMA) correlated with either disease progression or disease-free survival. Moore and coworkers[4] reported a survival rate of 60% for 10 infants with neuroblastomas. Parkes and coworkers[3] reported a survival rate of 35% for 31 neonates with neuroblastomas.

The prognosis for infants with cystic neuroblastomas is excellent. Of the reported cases complete surgical resection was possible in 86% of the patients, and none of these suffered recurrent disease.[41] It is clear that this form of neuroblastoma has biologic characteristics dramatically different from those of its more common solid counterpart.

Soft-Tissue Sarcomas

Soft-tissue sarcomas are the third most common solid tumor in neonates, accounting for 8% to 11% of newborn neoplasms (see Table 19–1).[3, 4, 49] Among all soft-tissue sarcomas only 2% are diagnosed in the newborn period.[50] It must be remembered that in infants up to 1 year of age over 75% of all soft-tissue lesions are benign and of either vascular, lymphatic, or fibromuscular origin. Malignant tumors are extremely rare.

In the CCG study the most common presentation was of an obvious soft-tissue mass on physical examination with half (50%) of the tumors evident at birth.[49] The most common site was the head and neck region (34%), followed by the extremities (29%) and the trunk (25%). Pathologic classification was equally divided into three groups: congenital fibrosarcoma (38%), rhabdomyosarcoma (34%), and nonrhabdomyosarcoma soft-tissue sarcomas (28%).

It has been well documented that congenital fibrosarcoma is a soft-tissue malignancy with a favorable prognosis no matter what its neonatal presentation.[51–53] It tends to be locally aggressive, with the predominant site of presentation being the extremities. Metastatic disease is uncommon, but local tumor control can be difficult after initial therapy; reported recurrence rates vary from 17% to 43%. Prognosis does not appear to be affected by tumor recurrence, but deaths in patients with primary-site recurrence and metastatic spread have been reported.[54]

In the past, treatment for these tumors involved aggressive surgical excision including amputation to ensure local tumor control. It is now recommended that chemotherapy be included in treatment protocols for this tumor. Such adjuvant therapy can alter the surgical approach to a large bulky lesion. If surgical resection is likely to result in significant morbidity or mutilation, preoperative chemotherapy should be used to try to consolidate the tumor and decrease the extent of the excision required.[55-58] Overall survival rates are excellent, from 90% to 100%.[49]

Very little is known about neonatal rhabdomyosarcomas, as these tumors tend to occur in older infants and children.[59] The Intergroup Rhabdomyosarcoma Study Group (IRS) has reported that less than 5% of all rhabdomyosarcomas are found before patients reach the age of 1 year.[60, 61] An IRS review found only 14 infants with neonatal rhabdomyosarcomas in an entire study group of 3217 patients, for an incidence of 0.4%.[62]

As in older patients, the predominant histologic cell type in neonatal rhabdomyosarcomas is embryonal or embryonal/botryoid.[49, 62] In the IRS study one half of the tumors arose in the lower pelvic region: buttock/sacrococcygeal area, perirectal, bladder, and vagina. Other sites included the head and neck area, upper trunk, and proximal lower extremity.[62] When classified by clinicopathologic groups, 60% were Stage 3 or 4. A characteristic of the neonatal rhabdomyosarcomas in the CCG study was their apparent aggressive biologic behavior, as almost half of the patients had evidence of widespread disease at the time of diagnosis.[49]

Multimodal therapy for these tumors has been well defined in the IRS studies of older children.[63] Lobe and coworkers[62] reported that half of the infants underwent complete resections. Dillon and coworkers[49] reported that only 18% of the infants underwent complete resections. Other surgical procedures included incisional biopsies or partial excisions. Adjuvant chemotherapy was utilized in almost all of the neonates. In contrast, the use of radiotherapy was quite variable. Despite reductions in the doses of various chemotherapeutic agents, related toxicity was still significant.[62]

The overall survival rate for soft-tissue rhabdomyosarcomas in neonates is disappointing. Lobe and coworkers[62] noted a 3-year survival rate of 49%, but found that anatomic site was a crucial prognostic factor regardless of the type of treatment administered. The 3-year survival rate for tumors arising in the pelvic area (caudal sites) was 86% compared with only 14% for all other

areas.[62] Only two patients in the CCG study were long-term survivors, and the sole infant with no evidence of disease at 9-year follow-up had had a tumor originating from the bladder.[49] Thus, despite standard multimodal therapy, the survival rate for neonates with rhabdomyosarcoma is dismal unless the tumors originate from a caudal site.

Nonrhabdomyosarcoma soft-tissue sarcomas (NRSTSs) in the pediatric age group have always been a difficult set of tumors to study effectively. Experience with neonatal NRSTSs appears to be limited to case reports. Salloum and coworkers[54] reported five infants with undifferentiated sarcomas diagnosed in the neonatal period, Dillon and coworkers[49] reported nine. In the CCG study males predominated, and seven of the nine tumors (78%) were evident at birth. Metastatic disease was noted at the time of diagnosis in four infants (44%). Anatomic sites included head and neck, trunk, and extremities.[49]

No consensus exists as to the optimum strategy of multimodal therapy for patients with these tumors. Complete surgical resection was possible in fewer than half of the CCG study infants, and so the others underwent incisional biopsies. Adjuvant therapy consisted of chemotherapy in five cases and radiotherapy in three. In this group, five patients (56%) survived at a mean follow-up of just over 9 years. These patients had no evidence of regional or metastatic disease at the time of the initial surgery. All patients with unresectable regional or metastatic disease died despite adjuvant therapy.[49] It appears that the ability to achieve a cure in patients with neonatal NRSTSs depends on the biologic nature of the tumor and the ability of the surgeon to eradicate it, because adjuvant therapy as it is currently employed appears to be ineffective against persistent disease.

Renal Neoplasms

Unlike cystic lesions of the kidney, solid renal neoplasms are extremely rare within the first month of life, accounting for 8% or less of all neonatal tumors (see Table 19-1).[3] The most common solid tumor is the benign *congenital mesoblastic nephroma* (CMN), also known as fetal renal hamartoma, followed by the nephroblastoma, or Wilms' tumor. In the CCG neonatal study there were 25 neonatal renal neoplasms, of which 17 (68%) were mesoblastic nephromas. The others were nephroblastomas (32%). Mesoblastic nephromas have dominated other neonatal studies as well.[3, 4, 64, 65] Underscoring just how rare malignant neoplasms are, Ritchey and co-workers[66] reviewed neonatal Wilms' tumors in the National Wilms' Tumor Study (NWTS) data bank and found 15 cases in a total of 6832 patients—an incidence of 0.16%.

As with other neoplasms, solid renal tumors can be diagnosed on prenatal ultrasound.[66, 67] No specific sonographic characteristics can differentiate a CMN from a Wilms' tumor, however, and subsequent evaluation must be undertaken following delivery. On physical examination both lesions usually appear as palpable abdominal masses. Among CMN cases, males outnumber females by 2:1. Among neonatal Wilms' tumor cases, males and females are affected equally, as are both the left and right kidneys. One case has been reported of an infant with Beckwith-Wiedemann syndrome who had a screening ultrasound done at 4 days of age in which a renal mass was found.[67]

All patients should undergo surgical excision of the tumor. For those with CMN, surgical excision is the only treatment necessary. Although these tumors are classified as benign, their growth pattern is one of local invasion and extension through the renal capsule. During the course of surgery, CMN tumors may be friable and prone to rupture. Local recurrences have been reported as well as case reports of metastases.[68, 69] Nephrectomy with wide local excision is advised. Among the 17 patients with CMN in the CCG study were one intraoperative death and 16 (94%) long-term survivors. One of the infants developed a local recurrence with intraperitoneal implants.

Of the 15 neonatal Wilms' tumors in the NWTS, 12 were Stage 1 at the time of surgery. The other three were Stage 2. All were of favorable histology.[66] In addition to nephrectomy, treatment of these infants included postoperative chemotherapy in 10 cases. Only one infant received radiation. Five received no additional therapy, and one subsequently died as a result of metastatic disease. The remaining infants (93%) were reportedly long-term survivors. In the CCG study seven of eight patients had Stage 1 or 2 disease, and one had Stage 4 disease with metastases. Current recommendations for patients with neonatal Wilms' tumors include primary excision of the tumor as the mainstay of therapy. It has been proposed that infants with small Stage 1 tumors be observed very closely following surgery with no adjuvant chemotherapy.[66, 70] In neonates receiving chemotherapy, the dosage should be reduced by 50%.

References

1. Bader JL, Miller RW: U.S. cancer incidence and mortality in the first year of life. *Am J Dis Child* 133:157–159, 1970.
2. Miller RW: Relation between cancer and congenital defects in man. *N Engl J Med* 275:87–93, 1985.
3. Parkes SE, Muir KR, Southern L, Cameron AH, Darbyshire PJ, Stevens MCG: Neonatal tumors: A thirty-year population-based study. *Med Pediatr Oncol* 22:309–317, 1994.
4. Moore SW, Kaschula ROC, Albertyn R, Rode H, Millar AJW, Karabus C: The outcome of solid tumours occurring in the neonatal period. *Pediatr Surg Int* 10:366–370, 1995.
5. Xue H, Horwitz JR, Smith MB, Lally KP, Black CT, Cangir A, Takahashi H, Andrassy RJ: Malignant solid tumors in neonates: A 40-year review. *J Pediatr Surg* 30:543–545, 1995.
6. Gale GB, D'Angio G, Uri A, et al: Cancer in neonates: The experience at the Children's Hospital of Philadelphia. *Pediatrics* 70:409–413, 1982.
7. Crom DB, Wiliman JA, Green AA, et al: Malignancy in the neonate. *Med Pediatr Oncol* 17:101–104, 1989.
8. Campbell AN, Chan HSL, O'Brien A, et al: Malignant tumors in the neonate. *Arch Dis Child* 62:19–23, 1988.
9. Davis CR, Carachi R, Young DG: Neonatal tumors: Glasgow 1955–1986. *Arch Dis Child* 63:1075–1078, 1988.
10. Werb P, Scurry J, Ostor A, Fortume D, Attwood H: Survey of congenital tumors in perinatal necropsies. *Pathology* 24:247–253, 1992.
11. Teal LN, Angtuaco TL, Jimenez JF, et al: Fetal teratomas: Antenatal diagnosis and clinical management. *J Clin Ultrasound* 16:329–332, 1988.
12. Azizkhan RG, Haase GM, Applebaum H, et al: Diagnosis, management, and outcome of cervicofacial teratomas in neonates: A Children's Cancer Group Study. *J Ped Surg* 30:312–316, 1995.
13. Giulian BB, Chang CCN, Yoss BB: Prenatal ultrasonographic diagnosis of fetal adrenal neuroblastoma. *J Clin Ultrasound* 14:225–227, 1986.
14. Ho PTC, Estroff JA, Kozakewich H, et al: Prenatal detection of neuroblastoma: A ten-year

experience from the Dana-Farber Cancer Institute and Children's Hospital. *Pediatrics* 92:358–364, 1993.

15. De Lorimier AA, Harrison, MR: Surgical treatment of tumors in the newborn. *Am J Pediatr Hematol Oncol* 3:271–277, 1981.

16. Littman P, D'Angio GJ: Radiation therapy in the neonate. *Am J Pediatr Hematol Oncol* 3:279–285, 1981.

17. Reaman GH: Special considerations for the infant with cancer. In Pizzo PA, Poplack DG (eds): *Principles and Practice of Pediatric Oncology*. Philadelphia: JB Lippincott Co., 1989, pp. 263–274.

18. Meadows AT, Gallagher JA, Bunin GR: Late effects of early childhood cancer therapy. *Br J Cancer Suppl* 66 (XVIII):S92–S95, 1992.

19. Miller DR: Late effects of childhood cancer. *Am J Dis Child* 142:1147–1151, 1988.

20. Silber JH, Littman PS, Meadows AT: Stature loss following skeletal irradiation for childhood cancer. *J Clin Oncol* 8:304–312, 1990.

21. Meadows AT, Gordon J, Massari DJ, et al: Declines in IQ scores and cognitive dysfunctions in children with acute lymphocytic leukaemia treated with cranial irradiation. *Lancet* 2:1015–1018, 1981.

22. Farwell J, Dohrmann G, Flanery JT: Intracranial neoplasms in infants. *Arch Neurol* 35:533–557, 1978.

23. Littman P, D'Angio GJ: Growth considerations in the radiation therapy of children with cancer. *Annu Rev Med* 30:405–415, 1979.

24. Maier JG: Effects of radiation on kidney, bladder and prostate. In Vaeth JM (ed): *Frontiers of Radiation Therapy and Oncology*, vol. 6. Basel: Karger, 1972, pp. 196–207.

25. Kraut JW, Bagshaw MA, Glatstein E: Hepatic effects of irradiation. In Vaeth JM (ed): *Frontiers of Radiation Therapy and Oncology*, vol. 6. Basel: Karger, 1972, pp. 182–195.

26. Allen JC: The effects of cancer therapy on the nervous system. *J Pediatr* 93:642–645, 1978.

27. Jones B, Breslow N, Takashima J: Toxic deaths in the Second National Wilms' Tumor Study. *J Clin Oncol* 2:1028–1033, 1984.

28. *Informational Bulletin*, National Wilms' Tumor Study II, February 16, 1977.

29. Reaman G, Zeltzer P, Bleyer WA, et al: Acute lymphoblastic leukemia in infants less than one year of age: A cumulative experience of the Children's Cancer Study Group. *J Clin Oncol* 3:1513–1521, 1985.

29a. Billmire DF, Grossfeld JL: Teratomas in childhood: Analysis of 142 cases. *J Pediatr Surg* 21:548–551, 1986.

30. McLeod HL, Relling MV, Crom WR, et al: Disposition of antineoplastic agents in the very young child. *Br. J. Cancer Suppl* 66 (XVIII), S23–S29, 1992.

31. Isaacs H Jr: Perinatal (congenital and neonatal) neoplasms: A report of 110 cases. *Pediatr Pathol* 3:165–216, 1985.

32. Altman RP, Randolph JG, Lilly JR: Sacrococcygeal teratoma: American Academy of Pediatrics Surgical Section Survey, 1973. *J Ped Surg* 9:389–398, 1974.

33. Rosenfeld CR, Coln CD, Duenhoelter JH: Fetal cervical teratoma as a cause of polyhydramnios. *Pediatrics* 64:176–179, 1979.

34. Berry CL, Keeling J, Hilton C: Teratomata in infancy and childhood: A review of 91 cases. *J Pathol* 98:241–252, 1969.

35. Tapper D, Lack EE: Teratoma in infancy and childhood. *Ann Surg* 1:398–410, 1983.

36. Dehner LP: Neoplasms of the fetus and neonate. In Naeye RL, Kissane JM, Kaufman N (eds): *Perinatal Diseases. International Academy of Pathology Monograph No. 22*, Baltimore: Williams & Wilkins, 1981, pp. 286–345.

37. Langer JC, Tabb T, Thompson P, et al: Management of prenatally diagnosed tracheal obstruction: Access to the airway in utero prior to delivery. *Fetal Diagn Ther* 7:12–16, 1992.

38. Beckwith JB, Perrin EV: In situ neuroblastoma: A contribution to the natural history of neural crest tumors. *Am J Pathol* 43:1089–1104, 1963.

39. Ikeda Y, Lister J, Bouton JM, et al: Congenital neuroblastoma, neuroblastoma in situ, and the normal fetal development of the adrenal. *J Pediatr Surg* 16:636–644, 1981.

40. Jennings RN, LaQuaglia MP, Leong K, et al: Fetal neuroblastoma: Prenatal diagnosis and natural history. *J Pediatr Surg* 28:1168–1174, 1993.

41. Richards ML, Gundersen E, Williams MS: Cystic neuroblastoma of infancy. *J Pediatr Surg* 30:1354–1357, 1995.

42. Janetschek G, Weitzel D, Stein W, et al: Prenatal diagnosis of neuroblastoma by sonography. *Urology* 24:397–402, 1984.

43. Dominici C, Berthold F, Brodeur GM, et al: Prenatal neuroblastoma: A report by the prenatal neuroblastoma study group. *Cancer Res* 35:329–332, 1994.

44. Laug W, Siegel S, Shaw K, et al: Initial urinary catecholamine metabolite concentrations and prognosis in neuroblastoma. *Pediatrics* 62:77–83, 1978.

45. Hosoda Y, Miyano T, Kimura K, et al: Characteristics and management of patients with fetal neuroblastoma. *J Pediatr Surg* 27:623–625, 1992.

46. Newton ER, Louis F, Dalton ME, et al: Fetal neuroblastoma and catecholamine-induced maternal hypertension. *Obstet Gynecol* 65(suppl.):49S–52S, 1985.

47. Voute PA Jr, Wadman SK, van Putten WJ: Congenital neuroblastoma—Symptoms in the mother during pregnancy. *Clin Pediatr* 9:206–207, 1970.

48. Suita S, Zaizen, Y, Sera H, et al: Neuroblastoma in infants aged less than 6 months: Is more aggressive treatment necessary? A report from the Pediatric Oncology Group of the Kyushu area. *J Pediatr Surg* 30:715–721, 1995.

49. Dillon PW, Whalen TV, Azizkhan RG, et al: Neonatal soft tissue sarcomas: The influence of pathology on treatment and survival. *J Pediatr Surg* 30:1038–1041, 1995.

50. Coffin CM, Dehner LP: Soft tissue tumors in the first year of life: A report of 190 cases. *Pediatr Pathol* 10:509–526, 1990.

51. Chung EB, Enzinger FM: Infantile fibrosarcoma. *Cancer* 38:729–739, 1976.

52. Soule EL, Pritchard DJ: Fibrosarcoma in infants and children: A review of 110 cases. *Cancer* 40:1711–1721, 1977.

53. Blocker S, Koenig J, Ternberg J: Congenital fibrosarcoma. *J Pediatr Surg* 22:665–670, 1987.

54. Salloum E, Flamont F, Caillaud JM, et al: Diagnostic and therapeutic problems of soft tissue tumors other than rhabdomyosarcoma in infants under 1 year of age: A clinicopathological study of 34 cases treated at the Institute Gustabe-Roussy. *Med Pediatr Oncol* 18:37–43, 1990.

55. Grier HE, Perez-Atayade AR, Weinstein HJ: Chemotherapy for inoperable infantile fibrosarcoma. *Cancer* 56:1507–1510, 1985.

56. Ninane J, Gosseye S, Panteon E, et al: Congenital fibrosarcoma: Preoperative chemotherapy and conservative surgery. *Cancer* 58:1400–1406, 1986.

57. Robinson W, Crawford AH: Infantile fibrosarcoma: Report of a case with long-term follow-up. *J Bone Joint Surg* 72A:291–294, 1990.

58. Kynaston JA, Malcolm AJ, Craft AW, et al: Chemotherapy in the management of infantile fibrosarcoma. *Med Pediatr Oncol* 21:488–493, 1993.

59. Raney Jr RB, Hays DM, Tefft M, et al: Rhabdomyosarcoma and the undifferentiated sarcomas. In Pizzo PA, Poplack DG (eds): *Principles and Practice of Pediatric Oncology.* Philadelphia: JB Lippincott Co., 1989, pp. 635–658.

60. Maurer HM, Beltangady M, Gehan EA: The Intergroup Rhabdomyosarcoma Study I: A final report. *Cancer* 61:209–220, 1988.

61. Ragab AH, Heyn R, Tefft M, et al: Infants younger than 1 year of age with rhabdomyosarcoma. *Cancer* 58:2606–2610, 1986.

62. Lobe TE, Wiener ES, Hays DM, Lawrence WH, et al: Neonatal rhabdomyosarcoma: The IRS experience. *J Pediatr Surg* 29:1167–1170, 1994.

63. Wiener ES: Rhabdomyosarcoma: New dimensions in management. *Semin Pediatr Surg* 2:47–58, 1993.

64. Bolande RP, Brough JA, Izant R: Congenital mesoblastic nephroma: A report of eight cases and the relationship to Wilms' tumor. *Pediatrics* 40:272–278, 1967.

65. Beckwith JB: Mesenchymal renal neoplasms of infancy. *J Pediatr Surg* 5:405–406, 1970.

66. Ritchey ML, Azizkhan RG, Beckwith JB, et al: Neonatal Wilms' tumor. *J Pediatr Surg* 30:856–859, 1995.

67. Giulian BB: Prenatal ultrasonographic diagnosis of fetal renal tumors. *Radiology* 152:69–70, 1984.

68. Howell CG, Othersen HB, Kiviat NE, et al: Therapy and outcome in 51 children with mesoblastic nephroma: A report of the National Wilms' Tumor Study. *J Pediatr Surg* 17:826–830, 1982.

69. Joshi VV, Kay S, Milstern R, et al: Congenital mesoblastic nephroma of infancy: Report of a case with unusual clinical behavior. *Am J Clin Pathol* 60:811–816, 1973.

70. Green DM, Breslow NE, Beckwith JB, et al: Treatment outcomes in patients less than two years of age with small, stage I/favorable histology Wilms' tumors: A report from the National Wilms' Tumor Study. *J Clin Oncol* 11:91–95, 1993.

Chapter

20

Melanomas and Other Rare Tumors

• *Cynthia A. Corpron, M.D.* • *Richard J. Andrassy, M.D.*

MELANOMA

Incidence, Risk Factors, and Associated Syndromes

Melanomas account for 3% of all pediatric malignancies.[1] Approximately 2% of melanomas occur in patients younger than 20 years, and 0.3% to 0.4% occur in prepubertal children.[1] The incidence of malignant melanoma has been estimated to be 2 per million population in children younger than 15 years old.[2] Reported risk factors for development of melanoma include light skin and eye color, sun sensitivity, excessive sun exposure, and family history of melanoma.

Several syndromes are associated with development of melanomas. The frequency of melanomas is 2000 times greater in children with xeroderma pigmentosum than in those without.[3] Giant *congenital melanocytic nevi* (CMN) are rare, occurring in fewer than 1 in 20,000 infants. Lesions are most common on the posterior trunk and may be associated with coarse hair, nodularity, and limb hypoplasia. Giant CMN overlying the head or posterior midline trunk may be associated with neural melanosis and leptomeningeal melanoma. An example of a CMN is shown in Figure 20–1.

The reported lifetime risk of melanomas developing in giant CMNs is estimated to be 5% to 15%.[4, 5] Although excision of all giant CMNs has been recommended to decrease the risk of subsequent development of melanomas, resection is often limited by the small size of the

349

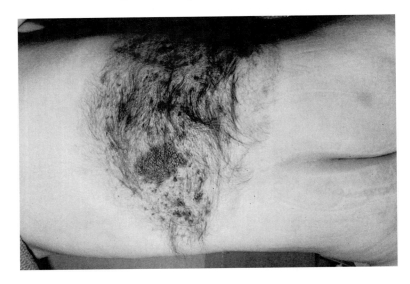

Figure 20–1 • Child with giant congenital melanocytic nevus.

child compared with the large size of the CMN. Techniques such as serial excisions and tissue expanders may allow successful resection, but the implications of such resection and the risk of malignant transformation must be carefully discussed with the child's parents before surgery is planned. These patients should be carefully followed, especially if the CMN is not resected.

The risk of melanomas developing in small CMNs is less clear. MacKie[6] suggests that as many as 50% of melanomas in young patients may develop at the site of a CMN, but no large prospective studies are available, and it is not clear whether resection of small CMNs will reduce the risk of melanomas developing.

Patients with *familial atypical mole/melanoma* (FAMM) syndrome account for approximately 5% of all melanoma cases.[7] FAMM is an autosomal dominant trait characterized by increased numbers of melanocytic nevi, development of melanomas at early ages, and multiple primary melanomas. Linkages to chromosome 1(1p36) and 9(9p13-p22) have been reported in FAMM kindreds.[8] Family members with atypical nevi have an estimated 100% lifetime risk of acquiring melanoma. First melanomas will develop before the age of 20 in 10% of patients with FAMM. Children from FAMM families should be strongly encouraged to make maximal efforts to reduce sun exposure.

Atypical mole syndrome is the name suggested for a condition of increased numbers (>50) of atypical nevi. A prospective study showed that patients with this syndrome had a 35-fold risk of acquiring melanoma.[9] Increased numbers of atypical nevi have been described as occurring after chemotherapy in children with malignancy and in adults with acquired immunodeficiency syndrome.[10] Immunosupressed patients should be counseled on sun avoidance and on the signs of melanoma. They should be regularly screened.

Melanomas have been reported to occur as second malignant tumors in patients with lymphomas, osteosarcomas, and, most commonly, retinoblastomas.[11] The occurrence of melanomas in irradiated fields suggests a role for radiation in the etiology of melanomas. Their occurrence after treatment for bilateral retinoblastomas suggests a genetic role for retinoblastomas in the development of melanomas.

Congenital melanoma has been described in neonates who acquired melanomas transplacentally from their mothers, who usually had disseminated melanomas.[12]

Differential Diagnosis

Differential diagnosis of pigmented lesions in children include café-au-lait spots, postinflammatory pigment changes, basal cell nevi, syringomas, dermatofibromas, and basal and squamous cell carcinomas as well as melanomas.

Signs and Symptoms

Symptoms suggestive of melanoma developing in a nevus include growth in the size of the nevus, changes in its color or contour, and associated bleeding, itching, or ulceration. Signs of melanoma include variation in color, irregular and raised surface, irregular contour, and ulceration. Diagnosis of melanoma is most often based upon changes in a preexisting skin lesion. The development of a melanoma de novo in uninvolved skin is less frequent.

Biopsy Techniques

Although melanomas are rare in children, pigmented lesions should be viewed with suspicion of malignancy. Inappropriate biopsy technique may prevent adequate staging and may require compromised treatment. Initial biopsy can be either incisional or excisional. Full-thickness biopsy must be performed to allow accurate microstaging of the lesion. Shave or curette biopsies are contraindicated. In children, Spitz nevi may be difficult to distinguish from melanomas,[13] so that a biopsy should be performed initially. Definitive surgical treatment is delayed until the diagnosis is confirmed and staging is possible.

Lesions less than 1.5 cm in diameter may be excised with a narrow (1 mm to 2 mm) margin of normal skin. Wider margins are inadvisable, especially in children, as re-excision may result in the need for a skin graft where primary closure might have been possible instead. If the lesion is benign, excision with margins of 1 mm to 2 mm is adequate treatment. The biopsy incision should be carefully oriented in such a way that a second surgical excision can be performed with maximal margins and minimal skin loss.

Staging

Current staging systems for melanomas incorporate microscopic depths of invasion of the primary lesions with presence of nodal and distal metastases. Clark and associates[14] described a system by which melanomas are classified by depth of invasion, as shown in Table 20–1. Microstaging by tumor thickness was originally described by Breslow.[15] The American Joint Committee on Cancer (AJCC) combined these two systems with evaluation for nodal and distant metastasis to develop the current staging system shown in Table 20–2.[16]

Table 20–1 • Clark Staging by Melanoma Depth

Level I	All tumor cells are confined to epidermis with no invasion through basement membrane.
Level II	Tumor cells penetrate through basement membrane into papillary dermis but do not extend to reticular dermis.
Level III	Tumor cells fill papillary dermis and abut against reticular dermis without invasion of reticular dermis.
Level IV	Extension of tumor cells between bundle of collagen characteristic of reticular dermis.
Level V	Invasion into subcutaneous tissue.

From Clark WH Jr, Ainsworth AM, Bernadino EA, et al: The developmental biology of primary human malignant melanomas. *Semin Oncol* 2:83, 1975, with permission.

Surgical Excision

For melanoma in situ, excision should involve a margin of normal skin 0.5 cm around the lesion. More limited excisions are associated with a local recurrence rate of up to 60%.[17] Prospective analysis has shown that lesions less than 1 mm thick can be excised with 1 cm margins instead of the previously used 3 cm margins with no effect on local recurrence or long-term survival.[18] Another randomized study showed no significant difference in disease-free or overall survival with 2 cm margins as opposed to 4 cm margins of melanomas 1 mm to 4 mm in depth.[19] For lesions of more than 4 cm, excision margins of at least 3 cm are recommended.

The site of the melanoma may compromise resection margins. For example, facial lesions may not be able to be excised with more than a 1 cm margin without significant morbidity. Subungual melanomas should be treated with amputation at either the metatarsophalangeal or metacarpophalangeal joint so that skin closure can be achieved. Plantar melanomas may require wide excisions and split-thickness skin grafts.

Lymph Node Dissection

Retrospective studies have shown no survival advantage for elective lymph node dissection in patients with melanomas less than 1 mm in thickness because cure rate is high with local excision alone.[20] Nor is there any survival advantage for elective lymph node dissections in patients with

Table 20–2 • Staging of Melanomas

Primary Tumor (T)

pTX	Primary tumor cannot be assessed
pT0	No evidence of primary tumor
pTis	Melanoma in situ
pT1	Tumor 0.75 mm or less in thickness, or Clark Level II
pT2	Tumor greater than 0.75 mm but no more than 1.5 mm in thickness, or Clark Level III
pT3	Tumor greater than 1.5 mm but no more than 4 mm in thickness, or Clark Level IV
pT4	Tumor greater than 4 mm in thickness, or Clark Level V, or satellites present within 2 cm of primary tumor.

Regional Lymph Nodes (N)

NX	Regional lymph nodes cannot be assessed
N0	No evidence of regional lymph node metastasis
N1	Metastasis 3 cm or less in greatest dimension in any regional lymph node or nodes
N2	Metastasis greater than 3 cm in greatest dimension in any regional lymph node or nodes and/or in transit metastasis.

Distant Metastasis (M)

MX	Presence of distant metastasis cannot be assessed
M0	No evidence of distant metastasis
M1	Distant metastasis present

Stage Grouping

Stage 1	pT1	N0	M0
	PT2	N0	M0
Stage 2	pT3	N0	M0
Stage 3	pT4	N0	M0
	Any pT	N1,N2	M0
Stage 4	Any pT	Any N	M0

From Beahrs OH, Henson DE, Hutter RVP, et al (eds): *American Joint Committee on Cancer: Manual for Staging of Cancer*, 3rd ed. Philadelphia: J. B. Lippincott, 1988, with permission.

melanomas greater than 4 mm in thickness, in this case because of the high rate of metastases.[21] Controversy exists regarding the role of elective lymph node dissections in patients with melanomas of intermediate thicknesses (1 mm to 4 mm). Although two prospective randomized studies failed to demonstrate any improvement in survival after elective lymph node dissection,[22, 23] the Melanoma Intergroup Trial reported that patients younger than 60 years of age with melanomas of 1 mm to 2 mm had significantly improved survival after elective lymph node dissections.[24]

When lymph node involvement is evident on clinical examination or biopsy, full regional lymph node dissection should be performed. But because lymph node dissection can be associated with complications such as postoperative edema, a method is needed to identify those patients with nodal metastases who are most likely to benefit from nodal dissections. Morton and co-workers[25] first described a method of intraoperative mapping of the regional lymphatics with selective lymphadenectomy. In this method, cutaneous lymphoscintigraphy was utilized to identify areas of primary lymphatic drainage of ambiguous sites such as the trunk and shoulders. A vital blue dye was used for intraoperative mapping of the regional lymphatics. This technique is performed in the following manner:

1. Patients undergo preoperative lymphoscintigraphy of the site of the melanoma with technetium-labeled sulfur colloid to identify draining nodal basins.
2. In the operating room, the area of the melanoma is injected with 0.5–2.0 ml of the vital blue dye, isosulfan blue.
3. Incision is made over the suspected location of the sentinel node, and the afferent lymphatic is traced to the sentinel node.
4. The sentinel node is excised and sent for pathologic examination.
5. If nodal metastases are identified histologically, formal lymph node dissection is necessary.

In Morton's[25] large series of lymphatic mapping for melanoma, 82% of patients had a sentinel node identified. This series showed a learning curve for this technique in that the most experienced surgeon identified a sentinel node in 96% of patients. Newer techniques employing the technetium-labeled colloid and intraoperative isotope detector are even more promising. We have reported on lymphatic mapping in six pediatric patients.[26] Sentinel nodes with micrometastases were identified in three of these. An example of a sentinel node identified by lymphatic mapping is shown in Figure 20–2.

Adjuvant Treatment

One prospective, randomized trial showed that treatment with interferon alfa-2b prolonged re-

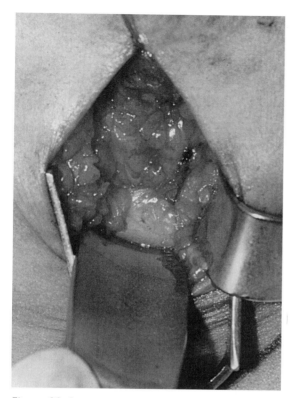

Figure 20–2 • Sentinel node identified by lymphatic mapping.

lapse-free interval and overall survival of patients with Stage 2b and 3 melanomas (those greater than 4 mm in thickness or those with lymphatic metastases).[27] No other adjuvant chemotherapy or biologic therapy has been shown to affect survival in prospective trials. Although several chemotherapeutic agents (DTIC (dacarbazine) and the nitrosoureas) have demonstrated varying activity against advanced melanoma,[28–32] no survival advantage has been seen in prospective randomized studies.[33–36]

Small series have described responses of children with metastatic melanoma to treatment with DTIC or cyclophosphamide, vincristine, and dactinomycin.[37–38] But these therapies have not been evaluated in randomized trials. Similarly, immunomodulators such as bacille Calmette-Guérin (BCG) and *Corynebacterium* have produced responses as compared with historical controls,[39, 40] but these responses have not been confirmed by any prospective, randomized studies.

Another promising treatment uses tumor-cell vaccines.[41] Phase II trials of melanoma-specific tumor-cell vaccines are in progress at the time of this writing. Some studies have suggested that the concomitant use of interleukin-2 with interferon alfa-2b might enhance antitumor activity.[42] Still another technique of adjuvant therapy that has been given for recurrent disease and in-transit metastases is isolated limb perfusion. The goal here is to isolate the extremity from systemic circulation and then deliver a high concentration of a chemotherapeutic agent. Isolated limb perfusion has been shown effective in reducing the incidence of in-transit disease in patients at high risk for relapse.[43] The effect of isolated hyperthermic perfusion with melphalan (LPAM) upon disease-free and overall survival rates is at the time of this writing being evaluated in a Phase I trial. A small series has described isolated limb perfusion in extremity melanomas in children.[44] The current treatment guidelines for melanoma at the University of Texas M. D. Anderson Cancer Center are summarized in Figure 20–3.

Follow-up

Patients who undergo resection of a melanoma should be carefully counseled regarding sun avoidance and sunscreen use. Follow-up should include instruction on patient's self-examination of skin (or parental examination in pediatric cases) every month, examination of skin by the physician every 3 months for 1–2 years, and chest radiographs and liver function tests every 3 months.[45] Any neurologic complaints or symptoms should be evaluated to rule out brain metastases.

Prognosis

Some have suggested that prognosis is worse for children with melanoma than for adults,[46–50] but others have suggested that children have a better response to treatment then do adults.[37, 38] The only series employing a multivariant analysis failed to identify age as an independent predictor of survival.[51] This study was also somewhat hampered by small numbers of younger (<13 years old) patients. It concluded that prognosis was similar for same-stage pediatric and adult melanoma patients.

Reported 5-year survival is 89% for adults with melanomas less than .75 mm in thickness, 46% to 75% for adults with melanomas .75 mm to 4 mm in thickness, and only 25% for adults with

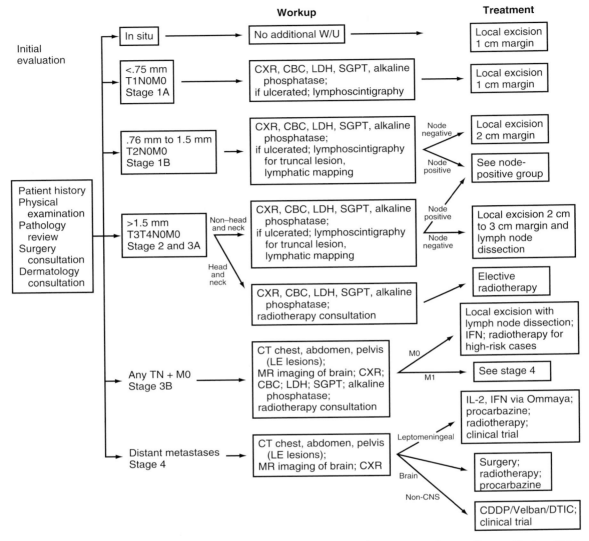

Figure 20–3 • Current guidelines for treatment of melanoma from the M. D. Anderson Cancer Center. CXR = chest x-ray; CBC = complete blood count; LDH = lactate dehydrogenase; SGPT = serum glutamate pyruvate transaminase; LE = lower extremity; IFN = interferon alpha 2a; CDDP/Velban/DTIC = cisplatin, Velban, DTIC (chemotherapy drugs).

melanomas greater than 4 mm in thickness.[52] Comparable figures for pediatric patients are not available. The 5-year survival for patients with multiple lymph node metastases is 8% to 26%.[53–55] The median survival for patients with disseminated metastases is less than 1 year.[56]

COLON CANCER

Incidence and Risk Factors

SEER (Surveillance, Epidemiology, and End Results) estimate that only about 80 cases per year

of colorectal cancer occur in patients younger than 20 years of age in the United States.[57] Several syndromes and diseases are associated with development of colon cancer: familial polyposis coli, Peutz-Jeghers syndrome, Gardner's syndrome, Turcot syndrome, ulcerative colitis, and Crohn's disease. The presence of a ureterosigmoidostomy is also associated with colon cancer. Most patients with these associated diseases have colon cancer as young adults; only 10% of these patients have colon cancer in childhood.[58] The incidence of pediatric colon cancer in this age group is about 1 in every million patients.[59] Caldwell and coworkers[60] identified 10 pediatric patients with colon cancer who resided in an area of high pesticide use, but levels of pesticide residues were no higher in these patients and their families than in controls, so that the role of pesticides as a causative factor was unclear.

Signs and Symptoms

In various series of pediatric patients, abdominal pain was the most common presenting symptom of colon cancer. Other reported symptoms include nausea and vomiting, diarrhea, rectal bleeding, hematochezia, and weight loss.

Differential Diagnosis

Differential diagnosis of colon masses in children may include benign polyps, lymphoid polyps, hyperplastic polyps, hamartomas, hemangiomas, lymphomas, carcinoid tumors, smooth-muscle tumors, and sarcomas.

Imaging and Staging

Most patients with colon cancer will have positive results on stool guaiac examinations.[61] Workup for a suspected colon cancer in a child should include barium enema and/or colonoscopy to evaluate for synchronous primary tumors. Colonoscopic biopsy can provide histologic confirmation of the diagnosis. Computed tomography of the abdomen should be performed to look for extracolonic spread and metastases to the liver. Transrectal ultrasound may help determine the extent of invasion and resectability of cancer.[62] Intraoperative ultrasound of the liver may reveal metastasis not seen by other imaging studies.

Although elevated carcinoembryonic antigen (CEA) can be useful in identifying recurrent disease after resection, Angel and coworkers[63] reported that 7 of 13 patients with advanced disease had normal or only minimally elevated CEA levels. CEA may not be a helpful tumor marker in pediatric patients with colon cancer.

The most important prognostic factor in colorectal cancer is depth of invasion of the primary tumor. This was first described by Dukes. Correlation of the AJCC/UICC staging system (International Union Against Cancer) with Dukes staging and the more common Astler-Coller

Table 20–3 • Staging of Colorectal Cancer

Primary Tumor

TX	Primary tumor cannot be assessed
T0	No evidence of primary tumor
Tis	Carcinoma in situ
T1	Tumor cells invade submucosa
T2	Tumor cells invade muscularis propria
T3	Tumor cells invade muscularis propria and penetrate into subserosa, or into nonperitonealized pericolic or perirectal tissues
T4	Tumor cells perforate the visceral peritoneum or directly invade other organs or structures

Nodal Involvement

NX	Regional lymph nodes cannot be assessed
N0	No evidence of regional lymph node metastasis
N1	Metastasis in one to three pericolic or perirectal lymph nodes
N2	Metastasis in four or more pericolic or perirectal lymph nodes
N3	Metastasis in any lymph node along the course of a named vascular trunk

Distant Metastasis

MX	Presence of distant metastasis cannot be assessed
M0	No evidence of distant metastasis
M1	Distant metastasis present

TNM Staging				Modified Astler-Coller Stage
Stage 0	Tis	N0	M0	A
Stage 1	T1	N0	M0	
	T2	N0	M0	B1
Stage 2	T3	N0	M0	B2
	T4	N0	M0	B3
Stage 3	Any T	N1	M0	C
	Any T	N2,N3	M0	C
Stage 4	Any T	Any N	M1	

From Beahrs OH, Henson DE, Hutter RVP, et al (eds): *American Joint Committee on Cancer: Manual for Staging of Cancer*, 3rd ed. Philadelphia: J. B. Lippincott, 1988, with permission.

modification of the Dukes staging is shown in Table 20–3.

Surgical Therapy

Anatomic location of a colon cancer determines the extent of surgical resection. Cecal or right colon cancers are treated with right hemicolectomy, transverse colon lesions with transverse colectomy lesions from the splenic flexure to the sigmoid colon, with left hemicolectomy, and sigmoid lesions with sigmoid colectomy. Low anterior resections can be performed in patients with tumors located 5 cm or more above the anal verge. Intraoperative ultrasound is helpful in identifying liver metastasis not found with preoperative imaging.[64] If present, liver metastases can be resected at the time of intestinal resection or at a later time. Although the majority of patients who undergo resection of liver metastases will not be cured, they have a better chance of complete response than patients treated with regional hepatic artery chemotherapy or systemic chemotherapy.[65, 66] The goal of resection is removal of metastatic disease with a margin of 1.0 cm to 1.5 cm of normal hepatic parenchyma. Lobectomy is not necessary if margins can be preserved with a lesser resection.

Adjuvant Therapy

As many as 20% to 50% of patients with transmural invasion or node-positive disease have local recurrence.[67] Postoperative radiation therapy is recommended for these patients with T3–4,N0, or Stage 3 adenocarcinomas. Fluorouracil (5-FU) is included in adjuvant radiation therapy as a radiosensitizer. Some investigations have suggested a role for preoperative radiation to reduce distal rectal cancers in an attempt to allow curative and sphincter-sparing resections.[68, 69] Patients are treated with 5000–6000 cGY. One series of pediatric colon cancer patients reported a 57% response rate to a regimen including vincristine, lomustine, and 5-FU[70]; however, only 5-FU with levamisole has shown a survival advantage in treatment of adult patients with node-positive colon cancers.[71–73] Adjuvant therapy for patients with earlier-stage disease is still under investigation.

Prognosis

LaQuaglia and coworkers[74] examined prognostic factors in patients younger than 21 years old with colon cancer. In multivariant analysis of patients who underwent resection for cure, positive nodal involvement or high histologic grade predicted decreased survival with a significant degree of accuracy. Patients with metastatic disease at the time of presentation had the worst prognosis.

Multiple investigators have reported a high incidence of high-grade tumors in pediatric colon cancer.[75, 76] In the series reported by LaQuaglia,[74] 45% of patients had signet-ring carcinomas. Signet-ring carcinomas are seen in only 5% of adult patients with colon cancer but have been reported in 20% to 43% of young adults with colon cancer and in up to 50% of pediatric patients with this cancer. Signet-ring histology is associated with early extension along peritoneal surfaces. Vascular invasion has also been reported to be increased in patients younger than 30 years of age.[77]

Overall survival of pediatric patients with colon cancer is inferior to that of adults. It is not clear whether this lower survival rate is a result of the aggressive histologic types and later-stage presentation characteristic of pediatric cases. Multivariant analysis of age as an independent prognostic factor is not available. Estimated 3-year survival in one large series of pediatric patients was 28%.[74] Expected 5-year survival in adult patients is approximately 90% for patients with tumors confined to the mucosa, 77% for patients with tumors extending through the bowel wall without lymphatic metastases, 47% for patients with tumors with lymphatic metastases, and less than 20% for those with disseminated disease at time of diagnosis.[78]

BREAST CANCER

Incidence and Risk Factors

Patients younger than 20 years old account for less than 1% of all breast cancers.[78] Many large series reporting the results of evaluation of breast masses in pediatric patients fail to show any primary breast cancers.[79] Malignancies are more commonly metastases to the breast from sarcomas or leukemic tumor involvement. Nevertheless, some primary breast carcinomas have been reported in both male and female children, and so breast cancer should remain part of the differential diagnosis in pediatric patients with breast masses. A report from M.D. Anderson Cancer Center on a series of patients younger than age 21 with breast cancer showed that a majority had suffered significant delay in diagnosis because breast cancer had not been included in the differential diagnosis of the breast masses evaluated at an earlier time.[80]

Risk factors for development of pediatric breast cancer are not well described. Suggested risk factors for development of breast cancer in adult patients include obesity, increased dietary fat, alcohol consumption, and early menarche.[81] Radiation exposure is a significant risk factor for development of breast cancer; a report on patients with breast cancer who had previously undergone mantle irradiation for Hodgkin's disease estimated the incidence as approaching 35% by age 40.[82]

Breast cancer as a second malignancy has also been reported in survivors of osteosarcoma, thyroid cancer, Wilms' tumor, and soft-tissue sarcoma.[83] Although most of these patients are young adults when breast cancer occurs, the pediatric oncologist and pediatric surgeon have an important role in educating childhood cancer survivors about this risk and about the need for close surveillance, including breast self-examinations and frequent physician examinations with early diagnostic imaging (mammogram and/or ultrasound).

It has long been recognized that a family history of a first-degree relative with breast cancer confers an increased risk for breast cancer. Several specific hereditary breast cancer syndromes have been identified. Li-Fraumeni syndrome is attributed to germline p53 tumor-supressor gene mutations and includes multiple types of cancers, including childhood sarcomas and maternal breast cancer.[84] The *BRCA1* gene has been localized to chromosome 17 by linkage analysis.[85] Germline mutations in *BRCA1* may be involved in as many as 5% of all breast cancers in the United States. The gene is characterized by autosomal dominant inheritance with a high degree of penetrance. The mutation is also associated with development of ovarian cancer.

A second gene, *BRCA2*, has been identified on chromosome 13q12-13.[86] Lifetime breast cancer risk approaches 90% in carriers of *BRCA2* and may also be associated with increased risk of male breast cancer. Implications and recommendations for screening and genetic counseling are still being evaluated. Patients with these syndromes tend to present at relatively young ages compared with the overall population, but as of yet the role of these mutations in the develop-

ment of breast cancer in pediatric patients has not been determined.

Signs and Symptoms

The majority of pediatric patients with breast cancer present with a mass.[87] Some may present with breast pain and some with nodal metastases. Adult patients may present with unilateral nipple discharge, but children rarely do. As few children undergo breast imaging prior to development of a mass, the finding of an asymptomatic mass in them is unusual.

Differential Diagnosis

Differential diagnosis of breast masses in pediatric patients includes fibroadenoma, cystosarcoma phyllodes, gynecomastia, fibrocystic disease, unilateral thelarche, abscess, and metastatic lesion.

Imaging and Biopsy Techniques

The valve of mammography in detecting breast cancers in children and adolescents is unclear. Some suggest that mammography may be helpful,[88, 89] but in one series of pediatric breast cancer patients, few of the cancers were identified by mammography.[81] Ultrasound may be more helpful in pediatric patients with dense breast tissue. Abnormalities or dominant masses found on mammography or ultrasound should be biopsied. A good initial approach is fine-needle aspiration of dominant masses. Aspiration may confirm the diagnosis of breast cyst if the aspirated fluid is clear or green. Bloody fluid indicates a need for pathologic examination and excisional biopsy. Diagnosis of fibroadenoma by an experienced cytopathologist may eliminate the need for surgical biopsy. Any questionable finding on fine-needle aspiration requires excisional biopsy.

Because the majority of breast lesions in children are benign, excisional biopsy to negative margins is the initial procedure. Newer techniques such as needle localization and stereotactically guided biopsies will probably not be widely utilized in pediatric patients as most of them present with dominant lesions. Biopsy specimens should be obtained and handled in such a manner that tumor size, hormone receptor status, and excision margin status can be identified. Because breast cancer is often an unexpected diagnosis in pediatric patients, special attention to proper handling of the specimen is important in all resections.

Staging

Pretreatment staging in all patients with breast cancer should include imaging of the contralateral breast to rule out ipsilateral disease, liver function tests to rule out liver metastases, and chest radiograph to rule out lung metastases. Hepatic imaging and bone scans are not routinely indicated in asymptomatic patients with normal laboratory values. In patients with locally advanced tumors or multiple involved nodes, radionuclide bone scan and CT of the chest and liver may detect occult metastasis. The AJCC/IUCC staging method for breast cancer is shown in Table 20-4.

Local Treatment

Local treatment for early-stage breast cancer consists of modified radical mastectomy or segmental resection with a margin of 1 cm to 2 cm of surrounding normal tissue, followed by radiation therapy. Prospective, randomized trials comparing these two approaches have shown no significant differences in local recurrence or overall survival.[91-93] Contraindications to breast-conserving therapy are pregnancy, collagen vascular disease history, multifocal disease, diffuse calcifications shown on mammogram, irradiation history, and diffusely positive margins after re-resection. Relative contraindications include patients with small breasts and large tumors in whom cosmetic results may be unacceptable and patients with associated intraductal carcinomas.

Local excision of more advanced-stage tumors may be facilitated by preoperative systemic therapy. Breast reconstruction can be performed at the time of mastectomy or can be delayed until after systemic treatment. Options for reconstruction include prosthetic implants, latissimus dorsi flaps, and pedicled or free *transverse rectus abdominis myocutaneous* (TRAM) flaps. Axillary dissection is included for staging purposes. Increasing the use of adjuvant systemic therapy regardless of nodal status may raise questions about the need for axillary dissection.

Table 20-4 • Staging of Breast Cancer

Primary Tumor

TX	Primary tumor cannot be assessed
T0	No evidence of primary tumor
Tis	Carcinoma in situ
T1	Tumor less than 2 cm in greatest dimension
T2	Tumor 2 cm to 5 cm in greatest dimension
T3	Tumor greater than 5 cm in greatest dimension
T4	Tumor extends into chest wall, or skin edema or skin ulceration, or satellite skin nodules are confined to the same breast, or inflammatory carcinoma.

Nodal Involvement

NX	Regional lymph nodes cannot be assessed
N0	No regional lymph node metatasis
N1	Metastasis in movable ipsilateral axillary lymph nodes
N2	Metastasis in ipsilateral axillary lymph nodes fixed to one another or other structures
N3	Metastasis to ipsilateral internal mammary nodes

Distant Metastasis

MX	Presence of distant metastasis cannot be assessed
M0	No evidence of distant metastasis
M1	Distant metastasis present

TNM Staging

Stage 0	Tis	N0	M0
Stage 1	T1	N0	M0
Stage 2a	T0-1	N1	M0
	T2	N0	M0
Stage 2b	T2	N1	M0
	T3	N0	M0
Stage 3a	T0-2	N2	M0
	T3	N1-2	M0
Stage 3b	T4	N1-2	M0
	Any T	N3	M0
Stage 4	Any T	Any N	M1

From Beahrs OH, Henson DE, Hutter RVP, et al (eds): *American Joint Committee on Cancer: Manual for Staging of Cancer*, 3rd ed. Philadelphia: J. B. Lippincott, 1988, with permission.

Adjuvant Therapy

Systemic therapy with regimens such as FAC (5-FU, Adriamycin [doxorubicin], and Cytoxan [cyclophosphamide]) and CMF (Cytoxan, methotrexate, and 5-FU) has produced significantly improved survival rates in patients with node-positive breast and metastatic breast cancers.[94, 95] The role of chemotherapy in treating node-negative breast cancer is less clear. Although disease-free survival has been shown to be significantly increased, the effect on overall survival is not yet clear.[96]

Treatment of metastatic disease has been less successful. New approaches include agents such as docetaxel and vinorelbine and high-dose chemotherapy with stem-cell transplantation.[97–99] Patients with estrogen and progesterone receptor-positive tumors have the highest likelihood of response to hormonal interventions such as oopherectomy, adrenalectomy, hypophysectomy, and antiestrogen drugs such as tamoxifen. The role of hormonal manipulation in premenopausal patients is unclear. The incidence of receptor-positive tumors in pediatric patients is not reported.

Prognosis

Studies have suggested that younger patients with breast cancer have decreased survival compared with older patients with cancer of the same stages.[100, 101] Although the small number of pediatric patients with breast cancers does not allow statistical evaluation, it appears that pediatric patients have a similar survival to that of same-stage adult patients. Five-year survival is approximately 90% for adult patients with Stage 1 breast cancer, 75% for those with Stage 2, 50% for those with Stage 3, and only 15% for those with Stage 4 disease.[102]

Cystosarcoma Phyllodes and Other Breast Sarcomas

Cystosarcoma phyllodes are manifested as painless breast masses. Skin and nodal involvement is rare even with large tumors of this type. Imaging studies usually reveal well-circumscribed lesions similar to fibroadenomas. Approximately 25% of these tumors are malignant by histologic criteria, but metastatic disease is present in only a small percentage of cases.[103] The optimal treatment for both benign and malignant tumors is wide resection with a margin of normal breast tissue.[104] This margin must be histologically clear because local recurrence can occur even with benign lesions. Lymph node dissection is not performed in the absence of biopsy-proven nodal involvement. Primary breast sarcomas have been reported in

pediatric patients and should be treated as recommended for the histologic subtype; this usually involves wide local excision with or without adjuvant therapy.[105]

HEMANGIOMA

Incidence and Natural History

Hemangiomas are the most common benign tumor of infancy, occurring in 10% to 12% of white children.[106] Superficial lesions usually appear in the first few weeks of life as a raised erythematous lesion, localized telangiectasia, or spot. Deep tumors may appear several months later as a discrete mass or an enlargement of an extremity. Hemangiomas most often show rapid growth for 8–18 months followed by slow regression for 5–8 years. Complete regression takes place in over 50% of children by age 5 and in over 70% of children by age 7.[107] Less than 10% of hemangiomas cause significant complications such as obstruction of ear, eye, or airway; ulceration; hemorrhage and infection; high-output congestive heart failure; and thrombocytopenic coagulopathy (Kasabach-Merritt syndrome).

Imaging

Ultrasound of hemangiomas typically shows an irregular mass with variable internal reflectivity on B scan and high flow on Doppler imaging. MR imaging typically shows high-flow characteristics, evidence of areas of intermediate intensity on T1-weighted images, and high-intensity signals on T2-weighted images.[108] MR imaging is the most sensitive study to distinguish these tumors from arteriovenous, lymphatic, and venous malformations.

Treatment

The majority of hemanigiomas require no treatment. Therapy should be considered for the less than 10% of lesions that (1) cause ulceration, infection, or hemorrhage; (2) put patients at risk for compromising auditory or visual systems; or (3) accompany high-output congestive heart failure, thrombocytopenic coagulopathy, or airway obstruction. The initial medical management usually consists of high-dose systemic corticosteroids. Prednisone or prednisolone is given 2–3 mg/kg/day orally for 2–3 weeks. A response to therapy is indicated by changes in color and consistency of the lesion with slowing of growth within 7–10 days of therapy.

With localized lesions, intralesional injections may be used. Steroid therapy creates dramatic response in 30% of patients.[109] Patients that are unresponsive to corticosteroid therapy should be treated with interferon alfa-2a.[110]

Surgical treatments, including laser ablation and coagulation produce many complications and have had varying results and thus should be reserved for residual defects or life-threatening lesions unresponsive to other medical treatment.[111]

NEUROFIBROMATOSIS

Incidence and Etiology

Neurofibromatosis is one of the most common dominantly inherited genetic disorders, occurring in about 1 of every 3000 live births. *NF1* is a result of a mutation of chromosome 17.[112] Gene products called *neurofibromins* have been identified with GTase-activating functions that negatively regulate *GTP-ras*.[113] Apparently the *NF* gene functions as a tumor-supressor gene that is mutated in patients with neurofibromatosis and may lead to development of neurofibromas by defective growth suppression.

The lifetime risk for *NF*-related malignancy is 5%.[114] The most common malignant tumor is neurofibrosarcoma, which usually appears after age 10. Other associated tumors are astrocytomas; rhabdomyosarcomas; melanomas; childhood leukemias; and breast, lung, and prostate cancers.[114] Half of all patients with neurofibrosarcomas present in the second decade of life. The age-adjusted risk for development of neurofibrosarcomas in patients with neurofibromatosis is 100,000 times the general population.[114] Neurofibrosarcomas must be excluded as a cause of acute or subacute onset pain in patients with neurofibromatosis. Any change in size of neurofibromas must be investigated carefully. Neurofibrosarcomas are generally resistant to therapy other than complete surgical excision.

Signs and Symptoms

The National Institutes of Health (NIH) criteria for *NF1* includes two of the following:[115] six or more café-au-lait spots; two or more neurofibromas or one plexiform neurofibroma; axillary or inguinal freckling; optic gliomas; Lisch's nodules (iris hamartomas); osseous lesions; a first-degree relative with *NF1*. The major morbidity from neurofibromatosis is the result of overgrowth of the peripheral nerve sheath, causing constriction of the nerve trunk or compression of adjacent organs. Neurofibromas are most adequately visualized by MR imaging.

Treatment

Chemotherapeutic agents, including ketotifen, alpha interferon, and *cis*-retinoic acid, have been ineffective in treating plexiform neurofibromas. Laboratory investigators have identified inhibitors of farnesil transferase and gerenyl transferase that offer promising theoretical systemic treatments, but these have not as yet been translated into clinical trials.

Surgical resection is limited by the diffuse nature of involvement and by the highly vascular nature of these tumors. For example, adjacent bone may be invested by plexiform neurofibromas. Many surgeons are reluctant to attempt resection of large plexiform neurofibromas, yet surgical resection is nevertheless an important tool in the management of neurofibromatosis. Radiation therapy is associated with increased development of second tumors, and these slowgrowing, benign tumors are not clearly responsive to radiation or chemotherapy; hence, surgical excision may offer the best functional result with the fewest associated complications of any treatment. Adkins and Ravitch[116] reported the results of surgical resection in 22 patients with head and neck neurofibromas and concluded that careful surgical resection often yielded adequate cosmetic and functional results even when margin-negative resection was not possible.

Indications for resection include intractable pain, functional compromise, and question of malignancy. Confirmation of malignant transformation is possible only by tissue sampling and pathologic analysis. Surgical resection of large plexiform neurofibromas involves extensive preoperative evaluation and coordinated planning among multiple surgical subspecialties. Anatomic relationships to peripheral nerve trunks is required before risks and potential benefits of surgical resection can be determined.

Seppala and coworkers[117] reported results of surgical resection in 32 patients with spinal neurofibromas. In their series, 69% of patients improved neurologically after resection, 12% remained unchanged, and 16% deteriorated. These findings emphasize the need for contemporary surgical techniques incorporating intraoperative motor and sensory nerve stimulated evoked potentials, microsurgical dissection, and soft-tissue flap closure. Such techniques may allow resection of neurofibromas previously thought unresectable. Pickard and Rose[118] describe successful application of these techniques in resection of a femoral nerve neurofibroma with successful preservation of nerve function.

References

1. Boddie A, Smith JL, McBride C: Malignant melanoma in children and young adults. *South Med J* 71:1074, 1978.
2. Lee JA, Kongchaiyuaha S: Incidence and mortality from malignant melanoma by anatomical site. *J Natl Cancer Inst* 47:253, 1971.
3. Kraemer KH, Lee MM, Scotto J: Xeroderma pigmentosum—Cutaneous, ocular and neurologic abnormalities in 830 published cases. *Arch Dermatol* 123:241, 1987.
4. Kaplan EN: The risk of malignancy in large congenital nevi. *Plast Reconstr Surg* 53:421, 1974.
5. Rhodes AR, Wood WC, Sober AJ, et al: Non-epidermal origin of malignant melanoma associated with giant congenital nevocellular nevus. *Plast Reconstr Surg* 67:782, 1981.
6. MacKie RM, Watt D, Doherty V, et al: Malignant melanoma occurring in those aged under 30 in the west of Scotland 1979–1986: A study of incidence, clinical features, pathological features and survival. *Br J Dermatol* 124:560, 1991.
7. Lynch HT, Frichot BC III, Lynch JF: Familial atypical multiple mole—Melanoma syndrome. *J Med Genet* 15:352, 1978.
8. Bale SJ, Dracopoli NC, Tucker MA, et al: Mapping the gene for hereditary cutaneous malignant melanoma—Dysplastic nevus to chromosome 1p. *N Engl J Med* 320:1367, 1989.
9. Greene MH, Clark WH Jr, Tucker MA, et al: High risk of malignant melanoma in melanoma-prone families with dysplastic nevi. *Ann Intern Med* 102:458–465, 1985.
10. DeWit PG, de Vaan GA, de Bo TM, et al: Prevalence of naevocytic naevi after chemotherapy for childhood cancer. *Med Pediatr Oncol* 18:336–338, 1990.
11. Corpron CA, Black CT, Ross MI, et al:

12. Potter JF, Schoeneman M: Metastasis of maternal cancer to the placenta and fetus. *Cancer* 25:380, 1970.
13. Crotty KA, McCarthy SW, Palmer AA, et al: Malignant melanoma in childhood: A clinicopathologic study of 13 cases and comparison with Spitz nevi. *World J Surg* 16:179–185, 1992.
14. Clark WH Jr, Ainsworth AM, Bernadino EA, et al: The developmental biology of primary human malignant melanomas. *Semin Oncol* 2:83, 1975.
15. Breslow A: Thickness, cross-sectional area and depth of invasion in prognosis of cutaneous melanoma. *Ann Surg* 172:902, 1970.
16. Beahrs OH, Henson DE, Hutter RVP, et al (eds): *American Joint Committee on Cancer: Manual for Staging of Cancer,* 3rd ed. Philadelphia: J.B. Lippincott, 1988.
17. Urist MM, Balch CM, Soong SJ, et al: The influence of surgical margins and prognostic factors predicting the risk of local recurrence in 3,445 patients with primary cutaneous melanoma. *Cancer* 55:1298, 1985.
18. Veronesi U, Cascinelli N, Adamus J, et al: Thin stage I primary cutaneous malignant melanoma: Comparison of excision with margins of 1 or 3 cm. *N Engl J Med* 318:1159, 1988.
19. Balch CM, Urist MM, Karakousis CP, et al: Efficacy of 2-cm surgical margins for intermediate-thickness melanomas (1 to 4 mm): Results of a multi-institutional randomized surgical trial. *Ann Surg* 218:262, 1993.
20. Balch CM: The role of elective lymph node dissection in melanoma: Rationale, results and controversies. *J Clin Oncol* 6:163, 1988.
21. Crowley NJ, Seigler HF: The role of elective lymph node dissection in the management of patients with thick cutaneous melanoma. *Cancer* 66:2522, 1990.
22. Veronesi U, Adamus J, Bandiera DC, et al: Delayed regional lymph node dissection in stage I melanoma of the skin of the lower extremities. *Cancer* 49:2420, 1982.
23. Sim FH, Taylor WF, Pritchard DJ, et al: Lymphadenectomy in the management of stage I malignant melanoma: A prospective randomized study. *Mayo Clin Proc* 61:697, 1986.
24. Balch CM, Soong SJ, Urist MM, et al: A prospective randomized surgical trial of 742 melanoma patients comparing the efficacy of elective (immediate) lymph node dissection versus observation. *Ann Surg* In press.
25. Morton DL, Wen DR, Foshag LJ, et al: Technical details of intraoperative lymphatic mapping for early-stage melanoma. *Arch Surg* 127:392, 1992.
26. Corpron CA, Ross MI, Black CT, et al:

Lymphatic mapping and sentinel node biopsy in pediatric melanoma patients. Surgical Section of the American Academy of Pediatrics, 47th Annual Meeting, San Francisco, CA, 1995 (poster presentation).

27. Kirkwood JM, Strawderman MH, Ernstoff MS, et al: Interferon alfa-2b adjuvant therapy of high-risk resected cutaneous melanoma: The Eastern Cooperative Oncology Group Trial EST 1684. *J Clin Oncol* 14:7, 1996.

28. Costanzi ME, Nathanson L, Schoenfeld D, et al: Results with methyl-CCNU and DTIC in metastatic melanoma. *Cancer* 40:1010, 1977.

29. Constanzi JJ, Vaitkevicius VK, Quagliana JM, et al: Combination chemotherapy for disseminated malignant melanoma. *Cancer* 35:342, 1975.

30. Fletcher WS, Green S, Fletcher JR, et al: Evaluation of *cis*-platinum and DTIC combination chemotherapy in disseminated melanoma. *Am J Clin Oncol* 11:589, 1988.

31. Banzet P, Jacquillat C, Civatte J, et al: Adjuvant chemotherapy in the management of primary malignant melanoma. *Cancer* 41:1240, 1978.

32. Del Prete SA, Maurer LH, O'Donnell J, et al: Combination chemotherapy with cisplatin, carmustine, dacarbazine, and tamoxifen in metastatic melanoma. *Cancer Treat Reports* 68:1984, 1984.

33. Hill GJ III, Moss SE, Golomb FM, et al: DTIC and combination therapy for melanoma: III. DTIC (NSC 45388) surgical adjuvant study COG protocol 7040. *Cancer* 47:2556, 1981.

34. Veronesi U, Adamus J, Auberg C, et al: A randomized trial of adjuvant chemotherapy and immunotherapy in cutaneous melanoma. *N Engl J Med* 307:913, 1982.

35. Wood WC, Cosimi AB, Carey RW, et al: Randomized trial of adjuvant therapy for "high risk" primary malignant melanoma. *Surgery* 83:677, 1978.

36. Knost JA, Reynold V, Greco FA, et al: Adjuvant chemoimmunotherapy: Stage I/II malignant melanoma. *J Surg Oncol* 19:165, 1982.

37. Hayes FA, Green AA: Malignant melanoma in childhood: Clinical course and response to chemotherapy. *J Clin Oncol* 2:1229, 1984.

38. Boddie AW Jr and Cangir A: Adjuvant and neoadjuvant chemotherapy with dacarbazine in high-risk childhood melanoma. *Cancer* 60:1720, 1987.

39. Eilber FR, Morton DL, Holmes EC, et al: Adjuvant immunotherapy with BCG in treatment of regional lymph node metastases from malignant melanoma. *N Engl J Med* 294:237, 1976.

40. Seigler JF, Cox E, Mutzner F, et al: Specific active immunotherapy for melanoma. *Ann Surg* 190:366, 1979.

41. Wallack MK, McNally KR, Leftheriotis E: A Southeastern Cancer Study Group phase I/II trial with vaccinia melanoma oncolysates. *Cancer* 57:649, 1986.

42. Lee KH, Talpaz M, Papadopoulos N, et al: Concomitant administration of recombinant human interleukin-2 and recombinant interferon-alfa-2a in cancer patients: A phase I study. *J Clin Oncol* 7:1726, 1989.

43. Cumberlain R, DeMoss E, Lassus M, et al: Isolation perfusion for malignant melanoma of the extremity: A review. *J Clin Oncol* 3:1022, 1985.

44. Baas PC, Hoekstra HJ, Schraffordt Koops H, et al: Hyperthermic isolated regional perfusion in the treatment of extremity melanoma in children and adolescents. *Cancer* 63:199, 1989.

45. Weiss M, Loprinzi CL, Creagan ET, et al: Utility of follow-up tests for detecting recurrent disease in patients with malignant melanomas. *JAMA* 274:1703, 1995.

46. Davidoff AM, Cirrincione C and Seigler HF: Malignant melanoma in children. *Ann Surg Oncol* 1:278, 1994.

47. Temple WJ, Mulloy RH, Alexander F, et al: Childhood melanoma. *J Pediatr Surg* 26:135, 1991.

48. Pratt CB, Palmer MK, Thatcher N, et al: Malignant melanoma in children and adolescents. *Cancer* 47:392, 1981.

49. Tate PS, Ronan SG, Feucht KA, et al: Melanoma in childhood and adolescence: Clinical and pathological features of 48 cases. *J Pediatr Surg* 28:217, 1993.

50. Rao BN, Hayes FA, Pratt CB, et al: Malignant melanoma in children: Its management and prognosis. *J Pediatr Surg* 25:198, 1990.

51. Reintgen DS, Vollmer R, Seigler HF: Juvenile malignant melanoma. *Surg Gynecol Obstet* 168:249, 1989.

52. Balch CM, Soong SJ, Milton GW, et al: A comparison of prognostic factors and surgical results in 1,786 patients with localized (stage I) melanoma treated in Alabama, USA, and New South Wales, Australia. *Ann Surg* 196:677, 1982.

53. Callery C, Cochran AJ, Roe DJ, et al: Factors prognostic for survival in patients with malignant melanoma spread to the regional lymph nodes. *Ann Surg* 196:69, 1982.

54. Calabro A, Singletary SE, Balch CM: Patterns of relapse in 1001 consecutive patients with melanoma nodal metastases. *Arch Surg* 124:1051, 1989.

55. Bevilacqua RG, Coit DG, Rogatko A, et al: Axillary dissection in melanoma: Prognostic variables in node-positive patients. *Ann Surg* 212:125, 1990.

56. Balch CM, Soong SJ, Murad TM, et al: A multifactorial analysis of melanoma: IV. Prognostic factors in 200 melanoma patients with distant metastases (Stage III). *J Clin Oncol* 1:126, 1983.

57. American Cancer Society: Cancer facts and figures—1992. New York, American Cancer Society, 1992.

58. Lynch HT, Giurgis H, Schwartz M, et al: Genetics and colon cancer. *Arch Surg* 106:669, 1973.

59. Young YL, Percy CL, Asire AJ (eds): *Surveillance, Epidemiology and End Results: Incidence and Mortality Data, 1973–1977.* NCI Monograph 57. Washington DC: U.S. Government Printing Office, 1981.

60. Caldwell GG, Cannon SB, Pratt CB, et al: Serum pesticide levels in patients with childhood colorectal carcinoma. *Cancer* 48:774, 1981.

61. Hardcastle JD, Farrands PA, Balfour TW: Controlled trial of faecal occult blood testing in the detection of colorectal cancer. *Lancet* 2:1, 1983.

62. Meade PG, Blatchford GJ, Thorson AG, et al: Preoperative chemoradiation downstages locally advanced ultrasound-staged rectal cancer. *Am J Surg* 170:612, 1995.

63. Angel CA, Pratt CB, Rao BN, et al: Carcinoembryonic antigen and carbohydrate 19-9 antigen as markers for colorectal carcinoma in children and adolescents. *Cancer* 69:1487, 1992.

64. Stone MD, Kane R, Bothe A Jr, et al: Intraoperative ultrasound imaging of the liver at the time of colorectal cancer resection. *Arch Surg* 129:431, 1994.

65. Steele G, Jr. Bleday R, Mayer RJ, et al: A prospective evaluation of hepatic resection for colorectal carcinoma metastases to the liver: Gastrointestinal Tumor Study Group Protocol 6584. *J Clin Oncol* 9:1105, 1991.

66. Patt, Charnsangavej C, Lawrence, et al: Hepatic arterial infusion of FUDR, leucovorin, Adriamycin and Platinol (FLAP): Effective pallation for nonresectable hepatocellular cancer. *Proc Am Soc Clin Oncol* 11:474, 1992.

67. Willitt CG, Tepper JE, Cohen AM, et al: Failure patterns following curative resection of colonic carcinoma. *Ann Surg* 200:685, 1984.

68. Gastrointestinal Tumor Study Group. Radiation therapy and fluorouracil with or without semustine for the treatment of patients with surgical adjuvant adenocarcinoma of the rectum. *J Clin Oncol* 10:549, 1992.

69. Aleman BM, Bartelink H, Gunderson LL: The current role of radiotherapy in colorectal cancer. *Eur J Cancer* 31A:1333, 1995.

70. Rao BN, Pratt CB, Flemming ID, et al: Colon carcinoma in children and adolescents: A review of 30 cases. *Cancer* 55:1322, 1985.

71. Moertel CG, Fleming TR, MacDonald JS, et al: Levamisole and fluorouracil for adjuvant therapy of resected colon carcinoma. *N Engl J Med* 322:353, 1990.

72. Wolmark N, Fisher B, Rockette H, et al: Postoperative adjuvant chemotherapy or BCG for colon cancer: Results from NSABP protol C-01. *J Natl Cancer Inst* 80:30, 1988.

73. Wolmark N, Rockette H, Fisther B, et al: The benefit of leucovorin-modulated fluorouracil as postoperative adjuvant therapy for primary colon cancer: Results from National Surgical Adjuvant Breast and Bowel Project Protocol C-03. *J Clin Oncol* 11:1879, 1993.

74. LaQuaglia MP, Heller HG, Filippa DA, et al: Prognostic factors and outcome in patients 21 years and under with colorectal carcinoma. *J Pediatr Surg* 27:1085, 1992.

75. Odone V, Chang L, Cacer J, et al: The natural history of colorectal carcinoma in adolescents. *Cancer* 49:1716, 1982.

76. Pratt CB, Rivera G, Shanks E, et al: Colorectal carcinoma in adolescents: Implications regarding etiology. *Cancer* 40:2464, 1977.

77. Recalde M, Holyoke ED, Elias EG: Carcinoma of the colon, rectum and anal canal in young patients. *Surg Gynecol Obstet* 139:909, 1974.

78. Noyes RD, Spanos WJ JR, Monatgue ED, et al: Breast cancer in women aged 30 and under. *Cancer* 49:1302, 1982.

79. West KW, Rescorla FJ, Scherer LR III, et al: Diagnosis and treatment of symptomatic breast masses in the pediatric population. *J Pediatr Surg* 30:186, 1995.

80. Stone AM, Shenker IR, McCarthy K: Adolescent breast masses. *Am J Surg* 134:275, 1977.

81. Corpron CA, Black CT, Singletary SE, et al: Breast cancer in adolescent females. *J Pediatr Surg* 30:322, 1995.

82. Bhatia S, Robison LL, Oberlin O, et al: Breast cancer and other second neoplasms after childhood Hodgkin's disease. *N Engl J Med* 334:745, 1996.

83. Smith MB, Xue H, Strong L, et al: Forty-year experience with second malignancies after treatment of childhood cancer: Analysis of outcome following the development of the second malignancy. *J Pediatr Surg* 2:1342, 1993.

84. Li FP, Fraumeni JF Jr, Mulvihill JJ, et al: A cancer family syndrome in 24 kindreds. *Cancer Res* 48:5358, 1988.

85. Hall JM, Lee MK, Newman B, et al: Linkage of early-onset familial breast cancer to chromosome 17q21. *Science* 250:1684, 1990.

86. Wooster R, Neuhausen SL, Mangion J, et al: Localization of a breast cancer susceptibility gene, BRCA2, to chromosome 13q12. *Science* 265:2088, 1994.

87. McDivitt RW, Stewart FW: Breast carcinoma in children. *JAMA* 195:388, 1966.

88. Yelland A, Grahan MD, Trott PA, et al: Diagnosing breast carcinoma in young women. *BMJ* 302:618, 1991.

89. Ashley S, Royle GT, Corder A, et al: Clinical, radiological and cytogenetic diagnosis of breast cancer in young women. *Br J Surg* 76:835, 1989.

90. Gupta RK, Buchanan A, Simpson J: Fine-needle aspiration cytology of breast: Its impact on surgical practice with an emphasis on the diagnosis of breast abnormalities in young women. *Diag Cytopathol* 4:206, 1988.

91. Ficher B, Redmond C, Poisson R, et al: Eight-year results of a randomized clinical trial comparing total mastecomy and lumpectomy with or without irradiation in the treatment of breast cancer. *N Engl J Med* 320:822, 1989.

92. Veronesi U, Banfi A, DelVecchio M, et al: Comparison of Halsted mastectomy with quadrantectomy, axillary dissection and radiotherapy in early breast cancer. *Eur J Cancer* 9:1085, 1986.

93. Grotting JC, Urist M, Maddox WA, et al: Convential TRAM flap versus microsurgical TRAM flap for immediate breast reconstruction. *Plast Reconstr Surg* 83:828, 1989.

94. Bonadonna G, Rossi A, Valagussa P: Adjuvant CMF chemotherapy in operable breast cancer: Ten years later. *World J Surg* 9:707, 1985.

95. NIH Consensus Conference: Treatment of early-stage breast cancer. *JAMA* 265:391, 1991.

96. Clinical alert from the National Cancer Institute, May 18, 1998. *Breast Cancer Res Treat* 12:3, 1988.

97. Peters WP: Autologous bone marrow transplantation for breast cancer. *Curr Opin Oncol* 16:129, 1992.

98. Reichman BS, Seidman AD, Crown JPA, et al: Paclitaxel and recombinant human granulocyte colony-stimulating factor as initial chemotherapy for metastatic breast cancer. *J Clin Oncol* 11:1943, 1993.

99. Lazarus H, Herzig GP, Grahan-Pole J, et al: Intensive melphalan chemotherapy and cryopreserved autologous bone marrow transplantation for the treatment of refractory cancer. *J Clin Oncol* 2:359, 1983.

100. De la Rochefordiere A, Asselain B, Campana F, et al: Age as prognostic factor in premenopausal breast carcinoma. *Lancet* 341:1039, 1993.

101. Lee CG, McCormick B, Mazumdar M, et al: Infiltrating breast carcinoma in patients age 30 years and younger: Long-term outcome for life, relapse, and second primary tumors. *Radiat Oncol Biol Phys* 23:969, 1992.

102. Beahrs IH, Henson DE, Juller RVP, et al: *Manual for Staging of Cancer*, 4th ed. Philadelphia: J.B. Lippincott, 1992, p. 149.

103. Raganoonan C, Fairbairn JK, Williams S, et al: Giant breast tumors of adolescence. *Aust N Z J Surg* 57:243, 1987.

104. Stromberg BV, Golladay ES: Cystosarcoma phyllodes in the adolescent female. *J Pediatr Surg* 13:423, 1978.

105. Gutman H, Pollock RE, Ross MI, et al: Sarcoma of the breast: Implications for extent of therapy. The M. D. Anderson experience. *Surgery* 116:505, 1994.

106. Jacobs AH: Strawberry hemangiomas: The natural history of the untreated lesion. *Calif Med* 86:7, 1957.

107. Bowers RE, Graham EA, Tomlinson KM: The natural history of the strawberry nevus. *Arch Dermatol* 82:667, 1960.

108. Greenspan A, McGahan JP, Vogel-sang P, et al: Imaging strategies in the evaluation of soft-tissue hemangiomas of the extremities: Correlation of the findings of plain radiography, CT, MRI, and ultrasonography in 12 histologically proven cases. *Skeletal Radiol* 21:11, 1992.

109. Zaren HA, Edgerton MT: Induced resolution of cavernous hemangiomas following prednisolone therapy. *Plast Reconstr Surg* 39:76, 1967.

110. Ezekowitz RAB, Mulliken JB, Folkman J: Interferon alfa-2a therapy for life-threatening hemangiomas of infancy. *N Engl J Med* 326:1456, 1992.

111. Garden JM, Makus AD, Paller AS: Treatment of cutaneous hemangiomas by the flashlamp-pumped dye laser: Prospective analysis. *J Pediatr* 12:555, 1992.

112. Barker D, Wright E, Nguyen K, et al: Gene for von Recklinghausen neurofibromatosis is in the pericentromeric region of chromosome 17. *Science* 236:1100, 1987.

113. DeClue JE, Cohen BD, Lowry DR: Identification and characterization of the neurofibromatosis type 1 protein product. *Proc Natl Acad Sci U S A* 88:9914, 1991.

114. Riccardi VM: Von Recklinghausen neurofibromatosis. *N Engl J Med* 305:1617, 1981.

115. National Institutes of Health Consensus Development Conference. Neurofibromatosis: Conference Statement. *Arch Neurol* 45:575, 1988.

116. Adkins JC, Ravitch MM: The operative management of von Recklinghausen's neurofibromatosis in children, with special reference to lesions of the head and neck. *Surgery* 9:342, 1977.

117. Seppala MT, Haltia MJ, Sankila RJ, et al: Long-term outcome after removal of spinal neurofibroma. *J Neurosurg* 82:572, 1995.

118. Pickard LR, Rose JE: Avoidable complications of resection of major nerve trunk neurofibromas and schwannomas. *Neurofibromatosis* 1:43, 1988.

Endocrine Tumors

• *John J. Doski, M.D.* • *Frank M. Robertson, M.D.* • *Henry W. Cheu, M.D.* °

Endocrine tumors represent approximately 5% of all pediatric tumors.[1–3] These tumors arise from a wide variety of endocrine tissues and may be either nonfunctional or hormonally active. Included in this definition of endocrine tumors are those of nonendocrine origin that secrete a varied array of hormonally active substances, producing unusual clinical findings. Such tumors are classified as "ectopic."

Approximately 400 pediatric endocrine cancers were reported by the National Cancer Institute over the 15-year period of 1973 to 1987.[3] Approximately 43% of these tumors were gonadal germ-cell tumors of trophoblastic origin. Thyroid carcinomas accounted for 33% of cases reported and pituitary tumors for approximately 13%. The remaining types of pediatric endocrine tumors are rarely encountered by any given physician. This chapter discusses parathyroid tumors, pheochromocytomas, adrenocortical carcinomas, so-called ectopic tumors producing adrenocorticotropic hormone (ACTH), tumors producing human chorionic gonadotropin (hCG) and growth-hormone-releasing hormone (GRH), tumors of the gastroenteropancreatic unit [insulinoma, glucagonoma, gastrinoma, and tumors secreting vasoactive intestinal peptide (VIP) and pancreatic polypeptide], pituitary tumors, and the *multiple endocrine neoplasia* (MEN) syndromes. Carcinoids are also discussed in this chapter. Thyroid tumors and neuroblastomas, which may produce hormonally active substances, are discussed in other chapters.

The majority of these tumors are sporadic in origin, but pheochromocytoma and the MEN syndromes have very characteristic patterns of

°Deceased

All the material in this chapter is in the public domain, with the exception of any borrowed figures or tables.

inheritance. These tumors also present unique pathology and diagnostic challenges that continue to evolve, including genetic analysis for RET proto-oncogene in children with medullary thyroid cancer. Surgery plays a major role in the therapy of endocrine tumors, often offering the only hope for prolonged disease-free survival. Most of these tumors are low-grade malignancies with low rates of metastases, thus, extended palliation and long-term survival are generally possible.

PITUITARY TUMORS

Pituitary adenomas constitute 2.0% to 2.7% of all intracranial tumors seen in children.[4, 5] Most children who have a pituitary adenoma—up to 94% in one series—will present with symptomatic endocrinopathy associated with pituitary hormonal hypersecretion.[6] The most common pediatric pituitary adenomas include corticotropinoma (excess ACTH), prolactinoma, and somatotropinoma (excess growth hormone). Nonfunctioning pituitary adenomas and adenomas producing thyroid-stimulating hormone (TSH) are rare in children.

Pituitary tumors may be contained exclusively within the sella turcica or may extend above the diaphragma sellae as a suprasellar mass. Microadenomas are less than 10 mm in size, and macroadenomas are more than 10 mm. The relative frequencies of pituitary adenomas in children are different from those in adults. Corticotropinomas in one study accounted for 54% of pediatric adenomas, followed by prolactinomas in 27% of patients, somatotropinomas in 12%, and nonfunctioning tumors in 6%.[6] A larger study, with breakdown into age groups, showed corticotropinomas as the most common pituitary adenomas seen prior to puberty, and prolactinomas as the most common during and after puberty.[4]

Pituitary adenomas may produce symptoms secondary to their space-occupying nature. Visual changes occur in up to 18% of children having suprasellar extension of the adenoma onto the optic chiasm. Quadrantanopsia, temporal hemianopsia, or diplopia may result.[7] Headaches are among the common, nonspecific findings associated with increasing mass effect. Growth arrest is likewise a common finding with all types of pituitary adenomas—except somatotropinomas. A significant percentage of patients (up to 36%)

present with deficiencies of one or more hypothalamic-pituitary hormones due to direct pressure from the tumor mass.[7]

The presentation of deficiency states depends on the hormone involved. ACTH deficiency leads to adrenal insufficiency with weakness, orthostatic hypotension, hyponatremia, and hypoglycemia. Menstrual changes in girls are common findings with all pituitary adenomas except with those causing Nelson's syndrome (delayed presentation of pituitary ACTH–secreting macroadenoma, hyperpigmentation, following adrenalectomy). These menstrual changes are believed to be related to impaired pituitary portal circulation and feedback.[4] Growth-hormone deficiency leads to short stature, poor growth, and hypoglycemia. Gonadotropin deficiency leads to pubertal delay, arrest, or regression. TSH deficiency leads to poor growth, diminished cognitive performance, constipation, cold intolerance, or dry skin. Hormonal deficiencies are most commonly associated with macroadenomas, rarely with microadenomas.[7]

Clinical presentation with subsequent laboratory confirmation will often provide the diagnosis of a functioning pituitary adenoma. Computed tomography (CT) and magnetic resonance imaging (MRI) scans are not especially accurate for detection or localization of pituitary adenomas; in one study their success rate was only 29%.[6] In this same study there was a higher detection rate with prolactinomas and somatotropinomas due to their generally larger size at time of presentation.

Studies have led to the conclusion that pediatric pituitary tumors are not more invasive or aggressive than adult pituitary tumors.[7] Invasiveness of pituitary adenomas correlates positively with tumor size. Macroadenomas often require aggressive adjuvant therapies and are associated with a higher rate of hypopituitarism—52% of patients in one study.[7]

Manifestations of Hormonal Secretion of Pituitary Adenomas

Adrenocorticotropic Hormone (ACTH)

Most corticotropinomas are microadenomas, with an occasional case being described of diffuse corticotropic-cell hyperplasia.[8] One study cited a female-to-male ratio of 3:1.[4] The diagnosis of Cushing's disease and existence of a corticotropinoma are established following dexamethasone suppression and corticotropin-releasing hormone tests. Lateralization of the ACTH-secreting pituitary adenoma can be assisted by bilateral petrosal sinus sampling and may be beneficial as the establishment of normal and pathologic pituitary tissues during surgery can be very difficult.

Because ACTH-secreting tumors are typically smaller than other adenomas, imaging studies frequently fail to reveal them.[5] Neither preoperative nor postoperative serum ACTH levels distinguish children who are at increased risk for tumor recurrence.[4] In one study, simple adenomectomy or subtotal hypophysectomy was followed by no immediate postoperative failures and produced a long-term symptomatic cure of 78% following reoperation.[6] Complications included transient hypocortisolism or diabetes insipidus. Adenomas leading to Nelson's syndrome occur more often in children and adolescents compared with adults.[4] In one study 83% of children with Nelson's syndrome were prepubertal.[4] In another study none of the children with Nelson's syndrome were successfully treated with surgery alone.[6]

Prolactin

Most prolactinomas are microadenomas, but there is a higher incidence of suprasellar extension of prolactinomas in children than in adults; in some studies it is as high as 72%.[6] Excess prolactin secretion causes the pituitary gonadal symptoms of galactorrhea and suppression of the reproductive system, with arrested growth. Girls are less likely to have galactorrhea than are women, and they almost always present with amenorrhea.[6] Boys often have macroadenomas at time of diagnosis, and they present with galactorrhea and delayed puberty.[4]

Surgical resection of prolactinomas is associated with a significant postoperative need for adjuvant therapies, in some studies as high as 67%.[6] A statistically significant positive correlation between the maximum preoperative serum prolactin level and tumor size shows macroadenomas associated with higher prolactin levels than microadenomas.[4] As a result, patients with smaller tumors, those associated with serum prolactin levels below 200 ng/l, have a higher rate of surgical cure.[6, 7] The 5-year recurrence-free survival rate is 90% in children with prolactin levels below 200 ng/l versus 51% in those with

prolactin levels above 200 ng/l.[7] In several studies boys were found to have larger tumors, and none of the boys with macroadenoma and clinical presentation of pubertal delay were cured surgically.[6, 7]

Growth Hormone

Most somatotropinomas are macroadenomas. A higher incidence of suprasellar extension is reported in children than in adults.[6] Elevations of growth hormone prior to epiphyseal plate closure results in gigantism, and if the growth plate is closed, the patient develops acromegaly. Carbohydrate intolerance progressing to diabetes, menstrual irregularities, arthropathy, and carpel tunnel syndrome is also seen with somatotropinomas.[8] In a study of pituitary tumors, 16% were seen in the prepubertal group, the youngest patient being 15 months of age.[4] In the majority of these children, diagnosis was made during puberty. Female-to-male ratio was 1:2. The mean time of onset of symptoms to diagnosis was shorter in children than in adults.[4]

Transsphenoidal resection of somatotropinomas controls the disease in a minority of children (12% in one study). Adjuvant therapies are frequently employed.[6] In contrast, surgical cure rates are 60% to 88% in adults with somatotropinomas, suggesting a more aggressive biologic nature of these tumors in children.[6] Elevated levels of growth hormone in the postoperative period have a statistically significant positive correlation with a higher rate of tumor recurrence, but preoperative levels have no significant correlation.[4]

Other Pituitary Adenomas

Pediatric pituitary adenomas that secrete TSH, luteinizing hormone (LH), or follicle-stimulating hormone (FSH) are scarce.[5] Elevations of LH or FSH in a child are more likely to represent a tumor with secretion of an alpha subunit.[5]

Endocrinologically silent tumors occur as significantly larger pituitary masses and are associated with focal neurologic findings in almost all patients.[4] Hypopituitarism is also common as a result of suprasellar expansion causing pituitary insufficiency.

Treatment and Prognosis of Pituitary Tumors

Transsphenoidal resection is the procedure of choice for pituitary adenomas. Patients with larger tumors and a significant suprasellar component may require either craniotomy or postoperative adjuvant therapy. In one study, 17% of children required drilling of an incompletely pneumatized sphenoid sinus as part of a transsphenoidal approach.[6] Complications of transsphenoidal surgery include panhypopituitarism, cavernous sinus hemorrhage, transient or permanent diabetes insipidus, cerebrospinal fluid (CSF) leak, or meningitis, or the need to perform total hypophysectomy.

Overall cure rates of 78% to 86% have been reported for corticotropinomas.[4, 6] Inability to find a very small lesion or to adequately remove a lesion are reasons commonly cited for surgical failures. Intraoperative exploration of the sellar contents must be very thorough, especially for corticotropinomas. Postoperative hypocortisolism is a favorable but not absolute sign of surgical cure for corticotropinomas.[6] Additional management options for recurrent ACTH excess include reexploration, radiation therapy (up to 5000 cGy), administration of adrenolytic agents (including mitotane, metyrapone, and ketoconazole), or, finally, bilateral adrenalectomy with its risk of precipitating Nelson's syndrome.[8]

In one study, patients with non-ACTH pituitary microadenomas had an operative cure rate of 70% and a long-term cure rate of 65%.[7] In the same study, patients with macroadenomas had an operative cure rate of 33% and long-term cure rate of 55%. Adjuvant therapy for patients with non-ACTH pituitary adenomas, particularly prolactinomas, included the long-term administration of bromocriptine, a dopamine agonist. Bromocriptine is the treatment of choice for prolactinomas, with doses of up to 15 mg/day required for years to effect a cure.[8] Patients with prolactin-secreting microadenomas are often cured by surgery, but those with macroadenomas may require bromocriptine and possibly radiation.[5] Postoperative levels of growth hormone are predictive of recurrence, and bromocriptine at higher doses (up to 25 mg/day) have been reported helpful. Sellar radiation therapy may also be utilized for patients with prolactinomas or somatotropinomas. Transsphenoidal reexploration is another modality indicated for recurrent disease.

Pituitary hormonal deficiencies call for replacement therapy, including the administration of growth hormone, hydrocortisone (with appropriate stress dosing), thyroxine, testosterone or estrogen, and DDAVP.

The overall prognosis for patients with pediatric pituitary adenomas is good. Most of the tumors are benign. A return to endocrine homeostasis is witnessed within 3 to 6 months and leads to normal growth, puberty, and conception, as well as to normal results on visual examination.[5] As outlined, some pediatric pituitary adenomas have a tendency toward recurrence or local invasion. In one large series there was no clear relationship between invasiveness and recurrent disease. Few ACTH-secreting tumors were invasive (up to 9.5%), but there was a high rate (up to 17%) of recurrent disease.[4] Growth-hormone-secreting adenomas had a 50% invasive rate but only a 17% recurrence rate. Prolactinomas had a 29% invasive rate and a 6% recurrence rate. It is therefore important to gauge the risks of recurrence of prolactinomas and somatotropinomas with examination of serum levels preoperatively and postoperatively, respectively. No other evidence exists that pediatric pituitary adenomas are more likely to be locally invasive or aggressive.[5, 7] Extended follow-up is indicated, with particular attention paid to growth, endocrine status, and careful neurologic examination with special emphasis given to the visual examination.

HYPERPARATHYROIDISM

Primary hyperparathyroidism (PHPT) in children is rare. Less than 130 cases are reported in the literature. PHPT in children occurs as three distinctive patterns based on the age at presentation and pathology involved.

Neonatal hyperparathyroidism is manifested as a "failure to thrive" syndrome with extremes of hypercalcemia within the first 3 months of life. It can be fatal unless treated early, and it has been reported in both autosomal dominant and recessive inheritance patterns.[9] Reviews cite 20% to 25% of all cases of childhood hyperparathyroidism occurring in the neonatal period.[10, 11]

PHPT in children may also be a component of inherited endocrinopathies. These include autosomal dominant MEN1 and MEN2A, autosomal dominant *familial hypocalcuric hypercalcemia* (FHH), and autosomal dominant *familial isolated hyperparathyroidism* (FIHP). Parathyroid disease is an almost universal finding in association with MEN1 syndrome and is often the first sign of the syndrome. Patients with MEN2A may also have elevations of *parathyroid hormone* (PTH), but have a clinically less severe course. Patients with MEN2B are not known to manifest parathyroid disease.[12]

In children and adolescents with no known familial association, PHPT is most often caused by a parathyroid adenoma.[10, 13] In pediatric studies, boys are affected more than girls, with some series reporting a 3:2 male-to-female ratio.[10, 14] In adult studies, women are affected up to twice as frequently as men, the majority of women developing the disease later in life.[15] Another difference between pediatric and adult series is the cause of hyperparathyroidism. In pediatric reviews, neonatal hyperparathyroidism is always due to parathyroid hyperplasia, and in children and adolescents who do not have a known inherited endocrinopathy, hyperparathyroidism is usually due to adenoma.[10, 11, 16] In adults, single-gland enlargement with adenoma is seen in 80% of hyperparathyroid cases, hyperplasia in 15% of cases, two-gland enlargement in 2.6% of cases, and intrathymic mediastinal adenoma in 2% of cases.[17] Patients who receive low-dose irradiation to the neck are at greater risk for development of hyperparathyroidism.[18]

Parathyroid carcinoma is the least common cause of hypercalcemia, accounting for 0.4% of cases in adult series, and only isolated cases reported in children.[17] Hypercalcemia can also be related to malignancy with either a humoral production of *parathyroid-related peptide* (PTHrP) or direct osteolytic effect on bone. *Humoral hypercalcemia of malignancy* (HHM) is seen in 5% to 20% of adults with cancer but is rare in children. In one large study of childhood cancers, it was found in 0.4% of children diagnosed with malignancy. Among these cases of malignancy, 44% were leukemias, 16% were rhabdomyarcomas, and the remainer included malignant rhabdoid, Hodgkin's disease, non-Hodgkin's lymphoma, hepatoblastoma, neuroblastoma, angiosarcoma, and brain tumor.[19]

In adults, mild to moderate hypercalcemia is often found incidentally in those undergoing routine screening, and as a result, the number diagnosed with hyperparathyroidism has dramatically increased over the last 20 years.[20] In contrast, hyperparathyroidism in children is most commonly diagnosed after symptoms become evident.[14]

Secondary hyperparathyroidism is related to chronic hypocalcemia and hyperphosphatemia in patients with renal failure, which increases parathyroid glandular activity. *Tertiary hyperparathyroidism* is caused by autonomous functioning of this chronically stimulated and hyperplastic parathyroid tissue.

Pathology of Hyperparathyroidism

The two principal histologic causes of hyperparathyroidism are parathyroid adenoma and hyperplasia, and it is generally not possible to distinguish these two on the basis of histologic examination of a single parathyroid gland.[21] The majority of adenomas are composed of chief cells, but some adenomas are composed of both oxyphilic and chief cells.[14, 17] The location of parathyroid adenomas is variable and includes an intrathyroid position (in 2.3% of clinical and autopsy studies) that is always associated with the inferior gland.[17]

Hyperparathyroidism associated with the endocrinopathies MEN1 and MEN2A is caused by chief-cell hyperplasia, with a very high incidence of multiglandular disease. Multiple glandular disease is observed in 90% of patients with MEN1 and in 83% of patients with MEN2A.[12] FIHP is caused by parathyroid adenomas and is thought to carry a high rate of malignant degeneration.[22] FHH is characterized by an elevated serum calcium level and an often normal PTH. These findings suggest either an abnormality of PTH suppression and cellular calcium transport or enhanced PTH action on the kidney. Hyperplasia is present in some parathyroid glandular tissue, but in more than 80% of patients the glands are within normal ranges of size and weight.[23]

The diagnosis of parathyroid carcinoma is made at the time of discovery of local invasion or metastatic disease. Metastases have been found in regional lymph nodes, lung, liver, pancreas, and bone. Mortality is related to the complications of hypercalcemia.[21] Parathyroid carcinoma is unusually firm and densely adherent to surrounding structures.

PHPT is characterized by catabolic activity

with increased osteoclastic and subperiosteal bone resorbtion. PHPT has also been shown to have anabolic activity, with osteosclerosis occurring in areas rich in cancellous bone, including long-bone metaphyses and vertebral bodies. As a result, the large increases in bone mass that take place during adolescence lead to increases in skeletal manifestations of PHPT in children.[24] HHM and the secretion of PTHrP cause intensive osteoclastic bone resorbtion but not the increased bone formation of PHPT.[20] Most adults experience no severe bone disease and present no radiologic abnormalities at time of diagnosis. Delayed parathyroid resection in neonatal hypercalcemic patients may cause metastatic calcifications in the lung, heart, and kidney.[9, 10]

Signs and Symptoms of Hyperparathyroidism

The constellation of symptoms is dependent on the patient's age at presentation. Neonates will commonly present with lethargy, hypotonia, diarrhea or constipation, poor feeding ability, respiratory distress, and overall failure to thrive.[10] Additionally, there can be significant bone demineralization leading to pathologic fractures of the extremities and ribs.[9]

In children and adolescents, symptoms may be vague and nonspecific. Abdominal pain, fatigue, anorexia, nausea and vomiting, constipation, and profound muscle weakness may be accompanied by significant weight loss.[14, 20, 24] Progressive parathyroid dependent bone loss poses a risk for development of pathologic extremity and rib fractures.[15] Radiologic findings include a salt-and-pepper appearance of the skull, subperiosteal resorbtion of long bones, and osteosclerosis of the long bones and spine.[24]

One review cited a 44% rate for children presenting with skeletal changes, whereas the corresponding rates for adults are significantly lower.[11] Other studies continue to emphasize skeletal lesions but cite a significant number of children who either had evidence of nephrocalcinosis preoperatively or developed sequelae necessitating treatment at a later date, including removal of renal calculi.[14, 16] Reviews of the literature showed renal lesions in 27% to 50% of children.[16, 20] Hypertension with and without accompanying headaches has been reported in pediatric reviews at rates of 3% to 8%. Cognitive difficulties and psychiatric symptoms can be very subtle and include worsening attention deficits, apathy, fatigue, drowsiness, depression, obtundation, and coma. Parathyroid carcinoma is usually associated with more profound clinical manifestations of hypercalcemia as compared with parathyroid adenoma.[25] In one adult series, 45% of patients with parathyroid carcinomas had a palpable tumor on clinical examination.[26]

Diagnosis of Hyperparathyroidism

The diagnosis of hyperparathyroidism is made biochemically following analysis of serum calcium and PTH concentrations.[20] Serum calcium level should be measured as a fasting value, obtained while the patient is off diuretics, and collected with minimal venous occlusion.[15] Marked elevations in serum calcium levels have been documented in neonates. One infant had a preoperative calcium level of 30.5 mg/dl.[9] Serum ionized calcium is a more sensitive indicator of abnormal parathyroid pathology in the presence of abnormal albumin concentrations. The appropriate measurement of parathyroid hormone is intact PTH, which must be analyzed with a two-site *immunoradiometric assay* (IRMA). IRMA offers an enhanced ability to distinguish hyperparathyroidism from PTHrP and HHM.[19] Additional biochemical abnormalities include a low serum phosphate and bicarbonate and an elevated serum chloride.

The differential diagnosis of hypercalcemia includes hyperparathyroidism (primary, secondary, and tertiary), malignancy, milk-alkali syndrome, hypervitaminosis D, sarcoid and other granulomatous disease, thyrotoxicosis, effect of administration of lithium or thiazide diuretics, FHH and maternal hypocalcemia stimulating fetal PTH production (Table 21–1).[10]

Preoperative localization studies are reserved for reoperation. Up to 70% of parathyroid tumors can be localized, but studies taken as a group are unreliable, with a 15% false-positive rate. In one adult series, only 20% of multiple gland enlargements were correctly identified.[15, 21] Localization techniques include ultrasound, CT scan, MRI, technetium-thallium subtraction, and technetium sestamibi scintigraphy. Ultrasound can be useful, but it is very operator dependent. Technetium-thallium scintigraphy is hindered by the requirement for subtraction techniques.

Table 21–1 • Hyperparathyroidism

Causes of Hypercalcemia

Hyperparathyroidism (1°, 2°, 3°)
Malignancy
Milk alkali syndrome
Hypervitaminosis D
Sarcoid/granulomatous diseases
Thyrotoxicosis
Thiazide diuretics or lithium
Familial hypocalciuric hypercalcemia
Maternal hypocalcemia

Sestamibi is a cationic lipophilic isonitrile derivative of technetium that is taken up and stored in abnormal parathyroid tissues. Sestamibi offers the advantage of obtaining planar images without subtraction techniques. It allows three-dimensional SPECT, affording much clearer images. One study examining sestamibi cited a sensitivity of 86% and a specificity range of 77% to 100%.[27]

Treatment of Hyperparathyroidism

Preoperative management of severe hypercalcemia includes correction of dehydration, enhancement of calcium excretion from the kidney with correction of sodium losses, and inhibition of osteoclastic bone resorbtion. Saline infusion and aggressive volume resuscitation should be followed by administration of a loop diuretic to increase urinary excretion of calcium. Both calcitonin and mithramycin have osteoclast-inhibiting activity, but resistance can develop with calcitonin, and mithramycin has significant toxic side effects. Etidronate disodium and pamidronate disodium are biphosphonates that bind to hydroxyapatite and are potent and effective inhibitors of osteoclastic bone resorption. These cause significant decreases in serum calcium concentration within 24 hours of intravenous administration.[20] Corticosteroids are effective with vitamin D intoxication and sarcoid but have no role in treating patients with PHPT.

Surgical intervention for cure is the current and accepted treatment for PHPT.[15] Most centers advocate complete neck exploration including identification of all four parathyroid glands for determination of hyperplastic versus normal tissue.[21] Children with adenomas should have normal-appearing parathyroid glands biopsied.[17]

If all four glands appear normal and give normal results on biopsy, the search should be extended for additional parathyroid tissue.

Neonatal hyperparathyroidism is a surgical emergency requiring immediate management. Delay can result in irreversible metastatic calcifications involving the lung, heart, and kidney. In one review, 8 of 17 infants with neonatal hyperparathyroidism died of disease prior to operation.[10] The choice of parathyroidectomy is either subtotal resection, leaving one fourth to one half of one gland with the significant risk of recurrence, or total resection, with lifelong supplementation necessary of vitamin D and calcium.[9]

Patients with MEN1 should undergo identification of all four parathyroid glands and at least subtotal parathyroid resection. Many researchers advocate total parathyroidectomy and transcervical thymectomy.[12, 21] Patients with MEN2A should undergo complete neck exploration, with resection of only those glands that are enlarged and hyperplastic.[12] Normal parathyroid tissue should be left alone, and routine transcervical thymectomy should not be performed in patients with MEN2A.[17] FIHP may represent a more aggressive course of parathyroid disease than MEN1, with an increased risk of malignancy. Surgical management includes adequate resection of the parathyroid tissue involved.[22]

The correct management of FHH is a point of controversy. Total parathyroidectomy is the only option for successful lowering of serum calcium, but it leaves the child requiring prolonged supplementation. With the pedigree for FHH established, and with a nonprogressive or falling serum calcium level, some researchers advocate close observation rather than surgery for the asymptomatic neonate or child. If the serum calcium level fails to fall after birth, or the neonate or child becomes symptomatic, surgery is recommended.[23]

The only curative therapy for parathyroid carcinoma is en bloc resection of the primary tumor with an effort to minimize seeding of tumor.[25] Some investigators advocate removal of the thyroid isthmus and ipsilateral thyroid lobe, excision of skeletal muscle intimately related to tumor, and excision of nodes in the tracheoesophageal groove.[26]

Surgical failure can result from abnormal gland location, multiglandular disease, supernumerary glands, or metastatic parathyroid carcinoma, and from surgical inexperience. Evaluation of vocal cord function should be performed prior to neck re-exploration.[21]

Postoperatively, the patient must be watched closely for signs or symptoms of hypocalcemia, which is the most common complication of parathyroidectomy.[28] Ischemic injury to remaining parathyroids after removal of adenoma results in transient hypocalcemia, which may last up to 6 months. Surgical removal of excessive parathyroid tissue can result in lifelong hypocalcemia requiring calcium and vitamin D supplementation.

Extensive skeletal remineralization in patients with severe PHPT produces low serum calcium and low phosphate levels and is referred to as *hungry bone syndrome*.[28] This syndrome reflects a brief period of intense deposition of extracellular calcium and phosphate into bone and is usually gone within 1 week.[21, 24, 28] Symptoms of hypocalcemia are related to abnormal neurologic sensation and neuromuscular excitability, including extremity and circumoral numbness, tetany, and seizures. The patient with hypocalcemia should be managed with aggressive calcium supplementation and administration of vitamin D.[28]

Parathyroid Malignancy

Residual or recurrent parathyroid carcinoma manifests with hypercalcemia as a result of PTH secretion from tumor mass. One adult series had a 5-year survival rate of 50%, and a 10-year survival rate of 13%.[20] Patients with metastatic disease generally die of complications resulting from hypercalcemia.[20, 25] Parathyroid carcinoma tends to recur in the operative site and may be cured or palliated for extended periods of time by re-excision with radical resection of the involved area. Isolated metastases have been reported to lung, adrenal, liver, brain, and bone, and if these lesions are well localized, resection may result in cure or palliation.[26]

Long-term survival has been reported as a result of multiple reoperations for excision of recurrent localized disease.[20] Radiation therapy and chemotherapy have been used in lieu of surgery with disappointing results.[26] Extended biphosphonate therapy can be used to control hypercalcemia.[20] Inactivation of the retinoblastoma gene can serve as a potentially useful molecular marker for parathyroid carcinoma. Application of this genetic marker of parathyroid carcinoma could allow identification of a subgroup of patients in whom early adjuvant therapy should be considered, or the marker could serve as a target for pharmacologic therapy.[25]

Prognosis for Patients with Hyperparathyroidism

The prognosis for patients with hyperparathyroidism following appropriate surgical management is excellent. Some series show a 100% rate of long-term normocalcemia.[14] Hungry bone syndrome with hypocalcemia and hypophosphatemia may be seen in the first postoperative week but is self-limited, with return of normocalcemia by 7 days. Skeletal manifestations are generally completely resolved by 3 months.[24]

Patients with MEN1 in one study had a surgical cure rate of up to 94%, but a 10-year follow-up showed recurrent hypercalcemia rates of up to 16%.[12] MEN2A patients in the same study who underwent resection of hyperplastic parathyroid were all cured, without recurrences. Total parathyroidectomy necessitates lifetime supplementation with calcium and vitamin D.

The causes of persistent hypercalcemia include residual or recurrent disease, missed adenoma or hyperplasia, or incorrect diagnosis. Sarcoid is diagnosed in 4% of cases of persistent hypercalcemia. The overall failure rate of cervical exploration in one report was 4%.[17] Mortality from metastatic or residual parathyroid cancer does not result from direct tumor effects but from excessive PTH production, with resultant hypercalcemia causing cardiac arrhythmias; nephrocalcinosis and renal failure; and metastatic calcium deposition in the heart, lungs, and brain.[26]

ADRENAL CORTICAL TUMORS

Adrenal cortical tumors account for approximately 5% of childhood endocrine tumors.[3] The incidence of *adrenal cortical carcinomas* (ACC) has a bimodal distribution with peaks in the first and fifth decades of life. Within the pediatric population, the median patient age at presentation is 4 years.[29] Annual estimated incidence ranges between 3 and 7 per million children.[30, 31] A study of 72 children with ACC revealed a peak incidence in the first year of life, tapering with increasing age, and an adolescent group with a more even distribution between 9 and 16 years.[32]

Approximately 25% of childhood adrenal cortical tumors are adenomas, the remainder are carcinomas. Although either type can secrete hormones or be inactive, adenomas are generally far more efficient than carcinomas in producing steroid hormones. Hence, carcinomas tend to be larger at discovery since they are less likely to produce symptoms of hormone excess.

Pathology of Adrenal Cortical Tumors

Adrenal adenomas are generally small, encapsulated, steroid-secreting tumors with characteristically increased smooth endoplasmic reticulum and lipid droplets within the cells.[33] Tumors infiltrate into adjacent tissues and spread locally. Cells are pleomorphic, with scant cytoplasm and frequent mitoses. Areas of tumor necrosis are common. Increased mitotic activity, vascular invasion, and extent of tumor necrosis are the most useful parameters in distinguishing benign from malignant neoplasms, but few histologic markers are diagnostic for malignancy.[34]

As a result of associations with congenital hemihypertrophy,[35] Li-Fraumeni syndrome,[36] and Beckwith-Wiedemann syndrome,[37] germline mutations of the p53 tumor-suppresser gene were discovered in a large percentage of ACC patients.[38, 39] These children may represent probands with which to identify Li-Fraumeni syndrome families. Loss of heterozygosity at chromosome 11p15 has been described in adrenal cortical tumors associated with Beckwith-Wiedemann syndrome.[40] Overexpression of IGF-II mRNA (from the 11p15.5 locus) was noted in 5 of 6 carcinomas and 2 of 17 adenomas.[41] DNA extraction studies have shown that most adrenal adenomas and carcinomas are monoclonal.[42]

Signs and Symptoms of Adrenal Cortical Tumors

Almost all children with adrenal cortical tumors present with signs and symptoms of endocrine excess. Cushing's syndrome in children less than 15 years old is caused by an adrenal cortical tumor in over 80% of cases.[43, 44] Adrenal tumors are the most frequent cause of Cushing's syndrome in infants.[45, 46, 47] The situation is reversed with adults, in whom pituitary-dependent ACTH overproduction (Cushing's disease) is the cause of Cushing's syndrome in 60% to 70% of cases.[48] In contrast to adults, over 90% of children with adrenal cortical neoplasms have endocrine manifestations or biochemical evidence of hypercorticalism. Large series of adults report the incidence of functionally active tumors to range from 24% to 96%.[49, 50] Rarely, children present with abdominal or flank pain, shock due to retroperitoneal hemorrhage, or hypertension.

ACCs are very inefficient in producing active hormones such as cortisol. About 50% will have attained palpable size by the time they result in an endocrine syndrome and thus may present late in the course of disease. ACCs are much more likely to be functional in children. In an exhaustive review, 85% of these carcinomas in children were functional compared with only 15% in adults over 30 years old.[29] In children less than 5 years old, 95% of ACCs are accompanied by virilization. In those older than 5 years, ACCs secrete cortisol (50% to 60%) and adrenal androgens but rarely secrete aldosterone, testosterone, or estrogen. Thus, patients may present with either virilization or mixed endocrine syndrome of virilization and Cushing's syndrome. ACCs have been reported to cause hypokalemic alkalosis in the absence of hypercortisolism by secreting deoxycorticosterone or corticosterone.[51] About 40% of adrenocortical carcinomas secrete no active hormones but produce inactive precursors such as pregnenolone, 17-hydroxypregnenolone, and 11-deoxycortisol detected in serum or as metabolites in urine.

The most common manifestations of hypercortisolism in younger children include hypertension, truncal obesity, moon facies, acne, hirsutism, and buffalo hump.[43, 47] Features of virilization include increased muscle mass, facial hair, voice deepening, pubic hair, and clitoral/penile enlargement. Virilization can also be caused by congenital adrenal hyperplasia. Three cases of ACC have occurred in children with congenital adrenal hyperplasia.[52] Severe thrombocytopenic purpura and Cushing's syndrome have been reported as symptoms in an infant with an adrenal cortical adenoma.[53]

Diagnosis of Adrenal Cortical Tumors

Ultrasound, CT, and MRI are all excellent modalities for evaluation of possible adrenal tumors.

In micronodular disease, the adrenals can be difficult to image, but they tend to appear rugged. Tumor extension into the inferior vena cava in patients with ACC is best demonstrated with ultrasound. Endocrine laboratory evaluation can confirm the underlying endocrinopathy, and in patients without a mass, can distinguish Cushing's syndrome resulting from micronodular dysplasia from Cushing's disease and ectopic ACTH production. A radioactive iodocholesterol scan allows imaging of cortisol-secreting adenomas and 50% of micronodular disease but not of carcinomas. Gallium-67 (Ga-67) scintigraphy was useful in detecting the recurrence of one case of adrenocortical carcinoma.[54] The tumor was Ga-67 avid at diagnosis.

Treatment of Adrenal Cortical Tumors

All primary adrenal tumors are treated by surgical resection. Micronodular dysplasia is cured by bilateral adrenalectomy. Adrenal adenomas should be removed with the entire ipsilateral gland. The contralateral gland should be examined for bilateral disease. Carcinomas require complete ipsilateral resection. If curative resection including metastatic disease is not possible, debulking should be performed. Treatment for recurrent carcinoma includes re-resection or redebulking if surgically feasible.[55] Solitary metastases should be resected. Long-term disease-free status has been achieved after resection of hepatic, cerebral, and pulmonary metastases; 5-year survival rates of up to 71% have been reported for patients with resected pulmonary metastasis.[56]

A period of adrenal insufficiency commonly follows removal of an autonomous adrenal adenoma or carcinoma. This hypothalamic-pituitary adrenal axis dysfunction lasts several weeks to a year. Stress doses of hydrocortisone (100 mg/m2) are given for 2 days postoperatively, followed by maintenance doses (15 mg/m2). These can be tapered over several weeks to every-other-day dosing. Steroid maintenance can be tapered off after an ACTH-stimulation test demonstrates a normal response (plasma cortisol >18 ug/kg at 1 hour after 10 ug/kg cosyntropin [Cortrosyn] IV). Patients should wear a medical alert bracelet for as long as they require steroid replacement.

Malignant Adrenal Cortical Tumors

Mitotane (*o,p'*-DDD) is the drug of choice for patients with inoperable, residual, or unresectable recurrent or metastatic disease. It is an adrenocytolytic agent that neutralizes endocrine excess in approximately two thirds of patients.[57] Given in maximal doses (up to 10 gm/m²/day), it has been shown to cause tumor regression or arrest in as many as one third of patients. In a series of 96 patients, those who achieved serum trough levels greater than or equal to 14 ug/ml demonstrated an independently favorable survival rate according to both univariate and multivariate analysis.[58]

Intestinal absorption of mitotane is maximized by using a lipid vehicle such as chocolate, milk-powder, or oil-emulsion preparations.[59] Adjuvant mitotane after total resection did not influence survival in one series.[58] Side effects of mitotane included nausea, vomiting, diarrhea, skin reactions, lethargy somnolence, muscle weakness, and dizziness. Cisplatin,[60] fluorouracil,[61] streptozotocin,[62] and etoposide have also shown some activity against ACC. Radiation therapy can also be helpful for palliation of metastasis.[63] Patients who have continued hypercortisolism can be palliated with aminoglutethimide, metyrapone, RU486, or ketoconazole. Those who develop hypoaldosteronism or hypocortisolism require replacement therapy.

Prognosis for Patients with Adrenal Cortical Tumors

Patients with adrenal adenomas and micronodular disease are cured by resection. Adult patients with ACC have a 20% to 25% 5-year survival rate. Patients who had complete resections of tumor have a 5-year survival rate of 49% compared with a 9% survival rate following subtotal resection and no survivors in patients who had no resection.[49, 50] Children seem to have a higher survival rate than adults. Humphrey and coworkers[32] reported a 53% 5-year survival rate for infants with ACC and a 17% 5-year survival rate for adolescents. Lack and coworkers[34] reported 70% survival rate for patients with ACC who were less than 5 years old at diagnosis and a 7% survival rate for those more than 5 years old. Mean follow-up was 9 years. All long-term survivors had complete resection.

In some patients, tumors are difficult to classify simply as benign or malignant. Furthermore, secondary malignancies occur in patients with ACC at an incidence of 12% to 37%.[29, 34, 64, 65]

Thus, patients with adrenal cortical tumors require careful clinical long-term follow-up.

PHEOCHROMOCYTOMA

Pheochromocytoma is an endocrine tumor arising from chromaffin cells of the adrenal medulla and sympathetic ganglia. It can occur anywhere from the neck to the pelvis, terminating in the organ of Zuckerkandl. Symptoms are related to autonomous secretion of catecholamines, and the most common presenting symptom is marked, sustained hypertension.[66] Pheochromocytoma is cited as the cause of high blood pressure in 0.05% to 1.7% of hypertensive children, with an equal male-to-female ratio.[67, 68, 75b]

The majority of pheochromocytomas occur as sporadic single tumors within the adrenal medulla. Pheochromocytoma may also occur in a familial form as a component of both MEN2A (*medullary thyroid cancer* [MTC], parathyroid hyperplasia and pheochromocytoma) and MEN2B (MTC, pheochromocytoma, skeletal abnormalities, and a characteristic facial and marfanoid appearance). As a result, it is important in patients with MTC and MEN2 to exclude the diagnosis of pheochromocytoma.

Adrenal medullary disease exists as pheochromocytoma or its presumed precursor, adrenal medullary hyperplasia, and is almost always found bilaterally in association with MEN2A and MEN2B.[69] Synchronous or metachronous pheochromocytomas have been reported in 33% to 90% of patients with MEN2.[68, 69]

Pheochromocytoma may be found in association with neurofibromatosis, Hippel-Lindau disease (retinal angioma, CNS hemangioblastoma, renal-cell carcinoma, pancreatic cyst, and epididymal cystadenoma), tuberous sclerosis, and Sturge-Weber syndrome (hemangioma of the trigeminal nerve). Nonendocrine familial cases of pheochromocytoma have been reported, often as being located in the same anatomic position.[70] One large study of unselected patients who presented with pheochromocytomas found that 23% were carriers of familial syndromes (19% with Hippel-Lindau disease and 4% with MEN2).[71]

Pathology of Pheochromocytoma

The adrenal medulla is ectodermal in origin and is derived from neural crest tissue. It is inner-vated by preganglionic sympathetic fibers that control secretory activity of chromaffin cells. Stimulation causes increased tyrosine hydroxylase activity, with the resultant release of metabolically active substances. Stimulation of the adrenal medulla results in predominantly epinephrine secretion, whereas stimulation of the sympathetic ganglia results in norepinephrine. This difference arises because phenylethanolamine N-methyl transferase is responsible for the conversion of norepinephrine to epinephrine and is found only in the adrenal medulla. Once released into the circulation, norepinephrine and epinephrine have short plasma half-lives. They are removed from the circulation by immediate reuptake into chromaffin cells, systemic neuronal uptake and degradation, enzymatic degradation during circulation, or excretion in the urine unchanged (Fig. 21–1).

Systemic neuronal degradation by the enzyme monoamine oxidase yields vanillylmandelic acid. Enzymatic degradation by carboxy-O-methyl transferase produces metanephrine and normetanephrine. Pheochromocytoma may produce both norepinephrine and epinephrine in an autonomous fashion. It has been known to also produce ACTH, and thus a concomitant Cushing's syndrome.[72] Other peptides produced by pheochromocytoma include calcitonin gene-related protein, atrial natriuretic peptide, and vasoactive intestinal protein.[68]

More than 90% of pheochromocytomas occur below the diaphragm.[68] They are located in the adrenal medulla in 70% to 95% of pediatric cases compared with 85% to 90% of adult cases.[68, 73] The majority of extra-adrenal tumors are found in the para-aortic region and the organ of Zuckerkandl.[68, 73] Sporadic pheochromocytoma in children is associated with bilateral disease in up to 24% of cases compared with 10% in adults.[73] Pediatric pheochromocytomas have a reported malignancy rate of 6% to 13%.[73, 74]

Pheochromocytomas appear tan-gray, with a soft, smooth consistency, and may have calcifications. Microscopic analysis reveals cells arranged in cords with abundant secretory granules within the cytoplasm. DNA flow cytometric studies have shown malignant cases to be tetraploid or aneuploid. This finding is nonspecific as large numbers of benign tumors have similar ploidy characteristics. Capsular extension into the cortex and

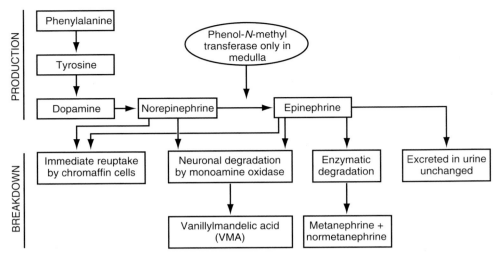

Figure 21–1 • Pheochromocytoma: Catecholamine production and breakdown sequence.

vascular invasion occur with equal frequency for both benign and malignant tumors.

Prognostic factors that have been identified for malignancy include large tumor size, local tumor infiltration and extension, and DNA ploidy.[68] Yet, neither histologic examination nor these prognostic factors are completely reliable in determining malignancy. Malignancy can be confirmed only by the presence of metastases, defined as disease found where the presence of chromaffin tissue is normally not found. Malignant tumors are seen more frequently with sporadic pheochromocytoma than with MEN2. They have been discovered as late as 28 years after resection.[75]

Histochemical and immunohistochemical identification of pheochromocytoma is achieved by focusing on the presence of chromogranin A, neuron-specific enolase, and S-100 protein. Chromogranin A is an acidic monomeric protein co-stored and co-released with catecholamines. Chromogranin A levels are not specific for pheochromocytoma, as they may be elevated any time excess catecholamine is released. One report cites the prognostic value of the serum chromogranin A level as a predictor of tumor size and overall catecholamine production.[73]

Signs and Symptoms of Pheochromocytoma

The signs and symptoms of pheochromocytoma are those of catecholamine excess. The most common presentation is sustained or paroxysmal hypertension; more than 90% of children with pheochromocytoma have sustained hypertension.[72] An abdominal mass may be palpable on physical examination but rarely cause the child to be brought to medical attention. The level of active hormone secretion is not related to tumor burden. Large tumors may be relatively inactive secondary to reuptake and metabolism of catecholamines.

Additional symptoms include headache, diaphoresis, palpitations with chest or epigastric pain, nausea, vomiting, diarrhea, hyperventilation, and attention deficit disorder. As a result of unopposed vasoconstriction, there may a nearly 15% reduction in circulating plasma volume, and the child may present with signs of hypovolemia or orthostatic hypotension.[73] Constipation may give rise to bowel obstruction. Hypertensive encephalopathy may cause intermittent visual disturbances, seizures, or coma. Elevated levels of circulating catecholamines may impair insulin response and lead to hyperglycemia, polyuria, polydipsia, or glycosuria.

Unusual presentation may suggest the location of the tumor, with pheochromocytomas of the bladder producing marked hypertension temporally associated with micturation. *Pheochromocytoma crisis* is a complication of unmanaged pheochromocytoma in which a massive release of catecholamines results in disseminated intravascular coagulopathy, seizures, rhabdomyolysis, acute renal failure, shock, and death.

The differential diagnosis includes hypertension associated with anxiety, severe migraine, hyperthyroidism, and reactions to medications, including illicit drugs, or withdrawal syndromes.[75b] Other causes of hypertension must also be considered, including coarctation of the aorta, renal artery stenosis, pyelonephritis, adrenogenital syndrome, renal and brain tumors, lead poisoning, and familial dysautonomia (Riley-Day syndrome).

Diagnosis of Pheochromocytoma

Biochemical and radiologic tests are complementary for the diagnosis and localization of pheochromocytoma. Biochemical testing includes analysis of plasma and urine for the presence of catecholamines and their metabolites. Pheochromocytomas secrete a heterogeneous group of substances, and many studies document varying sensitivities and specificities for plasma and urine analytes, with no single analyte achieving 100% sensitivity. Urine collection for 24 hours is evaluated for metanephrine, normetanephrine, vanillylmandelic acid, dopamine, epinephrine, and norepinephrine. A fasting blood specimen drawn intravenously is evaluated for epinephrine, norepinephrine, and chromogranin A.

A confirmatory test for patients who have intermediate levels of plasma catecholamines (500–2000 pg/ml) is the clonidine suppression test, which relies on the suppression of the sympathetic nervous system's production of norepinephrine.[72] Clonidine causes central inhibition of catecholamine release and has no effect on autonomous production of these substances. In a healthy individual there will be a >50% decrease in circulating plasma catecholamines but in a patient with pheochromocytoma there will be no change following clonidine administration.

Provocative tests previously utilized include metoclopromide and glucagon stimulation. These tests are now reserved for those patients highly suspect clinically of having pheochromocytoma but showing inconclusive results on all other biochemical and radiologic tests. Metoclopramide and glucagon stimulation are otherwise unnecessary and not indicated because of the risk of inducing hypertensive crisis.

Localization of pheochromocytoma is accomplished with CT, MRI, and metaiodobenzylguanidine (MIBG) scintigraphy. Tumors as small as 1 cm can be visualized using contrast-enhanced CT scan with thin cuts. The utility of CT is limited by the following factors: small (<1 cm) size; paucity of fat in the retroperitoneum of children, producing less surrounding contrast for tumors; oral contrast-obscuring, small adrenal tumors; inability to distinguish adenoma from metastatic disease; and effects of previous operation in the region.[70] MRI with T1-weighted images has increased sensitivity compared with CT, and T2-weighted images may distinguish pheochromocytoma from adenoma or carcinoma.[68] The expense of T2-weighted images, however, limits its standard use for screening.

MIBG is an iodinated norepinephrine analog that is accumulated in storage vesicles of chromaffin tissue. Potassium iodide is given before the test to saturate and therefore limit thyroid uptake of MIBG. Marked uptake of MIBG occurs in patients with pheochromocytoma, neuroblastoma, and carcinoid, with a specificity of up to 96%.[76] The distribution of MIBG in children differs from that in adults. Following administration, MIBG in pediatric patients shows marked activity in salivary glands, myocardium, liver, lungs, gut, and bladder.[76] Delayed images are obtained at 48 hours when normal adrenal is rarely visualized and gut activity is nearly absent. MIBG uptake is not related to histologic features of the tumor, tumor site, or tumor burden, or to urinary excretion of catecholamines and metabolites; it is not affected by the administration of antihypertensives.[75] A preoperative MIBG study is important because it reveals tumor uptake, identifies synchronous lesions, and postoperatively allows diagnosis of recurrence. With MIBG, it is no longer necessary to obtain arteriography or sequential caval sampling.[72]

Treatment of Pheochromocytoma

Preoperative screening recommendations to exclude other endocrinopathies include parathormone level, ophthalmoscopy, MRI of the brain, CT of the abdomen, ultrasound of the testes, pentagastrin-stimulation test, and careful pedigree history.[71] Cardiac status should be assessed with electrocardiogram and echocardiogram to diagnose cardiomyopathy, which may contribute to postoperative complications.[77]

Acceptable morbidity and mortality for patients undergoing surgical removal of pheochromocytoma is dependent on optimal preoperative preparation. Effective alpha-adrenergic blockade is begun 2–3 weeks before the anticipated surgery to control blood pressure and allow for gentle rehydration. This preparation can be done with phenoxybenzamine, starting at 1–2 mg/kg/ 24 hours given qid and titrated to effect. Beta-adrenergic blockade is given for resultant tachycardia, which may become very symptomatic but is started only after ensuring adequate alpha-adrenergic blockade. Calcium-channel blockers prevent the release of calcium-dependent catecholamines and may be of use in urgent situations. Metyrosine is also helpful, as it is a competitive inhibitor of tyrosine hydroxylase and can reduce catechol production by 50% to 80%.

Prior to induction of general anesthesia, phentolamine, sodium nitroprusside, esmolol or other adrenergic blocking agents, and antiarrhythmics should be readily available. Following tumor removal, dopamine and norepinephrine may be needed to maintain blood pressure. Central venous access and arterial catheterization are helpful in perioperative management.

The surgical procedure for pheochromocytoma is performed through a transabdominal approach. The right adrenal is exposed, with mobilization of the hepatic flexure followed by a Kocher maneuver. The left adrenal is exposed following mobilization of the splenic flexure. The tumor is mobilized with minimal manipulation, and the adrenal vein is ligated early in the operation to minimize the possibility of massive catecholamine release. Intraoperative manipulation of tumor has resulted in plasma catecholamine surges of up to 30,000 pg/ml.[77] Following removal of the tumor, a complete abdominal exploration is performed with particular attention paid to the contralateral adrenal, paraspinal, and para-aortic regions, the base of the mesentery, the urinary bladder, and the pelvis. Additional pathology should be examined if the blood pressure fails to decrease following tumor removal.

Unilateral adrenalectomy is the operation of choice for sporadic pheochromocytoma. Pheochromocytoma in patients with MEN2 is managed with bilateral adrenalectomy because of the high incidence of bilateral disease in those patients. The presence of synchronous bilateral tumors in patients with sporadic and nonendocrine familial pheochromocytoma calls for removal of the larger tumor by total adrenalectomy and of the smaller tumor by partial adrenalectomy. Controversy exists over management of the contralateral adrenal gland in nonendocrine familial patients with unilateral pheochromocytoma. One study with a 6-year follow-up saw no contralateral disease develop, and so the researchers advocate unilateral adrenalectomy with close observation of the other gland.[78] If bilateral adrenalectomy is indicated, some advocate adrenal cortical implantation of 1 mm cubes of tissue into the rectus or forearm.[78] The morbidity and mortality associated with this tumor lie in its hormonal activity, and justify resection of large primary tumors despite the presence of metastatic disease.[74]

The preoperative resolution of symptoms and normalization of blood pressure in one study were the only factors predictive of an uncomplicated outcome.[77] Postoperative complications occurred as a result of existing myocardial dysfunction and contributed to the development of pulmonary edema. Children with existing myocardial dysfunction were also found to require a greater (up to 10 ml/kg/hour) intraoperative volume (i.e., intravenous fluids, nonspecified crystalloid solutions) resuscitation.[77]

Malignant Pheochromocytoma

Treatment of malignant pheochromocytoma includes radiation therapy and chemotherapy, but only surgery is curative. Response rates are judged by tumor mass and biologic activity. Unresectable tumors may be made resectable by intensive chemotherapy similar to the protocols for neuroblastoma, including use of cyclophosphamide, vincristine, and dacarbazine. Adjuvant chemotherapy shoud be given for residual disease after surgery and for metastatic disease.[74]

Cure rates for metastatic disease range from 0% to 14% with the majority of patients having partial or minimal responses following chemotherapy.[75a] Some studies document 5-year survival rates of up to 44% with chemotherapy (streptozotocin, dacarbazine, 5-fluorouracil, vincristine, and cyclophosphamide) coupled with medical management of elevated catecholamines.[72] Other reviews report good palliation with a response rate of 50% following chemotherapy; however, cure requires complete surgical removal.[77]

Metastatic disease is more common to soft tissues (including pleura, lung, liver, brain) and bone, which produces osteolytic lesions. Resection of localized metastases should be considered because of the relatively slow growth or dormancy of pheochromocytoma coupled with the benefit of removing biochemically active tissues. Painful bony metastases may respond well to radiation therapy or chemotherapy.[72, 74]

The prognostic value of adrenal versus extra-adrenal location of a malignant primary tumor is disputed. One series documented statistically similar 5-year survival rates of 57% and 74% for adrenal and extra-adrenal malignancies, respectively.[79] Reported survival rates are significantly lower for extra-adrenal malignancies; in one study 5-year survival rates of 59% and 18% were reported for adrenal and extra-adrenal tumors.[79] Others have anecdotal reports of higher malignancy rates and lower survival rates for extra-adrenal tumors.[79] Most recurrences are within 3 years, but there are case reports of metastatic disease developing 28 years after primary resection.[75a]

Therapeutic administration of I^{131} MIBG in patients with tumors that localize MIBG has been undertaken, yielding a calculated local radiation delivery dose of up to several thousand cGy. Problems exist because of the heterogeneous delivery of isotope to tumor, particularly with marginal or minimal I^{131} uptake. Following two or more courses of I^{131} at 100 mCi, one study showed no cures, no impact on survival, and a 46% biochemical response.[75a] Side effects included myelosuppression.

Follow-up and Prognosis for Patients with Pheochromocytoma

Children with benign pheochromocytoma have a normal life expectancy postoperatively, with a cure rate approaching 100%. Because of the possibility of delayed metastatic disease, these children should be followed on a regular basis. Within the first week postoperatively, serum and urine catecholamine levels should be measured to obtain baseline readings. Patients should then be followed on a yearly basis. Blood pressures should be recorded on a frequent and regular basis. Long-term follow-up, including periodic CT, MRI, or MIBG studies, should be obtained as indicated. Patients with documented residual or metastatic disease must be followed closely and managed for catecholamine excess. With effective palliation, survival rates of up to 74% at 5 years have been reported.[79] Disease-free survival

rates of up to 75% have been reported, with variable 5-year survival rates of 45% to 82%.[74, 76]

PANCREATIC ENDOCRINE TUMORS

The true incidence of neuroendocrine tumors of the pancreas is unknown but has been estimated at less than 10 per million population year.[72, 80] These tumors arise from the pancreatic islet cells and share many cytochemical properties with other tumors from the APUD (amine precursor uptake and decarboxylation) cell line. Like other endocrine tumors, pancreatic tumors occur in either a sporadic form or a familial form associated with the MEN1 syndrome.

Pancreatic endocrine tumors are classified and described according to the clinical syndromes they produce. Clinical manifestations are secondary to excessive release of peptide hormones into the circulation. These hormones include insulin, gastrin, glucagon, somatostatin, vasoactive intestinal polypeptide, and others, in order of decreasing frequency. Pancreatic endocrine tumors contain dense secretory granules that may be visualized using electron microscopy. Although each tumor type produces a characteristic clinical syndrome, the majority of tumors contain multiple hormones as demonstrated by immunocytochemistry.[81, 82] The most common secondary hormone is pancreatic polypeptide, and the majority of tumors also contain somatostatin.

The heterogeneity of pancreatic polypeptides produced has allowed development of a number of common localization techniques for the detection of pancreatic endocrine tumors. Considerable controversy exists concerning indication, need, and accuracy, and there is no clear consensus on which method or combination of methods should be used. The more widespread use of and greater experience with intraoperative ultrasound may cause that technique to supplant many of the others. A brief discussion of these techniques is presented here, followed by a detailed discussion of the individual tumor types and their management.

Transabdominal Ultrasound

Transabdominal ultrasound is useful in the detection and localization of large intrapancreatic tumors. For tumors less than 2 cm in diameter the overall sensitivity of ultrasound is approximately

60%. In patients with gastrinoma or insulinoma the sensitivity of detecting primary pancreatic tumors has been reported at 20% to 30%[53, 54] and 20% to 70%,[85, 86] respectively. Transabdominal ultrasound can detect the presence of hepatic metastases with a sensitivity of about 60%. In this setting, it may be the only localization study required.

Computerized Tomography (CT)

The sensitivity of abdominal CT for pancreatic endocrine tumors has been reported at approximately 45% to 70%. CT can detect tumors as small as 1 cm in diameter and is slightly better than ultrasound in demonstrating hepatic metastases, with a sensitivity of 70%. In patients with primary gastrinoma or insulinoma, CT detected the lesion with a sensitivity of 30% to 60%[84, 87–89] and 30% to 75%,[13, 85, 90] respectively. Intravenous contrast material should be used, as most of these tumors appear as contrast-enhanced lesions. CT is also useful in detecting local spread to peripancreatic tissue.

Angiography

The reported sensitivity of angiography for the detection of primary pancreatic endocrine tumors varies widely and is dependent on the technique and the experience of the person performing the examination. Angiography can detect small tumors not found on ultrasound or CT. Angiography is most effective when contrast material is injected into branches of the celiac and superior mesenteric arteries following highly selective catheterization. In most cases the specificity approaches 100%; however, false-positive results have been reported.[88, 91] In patients with gastrinoma or insulinoma the sensitivity has been reported at 70% and 90%, respectively.[92]

Arterial-stimulated venous sampling is a technique in which a secretagogue is injected into branches of the celiac and superior mesenteric arteries and simultaneous hormone measurements are obtained from a catheter in the hepatic vein. This technique does not specifically localize a tumor but can determine the region in which it resides. As both arterial and venous cannulation are required for arterial-stimulated venous sampling, its utility in children is yet to be determined. Secretin injection with hepatic vein gas-

trin sampling has been successful in regionalizing gastrinoma in up to 92% of patients studied.[93] Selective arterial calcium injection has been utilized to identify tumors secreting insulin and pancreatic polypeptide.[94–96]

Transhepatic Portal Venous Sampling

This technique involves transhepatic cannulation of the portal vein and advancement of the catheter into the tributaries of the portal vein with sampling for hormone concentration. The maximum gradient of hormone between tributary and portal vein is used to regionalize the tumor.[97] The utility of this invasive technique in children is undetermined.

Endoscopic Ultrasound

Endoscopic ultrasound has been successful in detecting gastrinomas in the head of the pancreas as small as 6 mm in diameter.[98, 99] The technique is limited by the size of the scope, which is larger and more rigid than conventional adult endoscopes.

Somatostatin Analog Scintigraphy

The majority of pancreatic endocrine tumors contain somatostatin and somatostatin receptors. In vitro studies have demonstrated high affinity binding between radiolabeled somatostatin analogs and a variety of pancreatic tumors. Results of in vivo studies have been mixed. A study involving 25 adults who were intravenously injected with indium-111 DTPA-D-Phe-octreotide enabled the localization of a variety of pancreatic neurocrine tumors with a sensitivity of 80% and a positive predictive value of 100%.[100] This technique has also been employed to determine the extent of metastatic disease and to monitor the response to therapy.

Insulinoma

Insulinoma is the most common pancreatic endocrine tumor in the pediatric population.[101, 102] It is a tumor of beta-cell origin and occurs in sporadic and familial forms. The sporadic form accounts for 90% of cases and usually consists of a solitary, small (<2 cm), benign intrapancreatic tumor that has an equal distribution throughout the pancreas. Ten percent of patients with insulinomas have MEN1 syndrome. These patients typically have multiple pancreatic endocrine tumors. The management of this patient group differs from that of the sporadic group and is discussed in the section on Multiple Endocrine Neoplasm (MEN) Syndromes.

Signs and Symptoms of Insulinoma

The clinical syndrome of insulinoma is that of symptomatic hypoglycemia. Patients may experience a long history of hypoglycemic symptoms prior to diagnosis. Initial symptoms may occur following a fast as the patient tries to lose weight. Neuroglycopenic symptoms include limpness, twitching, apnea, diaphoresis, anxiety, dizziness, obtundation, seizures, and coma. In the newborn period, unrecognized persistent hypoglycemia can lead to severe neurologic compromise.

Diagnosis of Insulinoma

Documentation of Whipple's triad, which includes symptoms of hypoglycemia in the fasting state, serum glucose levels of less than 40 mg/dl, and resolution of hypoglycemic symptoms following glucose administration, is diagnostic of excessive insulin production.[103] This diagnosis is typically established during an in-hospital fast. Patients are given noncaloric fluids ad libitum, and serial serum glucose and insulin levels are obtained. The fast is continued for a total of 72 hours or until neuroglycopenic symptoms occur.[85] At this time, serum levels of glucose, insulin, proinsulin, and C-reactive protein are measured. Most patients have elevated levels of proinsulin and C-reactive protein. A normal or decreased C-reactive protein suggests exogenous insulin administration. The ratio of serum insulin to glucose may also be used as a diagnostic criterion for insulinoma, and a value of greater than 0.4 is diagnostic.[86] Suppression and stimulation tests are available for the diagnosis of insulinoma but are rarely necessary.

Treatment of Insulinoma

The mainstay of treatment of patients with sporadic insulinoma is surgical resection of the tumor. After the diagnosis of insulinoma is established, hypoglycemia may be treated by means of a variety of medical interventions. The diet is modified by increasing the frequency of meals. Diazoxide has been effective in increasing fasting glucose levels in approximately 60% of patients. Because of its long half-life, this drug should be discontinued 1 week prior to operation.[104] Octreotide has been effective in the management of infants with nesidioblastosis as well as patients with insulinoma.

Whether or not preoperative radiographic localization is needed in patients with sporadic insulinoma is unclear. Intraoperative palpation has a sensitivity of 75% to 95%, which rivals all preoperative localization studies. Without prior palpation, intraoperative sonography has a sensitivity of 75% to 90%, and the combination of palpation and intraoperative sonography has a sensitivity of 75% to 100%.[105] This high sensitivity exceeds the results of preoperative studies and makes it difficult to justify their cost and potential risks.

The goal of surgery is to locate and resect all tumor after a complete abdominal examination. The tumor may appear as a reddish-brown mass with increased vascularity. The pancreas is completely mobilized and inspected. Typically the tumor is within the pancreatic parenchyma and may be palpated as a firm, nodular mass. On intraoperative sonography, if employed, the tumor appears sonolucent compared with the more echo-dense normal pancreas. Insulinomas within the head or proximal body of the pancreas are enucleated. Tumors in the distal body or tail may be enucleated or removed as a distal pancreatectomy.

Results of Surgery for Insulinoma

Results of surgery for sporadic insulinoma are excellent. Following surgical resection of tumor, 96% to 100% of patients are reported cured of disease. Morbidity and mortality are low.[103]

Gastrinoma

Zollinger and Ellison described the association of intractable peptic ulcer disease, gastric acid hypersecretion, and pancreatic islet-cell tumor in 1955. They proposed that a substance produced by the tumor caused the ulcer disease.[105] This substance was subsequently identified as the peptide gastrin. Gastrinoma is the second most common pancreatic endocrine tumor found in children; overall incidence is approximately 0.5 to 1 per million population.[103] Of non-beta-cell origin, gastrinoma occurs in the sporadic form or as part of the MEN1 syndrome. Approximately 20% of patients with *Zollinger-Ellison syndrome* (ZES) have MEN1. Management of this subset of patients differs from that of patients with the sporadic form and is discussed in the section on Multiple Endocrine Neoplasm (MEN) Syndromes.

The majority of gastrinomas are found in the "gastrinoma triangle" centered on the first and second portion of the duodenum and the head of the pancreas. These tumors are often extrapancreatic. Up to 40% of patients have duodenal tumors without evidence of pancreatic disease. Other sites include the stomach, jejunum, liver, mesentery, spleen, and ovary. Primary tumors can be single or multiple. In cases of a single pancreatic tumor, it is usually greater than 1 cm in diameter and easily palpable. In cases of multiple tumors, particularly those in the duodenum and associated with MEN1, they may be very small, in the range of 1 to 3 mm. Approximately 30% to 60% of patients have liver metastases at the time of diagnosis. These tumors tend to be slow-growing. Patients with unresectable liver metastases have a 5-year survival rate of 20% to 40%.

Signs and Symptoms of Gastrinoma

Signs and symptoms of gastrinoma are secondary to gastric acid hypersecretion. Epigastric abdominal pain is the most common symptom of patients with ZES. This pain may be associated with indigestion caused by underlying esophagitis and may be relieved with antacids taken after meals. Up to 90% of patients have clinical, radiographic, or endoscopic evidence of peptic ulcer disease at the time of diagnosis. Often the ulcer disease is atypical. Ulcers may be in unusual locations, or may be multiple, or may recur after appropriate medical or surgical therapy. Patients may be referred only after an extended history of indolent peptic ulcer disease.

Up to 40% of patients with ZES do not have clinical evidence of peptic ulcer disease at the time of diagnosis.[106] Diarrhea is the second most common symptom and may be the only symptom in 20% of patients. Diarrhea is secondary to the excessive volume of gastric acid secreted. Weight loss is also common.

Diagnosis of Gastrinoma

The advent of an accurate immunoassay for serum gastrin has simplified the diagnosis of ZES. The diagnosis of ZES is established by the findings of an elevated fasting serum gastrin level and gastric acid hypersecretion.[103] Prior to testing, all ulcer medications must be discontinued. Basal acid output is then measured over a timed interval by determining the amount of sodium hydroxide required to neutralize gastric output. Gastric acid hypersecretion is defined as greater than 15 mEq/hour acid output. If previous antiulcer surgery has been performed, this number is reduced to 5 mEq/hour. A fasting serum gastrin level of greater than 500 pg/ml is diagnostic of ZES. Levels in the range of 200 pg/ml to 500 pg/ml are suggestive. Conditions that may produce a falsely elevated gastrin level include achlorhydria, hypochlorhydria, gastritis, prior gastric surgery, and failure to discontinue antacid medications. In these situations provocative tests, including either secretin administration or calcium infusion, may be useful. A rise in serum gastrin level to more than 1500 pg/ml following intravenous secretin administration (2 U/kg) is diagnostic. An upper gastrointestinal series or endoscopic evaluation may show ulceration of the duodenal bulb, prominent gastric rugal folds, or mucosal edema of the small bowel.

Treatment of Gastrinoma

Historically, removal of the end organ by total gastrectomy was the preferred treatment for patients with ZES. The development of effective medications that block gastric acid production has led to abandonment of this surgical approach. Histamine receptor antagonists such as cimetidine, ranitidine, and famotidine are effective in preventing gastric acid hypersecretion. Omeprazole has also been found effective. It has the advantage of requiring only once- or twice-daily dosing, which may improve patient compliance. The long-term side effects of these medications in the treatment of patients with ZES are unclear. Once control of gastric acid hypersecretion has been achieved, surgical intervention can be considered.

The goals of surgical intervention are to prevent gastric hypersecretion and limit the spread of disease by complete tumor excision. The operation for gastrinoma has evolved following recognition that many of these tumors are extrapancreatic in origin. A complete exploration of the entire abdomen is first performed. Gastrinoma generally appears as a small reddish nodule with increased vascularity. A Kocher maneuver is performed, and the pancreas is completely mobilized and inspected. Suspicious-looking nodules on the surface of the pancreas should be excised. Next the gland is bimanually palpated. Intraoperative ultrasound is then performed. Any intrapancreatic lesions are excised or removed by distal pancreatectomy.

The duodenum is evaluated by intraoperative endoscopy with transillumination. Intramural lesions are marked and excised. Regardless of the findings on endoscopy, duodenotomy is performed to rule out small medial-wall mucosal or submucosal lesions. This technique ensures little morbidity and no mortality, and gastrinomas can be found here in virtually all patients with nonfamilial disease. Antacid therapy should be continued postoperatively, as approximately 50% of patients continue to have elevated acid secretion due to increased parietal-cell mass. When basal acid output returns to normal, these medications can be stopped.[107]

The proper management of metastatic disease in patients with gastrinoma is debated. There is a poor response rate to chemotherapy, which includes doxorubicin, 5-fluorouracil, streptozotocin, and interferon. Medical control of acid hypersecretion allows symptom-free short-term survival in patients with metastatic disease, but many then die from malignant progression of disease. Many recommend aggressive surgical resection of localized metastatic disease, including resectable liver disease.[103] Decreased mortality and prolonged disease-free survival rates have been reported for this aggressive surgical approach.

Results of Surgery for Gastrinoma

Approximately 60% of patients are found to have metastatic disease at the time of diagnosis. Postoperative cure rates of up to 90% have been reported for patients in whom all disease has been removed. Long-term follow-up, however,
shows that at least 50% of these patients develop recurrence. Despite recurrences, the 10-year survival rate commonly exceeds 40%.[103, 106]

Other Pancreatic Endocrine Tumors

Other pancreatic endocrine tumors include glucagonoma, somatostatinoma, *vasoactive intestinal peptide* (VIP)–secreting tumor (VIPoma), and pancreatic polypeptide–secreting tumor. All of these tumors produce symptoms related to the hormone they secrete. They are rare, especially in children.

Glucagonomas are pancreatic tumors that secrete excessive amounts of glucagon. They produce a syndrome that is characterized by a distinctive skin rash, migratory necrolytic dermatitis, and weight loss, stomatitis, anemia, and hyperglycemia.[8] Glucagonomas are rare in older individuals and, to the authors' knowledge, have not been reported at all in children. Disease may be confined to the pancreas or be metastatic. Surgical removal is indicated when feasible. Octreotide has been given to control symptoms associated with metastatic disease.[108]

Somatostatinoma is also a disease of the adult population and is characterized by hyperglycemia, diarrhea, and malabsorption. Hepatic metastases are generally found at the time of diagnosis. Resection is indicated if possible, and chemotherapy with streptozotocin may be helpful.[8]

VIPoma is a pancreatic endocrine tumor that secretes excessive amounts of VIP and is associated with a syndrome of *watery diarrhea, hypokalemia, and achlorhydria* (WDHA). This syndrome, also referred to as pancreatic cholera syndrome and Verner-Morrison syndrome, has been reported in infants and children.[109, 110] Complete resection is curative but not always possible; 50% of patients have metastatic disease at the time of diagnosis.[111] Surgical debulking and streptozotocin and somatostatin analog therapy have been useful in the management of metastatic disease.

CARCINOID TUMORS

Carcinoid tumors arise from enterochromaffin cells, which are found throughout the gastrointestinal tract, biliary tree, thorax, and genitourinary tract. These tumors were initially called *car-*

cinoids because they resembled cancers but were thought to be benign. Carcinoids manifest in many ways including intussusception, obstruction, bleeding, metastatis, hormone secretion, or, most commonly, as an asymptomatic, incidental finding at exploration.[112]

The incidence of carcinoids in the pediatric population is estimated at 0.87 to 1.6 cases/100,000 children/year.[113] This estimate is based on clinical findings. True incidence is higher, because many people with carcinoids are asymptomatic.[72, 112] In one report of adults, 16% of carcinoids identified at a single institution were discovered at autopsy.[112]

In both adult and pediatric series, carcinoids are the most common gastrointestinal neuroendocrine tumor, the most common tumor of the appendix, and the most common form of bronchial adenoma.[113–115] A majority of carcinoids originate in the gastrointestinal tract.[72, 112] In one adult series of carcinoids occurring in the gastrointestinal tract, 35% were in the ileum, 31% in the appendix, 9% in the cecum, and 5% each in the duodenum, jejunum, and rectum.[112]

One review of pediatric appendiceal carcinoids cited a female-to-male ratio of 1.6:1 and a median patient age of 13.5 years at time of diagnosis.[115] In this same study most diagnoses were incidental, made at time of appendectomy for acute abdominal symptoms. In adults, a carcinoid is found in every 200 to 300 appendectomy specimens, and most of these are at the distal tip of the appendix.[72, 113] In children, a carcinoid is found in every 200 to 1000 appendectomy specimens.[113]

Pathology of Carcinoid Tumors

Carcinoid tumors have electron-dense neurosecretory granules and can synthesize a heterogeneous mix of biologic amines, peptides, and hormones. Products of carcinoid tumors include neuron-specific enolase, serotonin, chromogranin, insulin, gastrin, growth hormone (GH), growth hormone releasing hormone (GRH), human chorionic gonadotropin (hCG), adrenocorticotropin hormone (ACTH), and tachykinins (Table 21–2).[72]

Carcinoid has been found in the lungs, mediastinum, thymus, gastrointestinal tract, testes, ovaries, kidney, bladder, urethra, prostate, cervix, and vagina.[72, 114, 116] Large series of carcinoid tu-

---

Table 21–2 • Carcinoids

Hormones Known to Be Produced by Carcinoid Tumors

Adrenocorticotropic hormone (ACTH)
Chromogranin
Gastrin
Growth hormone (GH)
Growth hormone releasing hormone (GH-RH)
Human chorionic gonadotropin (hCG)
Insulin
Neuron specific enolase
Serotonin
Tachykinin

---

mors show most carcinoids as being appendiceal, small bowel, rectal, and bronchial in origin.[72, 112, 114, 115] Small bowel carcinoid often results in fibrosis and desmoplasia of surrounding mesentery, which can produce obstruction, necrosis, or perforation.[72]

The probability of regional nodal involvement is directly proportional to the size of the primary tumor. Tumors less than 1 cm are metastatic in 15% to 18% of small bowel cases and in less than 2% of appendiceal cases, whereas tumors greater than 2 cm are metastatic in 86% to 95% of small bowel cases and in 33% of appendiceal cases.[72, 117] Depth of invasion does not necessarily portend recurrence or metastatic disease. In one review of pediatric appendiceal carcinoids, 67% of tumors invaded to the subserosa, with 18% to appendiceal fat. No residual or recurrent disease was detected during extended follow-up, to 30 years, in these patients.[117] In this same review, 76% of tumors were at the tip of the appendix and only 6% at the base.

Carcinoid syndrome is a constellation of symptoms including flushing and diarrhea. Cardiac and retroperitoneal fibrosis occur when sufficient concentrations of hormonal products released by the carcinoid tumor reach the systemic circulation. Serotonin is directly and indirectly involved in producing the carcinoid syndrome. Serotonin has a direct role in the production of diarrhea and retroperitoneal fibrosis and a complementary role in causing asthma.[72] The role of serotonin in flushing is unexplained, but it is thought to provoke attacks through mediating release of other vasoactive substances, including kinins, prostaglandins, and histamine.[72] Serotonin is metabolized by monoamine oxidase to 5-hydroxyindole-acetic acid (5-HIAA), which is excreted in urine. Ovarian and bronchial carcinoids have rarely produced carcinoid syndrome without metastatic disease.

Additional hypersecretion states seen with carcinoids include excesses of ACTH and GRH. Carcinoids are the most common cause of ectopic ACTH syndrome, accounting for 54% of cases.[72, 118] Gastric carcinoids may be associated with hypergastrinemic states and pernicious anemia, duodenal carcinoids with the Zollinger-Ellison syndrome, and foregut carcinoids with MEN1.[72]

Signs and Symptoms of Carcinoid Tumors

Patients present with carcinoid tumors in different ways depending on the site of occurrence. The majority of children with appendiceal carcinoid present with acute abdominal symptoms of appendicitis. Carcinoid syndrome is extremely rare in this age group and type of presentation.[115, 117] Small bowel carcinoid, with or without regional extension, can cause the mesentery to become markedly fibrotic, with distortion of intestine and mesentery, and can cause clinical symptoms of small bowel obstruction or ischemia and bowel necrosis from mesenteric infarction. Additional symptoms of small bowel carcinoid include obstruction from tumor mass, intussusception, bleeding, and metastatic disease. Duodenal, gastric, and rectal carcinoids are usually found incidentally on endoscopy. In an adult series, up to 18% of patients with small bowel and rectal carcinoids presented with carcinoid syndrome.[112] Patients with bronchial and thoracic carcinoids may present with hemoptysis, but more commonly are detected on chest radiograph or suspected because of hormonal manifestations.

Carcinoid syndrome is characterized by asthma, diarrhea, flushing with deepening erythema of the upper body, unpleasant feelings of warmth, lacrimation, pruritus, and palpitations. Endocardial fibrosis produces predominantly right-sided cardiac disease, especially tricuspid regurgitation and pulmonic stenosis. *Carcinoid crisis* is a life-threatening emergency associated with intense flushing, diarrhea, abdominal pain, altered mental status progressing to coma, tachycardia, hypertension, or profound hypotension. Additional

presentations of hormonally active carcinoids include acromegaly from secretion of GH or GRH and Cushing's syndrome from secretion of ACTH.

Diagnosis of Carcinoid Tumors

No preoperative diagnostic workup is warranted with most cases of carcinoid. *Appendiceal carcinoids* in children are most often discovered incidentally by the surgeon at operation for acute appendicitis or postoperatively by the pathologist. *Duodenal and gastric carcinoids* are often found during esophagogastroduodenoscopy. They can rarely be detected on radiologic contrast studies. *Small bowel carcinoids* are often suspected on the basis of a desmoplastic mesenteric reaction or tumor mass or noted during laparotomy performed for acute abdominal pain. *Rectal carcinoids* are often discovered during proctoscopy. *Bronchial and thoracic carcinoids* are suspected because of (1) pulmonary or mediastinal mass and (2) secretion of hormonally active substances and can be confirmed with CT scan, MRI, or thoracotomy. *Ovarian and testicular carcinoids* are often detected as a mass on physical examination.

For patients with carcinoid syndrome, biochemical confirmation of carcinoid tumors should be obtained and can be followed by localization studies. Flushing and other symptoms of suspected carcinoid syndrome are evaluated with urinalysis for serotonin and 5-HIAA. Additional biochemical testing is indicated based on clinical suspicions. Localization studies for small bowel and metastatic carcinoid are successful with I^{123} MIBG. Carcinoids also possess somatostatin receptors, which allow effective tumor localization (>90%) with I^{123} Tyr-3 octreotide scintigraphy.[72, 119]

Treatment of Carcinoid Tumors

Surgery is considered to be the only potentially curative therapy for carcinoids. Resection of tumor with regional lymph node disease can result in long-term survival. For childhood appendical carcinoids <2 cm in size, appendectomy leaving disease-free margins is curative. For appendiceal tumors >2 cm, adult reviews advocate right hemicolectomy.[112] The pediatric literature cites long-term disease-free survival of patients with locally advanced tumors and tumors >2 cm following simple appendectomy leaving disease-free margins.[115, 117] Among children in these studies who underwent hemicolectomy because of tumor size, no residual tumor was seen. These investigators argue that appendectomy is curative for the great majority of children even when there is local invasion or larger tumor size.[115, 117] Careful consideration should be given to the small minority of patients at risk for metastatic disease before proceeding with right hemicolectomy. Jejunoileal tumors should receive wide en bloc resection because of their much stronger association with metastasis and carcinoid syndrome.[72, 120] Additionally, a thorough examination should be made of remaining bowel for additional carcinoids because of occasional multicentric disease.[112] Small gastric, duodenal, and rectal carcinoids up to 1 cm can be locally excised. Larger gastric and rectal tumors can be evaluated for anatomic resection, including gastrectomy and proctectomy, respectively.[72]

Surgical management of pulmonary and thoracic carcinoid includes complete exploration, anatomic resection of the involved lobe/structure, and lymph node dissection.[114, 121] Up to 54% of adult patients with bronchial carcinoids in one study had positive lymph nodes, and most of these experienced long-term survival.[121] Anecdotal reports on management of many different types of carcinoids suggest complete anatomic resection with lymph node dissection and postoperative radiation and chemotherapy as indicated.[72, 116, 121]

Malignant Carcinoids

Pathologists cannot distinguish benign from malignant carcinoids based on histologic examination, and they have difficulty differentiating pancreatic endocrine tumors, small-cell tumors of the lung, and carcinoids histologically. Malignancy is diagnosed when there is lymph node involvement or metastatic disease. Rare pediatric reports of metastatic disease or carcinoid syndrome cite primary tumors in the ileum and colon.[120] Postoperative treatment with conventional chemotherapy including 5-fluorouracil, streptozotocin, vincristine, or Adriamycin (doxorubicin) achieves limited success.[120] Radiation therapy has been used in patients having mediastinal and thoracic disease with metastases to

nodes and in those having symptomatic bone and skin metastases.[72, 121]

Octreotide has provided relief of symptoms from carcinoid syndrome by producing a decrease in serum and urine markers of carcinoid syndrome, and measurable shrinkage of tumor and metastatic disease.[72, 122] The most immediate life-threatening complication of carcinoid syndrome, carcinoid crisis, has also been successfully managed with octreotide.[72] Additional medical management of metastatic disease includes having the patient avoid stress and symptomatic therapies and administering diuretics to treat cardiac disease, bronchodilators to treat asthma, and antidiarrheals to treat diarrhea.

Prognosis for Carcinoid Tumors

Survival depends on the site of occurrence of the tumor and the extent of disease. Race, age, and sex do not affect survival.[117] Extended follow-up is vital; one lymph node recurrence was documented 29 years after an initial appendectomy in childhood.[115] Localized appendiceal disease with no metastatic disease results in 100% long-term survival.[115, 117] Jejunoileal disease is associated with decreased survival rates because of delayed presentation and higher likelihood of initial metastasis. Bronchial carcinoids are associated with an excellent prognosis in children.[114]

The presence of carcinoid syndrome is associated with decreased long-term survival rates, but flushing alone does not predict poor survival. There are reports of successful long-term survival in patients receiving octreotide.[72, 122]

ACTHoma (ECTOPIC ACTH SYNDROME)

The most common cause of hypercortisolism is adrenal production of corticosteroids stimulated by a pituitary tumor producing ACTH (Cushing's disease). A rare cause of Cushing's syndrome is the "ectopic" production of ACTH by tumors other than those of pituitary or adrenal origin.

In adults, ectopic ACTH syndrome accounts for 15% to 20% of cases of Cushing's syndrome, with 80% of these associated with medullary thyroid cancers, small-cell lung tumors, carcinoids, pancreatic islet-cell tumors, pheochromocytomas, or paragangliomas.[123]

In infants, adrenal tumors are the most fre-

Table 21–3 • Ectopic ACTH
Tumors Known to Produce ACTH
Carcinoid (bronchial, thymic) tumors   Medullary thyroid cancers   Neuroblastoma and other neural tissue tumors   Oat cell, lung cancers   Pancreatic islet cell cancers   Wilms' tumors (clear cell, stromal rich and poor)

quent cause of Cushing's syndrome, and they are accompanied by either virilism or signs of hypercortisolism. In patients older than age 7 years, hypercortisolism is predominantly the result of pituitary adenomas.[124] Ectopic ACTH secretion in children is very rare but has been documented in cases of Wilms' tumors, carcinoid tumors, neural tissue tumors (neuroblastoma and ganglioneuroblastoma), thymic tumors, pancreatic islet-cell tumors, and lung and bronchial tumors (Table 21–3). Case reports of ACTH-producing tumors include thymic carcinoids in 8- and 16-year-olds, an intrathymic parathyroid in a 10-year-old girl, and an oat-cell cancer in the thymus of an 11-year-old boy.[125, 126, 127] In patients with Wilms' tumor, epithelial or stromal elements, or both, may be responsible for the production of ACTH.[128] There is no significant age or sex predilection or any established incidence reported in the literature.

Pathology of ACTHoma

Ectopic ACTH syndrome is characterized by overexpression and aberrant post-translational processing of pro-opiomelanocortin (POMC) resulting in the elevation of ACTH or its precursors, not always ACTH alone.[129] Almost all tumors that have been associated with ectopic ACTH syndrome also secrete other hormones, including those associated with ZES, MEN syndromes, and pheochromocytoma. It is thought that the excess of ACTH is not a result of "ectopic" production of ACTH, but represents a preexisting capacity of tumor cells that undergo modification and amplification of protein production.[129]

The important clinical problems associated with ectopic ACTH-producing tumors include locating the source of ACTH production and managing the hypercortisol state.[72] Bronchial carcinoids are associated with a tendency toward local recurrence and can produce florid hypercortisolism in tumors as small as 5 mm in diameter.[125]

Signs and Symptoms of ACTHoma

Ectopic ACTH syndrome mirrors the hypercortisol state. Patients may present with moon facies, obesity, buffalo hump, longitudinal growth failure, hirsutism, hypertension, stria, skin hyperpigmentation, plethora, and renal stones. They may also present with manifestations of mineralocorticoid excess, including edema and hypokalemia. The duration of symptoms is variable, ranging from weeks to many years. Some have noted that more benign tumors present a gradual clinical picture of cortisol excess, whereas more malignant tumors produce symptoms much more rapidly.[129]

Diagnosis of ACTHoma

Several validation criteria have been advanced for the diagnosis of ectopic ACTH syndrome. These include one or more of the following: clinical and biochemical evidence of abnormal endocrine function, arteriovenous hormonal concentration gradient detected across a suspected tumor bed, elevated hormone concentrations in tumor tissues as compared with surrounding tissues, establishment of ACTH synthesis by tumor cells in culture, persistence of elevated ACTH levels after the removal of the pituitary, and disappearance of endocrine abnormalities following tumor removal.[129]

The diagnosis of hypercortisolism is made biochemically with documentation of elevated serum cortisol level, an elevated 24-hour excretion of urinary free cortisol, and elevated 17-hydroxycorticosteroids. Direct ACTH assay is useful to determine whether hypercortisolism is due to excess adrenal production (ACTH is suppressed) or is due to a pituitary or ectopic source (ACTH is elevated). Dexamethasone suppressibility can help to distinguish pituitary from ectopic ACTH sources. High-dose dexamethasone suppression is seen with pituitary sources. It causes serum cortisol levels to drop to less than 10% of baseline. In contrast, no suppression is noted with ectopic ACTH production.[124] Even with these

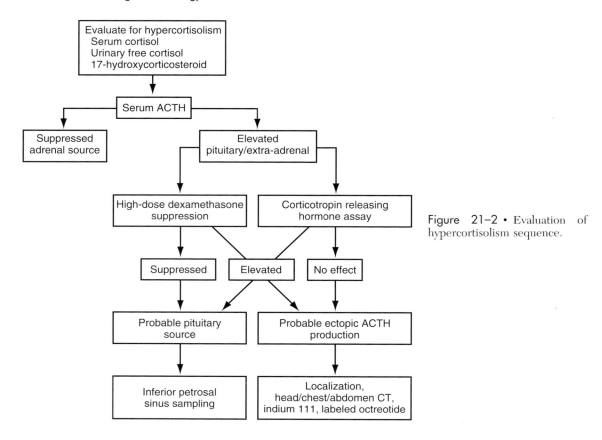

Figure 21–2 • Evaluation of hypercortisolism sequence.

tests, distinguishing between pituitary and ectopic origins of ACTH may be difficult (Fig. 21–2).[123]

With a suggested diagnosis of ectopic ACTH syndrome, localization becomes paramount. Radiologic studies should include chest, abdominal, and head CT scans and MRI. Inferior petrosal venous sampling is useful for the confirmation and lateralization of pituitary tumors. Selective venous sampling may confirm production of ectopic ACTH where a tumor mass has been localized.

Further localization efforts have benefited from the empiric finding of hormonal responsiveness to somatostatin. ACTH release was significantly reduced and symptoms improved by administration of somatostatin to patients with carcinoid tumors, medullary thyroid cancers, and pancreatic islet-cell tumors.[123] As a result, indium-111 labeled octreotide has been used with considerable success in adults to localize ectopic ACTH tumors. One report cites a 62% to 100% success rate in localizing medullary thyroid tu-

mors, small-cell cancers of the lung, carcinoids with metastases, and gastrinomas.

Somatostatin receptor status is important. It is believed that pituitary tumors, cortisol-producing adrenal adenomas, and some nonresponding ectopic ACTH tumors lack somatostatin receptors.[123] One report documenting successful localization of a 6 mm bronchial carcinoid, advocates radiolabeled octreotide for localization if a clinical hormonal response is seen after 3 days of octreotide administration.[130]

Treatment of ACTHoma

Once the diagnosis of ectopic ACTH syndrome is made, the goal is to localize and remove the neoplasm responsible for hormonal secretion. Benign ACTH-secreting tumors, including bronchial carcinoids and pheochromocytomas, can be surgically excised following principles of anatomic resection, with a good prospect for cure. Pancreatic endocrine tumors are notably slow-growing and are similarly cured with resection. Patients with more malignant tumors, including medullary thyroid tumors and thymic carcinoid with locally advanced or metastatic disease, often benefit from partial removal of tumor mass or radical local excision. Palliative therapy and debulking procedures may be helpful in the management of these tumors, particularly in the case of liver disease and hepatic metastases.[129]

A significant percentage of ectopic ACTH tumors possess the somatostatin receptor and are hormonally inhibited by somatostatin administration. Somatostatin has been given for periods of up to 1 month for the control of hypercortisolism, but with cessation, there was rapid return to elevated serum cortisol levels.[130] Long-term administration was found inadequate to maintain complete suppression of ACTH.[47]

Malignant ACTHoma

Malignant ACTHomas have a high local recurrence rate. Tumors may recur many years after initial resection. One series reported that 67% of carcinoids recurred up to 9 years after resection of all gross disease.[131a] Few data otherwise exist about the malignant potential of these rare tumors.

Chemotherapy and radiotherapy have both been administered for residual disease. Postoperative radiotherapy has been especially useful for residual or node positive thoracic and bronchial carcinoids. Chemotherapeutic regimens for carcinomas include FAC [5-fluorouracil, Adriamycin (doxorubicin), and Cytoxan (cyclophosphamide)] and streptozotocin, etoposide, and cisplatin.[129]

Medical management of mineralocorticoid and glucocorticoid excess becomes vital in cases of unlocalizable or unresectable tumors because the tumor continues to secrete ACTH and can cause significant morbidity. Mineralocorticoid excess is managed with potassium supplementation, spironolactone, and antihypertensives.

Hypercortisolism can be managed chemically with metyrapone, aminoglutethimide, or mitotane (Table 21–4).[72] Long-term control with drugs inhibiting steroidogenesis in children often proves unsatisfactory or impractical. Patients whose tumors cannot be localized or resected should be evaluated for bilateral adrenalectomy.

Table 21–4 • Medical Management of Hypercortisolism

Drug	Effect
Aminoglutethimide	Inhibits cytochrome P450–dependent enzymes
Ketoconazole	Inhibits cholesterol side chain cleavage
Metyrapone	Inhibits 11-beta hydroxylase
Mitotane	Inhibits steroidogenesis
RU 486	Competitive antagonistic effect on 19 "nor" steroids

Follow-up and Prognosis for Patients with ACTHoma

Extended follow-up is indicated for patients who have been treated for ACTHoma, with close monitoring for clinical manifestations of hypercortisolism and periodic surveillance of serum ACTH levels. A persistently elevated or rising ACTH level indicates residual or recurrent disease. As stated, long-term survival is possible for patients with ectopic ACTH disease amenable to complete surgical resection. Failing this, extended survival is possible with medical management of hypercortisolism. When medical management fails, bilateral adrenalectomy with cortisol and aldosterone replacement may be considered.

ECTOPIC GROWTH HORMONE RELEASING HORMONE (GRH)-PRODUCING TUMORS

Gigantism and acromegaly are caused by an excess of growth hormone (GH), which can result from direct pituitary production, pituitary stimulation by growth hormone releasing hormone (GRH), or nonpituitary stimulation from ectopic GRH. Plasma GH levels normally fluctuate widely in response to exercise, dietary intake, and sleep, as well as other normal physiologic events.[131b] Persistent hypersecretion of GH during childhood causes excessive linear growth and gigantism syndrome. Acromegaly results from the hypersecretion of GH after epiphyseal fusion.

GH secretion by pituitary adenomas is the most common cause of acromegaly in adults and gigantism in children.[132] Fewer than 1% of patients with gigantism or acromegaly have elevations of GRH levels from carcinoid tumor or islet-cell production, and no cases have been reported of ectopic GRH secretion in infancy or early childhood.[132, 133] Conversely, GH-secreting pituitary adenomas are rare in younger patients, and ectopic GRH should be suspected in these cases. In one study, 23% of patients found to have GRH hypersecretion were younger than 25 years.[134] Failure of clinical resolution or recurrence of tumor after pituitary surgery should also arouse the suspicion of the existence of a GRH-secreting tumor.

The most common tumor associated with ectopic GRH is carcinoid, accounting for 69% of cases in one study.[134] Carcinoids were pulmonary in 78% of cases and gastrointestinal in 11% of cases. The second most common tumor associated with ectopic GRH was islet-cell tumor of the pancreas. In patients with MEN1 syndrome, GRH production by pancreatic tumors can stimulate hypophyseal somatotrophs, resulting in GH excess, acromegaly, and reversible pituitary lesion.[135] It is extremely important that the cause of acromegaly be correctly determined before ablative pituitary therapy is rendered, lest the syndrome of GH excess continues. A 15-year-old girl with gigantism underwent pituitary resection and suffered recurrence of GH excess 8 weeks postoperatively. Further workup revealed a metastatic duodenal-jejunal carcinoid.[136]

Pathology of GRH-Producing Tumors

Circulating GRH cannot be detected in normal, healthy persons.[136] GRH immunoreactivity has been detected in highest concentration in the hypothalamus, septum, and substantia inominata in the brain. The normal gastrointestinal tract shows GRH immunoreactivity in the upper jejunum, which is localized to the mucosa.[137]

GRH immunoreactivity has also been analyzed in neoplasms and has been documented in a variety of tumors arising from and composed of peptide-hormone-producing endocrine cells. No GH was identified in any of these tumors. Immunohistochemical studies indicate that carcinoid tumors contain GRH frequently, even if it is not secreted in sufficient amounts to cause clinical or biochemical acromegaly. Many carcinoids produce more than one type of hormone. In one study of symptomatic carcinoids, 17% of pancreatic, 20% of bronchial, and 50% of thymic tumors showed GRH immunopositivity.[138]

Other tumors that have GRH activity include medullary thyroid, pheochromocytoma, small-cell tumor of the lung, adrenal pheochromocytoma, and endometrial cancer.[134, 137, 138] Very few of these tumors are associated with clinical signs of GH excess, presumably because of production of biologically inactive forms of GRH, inability to secrete the GRH produced, or death (prior to development of symptoms). In another study of patients with carcinoid tumors, 52% had disturbed regulation of serum GH, 30% had abnormal results on two or more tests, and 18% had clinical acromegaly.[139]

Chronic stimulation from ectopic GRH yields pituitary somatotroph hyperplasia and GH hypersecretion. Pituitary hyperplasia associated with MEN1 syndrome may be caused by releasing factors synthesized in carcinoids or islet-cell tumors.[135] Removal of ectopic GRH-producing tumors can result in normalization of pituitary GH secretion and cure of acromegaly. The amount of GRH released into the circulation must be greater than a set threshold because of rapid degradation of GRH into inactive metabolites.[134] Cases exist of precocious puberty associated with ectopic GRH, presumed secondary to gonadal stimulation by insulin-like growth factor-1 (IGF-1).[132]

Signs and Symptoms of GRH-Producing Tumors

The clinical features of ectopic GRH-producing tumors mirror those of GH excess and include gigantism in children prior to epiphyseal growth plate closure, plus acromegaly. Gigantism involves dramatic growth in both height and weight.[136] Children with gigantism may also have acromegalic physical features, including enlargement of hands and feet, soft-tissue thickening, coarse oily skin, prognathism, and coarse facial features.[132, 136, 140] Metabolic effects of GH excess include hyperglycemia and mineral metabolism abnormalities.

Diffuse enlargement of the pituitary from GRH stimulation may produce bitemporal hemianopsia, headaches, galactorrhea, and menstrual changes.[136] Presentation may also be related to mass effect or systemic neoplastic changes. A bronchial carcinoid in a 54-year-old man produced fever, chills, and hemoptysis when it bled into the distal bronchus intermedius and caused complete obstruction.[141]

Diagnosis of GRH-Producing Tumor

The criteria for diagnosis of GRH-producing tumor includes establishing an arteriovenous gradient across the tumor bed, rapid fall of GH and IGF-1 after tumor resection, tumor immunostaining for GRH, in vitro synthesis and release of GRH, and presence of hormone-specific mRNA.[134] Workup includes analysis of multiple baseline levels of GH, IGF-1, and GRH along with provocative testing. Provocative tests include the oral glucose tolerance test (OGTT), administration of thyroid-releasing hormone (TRH), and reaction to somatostatin (Table 21–5).[139] The oral administration of glucose normally produces a suppressive effect on serum GH, but this response is absent in patients with GH excess. TRH normally produces minimal change in serum GH levels, but it causes a marked stimulation in patients with GH excess. Somatostatin administration normally has no effect on GH, but it produces a marked decrease in GH and GRH in patients with ectopic GRH secretion.

Imaging studies may include CT, ultrasound, MRI, angiography, and selective venous sampling, along with the use of labeled somatostatin analogs. The definitive test in differentiating GH excess from ectopic GRH syndrome is radioimmunoassay for GRH.[141] Normal subjects have a GRH levels ≤10 pg/ml. A serum level of ≥300 pg/ml strongly suggests ectopic GRH hypersecretion.[132] Very rarely gigantism is caused by central production within the hypothalamus.[132] This diagnosis is suggested by intermediate serum concentration of GRH that are lower than peripheral concentrations because of the existence of the portal circulation to the pituitary. The serum GRH should be routinely measured in patients with gigantism or acromegaly who are being considered for pituitary surgery or radiation therapy.[141]

Treatment of GRH-Producing Tumors

Surgical excision of the tumor remains the treatment of choice for ectopic GRH syndrome. Plasma GRH levels should fall rapidly to undetectable levels following complete resection. The established criteria for cure include normalization and maintenance of normal GRH, GH, and IGF-1 levels, normal suppressibility with OGTT, and disappearance of the paradoxic GH response to TRH.[134]

These tumors are slow-growing, however, and patients usually present late with metastatic disease following the insidious development of gigantism or acromegaly. Residual and metastatic disease can be effectively managed by the administration of the somatostatin analog, octreotide.

Malignant GRH-Producing Tumors

The aim of managing residual or metastatic disease is to arrest progression of the neoplastic process and to control GH hypersecretion. Traditional chemotherapy has been ineffective.[134] Octreotide effectively neutralizes the biochemical and clinical syndromes of gigantism and acromegaly. It is also very effective in reducing GH levels, less so in reducing GRH levels.[142]

Somatostatin is a noncompetitive inhibitor of GRH-induced stimulation of GH secretion.[138] Tissue culture has established that the effect of somatostatin on plasma GRH is mediated by a direct immediate action on GRH-secreting cells of the tumor.[143] Bromocriptine has a direct inhibitory effect on pituitary secretion of growth hormone but fails to significantly lower serum GH and IGF-1 levels has not influenced the management of metastatic disease.[134, 142]

Long-term therapy with intravenous or subcu-

Table 24–5 • Ectopic Growth Hormone Releasing Hormone (GH-RH)

Provocative Testing

Oral glucose tolerance test
  Administration of glucose fails to suppress growth hormone (GH) levels (normal = positive suppression)
Thyroid-releasing hormone (TRH)
  Administration of TRH produces marked elevation of GH levels (normal = no response)
Somatostatin
  Administration of somatostatin produces marked GH suppression (normal = no response)

Additional Testing

GH-RH radioimmunoassay (determine GH excess vs. GH-RH elevation)

taneous injection of somatostatin offers clinical improvement with resolution of acromegaly or cessation of rates of growth in gigantism. GH and IGF-1 can be significantly reduced, in one report to normal, and GRH can be reduced 50% to 75%.[136, 142, 143] Long-term octreotide therapy has also been found to either arrest neoplastic progression or cause tumor and metastatic regression as documented by CT and ultrasound.[134, 136]

Prognosis for Patients with GRH-Producing Tumors

Long-term survival for patients with GRH-producing tumors is achieved with effective surgical resection or ongoing management with octreotide. Several case reports extending beyond 2 years show normalization of symptoms from hormonal excess and stabilization or regression of disease for up to 44 months.[134, 136] Normalization of GH excretion after operation or with long-term administration of octreotide should be ensured, and surveillance should be maintained.

HUMAN CHORIONIC GONADOTROPIN (hCG)-PRODUCING TUMORS

Human chorionic gonadotropin (hCG) is a 45kd glycoprotein normally produced by trophoblasts in the placenta. Germ-cell tumors often contain these trophoblastic cells, making hCG a useful marker for diagnosis, treatment, and follow-up of germ-cell tumors. Germ-cell tumors are classified as germinomas or nongerminomas, which include embryonal-cell tumors, teratomas, yolk-sac or endodermal sinus tumors, choriocarcinomas, and tumors with mixed components. Secretion of hCG can be seen with all of these tumor types (Table 21–6), but it is more common with nongerminoma tumors. Up to 70% of tumors containing yolk-sac elements secrete hCG.[144] Tumors producing hCG are believed to arise from aberrant migration of cells in the fetus. These tumors can be gonadal or extragonadal.[145] Hepatoblastoma is morphologically similar to syncytiotrophoblast cells, and it also contains and secrets hCG.[146]

Locations of germ-cell tumors vary in reported studies, with estimated rates of 33% to 50% for ovarian tumors, 18% to 25% for testicular tumors, 12% to 23% for presacral tumors, 2% to 9% for intracranial tumors, and 2% to 6% for mediastinal tumors.[147, 148] Other, rarer locations include the stomach, bowel, liver, retroperitoneum, umbilicus, urinary bladder, and vagina.[148] Certain germ-cell tumor types are more common in specific areas. Teratomas are the most common germ cell tumors found in the mediastinum, followed by yolk sac tumors.[145, 148] Testicular germ cell tumors occur early as masses, and are most commonly seminomas or yolk sac tumors.[145, 147]

A very strong association exists between mediastinal germ-cell tumors, especially teratomas, and Klinefelter's syndrome. A boy with Klinefelter's syndrome, usually 47,XXY, is 30 to 50 times more likely to have a mediastinal teratoma than the rest of the male population.[150]

Pathology of hCG-Producing Tumors

The two subunit proteins of hCG are an alpha unit (alpha-fetoprotein), nearly indistinguishable from other hormones, and a beta unit (β-hCG). Elevations of either or both are seen in up to 90% of patients with nonseminomatous testicular tumors.[151] β-hCG can be detected in serum or urine by radioimmunoassay.[146] A majority of patients with ovarian tumors present with multiple markers.[148]

Precocious puberty is caused by testosterone in boys and estradiol in girls. The production of testosterone is stimulated by LH, which causes hyperplasia of Leydig's cells. The production of estradiol is dependent on both LH and FSH. The development of precocious puberty can be linked to high circulating levels of hCG, which is known to have LH bioactivity and weak FSH bioactivity. As a result, precocious puberty in boys does occur, but without stimulation of Sertoli cells (FSH-dependent), resulting in the absence of spermatogenesis.[145] Precocious puberty in girls is extremely rare; the theory is that hCG cannot produce precocious puberty in girls in the

---

Table 24–6 • Tumors That May Produce Human Chorionic Gonadotropin

Hepatoblastomas
Intracranial tumors
Mediastinal tumors (teratoma, yolk sac)
Ovarian tumors (teratoma, yolk sac)
Testicular tumors (seminoma, yolk sac)

absence of FSH.[152] One case of a girl with an hCG-secreting suprasellar teratoma who did present with precocious puberty was reported with the researchers' speculation that very high levels of hCG allowed for sufficient FSH stimulation and precocious puberty.[152]

The most common hCG-secreting tumor causing precocious puberty is hepatoblastoma, accounting for 50% of cases in one large series.[146] Other tumors causing precocious puberty in this study included mediastinal teratomas (26%) and intracranial tumors (17%).

Signs and Symptoms of hCG-Producing Tumors

Symptoms of hCG-producing tumors depend on the location of the tumor as well as the level of production of hCG. As described earlier, precocious puberty may be the first clinical manifestation reported, more commonly in boys than in girls. Precocious puberty involves accelerated height and weight gain, advanced osseous maturation, and secondary sex characteristics. In boys this includes the appearance of pubic hair, acne, voice coarsening and genital growth. Minimal or modest increases in testicular size may also occur.[146] With Klinefelter's syndrome, testicular enlargement may be secondary to hyalinization.[146, 150] In girls there is breast budding, pubic hair, and external genitalia development.

Patients with germ-cell tumors may also have symptoms related to tumor mass or location, concurrent with or preceding hormonal effects. A palpable liver mass with splenomegaly and anemia has been reported to accompany both hepatoblastoma and choriocarcinoma.[153] Patients with ovarian tumors may present with a vague abdominal mass with pain and distention, generally occurring around the onset of normal puberty. Testicular tumors are detected at an earlier age and are associated with pain and swelling. Patients with presacral tumors may present with constipation, pain after defecation, weight loss, difficulty with ambulation, urinary incontinence, or palpation on rectal examination.[148]

Diagnosis of hCG-Producing Tumors

The diagnosis of functional germ-cell tumors secreting hCG is made when precocious puberty is determined and elevation of hCG is established.

A suppressed gonadotropin response to the administration of *gonadotropin-releasing hormone* (Gn-RH) should be observed. With Gn-RH stimulation, pubertal changes due to hypothalamic or pituitary causes allow elevation of FSH and LH, whereas production of hCG has no effect on LH or FSH.[150] The detection of the ongoing presence of hCG in the serum can accurately reflect the activity and course of the tumor.[151]

Localization of a functioning germ-cell tumor should include exclusion of an intracranial tumor. Head CT/MRI and hCG determinations in serum and CSF allow for accurate determination. The serum/CSF hCG ratio should be less than 1 for intracranial lesions, in marked contrast to the very large ratios seen in patients with choriocarcinoma or teratocarcinoma.[154]

Chest radiographs performed for vague complaints may reveal a mediastinal mass or an intrathoracic calcification consistent with teratoma. Workup should include serum analysis for β-hCG and performance of CT imaging. Because of the strong association of Klinefelter's syndrome with functional mediastinal teratomas, β-hCG analysis should be performed on children with Klinefelter's syndrome when early pubertal changes or when testosterone production is detected.[150] Males with hCG-producing mediastinal teratomas should undergo chromosomal analysis.[145]

Treatment of hCG-Producing Tumors

Total extirpation of functional germ-cell tumors secreting hCG is the treatment of choice. Generally, Stage 1 germ-cell tumors should be removed completely and tumor markers followed postoperatively, with chemotherapy considered after evaluation of histology, type, size, and location. Higher-stage tumors should be managed with aggressive surgery, chemotherapy (possibly both preoperative and postoperative) and radiation therapy.[148] Failing complete removal, initial debulking along with multimodal intensive chemotherapy may allow extended survival with normal body growth and normalization of sexual maturity. Chemotherapy regimens are cisplatin-based and may include dactinomycin, doxorubicin, vincristine, bleomycin, or cyclophosphamide.[148]

Survival rate after surgical resection is related to the rate of disappearance of tumor marker, with a half-life for β-hCG of up to 3 days.[151]

Following removal of tumor and disappearance of hCG, pubertal changes regress.[146] When a child presents with elevated tumor markers for initial resection, tumor markers should be followed in the postoperative period. Second-look surgery in patients who had elevated markers before resection but not afterwards is now disfavored. Second look surgery is recommended when there is a possibility of residual mass and when tumor markers were not elevated preoperatively.[144]

One report on dysgerminomas cites a 15% incidence of bilateral disease and recommends consideration of wedge biopsy of the contralateral ovary.[149] With other primary ovarian tumors, a contralateral biopsy is not recommended because of a related incidence of postoperative infertility of up to 14%.[149]

Malignant hCG-Producing Tumors

As mentioned earlier, chemotherapy regimens are based on cisplatin, and there have been some successes in preoperative delivery.[153] Successful management of metastatic choriocarcinoma of the liver has been known with preoperative chemotherapy [bleomycin, VP (vincristine and prednisone) 16, and cisplatin] followed by profound hypothermic arrest with trisegmentectomy allowing for complete resection of the tumor.[153] A case report of ovarian germ-cell tumors suggests that only 3% of such tumors are malignant.[149] Transient elevations of hCG may be observed after the initiation of chemotherapy and is presumed to result from tumor lysis.[151] One study found that patients with persistent elevation of tumor markers eventually had measurable disease.[144]

Prognosis for Patients with hCG-Producing Tumors

Patients with gonadal germ-cell tumors in one study had an 85% disease-free survival at 38 months, whereas those with extragonadal tumors had a 93% disease-free survival.[148] Pubertal changes generally regress slowly following resection, with resolution by 3 months.[146] Survival rate is related to tumor size, stage at time of diagnosis, and concentrations of circulating alpha-fetoprotein and β-hCG.[148, 151] Patients with small tumors and low marker levels had a 3-year survival rate of 91%, whereas those with small tumors

and high marker concentrations had a 3-year survival rate of 69%.[151] In another study, patients with Stage 1 ovarian and testicular tumors had a 100% survival rate, whereas those with Stage 3 tumors had an 82% survival rate and those with Stage 4 tumors had a 75% survival rate. Most recurrences (estimated as up to 80%) are within 12 to 16 months; longer disease-free periods are considered curative.[148] Delays in recognizing recurrences can negatively affect disease-free and long-term survival. Yolk-sac tumors are associated with a poorer prognosis, especially those of ovarian origin.[147]

MULTIPLE ENDOCRINE NEOPLASIA (MEN) SYNDROMES

MEN syndromes are composed of hereditary neoplastic transformations in more than one endocrine gland. These transformations occur as three distinctive, autosomal dominant patterns of inheritance and have been labeled MEN1, MEN2A, and MEN2B (Table 21–7). MEN1 includes pancreatic islet-cell, pituitary, and parathyroid tumors and is also known as Wermer's syndrome. MEN2A includes MTC, pheochromocytoma, and parathyroid tumors and is known as Sipple's syndrome. MEN2B is characterized by a complex marfanoid habitus and is associated with MTC, pheochromocytoma, mucosal neuroma, and intestinal ganglioneuroma.[155]

Patients are diagnosed with MEN based on the occurrence of two or more primary features or one primary feature along with the existence of a first-degree relative with MEN.[12] Neoplastic changes can include hyperplasia, microadenoma, adenoma, and carcinoma.

Case of MEN1, MEN2A, and approximately one half of MEN2B cases demonstrate an autosomal dominant mode of transmission. More than 50 families on six continents have been identified as having MEN2A.[156] Kindreds with MEN2A demonstrate near complete penetrance with variable expressivity.[157] Some kindreds within affected MEN1 families demonstrate identical hormone secretion profiles and a similar malignant course.[158] Other affected families have variable pathologic findings of hormonal secretion and neoplastic change.

Much research has gone into the elucidation of MEN syndromes on a cellular and genetic level. Mutations may confer a predisposition to-

Table 21–7 • Multiple Endocrine Neoplasia Syndromes

Multiple Endocrine Neoplasia (MEN)	Neoplasia	Genetic Defect	Penetrance (%)	Additional Associations	Screening
MEN I Wermer's	Pancreatic (gastrinoma, insulinoma, nonfunctioning pleurihormonal)	Chromosome 11q13	38–75	Thymic, bronchial carcinoids	Serum calcium Parathyroid hormone Glucose Gastrin Prolactin
	Pituitary GH, ACTH, prolactin		19–47	Single, multiple lipomas	
	Parathyroid		90–100		
MEN IIA Sipple's	MTC	Chromosome 10 RET proto-oncogene	Near 100		Basal and stimulated plasma calcitonin Serum calcium Urinary catecholamine DNA analysis—RET proto-oncogene
	Pheochromocytoma		38–42		
	Parathyroid	Mutation	24–35		
MEN IIB	MTC		Near 100		Basal and stimulated plasma calcitonin DNA analysis—RET proto-oncogene
	Pheochromocytoma	Chromosome 10 RET proto-oncogene	44	Marfanoid phenotype	
	Mucosal neuroma		Near 100	GI motility problems	
	Intestinal ganglioneuroma		75		

GH = growth hormone; ACTH = adrenocorticotropic hormone; MTC = medullary thyroid carcinoma

ward malignancy, specifically in tissues of neural crest origin.[155] The MEN1 gene has been mapped to chromosome 11q13, and it is believed that this region codes for an inactivated suppressor gene.[158] Detection of this chromosomal abnormality could allow identification of individuals at risk for development of MEN1 with a high degree of accuracy.[158]

The MEN2A gene has been mapped to the pericentromeric region of chromosome 10.[155, 157] This region codes for the RET proto-oncogene, a transmembrane tyrosine kinase, which when mutated may be responsible for the development of neoplasia in these inherited disorders.[155] Evidence suggests that the RET proto-oncogene is responsible for at least two of the three inherited forms of MTC MENIIA and familial MTC. Initially no genomic variants or deletions were detected in analyzed MEN2B kindreds nor sporadic MTC.[155] Some researchers have now documented mutations in the RET proto-oncogene for both MEN2A and 2B.[162b] Direct DNA analysis with polymerase chain reaction now permits the unambiguous identification of RET proto-oncogene carriers, allowing for earlier identification of children at risk for MTC.[159, 160] The rationale is

that early detection will significantly increase the number of children surgically cured at first operation who had no biochemical evidence of disease.[160] Nevertheless, no causal relation has yet been established between specific RET mutations and the presence of MTC or pheochromocytoma as revealed on functional testing.[159]

MEN1

The mean patient age at diagnosis of MEN1 is 35 years, with a female-to-male ratio of 1.72:1.[12] Hyperparathyroidism is an almost universal finding in patients with MEN1, approaching 90% to 100%.[12, 158] Pancreatic islet-cell tumors are seen in 38% to 75% of patients, pituitary adenomas in 19% to 47%, and benign adrenal disease in up to 12%.[12, 158, 160] Benign and malignant thymic and bronchial carcinoids may also accompany MEN1. Lipomas, either single or multiple, are found in up to one half of patients with MEN1.[8] Presentation is varied and is related to specific neoplastic changes. These changes can include hyperparathyroidism from adenoma or hyperplasia, ZES from gastrinoma, hypoglycemia from insulinoma, migratory necrolytic erythema with glucagonoma, gigantism, acromegaly and nonspecific symptoms from pituitary adenoma, and Cushing's syndrome from cortisol-secreting tumors and ectopic ACTH.[8]

Screening tests for patients at risk for development of MEN1 include serum calcium, PTH, glucose, gastrin, and prolactin levels.[8] Prospective screening of calcium and PTH levels in patients at risk can provide a much earlier diagnosis and in clinical practice has decreased patient age at diagnosis from 38 to 19 years.[158] One report cites enhanced early detection of endocrine pancreatic tumors using the measurement of serum pancreatic polypeptide (PP) and gastrin following meal stimulation.[158]

Pancreatic Islet-Cell Tumors in Association with MEN1

Nearly all patients with MEN1 have multiple pancreatic tumors that can be located in extrapancreatic positions.[161] The range of islet-cell tumors seen includes gastrinomas (45% to 75%), insulinomas (35%), nonfunctional tumors (10%), and pleurihormonal tumors (7%).[8, 160] These multiple, usually benign islet-cell tumors can cause ZES, hypoglycemic hyperinsulinism seen with fasting, or watery diarrhea.[8, 160, 161]

The effects of hypoglycemia in patients with insulinomas can be much more difficult to manage than the hypergastrinemic state in patients with ZES. Pancreatic islet-cell tumor resection, particularly for gastrinomas, includes careful exploration of the entire region and intraoperative palpation, endoscopy, and ultrasound for locating tumors that may be extrapancreatic and malignant.[161] For patients with hyperparathyroidism and ZES, parathyroidectomy as an initial procedure can effectively lower serum gastrin levels and should be pursued prior to abdominal exploration.[161] Up to one half of gastrinomas, VIPomas, glucagonomas, and tumors secreting pancreatic polypeptide (PPomas) are malignant.[8, 161] Prospective screening of family members in one report lowered the occurrence of metastatic disease at initial exploration to around 10%.[158]

Surgery is the only effective therapy for the insulinomas in patients with MEN1. All gross disease and a portion of normal pancreas, usually to the portal vein, are removed.[160] One study cited an overall 10% rate of malignant disease for insulinoma.[160] Another study reported up to one third of patients with islet-cell tumors as having metastatic disease at the time of diagnosis.[158]

Pituitary Tumors in Association with MEN1

Pituitary tumors generally consist of hormonally active adenomas, with prolactinomas being the most frequently encountered pathology.[8] Additional hormonally active substances secreted by pituitary adenomas include ACTH and GRH. Adenomas may also occur, which are clinically silent.

Hyperparathyroidism in Association with MEN1

The incidence of multiglandular disease in patients with MEN1 ranges from 63% to greater than 90%.[8, 12] Parathyroid hyperplasia is seen in more than 80% of cases. Surgical management of hyperparathyroidism includes identification of all four glands, subtotal or total parathyroidectomy, and routine cervical thymectomy. There is a high rate of recurrent parathyroid hyperplasia in residual glandular tissues.[12]

MEN2A

MEN2A is associated with virtually all affected kindred members having MTC. Penetrance of pheochromocytoma and parathyroid tumors is variable.[8, 156] One large study of patients with MTC and MEN2A detected pheochromocytoma in 42% and hyperparathyroidism in 35% of the cohort group. A review of the literature cited prevalence rates of 38% for pheochromocytoma and 24% for hyperparathyroidism. The average patient age at diagnosis was 29 years for MTC, 37 years for pheochromocytoma, and 36 years for hyperparathyroidism.[156]

Biochemical manifestations of MTC generally appear between 5 and 25 years of age, with a mean of 15 years, most often preceding pheochromocytoma.[159] Screening should be undertaken in identified families and should include basal and stimulated plasma calcitonin levels, serum calcium level, and urinary excretion of catecholamines.[8, 159] An updated evaluation of patients who underwent total thyroid resection for MTC based on detection of the RET proto-oncogene found more than half of these children had normal serum calcitonin but with a small foci of MTC on histologic examination and no false-positives.[159]

Medullary Thyroid Cancer (MTC) in Association with MEN2

Serum analysis of calcitonin at basal and stimulated levels is able to detect otherwise occult, subclinical disease. The occult disease of MTC seen in children with MEN2 who are also positive for the RET proto-oncogene has led some to advocate thyroidectomy as early as 1 year of age.[162a] In one study, 50% of patients with MEN2A who presented clinically with a palpable neck mass or an elevated basal level of calcitonin had either persistent or recurrent MTC documented over a 10-year follow-up.[156] Literature reviews show that the youngest reported child with C-cell hyperplasia was 20 months of age and the youngest child with MTC was 3 years.[162a]

Management of MTC in patients with MEN includes total thyroidectomy with central neck dissection at initial operation and emphasis on early diagnosis and treatment.[156, 162b] Timing of the resection is a point of controversy. Advocates of early operation cite improved detection of C-cell hyperplasia and improved disease-free survival rates when the operation is done in children who are RET proto-oncogene positive and have normal serum calcitonin levels.[162b, 162] Others base the indication for operation on a positive calcitonin assay or adolescent age, arguing an increased risk of hypothyroidism and recurrent laryngeal nerve injury exists with earlier intervention.[159] The incidence of metastatic disease at initial exploration is low, but the recurrence rate in patients who were symptomatic is above 20%.[162b]

Pheochromocytoma in Association with MEN2

Most pheochromocytomas that occur in association with MEN2A are bilateral and only in rare cases develop before MTC.[156, 159] In one unselected study of patients with pheochromocytoma, 23% were found to have familial associations, 19% with Hippel-Lindau disease and 4% with MEN2A.[71] In this same study, significant differences were appreciated between familial and sporadic occurrence, with familial disease appearing at a younger age (a mean of 32 years) and having a higher incidence of multifocal disease (55% of cases) and a lower rate of progression to malignancy. In another study, the mean interval of diagnosis between MTC and pheochromocytoma was 7.4 years. Rarely was the pheochromocytoma extra-adrenal in origin.[156]

Treatment involves surgical resection of the affected adrenal gland. Based on a series from the Mayo Clinic, however, researchers maintained that the uninvolved, normal-appearing adrenal was always abnormal on pathologic review and therefore recommended bilateral adrenalectomy.[69] In a review of the literature, 88% of patients required bilateral adrenalectomy.[163] Of those who had unilateral adrenalectomy, 55% required completion total adrenalectomy within 5 years. Because of the high incidence of bilateral disease and low morbidity for total resection, many researchers agree in recommending bilateral adrenalectomy.

Hyperparathyroidism in Association with MEN2

Compared with MEN1 patients, MEN2A in children produces lower preoperative serum calcium levels and fewer symptoms related to hypercalcemia.[12] In one study the mean interval between diagnosis of MTC and clinical hyperparathyroidism was 5.8 years.[156] Management of hyperparathyroidism in children with MEN2A generally occurs concurrently with thyroid resection. Total, subtotal, or partial parathyroid resections for abnormal tissue offer similar results, having a 100% cure rate regardless of the technique.[12]

MEN2B

MEN2B is inherited as an autosomal dominant trait with variable penetrance—50% of offspring in one study.[164] The mean patient age at diagnosis in one study was 18 years, and most often the patient initially presented with MTC.[163] In the same study 44% had pheochromocytomas, 75% had gastrointestinal abnormalities, 87% had skeletal manifestations, and 43% of girls experienced delayed puberty. MTC is seen 10 to 15 years earlier in patients with MEN2B than in those with MEN2A.[8]

Surgical management of patients with MEN2B is similiar to that outlined for those with MTC and pheochromocytoma.[8] MTC with MEN2B is seen at a much earlier age compared with disease with MEN2A. As a result, there is an increased incidence of metastatic disease at initial presentation—believed to be more virulent.[162b] One long-term study, however, found the MTC with MEN2B to be biologically less aggressive than sporadic MTC and produced less morbidity than other components of the phenotype.[164] MTC patients with MEN2B have an earlier age of development and presentation of neoplasia and as a result have recurrence rates of MTC of up to 64%.[160] The natural course of patients with metastatic disease is comparable between MEN2A and MEN2B.[163]

Patients with MEN2B have a distinctive marfanoid phenotype that includes slender body build, long and thin extremities, abnormal laxity of joints, high-arched palate, and chest wall deformities including pectus excavatum.[8] Thickened lips are a result of embedded mucosal neuromas, which are also found on the eyelids, tongue, and arytenoid cartilege.[8, 164] Superficial mucosal neuromas can be resected for functional or cosmetic indications.[8] Corneal nerve fibers may become significantly thickened.[164] Ganglioneuromas may be present at any level of the gastrointestinal tract and contribute to abnormalities of gastrointestinal motility, including constipation, diarrhea, and megacolon.[8] Up to 30% of patients may require laparotomy with colon resection. Hyperparathyroidism is not seen with MEN2B. No occurrences were found in kindreds of multiple affected families.[12, 164] Following operation for thyroidectomy, parathyroid tissue in patients with MEN2B has been found to be macroscopically and microscopically normal.[164]

Prognosis for Patients with MEN Syndromes

Patients with MEN1 have a favorable prognosis when pathology is limited to discrete adenomas of the parathyroid, islet-cell, or pituitary glands. Parathyroid hyperplasia requires near total parathyroidectomy or recurrence is likely. Islet-cell and carcinoid tumors are slowly progressive. Rarely can ZES be cured in patients with MEN1 by abdominal exploration and resection of tumor because of the multicentric nature of disease.[161] Insulinoma can be cured in patients with MEN1 by pancreatic or tumor resection.[161]

Patients with MEN2A also have an overall good prognosis. In one study, extended follow-up, beyond 10 years, showed cause of death as MTC in 50%, with 14 of 86 kindred deceased.[156] Early resection of thyroid and adrenal disease markedly decreases the risk of recurrence. Hyperparathyroidism in patients with MEN2A is not associated with recurrence and is cured by resection of abnormal tissue.

MEN2B kindred have a 10-year survival of 50%.[8] Morbidity and mortality for MEN2B are related to other components of the phenotype, especially gastrointestinal problems.[8, 164]

Screening is of vital importance to outcome, because earlier diagnosis and therapy can significantly affect disease-free survival rate and lifespan.

References

1. Correa P, Chen VW: Endocrine gland cancer. *Cancer* 75:338, 1994.
2. Gurney JG, Severson RK, Davis S, et al: Incidence of cancer in children in the United States. *Cancer* 75:2186, 1995.
3. Miller RW, Young JL, Novakovic B: Childhood cancer. *Cancer* 75:395, 1994.
4. Mindermann T, Wilson CB: Pediatric pituitary adenomas. *Neurosurgery* 36(2):259, 1995.
5. Partington MD, Davis DH, Laws ER Jr, et al: Pituitary adenomas in childhood and adolescence. Results of transsphenoidal surgery. *J Neurosurg* 80(2):209, 1994.
6. Dyer EH, Civit T, Visot A, et al: Transsphenoidal surgery for pituitary adenomas in children. *Neurosurgery* 34(2):207, 1994.
7. Kane LA, Leinung MC, Scheithauer BW, et al: Pituitary adenomas in childhood and adolescence. *J Clin Endocrinol Metab* 79(4):1135, 1994.
8. Chrousos GP: Endocrine Tumors. In Pizzo PA, Poplack DG (eds): *Principles and Practice of Pediatric Oncology*, 2nd ed. Philadelphia: J. B. Lippincott Co., 1993, p. 889.
9. Thompson NW, Carpenter LC, Kessler DL, et al: Hereditary neonatal hyperparathyroidism. *Arch Surg* 113:100, 1978.
10. Girard RM, Belanger A, Hazel B: Primary hyperparathyroidism in children. *Can J Surg* 25:11, 1982.
11. Huang CB, Huang SC, Chou FF, et al: Primary hyperparathyroidism in children: Report of a case and a brief review of the literature. *J Formos Med Assoc* 92:1095, 1993.
12. O'Riordain DS, O'Brien T, Grant CS, et al: Surgical management of primary hyperparathyroidism in multiple endocrine

neoplasia types 1 and 2. *Surgery* 114:1031, 1993.

13. Bottger TC, Weber W, Beyer J, et al: Value of tumor localization in patients with insulinoma. *World J Surg* 14:107, 1990.

14. Rapaport D, Ziv Y, Rubin M, et al: Primary hyperparathyroidism in children. *J Pediatr Surg* 21:395, 1986.

15. Consensus Development Conference Panel: Diagnosis and management of symptomatic primary hyperparathyroidism. *Ann Intern Med* 114:593, 1991.

16. Allo M, Thompson NW, Harness JK, et al: Primary hyperparathyroidism in children, adolescents, and young adults. *World J Surg* 6:771, 1982.

17. Thompson NW, Eckhauser FE, Harness JK: The anatomy of primary hyperparathyroidism. *Surgery* 92:814, 1982.

18. Tezelman J, Rodriguez JM, Shen W, et al: Primary hyperparathyroidism in patients who have received radiation therapy and in patients who have not received radiation therapy. *J Am Coll Surg* 180:81, 1995.

19. McKay C, Furman L: Hypercalcemia complicating childhood malignancies. *Cancer* 72:256, 1993.

20. Tisell LE, Hedback G, Jannson S, et al: Management of hyperthyroid patients with grave hypercalcemia. *World J Surg* 15:730, 1991.

21. Kaplan EL, Yashiro T, Salti G: Primary hyperparathyroidism in the 1990s. *Ann Surg* 215:300, 1992.

22. Wassif WS, Moniz CF, Friedman E, et al: Familial isolated hyperparathyroidism: A distinct genetic entity with an increased risk of parathyroid cancer. *J Clin Endocrinol Metab* 77:1485, 1993.

23. Heath H: Familial benign (hypocalciuric) hypercalcemia. *Endocrinol Metab Clin North Am* 18:723, 1989.

24. Boechat MI, Westra SJ, Van Dop C, et al: Decreased cortical and increased cancellous bone in two children with primary hyperparathyroidism. *Metabolism* 45:76, 1996.

25. Cryns VL, Thor A, Xu HJ, et al: Loss of the retinoblastoma tumor-suppressor gene in parathyroid carcinoma. *N Engl J Med* 330:757, 1994.

26. Flye MW, Brennan MF: Surgical resection of metastatic parathyroid carcinoma. *Ann Surg* 193:425, 1981.

27. Mitchell BK, Merrell RC, Kinder BK: Localization studies in patients with hyperparathyroidism. *Surg Clin North Am* 75:483, 1995.

28. Kale N, Basaklar AC, Sonmez K, et al: Hungry bone syndrome in a child following parathyroid surgery. *J Pediatr Surg* 27:1502, 1992.

29. Wooten MD, King DK: Adrenal cortical carcinoma. *Cancer* 72:3145, 1993.

30. Hartley AL, Birch JM, Marsden HB, et al: Adrenal cortical tumors: Epidemiological and family aspects. *Arch Dis Child* 62:683, 1987.

31. Young JL Jr, Miller RW: Incidence of malignant tumors in U.S. children. *J Pediatr* 86:254, 1975.

32. Humphrey GB, Pysher T, Holcombe J, et al: Overview on the management of adrenocortical carcinoma. In Humphrey GB (ed): *Adrenal and Endocrine Tumors in Children*. Boston: Martinus Nijhoff, 1983, p. 349.

33. VanSlooten H, Schaberg A, Smeenk D, et al: Morphological characteristics of benign and malignant adrenocortical tumors. *Cancer* 55:776, 1985.

34. Lack EE, Mulvihill JJ, Travis WD, et al: Adrenal cortical neoplasms in the pediatric and adolescent age group. *Pathol Annu* 27(1):1, 1992.

35. Miller RW: Peculiarities in the occurrence of adrenal cortical carcinoma. *Am J Dis Child* 132:235, 1978.

36. Fraumeni JF, Miller RW: Adrenocortical neoplasms with hemihypertrophy, brain tumors, and other disorders. *J Pediatr* 70:129, 1967.

37. Tank ES, Kay R: Neoplasms associated with hemihypertrophy, Beckwith-Wiedemann syndrome and aniridia. *J Urol* 124:266, 1980.

38. Mark S, Clark OH, Kaplan RA: A virilized patient with congenital hemihypertrophy. *Postgrad Med J* 70:752, 1994.

39. Wagner J, Portwine C, Rabin K, et al: High frequency of germline p53 mutations in childhood adrenocortical cancer. *J Natl Cancer Inst* 86(22):1707, 1994.

40. Koufos A, Grundy P, Morgan K, et al: Familial Wiedemann-Beckwith syndrome and a second Wilms' tumor locus both map to 11p15.5. *Am J Hum Genet* 44:711, 1989.

41. Gicquel C, Bertagna X, Schneid H, et al: Rearrangements at the 11p15 locus and overexpression of insulin-like growth factor-II gene in sporadic adrenocortical tumors. *J Clin Endocrinol Metab* 78(6):1444, 1994.

42. Beuschlein F, Reincke M, Karl M, et al: Clonal composition of human adrenocortical neoplasms. *Cancer Res* 54(18):4927, 1994.

43. Bickler SW, Thomas JM, Campbell JR, et al: Preoperative diagnostic evaluation of children with Cushing's syndrome. *J Pediatr Surg* 29:671, 1994.

44. Gilbert MG, Cleveland WW: Cushing's syndrome in infancy. *Pediatrics* 46:217, 1970.

45. Hayles AB, Hahn HB: Hormone-secreting tumors of the adrenal cortex in children. *Pediatrics* 37:19, 1966.

46. McArthur RG, Cloutier MD, Hayles AB, et al: Cushing's disease in children. *Mayo Clin Proc* 47:318, 1972.

47. Thomas CG, Smith AT, Griffith JM, et al: Hyperadrenalism in childhood and adolescence. *Ann Surg* 199:538, 1984.

48. Gold EM: The Cushing's syndromes: Changing

views of diagnosis and treatment. *Ann Intern Med* 90:829, 1979.

49. Cohn K, Gottesman L, Brennan M: Adrenal cortical carcinoma. *Surgery* 100:1170, 1986.

50. Henley DJ, van Heerden JA, Grant CS, et al: Adrenal cortical carcinoma: A continuing challenge. *Surgery* 94:926, 1983.

51. Powell-Jackson JD, Calin A, Fraser R, et al: Excess deoxycorticosterone secretion from adrenocortical carcinoma. *Br Med J* 2:32, 1974.

52. Pang S, Becker D, Cotelingham J, et al: Adrenocortical tumor in a patient with congenital adrenal hyperplasia due to 21-hydroxylase deficiency. *Pediatrics* 68:242, 1981.

53. Magbool GM: Acute thrombocytopenic purpura in an infant with Cushing's syndrome: A case report. *Am J Hematol* 43(1):54, 1993.

54. Howman-Giles R, Dalla Pozza L, Uren R: Ga-67 scintigraphy in a child with adrenocortical carcinoma. *Clin Nucl Med* 18(8) 642, 1993.

55. al-Salem AH, Abu-Srair HA: Recurrent adrenocortical carcinoma in a 4-year-old girl. *Aust N Z J Surg* 64(10):723, 1994.

56. Kwauk S, Burt M: Pulmonary metastases from adrenal cortical carcinoma: Results of resection. *J Surg Oncol* 53(4):243, 1993.

57. Loriaux DL, Cutler GB Jr: Diseases of the adrenal glands. In Kohler PO (ed): *Clinical Endocrinology*. New York: John Wiley & Sons, 1986, p. 157.

58. Haak HR, Hermans J, van de Velde CJ, et al: Optimal treatment of adrenocortical carcinoma with mitotane: Results in a consecutive series of 96 patients. *Br J Cancer* 69(5):947, 1994.

59. Moolenaar AJ, vanSlooten H, vanSetters AP, et al: Blood levels of o,p'-DDD following administration in various vehicles after a single dose and during long-term treatment. *Can Chemother Pharmacol* 7:51, 1981.

60. Bukowski RM, Montie J, Crawford D, et al: Cisplatin and mitotane in metastatic adrenal cortical carcinoma: A southwest oncology group study. *Proc Am Soc Clin Oncol* 9:136, 1990.

61. Ostuni JA, Roginsky MS: Metastatic adrenal cortical carcinoma: Documented cure with combined chemotherapy. *Arch Intern Med* 135:1257, 1975.

62. Eriksson B, Oberg K, Curstedt T, et al: Treatment of hormone-producing adrenocortical cancer with o,p'-DDD and streptozocin. *Cancer* 59:1398, 1987.

63. Percarpio B, Knowlton AH: Radiation therapy of adrenal cortical carcinoma. *Acta Radiat Ther Biol* 15:288, 1976.

64. Didolkar MS, Bescher RA, Elias EG, et al: Natural history of adrenal cortical carcinoma. *Cancer* 47:2153, 1981.

65. Ventakesh S, Hickey RC, Sellin RV, et al: Adrenal cortical carcinoma. *Cancer* 64:765, 1989.

66. Caty MG, Coran AG, Geagen M, et al: Current diagnosis and treatment of pheochromocytoma in children. *Arch Surg* 125:978, 1990.

67. Londe S: Causes of hypertension in the young. *Pediatr Clin North Am* 25:55, 1978.

68. Werbel SS, Ober KP: Pheochromocytoma update on diagnosis, localization, and management. *Med Clin North Am* 79:131, 1995.

69. van Heerden JA, Sizemore GN, Carney JA, et al: Surgical management of the adrenal glands in the multiple endocrine neoplasia type II syndrome. *World J Surg* 8:612, 1984.

70. Levine C, Skimming J, Levine E: Familial pheochromocytomas with unusual associations. *J Pediatr Surg* 27:447, 1992.

71. Neumann HP, Berger DP, Sigmund G, et al: Pheochromocytomas, multiple endocrine neoplasia type 2, and von Hippel-Lindau disease. *N Engl J Med* 399:1531, 1993.

72. Norton JA, Jensen RT, Doppman JL: Cancer of the endocrine system. In DeVita VT, Hellman S, Rosenberg SA (eds): *Cancer: Principles and Practice of Oncology*, 4th ed., vol 2. Philadelphia: J. B. Lippincott Co, 1993, p. 1269.

73. Fonkalsrud E: The adrenal glands. In Welch KJ, Randolph JG, Ravitch MM, et al (eds): *Pediatric Surgery*, 4th ed., vol 2. Chicago: Yearbook Medical Publishers Inc, 1986, p. 1113.

74. Ein SH, Weitzman S, Thorner P, et al: Pediatric malignant pheochromocytoma. *J Pediatr Surg* 29:1197, 1994.

75a. Schlumberger M, Gicquel C, Lumbroso J, et al: Malignant pheochromocytoma: Clinical, biological, histologic and therapeutic data in a series of 20 patients with distant metastases. *J Endocrinol Invest* 15:631, 1992.

75b. Wyszynska T, Cichocka E, Wieteska-Klimczak A, et al: A single pediatric center experience with 1025 children with hypertension. *Acta Pediatr* 81:244, 1992.

76. Paltiel HJ, Gelfand MJ, Elgazzar AH, et al: Neural crest tumors: I 123-MIBG imaging in children. *Radiology* 190:117, 1994.

77. Turner MC, Lieberman E, DeQuattro V: The perioperative management of pheochromocytoma in children. *Clin Pediatr* 10:583, 1992.

78. Albanese C, Wiener ES: Routine total bilateral adrenalectomy is not warranted in childhood familial pheochromocytoma. *J Pediatr Surg* 28:1248, 1993.

79. Pommier RF, Vetto J, Billingsly K, et al: Comparison of adrenal and extra-adrenal pheochromocytoma. *Surgery* 114:1160, 1993.

80. Buchanan KD, Johnson CF, O'Hare, et al: Neuroendocrine tumors: A European view. *Am J Med* 81(68s):14, 1986.

81. Koppel G, Heitz PU: Pancreatic endocrine tumors. *Pathol Res Pract* 135:155, 1988.

82. Mukia K, Greider MH, Grotting JC, et al: Retrospective study of 77 pancreatic endocrine tumors using the immunoperoxidase method. *Am J Surg Pathol* 6:387, 1982.

83. London JF, Shawker TH, Doppman JL, et al: Zollinger-Ellison syndrome: Prospective

assessment of abdominal US in the localization of gastrinomas. *Radiology* 178:763, 1991.

84. Wise SR, Johnson J, Sparks J, et al: Gastrinoma: The predictive value of preoperative localization. *Surgery* 106:1087, 1989.

85. Doherty GM, Doppman JL, Shawker TH, et al: Results of a prospective strategy to diagnose, localize, and resect insulinomas. *Surgery* 110:989, 1991.

86. Pasieka JL, McLeod MK, Thompson NW, et al: Surgical approach to insulinomas: Assessing the need for preoperative localization. *Arch Surg* 127:442, 1992.

87. Daggett PR, Goodburn EA, Kurtz AB, et al: Is preoperative localization of insulinomas necessary? *Lancet* I:483, 1981.

88. Maton PN, Miller DL, Doppman JL, et al: Role of selective angiography in the management of patients with Zollinger-Ellison syndrome. *Gastroenterology* 92:913, 1987.

89. Wank SA, Doppman JL, Miller DL, et al: Prospective study of the inability of computed axial tomography to localize gastrinomas in patients with Zollinger-Ellison syndrome. *Gastroenterology* 92:905, 1987.

90. Liessi G, Pasquali C, D'Andrea AA, et al: MRI in insulinomas: Preliminary findings. *Euro J Radiol* 14:46, 1992.

91. Geoghegan JG, Jackson JE, Lewis MP, et al: Localization and surgical management of insulinoma. *Br J Surg* 81:1025, 1994.

92. Hammond PJ, Jackson JA, Bloom SR: Localization of pancreatic endocrine tumors. *Clin Endocrinol* 40:3, 1994.

93. Imamura M, Takahashi K: Use of selective arterial secretion injection test to guide surgery in patients with Zollinger-Ellison syndrome. *World J Surg* 17:433, 1993.

94. Doppman JL, Miller DL, Chang R, et al: Insulinomas: Localization with selective intra-arterial injection of calcium. *Radiology* 178:237, 1991.

95. Fedorak IJ, Ko TC, Gordon D, et al: Localization of islet cell tumors of the pancreas: A review of current techniques. *Surgery* 113:242, 1993.

96. Schwartz DL, White JJ, Saulsbury F, et al: Gastrin response to calcium infusion: An aid to the improved diagnosis of Zollinger-Ellison syndrome in children. *Pediatrics* 54(5):599, 1974.

97. Vinik AI, Delbridge L, Moattari R, et al: Transhepatic portal vein catheterization for localization of insulinomas: A ten-year experience. *Surgery* 113:242, 1991.

98. Palazzo L, Roseau G, Salmeron M: Endoscopic ultrasonography in the preoperative localization of pancreatic endocrine tumors. *Endoscopy* 24(S1):350, 1992.

99. Rosch T, Lightdale CJ, Botet JF, et al: Localization of pancreatic endocrine tumors by endoscopic ultrasonography. *N Engl J Med* 326:1721, 1992.

100. Van Eyck CH, Braining HA, Reubi JC, et al: Use of isotope-labelled somatostatin analogs for visualization of islet cell tumors. *World J Surg* 17:444, 1993.

101. Grosfeld JL, Vance DW, Rescorla FJ, et al: Pancreatic tumors in childhood: Analysis of 13 cases. *J Pediatr Surg* 25:1057, 1990.

102. Jaksic T, Yaman M, Thorner P, et al: A 20-year review of pediatric pancreatic tumors. *J Pediatr Surg* 27(10):1315, 1992.

103. Norton JA: Neuroendocrine tumors of the pancreas and duodenum. *Curr Probl Surg* 31(2):79, 1994.

104. Comi RJ, Gordon P, Doppman M5HL, et al: Insulinoma. In Go VL, Gardner JD, Brooks FP, et al (eds): *The Exocrine Pancreas: Biology, Pathology, and Diseases.* New York: Raven Press, 1986, p. 745.

105. Zollinger RM, Ellison EH: Primary peptic ulceration of the jejunum associated with islet cell tumors of the pancreas. *Ann Surg* 142:709, 1955.

106. Norton JA, Doppman JL, Jensen RT: Curative resection in Zollinger-Ellison syndrome: Results of a 10-year prospective study. *Ann Surg* 215:8, 1992.

107. Fraker DL, Norton JA, Saeed ZA, et al: A prospective study of perioperative and postoperative control of acid hypersecretion in patients with Zollinger-Ellison syndrome undergoing gastrinoma resection. *Surgery* 104:1054, 1988.

108. Rosenbaum A, Flourie B, Chagnan S, et al: Octreotide in the treatment of metastatic glucogonoma: Report of one case and review of the literature. *Digestion* 42(2):116, 1989.

109. Brenner RW, Sank LI, Kerner MB, et al: Resection of a VIPoma of the pancreas in a 15-year-old girl. *J Pediatr Surg* 21:983, 1986.

110. Ghishan FK, Soper RT, Nassif EG, et al: Chronic diarrhea of infancy: Non-beta islet cell hyperplasia. *Pediatrics* 64(1):46, 1979.

111. Krejs GJ: VIPoma syndrome. *Am J Med* 82(5B):37, 1987.

112. Marshall JB, Bodnarchuk G: Carcinoid tumors of the gut. *J Clin Gastroenterol* 16:123, 1993.

113. Newton JN, Swerdlow IM, dos Santos Silva IM, et al: The epidemiology of carcinoid tumours in England and Scotland. *Br J Cancer* 70:939, 1994.

114. Hancock BJ, Di Lorenzo M, Youssef S, et al: Childhood primary pulmonary neoplasms. *J Pediatr Surg* 28:1133, 1993.

115. Moertel CL, Weiland LH, Telander RL: Carcinoid tumor of the appendix in the first two decades of life. *J Pediatr Surg* 25:1073, 1990.

116. Whelan T, Gatfield CT, Robertson S, et al: Primary carcinoid of the prostate in conjunction with Multiple Endocrine Neoplasia IIB in a child. *J Urol* 153:1080, 1995.

117. Parkes SE, Muir KR, Al Sheyyab M, et al: Carcinoid tumors of the appendix in children

1957–1986: Incidence, treatment, and outcome. *Br J Surg* 80:502, 1993.

118. Otsuka T, Ohshima Y, Sunaga Y, et al: Primary pulmonary choriocarcinoma in a four month old boy complicated with precocious puberty. *Acta Paediatr Jpn* 36:404, 1994.

119. Lamberts SW, Barker WH, Reubi JC, et al: Somatostatin-receptor imaging in the localization of endocrine tumors. *N Engl J Med* 323:1246, 1990.

120. Chow CW, Sane S, Campbell PE, et al: Malignant carcinoid tumors in children. *Cancer* 49:802, 1982.

121. Pass HI, Doppman JL, Nieman L, et al: Management of the ectopic ACTH syndrome due to thoracic carcinoids. *Ann Thorac Surg* 50:52, 1990.

122. Barkan AL, Shenker Y, Grekin RJ, et al: Acromegaly from ectopic growth-hormone-releasing hormone secretion by a malignant carcinoid tumor. *Cancer* 61:221, 1988.

123. DeHerder WW, Krenning EP, Malchoff CD, et al: Somatostatin receptor scintigraphy: Its value in tumor localization in patients with Cushing's syndrome caused by ectopic corticotropin or corticotropin-releasing hormone secretion. *Am J Med* 96:305, 1994.

124. Bickler SW, Mc Mahon TJ, Campbell JR, et al: Preoperative diagnostic evaluation of children with Cushing's syndrome. *J Pediatr Surg* 29:671, 1994.

125. Doppman JL, Nieman L, Miller DL, et al: Ectopic adrenocorticotropic hormone syndrome: Localization studies in 28 patients. *Radiology* 172:115, 1989.

126. Doppman JL, Pass HI, Nieman LK, et al: Corticotropin-secreting carcinoid tumors of the thymus: Diagnostic unreliability of thymic venous sampling. *Radiology* 184:71, 1992.

127. Omenn GS: Ectopic hormone syndromes associated with tumors in childhood. *Pediatrics* 47:613, 1971.

128. Cummins GE, Cohen D: Cushing's syndrome secondary to ACTH-secreting Wilms' tumor. *J Pediatr Surg* 9:535, 1974.

129. Wajchenberg BL, Mendonca BB, Liberman B, et al: Ectopic adrenocorticotropic hormone syndrome. *Endocrinol Rev* 15:752, 1994.

130. Philipponneau M, Nocaudie M, Epelbaum J, et al: Somatostatin analogs for the localization and preoperative treatment of an adrenocorticotropin-secreting bronchial carcinoid tumor. *J Clin Endocrinol Metab* 78:20, 1994.

131a. Hsiao JC, Yang CP, Lin CJ, et al: Ectopic ACTH syndrome due to clear cell sarcoma of the kidney. *Child Nephrol Urol* 11:103, 1991.

131b. Sano S, Asa S, Kovacs K: Growth-hormone-releasing hormone–producing tumors: Clinical, biochemical, and morphological manifestations. *Endocrine Rev* 9(3):357, 1988.

132. Zimmerman D, Young WF, Ebersold MJ, et al:

Congenital gigantism due to growth-hormone-releasing hormone excess and pituitary hyperplasia with adenomatous transformation. *J Clin Endocrinol Metab* 76:216, 1993.

133. Thorner M, Frohman LA, Leong DA, et al: Extrahypothalamic growth-hormone-releasing factor (GRF) secretion is a rare cause of acromegaly: Plasma GRF levels in 177 acromegalic patients. *J Clin Endocrinol Metab* 59:846, 1984.

134. Faglia G, Arosio M, Bazzoni N: Ectopic acromegaly. *Endocrinol Metabol Clin North Am* 21(3):575, 1992.

135. Ramsay JA, Kovacs K, Asa S, et al: Reversible sellar enlargement due to growth-hormone-releasing hormone production by pancreatic endocrine tumors in an acromegalic patient with multiple endocrine neoplasia type 1 syndrome. *Cancer* 62:445, 1988.

136. Von Werder K, Losa M, Stalla GK, et al: Long-term treatment of a metastasizing GRFoma with a somatostatin analogue (SMS 201–995) in a girl with gigantism. *Lancet* 2:282, 1984.

137. Christofides ND, Stephanou A, Yiangou Y, et al: Distribution of immunoreactive growth-hormone-releasing hormone in the human brain and intestine and its production by tumors. *J Clin Endocrinol Metab* 59(4):747, 1984.

138. Asa S, Kovacs K, Thorner MO, et al: Immunohistological localization of growth-hormone-releasing hormone in human tumors. *J Clin Endocrinol Metab* 60(3):423, 1985.

139. Oberg K, Norheim I, Wide L: Serum growth hormone in patients with carcinoid tumours: Basal levels and response to glucose and thyrotropin-releasing hormone. *Acta Endocrinol* 109:13, 1985.

140. Moran A, Asa S, Kovacs K, et al: Gigantism due to pituitary mammosomatotroph hyperplasia. *N Engl J Med* 323(5):322, 1990.

141. Garcia-Luna PP, Leal-Cerro A, Montero C, et al: A rare cause of acromegaly: Ectopic production of growth hormone-releasing factor by a bronchial carcinoid tumor. *Surg Neurol* 27:563, 1987.

142. Moller DE, Moses AC, Jones K, et al: Octreotide suppresses both growth hormone (GH) and GH-releasing hormone (GHRH) in acromegaly due to ectopic GHRH secretion. *J Clin Endocrinol Metab* 68(2):499, 1989.

143. Glikson M, Gil-Aid I, Galun E, et al: Acromegaly due to ectopic growth-hormone-releasing hormone secretion in a bronchial carcinoid tumor: Dynamic hormonal responses to various stimuli. *Acta Endocrinol* 125:366, 1991.

144. Marina NM, Rao B, Etcubanas E, et al: The role of second-look surgery in the management of advance germ cell malignancies. *Cancer* 68:309, 1991.

145. Englund AT, Geffner ME, Nagel RA, et al: Pediatric germ cell and human chorionic

gonadotropin-producing tumors. *Am J Dis Child* 145:1294, 1991.

146. Navarro C, Corretger JM, Sancho A, et al: Paraneoplastic precocious puberty. *Cancer* 56:1725, 1985.

147. Marsden HB, Birch JM, Swindell R: Germ cell tumours of childhood: A review of 137 cases. *J Clin Pathol* 34:879, 1981.

148. Wollner N, Ghavimi F, Wachtel A, et al: Germ cell tumors in children: Gonadal and extragonadal. *Med Pediatr Oncol* 19:228, 1991.

149. Deleted in print.

150. Derenoncourt AN, Castro-Magana M, Jones KL: Mediastinal teratoma and precocious puberty in a boy with mosaic Klinefelter syndrome. *Am J Med Genet* 55:38, 1995.

151. Schwartz MK: Cancer Markers: In DeVita VT, Hellman S, Rosenberg SA (eds): *Cancer: Principles and Practice of Oncology*, 4th ed. Philadelphia: J. B. Lippincott Co, 1993, p. 533.

152. Kitanaka C, Matsutani M, Sora S, et al: Precocious puberty in a girl with an hCG-secreting suprasellar immature teratoma. *J Neurosurg* 81:601, 1994.

153. Fraser GC, Blair GK, Hemming A, et al: The treatment of simultaneous choriocarcinoma in mother and baby. *J Pediatr Surg* 27(10), 1992.

154. Lippe BM, Edwards MS, Braunstein GD, et al: A non-malignant teratoma secreting hCG: Expanding the spectrum of ectopic hormone production. *J Pediatr* 105(5):765, 1984.

155. Donis-Keller H, Dou S, Chi D: Mutations in the RET proto-oncogene are associated with MEN2A and FMTC. *Hum Mol Genet* 2:851, 1993.

156. Howe JR, Norton JA, Wells SA: Prevalence of pheochromocytoma and hyperparathyroidism in multiple endocrine neoplasia type 2A: Results of long-term follow-up. *Surgery* 114:1070, 1993.

157. Wells Jr SA, Chi DD, Toshima K, et al: Predictive DNA testing and prophylactic thyroidectomy in patients at risk for multiple endocrine neoplasia type 2A. *Ann Surg* 220:237, 1994.

158. Skogseid B, Oberg K: Prospective screening in multiple endocrine neoplasia type 1. *Henry Ford Hosp Med J* 40:167, 1992.

159. Lips CJ, Landsvater RM, Hoppener JW, et al: Clinical screening as compared with DNA analysis in families with multiple endocrine neoplasia type 2A. *N Engl J Med* 331:828, 1994.

160. O'Riordain DS, O'Brien T, van Heerden JA, et al: Surgical management of insulinoma associated with multiple endocrine neoplasia type I. *World J Surg* 18:488, 1994.

161. Sheppard BC, Norton JA, Doppman JL, et al: Management of islet cell tumors in patients with multiple endocrine neoplasia: A prospective study. *Surgery* 106:1108, 1989.

162a. Telander RL, Zimmerman D, van Heerden JA, et al: Results of early thyroidectomy for medullary thyroid carcinoma in children with multiple endocrine neoplasia type 2. *J Pediatr Surg* 21:1190, 1986.

162b. Skinner MA, DeBenedetti MK, Moley JF, et al: Medullary thyroid carcinoma in children with multiple endocrine neoplasia types 2A and 2B. *J Pediatr Surg* 31:177, 1996.

163. Vasen HF, van der Feltz M, Raue F, et al: The natural course of multiple endocrine neoplasia type IIB: a study of 18 cases. *Arch Intern Med* 152:1250, 1992.

164. Sizemore GW, Carney JA, Gharib H, et al: Multiple endocrine neoplasia type 2B: Eighteen-year follow-up of a four-generation family. *Henry Ford Hosp Med J* 40:236, 1992.

165. Zeiger MA, Shawker TH, Norton JA: Use of intraoperative ultrasonography to localize islet cell tumors. *World J Surg* 17:448, 1993.

Chapter

22

Metastases from Solid Tumors

• *Nicholas C. Saenz, M.D.* • *Michael P. LaQuaglia M.D.*

Local tumor control first became possible with the development of radical resections. Multidisciplinary approaches that utilized surgical resection combined with local radiation therapy followed, reducing morbidity (such as that requiring amputation) while preventing growth of solid malignancies in the primary site. As techniques and understanding of principles for local control developed, surgeons addressed the problem of metastatic disease. Weinlechner[1] reported one of the first successful pulmonary resections for a primary sarcoma of the chest wall in 1892. In 1927 and 1930 Divis[2] and Torek[3] detailed their experiences with pulmonary resections for metastatic disease. Barney and Churchill[4] did a successful partial lobectomy for metastatic adenocarcinoma of the kidney in 1933, and the patient survived for more than 23 years. In 1978 Mountain and coworkers[5] compiled data from nine reported series, including 660 patients with pulmonary metastases, and reported a 5-year survival rate of 30% (range: 25% to 40%). In comparison, the natural history of 78 patients with lung metastases was studied by Farrel,[6] who reported that 44% died within 6 months and only 9% survived more than 2 years. Farrel[6] also found that in adult autopsy series close to 10% of those who died from cancer had only lung metastases and no other sites of dissemination.

In the last two decades, most investigators have shown that resection of hepatic metastases in selected situations (appropriate primary tumor histology, limited extent of metastatic disease, and satisfactory patient status) is the treatment of choice. Patients undergoing hepatic resections for metastases from colorectal carcinomas have a

5-year survival rate of 33% and a disease-free survival rate of 25%.[7–10] Galicich and coworkers[11] reported that in highly selected adults with solitary cerebral metastases, metastasectomy was associated with a 44% survival rate at 1 year. The patients also received postoperative cerebral radiotherapy but did better than reported series of patients who received radiation alone. Thus, active surgical intervention in metastatic disease has efficacy when the patient status and tumor type are favorable.

The focus of this chapter is the role of the pediatric surgical oncologist in the management of metastatic tumors. A survey of the extent of the clinical problem of interest to pediatric surgeons may be useful. Table 22–1 lists the six most common non–central nervous system solid tumors of childhood in decreasing order of incidence, along with the percentage of patients who present with synchronous metastases. The average reported disease-free survival rate at 2 or 3 years for patients with disseminated disease at time of diagnosis is also listed.[12, 13] Clearly, tumor dissemination is a major obstacle to cure in these patients. The challenge for the surgical member of the interdisciplinary oncology team is to decide on the efficacy and morbidity of metastasectomy in a given case and determine conditions warranting its application.

BIOLOGIC PRINCIPLES

A metastasis can be defined as the transfer of disease from one organ or part to another not directly connected with it. The idea of metastasis is intimately linked with invasion. The ability to metastasize is a defining quality for malignant cells and causes most therapeutic failures in patients with solid tumors.[14–16] A simplified but generally accepted model describing the cellular events in the development of metastases is depicted in Figure 22–1.[17–19] An initial expansion of the malignant population in the primary site is necessary for tumor development. During this expansion the tumor consists of phenotypically distinct subclones, some of which will possess the ability to invade through the various restraining basement membranes enclosing the primary site. Malignant cells must then penetrate through the vascular basement membrane and into the vascular space, traveling through the veins or lymphatics to enter the target organ. This target will be determined by the lymphaticovenous drainage of the primary site and by the compatible receptors on both the metastatic cells and the target organ cells. These receptors allow tumor cell adherence and a second invasive process away from the vascular tree. Once the second invasion has been completed, the metastatic cell must divide, recruit a new blood supply, and produce a macroscopic tumor.

This model suggests that simple anatomic or hemodynamic factors do not adequately explain the frequency or specificity of metastases for a particular malignancy. For example, neuroblastoma often spreads to bone, bone marrow, or lymph nodes, whereas osteogenic sarcoma specifically spreads to lungs. The implication is that tumor cell and host factors are operative in the occurrence and specificity of metastases. This "fertile seed and soil" hypothesis, first proposed by Paget, is supported by experimental data. For

---

Table 22–1 • Impact of Metastases on Outcome in Patients with Pediatric Solid Tumors

Tumor Type	Percent of Patients with Metastases at Diagnosis	Common Metastatic Sites	Survival Rate for Stage 4 Patients (%)
Neuroblastoma	60	bone, liver, marrow	25[a]
Wilms' tumor	15	lung, liver	63–69[b]
Rhabdomyosarcoma	10–20	lung, bone, liver	43–62[c]
Osteogenic sarcoma	10–20	lung, bone	30–40[d]
Ewing's sarcoma	14–50	lung, bone	33[a]
Primary hepatic tumors	20	lung, bone	0

[a] Three-year survival
[b] Two-year survival
[c] Of those responding to therapy

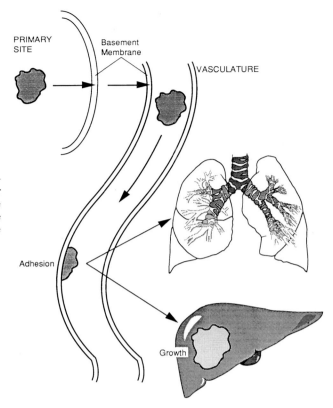

Figure 22–1 • The metastatic cascade is depicted, with invasion through tissue and vascular basement membranes followed by entry into the vascular tree. Transit through the vasculature is followed by adhesion and invasion into the target site.

instance, striated muscle has an excellent blood supply but is almost never the site of distant metastases. One may speculate that specific receptors that allow tumor cells to initially adhere do not exist on the vascular endothelium in striated muscle. Furthermore, distribution studies using radiolabeled tumor cells have shown in animal models that initial tumor cell adherence does not always result in macroscopic tumor growth. Necessary trophic factors that allow cell multiplication may not be present with subsequent population failure.

Interestingly, the major steps in metastasis development just described, when examined at the molecular biologic and protein level, reveal a number of correlations between oncogene activation in primary tumors and occurrence of distant metastases. As an example, N-*myc* amplification in neuroblastoma and *int*-1 activation in retinoblastoma are positively correlated with the presence of metastases. In another area of research, workers are beginning to understand the molecular basis of metastasis specificity. For lymphoma cells metastasizing to liver, the initial adherence

and invasion may rest on expression by the tumor cells of the adhesion molecule, LFA-1. Similarly, endothelial binding of colorectal carcinoma cells may sometimes depend on expression of ELAM-1.

THE CLINICAL PROBLEM

Clinical management of metastatic disease in childhood is rationally determined by (1) the underlying disease process and its responsiveness to other forms of treatment and (2) the affected target organ (e.g., lung, liver, bone, brain). In view of this approach, discussion of the clinical management is categorized by specific solid tumor and metastatic site. Usually, operative removal of metastatic disease should be undertaken in the context of a significant tumor response in the primary site. Ideally, it should also be shown that the metastases have responded to systemic chemotherapy before the resection. Such response ensures that undetectable micrometastases will not result in the patient's early re-relapse. It must be emphasized, however, that all the data on the resection of metastases are nonrandomized and retrospective. Often reports are concerned with the total number of patients undergoing resections rather than the true denominator, which is the number of patients in whom metastases develop. Caution must therefore be used in interpreting data on surgical intervention for metastatic disease.

Osteogenic Sarcoma Metastatic to Lung

The paradigm for surgical removal of metastases is osteogenic sarcoma. More than 85% of recurrences of osteogenic sarcomas are in the lung. Many patients have only pulmonary metastases and are curable by resection of all metastatic disease. Part of the reason for the success of thoracotomy in this disease is the fact that effective chemotherapeutic agents are available and the metastatic deposits are calcified and detectable by palpation. Most of these lesions can be resected by wedge resections without sacrifice of significant amounts of adjacent normal lung tissue. At Memorial Sloan-Kettering Cancer Center, up to 20 lesions have been removed from one lung during thoracotomy because the lesions could be detected to 1 mm to 2 mm, owing to the calcifications. Soft-tissue tumors metastasizing to the lung cannot be so easily detected, and this is one reason for the diminished effectiveness of surgery in that setting.

Table 22–2 lists data obtained from 12 published series on the management of metachronous pulmonary metastases in patients with osteogenic sarcomas.[20–31] Of particular note in interpreting these results is that some studies include patients who did not undergo resection of pulmonary metastases because of technical unresectability (mediastinal extension) or use of alternative treatments (pulmonary irradiation or chemotherapy). Disease-free survival rate was zero for the unresected group. It can be seen from this table that pulmonary metastasectomy can result in long-term disease-free survival in about one third of patients who develop metachronous pulmonary metastases. It must be recognized, however, that these are nonrandomized patients. A resection might be better avoided in patients with diffuse or extensive disease or those in poor general condition. These prognostic variables should be kept in mind when interpreting retrospective patient reviews.

Roth and coworkers[32] analyzed the effect of metastasis number, length of disease-free interval from first remission to development of pulmonary metastases, and tumor-doubling time on the outcome. For osteogenic sarcomas they found that patients with four or fewer pulmonary nodules had a post-thoracotomy median survival of 37 months compared with 10 months for patients with more than four lesions. Goorin and coworkers[27] showed that complete resection of all pulmonary lesions is the most important determinant of the outcome. In their study, penetration through the parietal pleura or residual pulmo-

Table 22–2 • Experience with Pulmonary Metastasectomy for Osteogenic Sarcoma

Author and Year (ref.)	Number of Patients	Median Interval to Relapse in Months (Range)	Number of Procedures (No. Lesions)	Number and Percent of Patients with Disease-Free Survival	Median F/U for Survivors in Months (Range)
Martini 1971[20]	22	10 (2–25)	59 (113)	7 (32%)	33 (15–234)
Spanos 1976[21]	29	15.7 (4–30)	52 (124)	11 (37%)	36 (9–234)
Telander 1978[22]	28	9.6 (2–34)	60 (173)	13 (46%)	25 (6–48)
Giritsky 1978[23]	12	9 (1–21)	19	6 (50%)	17 (9–39)
Rosenberg 1979[24]	18			7 (39%)	
Burgers 1980[25]	12	13 (2–20)	9	5 (42%)	(36–72)
Schaller 1982[26]	17		34	7 (41%)	(12–192)
Goorin 1984[27]	32	12.5 (4–59)	26 (>63)	9 (28%)	55 (19–101)
Carter 1991[28]	43	13 (1–83)		4 (10%)	69 (59–80)
Saltzman 1993[29]	27	14	146 (147)	24% at 5 yrs.	
Heij 1994[30]	40	10.2 ± 9.2	10.2 ± 12.5/pt.	6 (15%) at 5 yrs.	(18–240)
Temeck[31]	76	7.2 (median)		45% at 5 yrs.	

F/U = follow-up.

nary disease adversely affected outcomes. Meyers and coworkers[33] reported that aggressive and total surgical resection of the tumor was necessary for survival in patients presenting with synchronous pulmonary metastases.

Of interest is a 20-year follow-up[34] on five patients initially reported by Martini and coworkers (see Table 22–2). One patient had no evidence of disease after 20 years, but three had died: one from recurrence, another from a second primary in the opposite knee, and a third from breast cancer. The fifth patient in this 20-year follow-up remained in remission both from osteogenic sarcoma and diffuse histiocytic lymphoma for which she had received an autologous bone marrow transplant. This report illustrates both the possibility for long-term survival after resections of pulmonary metastases and the necessity for careful follow-up.

Available data support an aggressive attempt at surgical resection of pulmonary metastases in patients with osteogenic sarcomas no matter what the number of lesions is or the interval to development of metastases.

Osteogenic Sarcoma Metastatic to Sites Other Than Lung

Osteogenic sarcomas can metastasize to other bones and, rarely, to liver and brain. Nevertheless, no large series have been reported upon which to base rational surgical treatment of metastases to these sites. Because the outlook for patients with residual gross disease is poor, selected attempts at the resection of bone, brain, and hepatic metastases are warranted when lesions are isolated and remain responsive to chemotherapy. A resection in the presence of resistant or progressive disease is futile.

Soft-Tissue Sarcoma Metastatic to Lung

Many reports support the efficacy of the resection of pulmonary soft-tissue sarcoma metastases.[35–39] These reports, however, are concerned with adult patients. Common histologies include tenosynovial sarcoma and malignant fibrous histiocytoma, tumors rarely seen in pediatric patients. No reports focus on the treatment of metastatic rhabdomyosarcoma or Ewing's sarcoma, childhood sarcomas sensitive to both chemotherapy

and radiation. Surgical detection of metastatic deposits, especially deep within lung parenchyma, is very difficult. In contrast, whole-lung radiation to doses of 1200 cGy along with systemic chemotherapy has been effective in controlling pulmonary metastases from these tumors. Surgery is useful in these cases only for diagnostic purposes and removal of a localized or nonresolving focus of gross disease.

Unfortunately, many childhood tumors are resistant to radiation and chemotherapy. These include liposarcoma, leiomyosarcoma, alveolar soft-parts sarcoma, synovial sarcoma, fibrosarcoma, neurogenic sarcoma, and epithelioid sarcoma. Pulmonary resections may be beneficial for patients with soft-tissue sarcomas whose primary tumor has been controlled. The disease-free interval, the number of lesions, and the tumor-doubling time are significant prognostic indicators for patients with the soft-tissue sarcomas (usually high-grade) in contrast to those with the osteogenic sarcomas, for which only lesion number is predictive of outcome.

Wilms' Tumor Metastatic to Lung

Resection of pulmonary metastases from a Wilms' tumor is often accompanied and confounded by whole-lung radiation and systemic chemotherapy. Certain observations can still be made from the literature. Figure 22–2 displays data from seven reports of pulmonary metastatic Wilms' tumor.[40–45] The figure includes only patients with metachronous pulmonary lesions that were either solitary or few at the time of treatment. The total number of patients undergoing treatment is plotted, and alongside this is the number surviving for at least 20 months after initial treatment (the smallest follow-up time in the seven reports). The proportion surviving at 20 months is the same for patients undergoing resection as those treated with chemotherapy alone or with chemotherapy plus radiation. If these data are combined, we find that there are 41 survivors of 53 patients (77%) treated with multiple modalities including surgery, whereas 13 of 19 (68%) patients who did not receive surgery also survived. Significance testing using Fisher's exact test (at 20 months' follow-up) reveals a p value of 0.84. This test result suggests that the addition of surgery does not offer a survival advantage over whole-lung radiation and

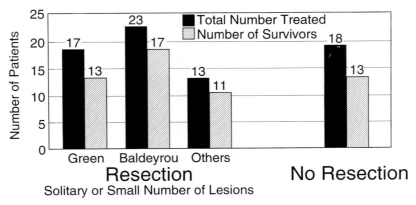

Figure 22–2 • Comparison of total data from two large series[42, 45] and a collection of three smaller ones[38b, 40, 41, 43, 44] regarding treatment of Wilms' tumor with pulmonary metastases. Patients were followed for a minimum of 20 months after metastasis treatment. Also compared are results of resection of pulmonary metastases versus chemotherapy and irradiation without such resection. It must be noted that many patients undergoing resection also received pulmonary irradiation or chemotherapy. The data show no benefit for the addition of surgical resection to the treatment of patients with Wilms' tumor and pulmonary metastases.

chemotherapy in the treatment of solitary or few pulmonary metastases from Wilms' tumor. Five of the seven reports, however, include nonsurgical patients, and exact comparison is hampered by different follow-up times. In addition, most of the patients undergoing surgery also were treated with pulmonary radiation and chemotherapy. Nevertheless, the addition of a surgical resection did not improve survival rates for patients with localized pulmonary metastases. In patients with diffuse pulmonary disease, complete extirpation of all foci becomes less feasible and surgery less effective.

Currently whole-lung radiation is administered at a dose of 1200 cGy and has the advantage of treating undetected micrometastases. But pulmonary irradiation is associated with significant and possibly lethal side effects on the growing lung. Wohl and coworkers[46] determined lung function on 12 patients treated for lung metastases compared with 8 treated for the primary tumor but who did not develop lung metastases and found that total lung capacity and diffusing capacity were reduced in the entire group of patients treated with pulmonary radiation. Green and coworkers,[45] in a report from the National Wilms' Tumor Study (NWTS), noted that diffuse pneumonitis developed in 15 of 153 (9.8%) patients receiving 1200 cGy for localized or diffuse pulmonary disease. Eleven of the 15 (73%) succumbed to progressive pulmonary failure despite institution of steroid therapy. A surgical resec-

tion, therefore, may have some advantage in treating patients with localized pulmonary metastases if the need for whole-lung irradiation is eliminated.

Five patients in NWTS 1 through 3 were treated with a resection of pulmonary metastases and chemotherapy but with avoidance of whole-lung irradiation. Four of these had a second recurrence; two survived more than 500 days after an initial relapse. Baldeyrou and coworkers[42] reported that 9 of 17 patients treated for solitary lesions avoided pulmonary irradiation. Specific survival times were not reported for these 9 patients. The overall survival rate after resection of Wilms' tumor metastases in this report was 51% (38 of 75 patients). Soper[40] reported one patient who survived 20 months after thoracotomy alone for a pulmonary relapse. Thus, some data support a role for surgery and chemotherapy in specific situations of localized, limited pulmonary disease. This approach seems most applicable in patients less than 2 years of age with favorable-histology lesions and lungs that might be more susceptible to radiation toxicity.

Few complications of thoracotomy were observed in children with Wilms' tumor. Baldeyrou and coworkers[42] reported that 2 of 75 patients (2.7%) undergoing thoracotomy for metastatic Wilms' tumor died during the perioperative period. Four additional patients died with interstitial pneumonitis during the months after surgery, but two of these had also received large doses of whole-lung radiation therapy. Operative or post-operative hemorrhage, empyema, bronchopleural fistula, and other complications have been reported for thoracotomy in patients in this age group but at a low incidence. Radiation-induced pneumonitis occurs in 8% to 10% of patients receiving 1200 cGy to the whole lung and is associated with a 70% mortality. In view of this finding, thoracotomy may warrant consideration in the treatment of metastases to the lung from Wilms' tumors.

The addition of pulmonary metastasectomy offers no advantage in the treatment of metastatic Wilms' tumor. As whole-lung irradiation and chemotherapy are uniformly given now and have the advantage of treating diffuse metastases, surgery should be reserved for special cases. Pulmonary resections may play a role in the treatment of very young patients with solitary or few metastases and favorable histology. Moreover, the resection of pulmonary lesions may be required to obtain tissue for diagnosis, determine the effects of therapy, or remove particularly large metastatic tumors that would be difficult to cure with the usual 1200 cGy dose.

Wilms' Tumor Metastatic to Liver, Brain, and Bone

Little data exist on the treatment of patients with Wilms' tumor metastases to sites other than the lungs. Foster[48] collected 15 cases undergoing hepatic resections for metastatic Wilms' tumor from the literature and reported a median survival of 24 months after metastasectomy (mean was 32 months). In this series there were two (13%) operative deaths; eight of thirteen patients survived 2 years; four of nine patients survived 5 years; and none died of recurrence after 5 years. Morrow and coworkers[49] reported on four patients undergoing hepatic resections for metastatic Wilms' tumor, and the cumulative five-year survival was 50%. These data support hepatic resection for metastatic Wilms' tumor as a part of protocol-based therapy, assuming some response to chemotherapy is evident.

Similar considerations hold for tumor recurrences in bone or brain. Surgical removal of favorably located metastases is more effective if initial response to chemotherapy is good. In situations in which the metastases are extensive and/or nonresponsive to salvage chemotherapy, heroic attempts at resection are not indicated.

Hepatoblastoma Metastatic to Lung

Approximately 24% of hepatoblastomas appear with metastatic disease, and about 10% spread to the lung.[50, 51] Bone and regional nodes are other common metastatic sites. Rare metastases to kidneys, epidural space, and other areas have been noted as well. Most researchers agree that a complete resection of the primary site is necessary for cure,[52, 53] but little data are available from which to infer the role of metastasectomy. Table 22–3[44, 50, 54–59] lists data from reported cases of pulmonary metastasectomy for metachronous disease that show resection of pulmonary metastases as feasible and associated with significant post-thoracotomy disease-free intervals. Yet, no account of the total number of patients developing metastases (only those undergoing surgery) or comparisons to alternative therapy (chemotherapy or radiotherapy) have been reported. Weinblatt and coworkers[60] reported one patient with a case of total resolution of pulmonary metastases from a hepatoblastoma with chemotherapy alone, and this patient remains disease-free 6 years after diagnosis. Significant resolution of synchronous pulmonary metastases with chemotherapy alone has been noted.[61] Therefore, pulmonary metastasectomy is recommended in patients with significant localized hepatoblastoma disease that has shown response to, but not total resolution after, induction chemotherapy. Figure 22–3 shows that the serum alpha-fetoprotein level can be used to detect relapses, and its determination helps to differentiate benign (scar, fungal infection) from malignant pulmonary nodules.

DIAGNOSTIC STUDIES

Patients at high risk for development of pulmonary metastases should be followed with monthly chest radiographs for the first year after diagnosis (the interval of highest risk). Computed tomography (CT) of the chest with lung windows is probably the most sensitive study and should complement plain chest radiographs, being done every 3 months for the first year of follow-up. The helical CT scanner performs tomography continuously, advancing in a helical fashion. In

Table 22–3 • Reports of Pulmonary Metastasectomy for Hepatoblastoma

Author and Year (Ref.)	Number of Patients	Interval to Metastases in Months	Number of Lesions (Site of Metastases)	Follow-up Time After Thoracotomy in Months	Outcome
Bradham 1965[54]	1	5.5	1 (lung) 1 (diaphragm)	36 +	NED[c]
Ballantine 1975[55]	1	5		6	DOD[d]
Lembke 1986[56]	2			17 + 41 +	NED NED
Feusner 1986[57]	2	13 5		13 + 10 +	NED NED
DiLorenzo 1988[44]	2				NED DOD
Borger 1989[58]	1	10	1 (lung)	9 +	AWD
Mildenberger 1989[59]	2	14 20		48 + 84 +	NED NED
Black[b] 1991[50]	1	17	2 (rt. lung) 5 (lt. lung)	83 +	NED
	2	8	1 (rt. lung)	36 +	NED
	3	14	1 (lt. lung)	8 + (2nd rel.)	NED
	4[1]	4	2	42 + (2nd rel.)	NED
	5	3	12	7 +	DOD

[a] Hepatocellular carcinoma
[b] Five patients
[c,d] NED = no evidence of disease; DOD = dead of disease.

comparison, standard CT advances discontinuously, usually at 1 cm intervals. Because of this misregistration effect, lesions of less than 1 cm may be missed. Thus, helical CT scanning is associated with a decreased frequency of false-negative results. For patients at risk for liver metastases, hepatic ultrasound should be done every other month for the first year and should be accompanied by magnetic resonance imaging (MRI) or CT at 3-month intervals.

TECHNIQUES

Surgeons treating metastatic disease in childhood must be versed in the techniques of lateral thora-

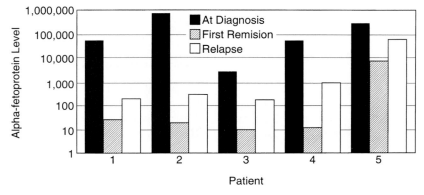

Figure 22–3 • The serum alpha-fetoprotein (AFP) level of four patients with hepatoblastoma and one with hepatocellular carcinoma graphed from diagnosis to remission to relapse. The figure illustrates the utility of serum AFP measurements in monitoring for relapse in these tumors.

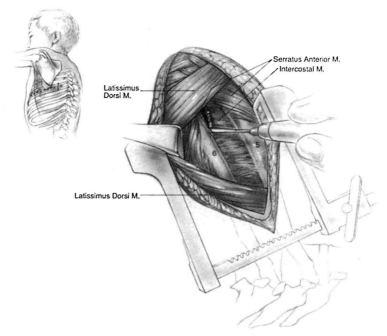

Figure 22–4 • Technique for posterolateral thoracotomy. In children the serratus anterior and often latissimus dorsi muscles can be mobilized and not cut to gain adequate exposure.

cotomy and sternotomy and able to do a wedge or anatomic resection of the lung, including pneumonectomy. Figures 22–4 and 22–5 illustrate the technique of posterolateral thoracotomy sparing the serratus anterior and latissimus dorsi muscle groups. Median sternotomy (Fig. 22–6) or transverse sternotomy (Fig. 22–7) gives good exposure to both lung fields, avoiding the need for staged procedures. Automatic stapling devices are standard equipment when doing wedge pulmonary resections.

Thoracoscopy was first shown to be useful for

Figure 22–5 • A stapling device can be used to perform pulmonary metastasectomy.

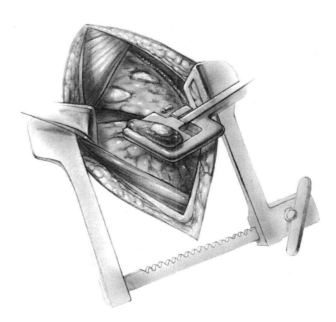

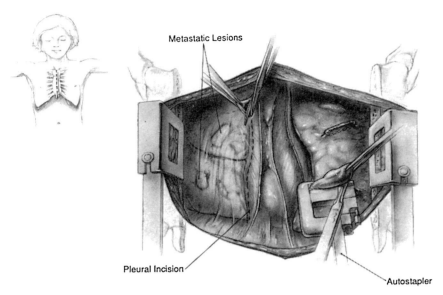

Figure 22–6 • Technique for pulmonary metastasectomy via median sternotomy.

diagnostic and therapeutic purposes in the adult population. Minimal-access surgery has expanded to include the pediatric patient as well. Currently thoracoscopy is an effective modality for diagnostic biopsies of lung nodules, pulmonary wedge resection, and both diagnosis and treatment of mediastinal masses in the pediatric population.[62, 63]

The resection of hepatic metastases requires familiarity with the techniques of anatomic and nonanatomic resections of the liver and obeys the basic principles of liver surgery. The underlying

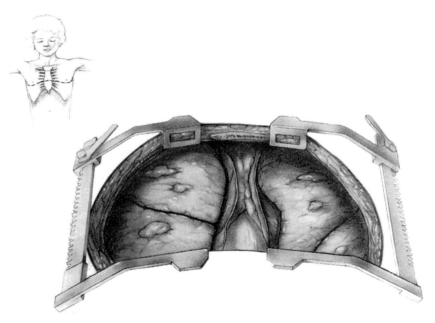

Figure 22–7 • Exposure can be gained by transverse sternotomy in the performance of pulmonary metastasectomy.

principle of all metastasis surgery is complete removal of disease, leaving margins free of disease on microscopic examination. This surgery requires adequate exposure, knowledge of the anatomy, technical expertise, and clarity in regard to the number and location of nodules as identified by imaging studies. Similar to thoracoscopy, laparoscopy is a good tool in the surgeon's armamentarium for the diagnosis of intraperitoneal metastatic lesions. These tumor deposits, however, do not lend themselves to curative resections as metastatic lesions confined to the thorax do.

CONCLUSIONS

The pediatric surgical oncologist who cares for patients with metastatic disease must understand metastasis biology and recognize the necessity of a multidisciplinary approach. Overall, metastasectomy should be undertaken only after control of the primary tumor and demonstration of a chemoresponsive metastatic disease. The most favorable results are obtained in patients with localized disease. A resection is more effective than other modalities when dealing with bulky deposits. When interpreting reported data, one should identify the total number of patients developing metastases versus the number undergoing surgery. Long-term survival of those undergoing resections must always be compared with survival of those undergoing nonoperative therapy, with particular attention to the morbidity of the two approaches.

References

1. Weinlechner: Tumoren an der Brustwand und deren Behandlung (Resection der Rippen) Eroffnung der Brusthohle und partielle Entfernung der Lunge. *Wien Med Wschr* 32:590, 1892.
2. Divis G.: Ein Beitrang zur operativen Behandlung der Lungengeschwulste. *Acta Chir Scand* 62:329–341, 1927.
3. Torek F: Removal of metastatic carcinoma of the lung and mediastinum. Suggestions to the technique. *Arch Surg* 21:1416–1930.
4. Barney JD, Churchill ED: Adenocarcinoma of the kidney with metastases to the lung cured by nephrectomy and lobectomy. *Trans Am Assoc Genitourin Surg* 31:71–79, 1938.
5. Mountain CF, Khalil KG, Hermes KE, Frazier OH: The contribution of surgery to the management of carcinomatous primary metastases. *Cancer* 41:833–840, 1978.
6. Farrel JT: Pulmonary metastases: A pathologic, clinical, recent study based on 78 cases of necropsy. *Radiology* 24:444–451, 1935.
7. Wilson SM, Adson MA: Surgical treatment of hepatic metastases from colorectal carcinoma. *Arch Surg* 111:330–333, 1976.
8. Adson MA, Van Heerdon JA: Major hepatic resections for metastatic colorectal cancer. *Ann Surg* 191:576–583, 1980.
9. Taylor I: A critical review of the treatment of colorectal liver metastases. *Clin Oncol* 8:149–158, 1982.
10. Hughes KS, Simon R, Songhorabodi S, et al: Resection of the liver for colorectal carcinoma metastases: A multi-institutional study of patterns of recurrence. *Surgery* 100:278–284, 1986.
11. Galicich JH, Sundaresan N, Thaler HT: Surgical treatment of single brain metastases. *J Neurosurg* 53:63–67, 1980.
12. Pizzo PA, Miser JS, Cassady JR, Filler RM: Solid tumors of childhood. In DeVita VT Jr, Hellman S, Rosenberg SA (eds): *Cancer: Principles and Practice of Oncology*, Philadelphia: J.B. Lippincott Co., 1985, pp. 1511–11589.
13. Schweizer P, Gauthier F: Resectability of liver tumors and principles of liver resection techniques. In Schweizer P, Schier F (eds): *Hepatobiliary Surgery in Childhood*, New York: Schattauer, 1991, pp. 101–115.
14. Sugarbaker EV, Ketcham AS: Mechanisms and prevention of cancer dissemination: An overview. *Semin Oncol* 4:19–31, 1977.
15. Sugarbaker EV: *Cancer Metastasis: A Product of Tumor-Host Interactions*, Chicago: Year Book Medical Publishers, 1979, pp. 1–59.
16. Fidler IJ, Hart IR: Principles of cancer biology: Cancer metastasis. In DeVita VT, Hellman S, Rosenberg SA (eds): *Cancer: Principles and Practice of Oncology*, Philadelphia: J.B. Lippincott Co., p. 113.
17. Poste G, Fidler IJ: The pathogenesis of cancer metastasis. *Nature* 283:141–146, 1980.
18. Fidler IJ, Hart IR: Biological diversity in metastatic neoplasms: Origins and implications. *Science* 217:998–1003, 1982.
19. Mareel MM, De Baetselier P, Van Roy FM: *Mechanisms of Invasion and Metastases*. Boca Raton, FL: CRC Press, 1991, pp. 7–21.
20. Martini N, Huvos AG, Mike V, Marcove RC, Beattie EJ Jr: Multiple pulmonary resections in the treatment of osteogenic sarcoma. *Ann Thorac Surg* 12:271–278, 1971.
21. Spanos PK, Payne WS, Ivins JC, Pritchard DJ: Pulmonary resection for metastatic osteogenic sarcoma. *J Bone Joint Surg* 58:624–628, 1976.
22. Telander RL, Pairolero PC, Pritchard DJ, et al: Resection of pulmonary metastatic osteogenic sarcoma in children. *Surgery* 84:335–341, 1978.
23. Giritsky AS, Etcubanas E, Mark JBD: Pulmonary resection in children with metastatic osteogenic

sarcoma. *J Thorac Cardiovasc Surg* 75:354–361, 1978.

24. Rosenberg SA, Flye MW, Conkle D, et al: Treatment of osteogenic sarcoma II: Aggressive resection of pulmonary metastases. *Cancer Treatment Reports* 63:753–756, 1979.

25. Burgers JM, Breur K, van Dobbenburgh OA, et al: Role of metastasectomy without chemotherapy in the management of osteosarcoma in children. *Cancer* 45:1664–1668, 1980.

26. Schaller RT Jr, Haas J, Schaller J, et al: Improved survival in children with osteosarcoma following resection of pulmonary metastases. *J Pediatr Surg* 17:546–550, 1982.

27. Goorin AM, Delorey MJ, Lack EE, et al: Prognostic significance of complete surgical resection of pulmonary metastases in patients with osteogenic sarcoma: Analysis of 32 patients. *J Clin Oncol* 2:425–431, 1984.

28. Carter SR, Grimer RJ, Sneath RS, Matthews HR: Results of thoracotomy in osteogenic sarcoma with pulmonary metastases. *Thorax* 46:727–731, 1991.

29. Saltzman DA, Snyder CL, Ferrell KL, Thompson RC, Leonard AS: Aggressive metastasectomy for pulmonic sarcomatous metastases: A follow-up study. *Am J Surg* 166:543–547, 1993.

30. Heij HA, Vos A, de Kraker J, Voute PA: Prognostic factors in surgery for pulmonary metastases. *Surgery* 115(6), 687–693, 1994.

31. Temeck BK, Wexler LH, Steinberg SM, Mclure LL, Horowitz M, Pass HI: Metastasectomy for sarcomatous pediatric histologies: Results and prognostic factors. *Ann Thorac Surg* 59:1385–1390, 1995.

32. Roth JA, Putnam JB, Wesley MN, Rosenberg SA: Differing determinants of prognosis following resection of pulmonary metastases from osteogenic and soft tissue sarcoma patients. *Cancer* 55:1361–1366, 1985.

33. Meyers PA, Heller G, Healey JH, et al: Osteogenic sarcoma with clinically detectable metastasis at initial presentation. *J Clin Oncol* 11:449–453, 1993.

34. Beattie EJ, Harvey JC, Marcove R, Martini N: Results of multiple pulmonary resections for metastatic osteogenic sarcoma after two decades. *J Surg Oncol* 46:154–155, 1991.

35. Jablons D, Steinberg SM, Roth J, et al: Metastasectomy for soft tissue sarcoma. *J Thorac Cardiovasc Surg* 97:695–705, 1989.

36. Casson AG, Putnam JB, Natarajan G, et al: Efficacy of pulmonary metastasectomy for recurrent soft tissue sarcoma. *J Surg Oncol* 47:1–4, 1991.

37. Pogrebniak HW, Roth JA, Steinberg SM, et al: Reoperative pulmonary resection in patients with metastatic soft tissue sarcoma. *Ann Thorac Surg* 52:197–203, 1991.

38a. Casson AG, Putnam JB, Natarajan G, et al: Five-year survival after pulmonary metastasectomy for adult soft tissue sarcoma. *Cancer* 69:662–668, 1992.

38b. White JG, Krivit W: Surgical excision of pulmonary metastases. *Pediatrics* 29:927–931, 1962.

39. Karakousis CP, Blumenson LE, Canavese G, Rao U: Surgery for disseminated abdominal sarcoma. *Am J Surg* 163:560–564, 1992.

40. Soper RT: Management of recurrent or metastatic Wilms' tumor. *Surgery* 50:555–560, 1961.

41. Bond JV, Martin EC: Pulmonary metastases in Wilms' tumor. *Clin Radiol* 27:191–195, 1976.

42. Baldeyrou P, Lemoine G, Zucker JM, Schweisguth O: Pulmonary metastases in children: The place of surgery. A study of 134 patients. *J Pediatr Surg* 19:121–125, 1984.

43. Omar R, Davidian MM, Marcus JR, Rose J: Significance of the "maturation" of metastases from Wilms' tumor after therapy. *J Surg Oncol* 33:239–242, 1986.

44. DiLorenzo M, Collin PP: Pulmonary metastases in children: Results of surgical treatment. *J Pediatr Surg* 23:762–765, 1988.

45. Green DM, Breslow NE, Ii Y, et al: The role of surgical excision in the management of relapsed Wilms' tumor patients with pulmonary metastases: A report from the National Wilms' Tumor Study. *J Pediatr Surg* 26:728–733, 1991.

46. Wohl MEB, Griscom NT, Traggis DG, Jaffe N: Effects of therapeutic irradiation delivered in early childhood upon subsequent lung function. *Pediatrics* 55:507–516, 1975.

47. Green DM, Finkelstein JZ, Tefft ME, Norkool P: Diffuse interstitial pneumonitis after pulmonary irradiation for metastatic Wilms' tumor. *Cancer* 63:450–453, 1989.

48. Foster JH: Survival after liver resection for secondary tumors. *Am J Surg* 135:389–394, 1978.

49. Morrow CE, Grage TB, Sutherland DER, Najarian JS: Hepatic resection for secondary neoplasms. *Surgery* 92:610–614, 1982.

50. Black CT, Luck SR, Musemeche CA, Andrassy RJ: Aggressive excision of pulmonary metastases is warranted in the management of childhood hepatic tumors. *J Pediatr Surg* 26:1082–1086, 1991.

51. King DR, Ortega J, Campbell J, et al: The surgical management of children with incompletely resected hepatic cancer is facilitated by intensive chemotherapy. *J Pediatr Surg* 26:1074–1081, 1991.

52. Exelby PR, Filler RM, Grosfeld JL: Liver tumors in children with particular reference to hepatoblastoma and hepatocellular carcinoma: American Academy of Pediatrics Surgical Section Survey 1974. *J Pediatr Surg* 10:329–337, 1975.

53. Giacomantonio M, Ein SH, Mancer K, Stephens CA: Thirty years' experience with pediatric primary malignant liver tumors. *J Pediatr Surg* 19:523–526, 1984.

54. Bradham RR, Paul JR, Thrower WB, et al:

Malignant hepatoma in a child: Survival following right hepatectomy, right pneumonectomy, and resection of diaphragmatic and parietal recurrence. *Surgery* 57:767–773, 1965.

55. Ballantine TVN, Wiseman NE, Filler RM: Assessment of pulmonary wedge resection for the treatment of lung metastases. *J Pediatr Surg* 10:671–676, 1975.

56. Lembke J, Havers W, Doetsch N, et al: Long-term results following surgical removal of pulmonary metastases in children with malignomas. *Thorac Cardiovasc Surg* 34:137–139, 1984.

57. Feusner J, Beach B, O'Leary M, et al: Pulmonary metastatic disease does not preclude survival in children with hepatoblastoma. *Proceedings of the Annual Meeting of the American Society of Clinical Oncology* 5:212(abstract), 1986.

58. Borger JA, Barbosa JL, Lehan CA: Chemotherapy combined with surgery in successful treatment of hepatoblastoma. *J Fla Med Assoc* 76:1023–1026, 1989.

59. Mildenberger H, Burger D, Weinel P: Hepatoblastoma: A retrospective study and proposal of a treatment protocol. *Zeitshrift Kinderchirurgie* 44:78–82, 1989.

60. Weinblatt ME, Siegel SE, Siegel MM, Stanley P, Weitzman JJ: Preoperative chemotherapy for unresectable primary hepatic malignancies in children. *Cancer* 50:1061–1064, 1982.

61. Pierro A, Langevin AM, Filler RM, et al: Preoperative chemotherapy in "unresectable" hepatoblastoma. *J Pediatr Surg* 24:24–29, 1989.

62. Kern JA, Daniel TM, Tribble CG, et al: Thoracoscopic diagnosis and treatment of mediastinal masses. *Ann Thorac Surg* 56:92–6, 1993.

63. Rodgers, BM: Pedatric thoractoscopy: Where have we come and what have we learned? *Ann Thorac Surg* 56:704–7, 1993.

Osteosarcoma and Other Bone Tumors

• *Alan W. Yasko, M.D.*

Primary bone neoplasms in children are rare. Consequently, most clinicians lack experience in the diagnosis and management of these diverse neoplasms. Coupled with a low index of suspicion, this lack of experience causes clinicians to often overlook bone tumors as the cause of a child's musculoskeletal symptoms. The diagnosis and treatment of bone tumors requires a multidisciplinary team of experts in orthopedic surgical oncology, pediatric oncology, pathology, radiation oncology, diagnostic and interventional radiology, physiatry, psychiatry, and nursing, all working together with other allied health personnel to coordinate patient management.

Current treatment strategies for malignant bone tumors have evolved over the past two decades with the emergence of effective chemotherapy, advances in diagnostic imaging modalities, and improvements in reconstructive techniques. Technically demanding yet more tissue-conserving surgical procedures have been successful in preserving function without compromising local tumor control or overall survival in selected patients. Refinements in surgical techniques and advances in bioengineering continue to overcome the limitations of current limb-sparing reconstructive approaches to preserve long-term function, particularly in the skeletally immature patient.

Similar efforts are directed at the management of benign neoplasms of bone. Local tumor control with minimal patient morbidity has been the goal. Minimally invasive techniques for diagnosis and treatment have been the focus of investigations to reduce short- and long-term morbidity through the preservation of normal bone stock, adjacent joint and soft-tissue structures, and growth plates. Tissue-engineered bone-graft substitutes used to reconstruct skeletal defects after tumor excision have been the subject of research in many centers. Such substitutes could be particularly important for pediatric patients because a limited supply of tissue is available for transplantation in these patients. Moreover, potential disease transmission, specifically hepatitis and HIV associated with allogeneic materials, remains a concern for pediatric patients.

The following discussion reviews current approaches to evaluation, diagnosis, and management of the most common primary malignant and benign bone tumors in children and adolescents, with an emphasis on reconstructive alternatives for optimizing function.

EVALUATION, DIAGNOSIS, AND STAGING

Most children and adolescents with musculoskeletal complaints seek medical attention because of pain. The character of the pain varies depending upon the pathologic process, the site and extent of involvement, and the presence of impending or established pathologic fracture. Pain is usually localized, dull and continuous, deep-seated, present at rest and at night, and is usually exacerbated by motion or weight-bearing of the affected limb. Typically, recent trauma prompts medical attention, at which time the underlying neoplasm is detected. Localized soft-tissue swelling, when present, is usually associated with tenderness and a palpable, firm, deep, fixed mass. Perilesional inflammation induced by the tumor may result in soft-tissue edema, synovitis, and joint effusion that may compromise the range of motion of the affected extremity.

The initial evaluation of any presenting musculoskeletal complaint should include conventional radiographs. Biplanar radiographs reveal the anatomical location of the abnormality within the affected bone and its relationship to the joint and growth plate, pattern of bone destruction, characteristics of a periosteal reaction, matrix production within the lesion, and presence of a soft-tissue mass. Often the diagnosis of the primary neoplasm can be made presumptively from this basic clinical and radiographic evaluation. Other studies are usually indicated to define more clearly the local and systemic extent of disease (Fig. 23–1). These staging studies usually include computed tomography (CT), magnetic resonance imaging (MRI), technetium Tc 99m bone scan, and, for patients with malignant neoplasms, a chest radiograph and CT scan of the chest.

The CT scan provides valuable information on the reactive response of the bone to the tumor. The scan also provides excellent detail of changes in the cortical and cancellous bone and mineralization within the lesion and surrounding soft tissues. The MRI complements the CT scan by demonstrating the relational anatomy between normal and diseased tissues. The extent of bone marrow and soft-tissue involvement are optimally visualized with this technique. The relation of the tumor to vital adjacent neural, vascular, and joint structures is best delineated by MRI. Cross-sectional images afforded by CT and MRI are critical to delineate the local extent of tumors arising in the spine and pelvis.

Technetium Tc 99m bone scans are performed primarily to screen the skeleton for polyostotic involvement and to enable early detection of skeletal metastases from malignant lesions. A skeletal survey is a more appropriate alternative to the bone scan to screen for hereditary multiple exostosis and Langerhans-cell histiocytosis. Chest radiographs and a CT scan of the chest are necessary to complete staging of any bone sarcoma to detect pulmonary metastases.

Peripheral blood studies have limited value for the evaluation of patients with primary bone neoplasms. Alkaline phosphatase and lactate dehydrogenase (LDH) may be elevated in patients with osteosarcoma and Ewing's sarcoma, respectively. A sedimentation rate and leukocyte count may be helpful if osteomyelitis is in the differential diagnosis.

The biopsy is a critical step in diagnosing primary bone neoplasms. Essential for performing a successful biopsy is a working knowledge of bone neoplasms and their treatment. Expertise in procuring bone tissue and analyzing limited samples of these rare tumors reduces errors in

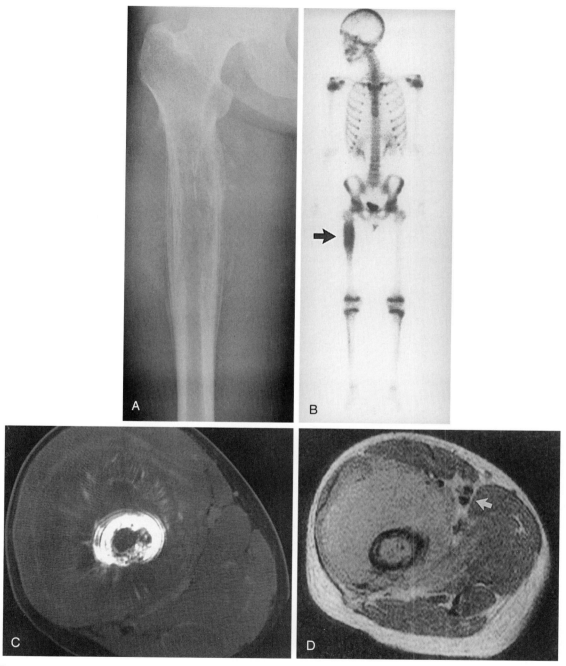

Figure 23–1 • Ewing's sarcoma of the right proximal femur diagnosed in a 17-year-old male. *A,* Plain radiographs demonstrate the characteristic permeative pattern of bone destruction with an associated lamellated periosteal reaction. *B,* Technetium bone scan demonstrates increased activity in the area of the lesion *(arrow). C,* CT scan delineates the degree of cortical destruction, periosteal reaction, and associated soft-tissue mass. *D,* MR imaging demonstrates the extent of the soft-tissue mass and its relationship to the major neurovascular structures *(arrow).*

diagnosis. The biopsy may be performed as a surgical (open) or percutaneous (closed) procedure. Currently, most biopsies are surgical. Skill is required to optimize the yield of diagnostic tissue without compromising the definitive surgical procedure for malignant tumors. Longitudinal skin incisions, limited tissue flaps, meticulous maintenance of hemostasis, avoidance of the joint and the plane of adjacent neurovascular structures are recommended.

The importance of a properly performed biopsy cannot be overstated. Biopsy-related problems occur three to five times more frequently when the biopsy is performed at the referring institution than when it is performed at the center where the definitive surgical resection is to be performed, according to a multi-institutional study.[1, 2] This study also revealed that approximately 5% of patients required what would have otherwise been an unnecessary amputation and approximately 9% experienced an adverse outcome because of a poorly executed biopsy.

Experience with percutaneous biopsies at large referral centers has led to increased application of fine needle aspiration and cutting core biopsy for the diagnosis of bone lesions. This minimally invasive procedure has proved a safe, highly accurate, and economic diagnostic method when performed by experts in percutaneous musculoskeletal biopsy techniques. Percutaneous biopsies are usually performed with the child under conscious sedation or under general anesthesia. The accuracy of percutaneous biopsy has reached 90% in some centers[3] but remains highly variable overall, reflecting the different levels of clinical experience and cytopathologic expertise available to diagnose these rare neoplasms on limited tissue samples. Biopsy-obtained tissue may be processed for standard histologic and cytologic preparations, immunohistochemical studies, electron microscopy, flow cytometry, and molecular studies as indicated. The histopathologic diagnosis should always be interpreted in the context of the clinical presentation and radiographic features of the primary lesion.

The staging system of the Musculoskeletal Tumor Society is used currently for both malignant and benign neoplasms of bone.[4] For malignant tumors, the stage is determined by tumor grade (I = low-grade, II = high-grade); tumor extent (A = intraosseous involvement only, B = extraosseous extension); and presence of distant metastases (III). Patients with localized tumor may have Stage IA, IB, IIA, or IIB disease. The presence of metastatic disease, regardless of the extent of the local disease, represents Stage III disease. For benign tumors, the stage of the lesion is defined by its level of activity as revealed by its radiographic characteristics: latent (Stage 1), active (Stage 2), or aggressive (Stage 3).

MANAGEMENT CONSIDERATIONS FOR PRIMARY SARCOMAS

The management approach to primary bone sarcomas depends upon the diagnosis and stage of disease at presentation. The treatment paradigm for high-grade bone sarcomas includes preoperative chemotherapy followed by tumor resection and adjuvant chemotherapy (which is tailored to the responsiveness of the tumor to the preoperative therapy). Multiagent chemotherapy is usually administered preoperatively for three or four cycles. Specific chemotherapy regimens, mode of delivery (intraarterial and/or intravenous), dose schedules, intensity, and duration are variable.

An increased understanding of tumor biology, the natural history of specific neoplasms, advances in diagnostic imaging modalities, and application of new technologies and techniques for surgical resection and reconstruction have all helped shape current surgical strategies. The single most important influence on the nature and extent of surgery, however, has been the development of effective multiagent chemotherapy regimens.

Satisfactory surgical resection of the tumor-bearing portion of the bone can be accomplished by limb ablation or by a limb-salvage procedure. The tumor, the reactive zone about the tumor, and a cuff of normal tissue in all planes constitute a satisfactory surgical margin. Local disease control is achieved in more than 90% of patients. Refinements in operative approaches, bone and joint reconstructive techniques, and soft-tissue coverage methods have increased the pool of patients with extremity sarcomas who are candidates for limb conservation without risk of local tumor recurrence. The timing of surgery must be coordinated with the patient's chemotherapy schedule and with bone marrow recovery to minimize interruption of systemic therapy.

Chemotherapy is reinitiated postoperatively

after wound healing has occurred (usually 2–3 weeks). Regimens vary depending upon response to chemotherapy. Response to chemotherapy is assessed according to the methodical histologic evaluation of the resected tumor specimen. For all low-grade malignant tumors, surgical excision with wide margins provides excellent local tumor control. The adequacy of surgery is the most significant predictor of outcome for these patients.

Radiotherapy has selected application in the treatment of primary malignant and benign bone tumors. It is most frequently administered as part of the multimodality treatment of malignant tumors such as Ewing's sarcoma, primitive neuroectodermal tumor (PNET), and lymphoma. Such treatment is for curative intent and for local symptom palliation in patients with metastatic disease. Radiation may be the primary therapy for certain benign lesions (such as localized Langerhans-cell histiocytosis), or it may be an adjunct for locally recurrent or unresectable aggressive lesions (such as osteoblastomas and aneursymal bone cysts).

Osteosarcoma

Osteosarcomas are the most common primary malignant bone tumor in children and adolescents constituting approximately 5% of all tumors in children. Osteosarcomas can occur at any age, but more than 75% of such tumors develop in patients between 12 and 25 years of age, with a peak incidence during the second decade of life. This age group of peak incidence parallels the period of rapid skeletal growth. Any bone and any site within a given bone can be affected by osteosarcoma. The overwhelming majority of these tumors (90%) arise near the end of the long bones in the metaphyseal region. In descending order of frequency, the tumors arise in the distal femur, proximal tibia, proximal humerus, and proximal femur. Most occur around the knee, which is the site of greatest contribution to skeletal growth of the extremities in children. Osteosarcomas of the spine and pelvis are much less frequently seen.

Osteosarcoma is classified by whether it is a primary or secondary process and by the site of origin. Approximately 95% of all osteosarcomas are primary tumors that develop de novo in a bone, that is, without preexisting lesion or prior

treatment of the affected bone with radiation. In contrast, secondary lesions may develop after local irradiation or at the site of a preexisting benign lesion. In general, both primary and secondary lesions present as unifocal, monostotic lesions. Rarely, a multifocal presentation is observed. Intraosseous and transarticular skip metastases are unusual.

Osteosarcomas can develop within the bone (central, intramedullary) or on the surface. Most osteosarcomas are high-grade central, intramedullary tumors. The subtypes of these conventional osteosarcomas reflect the predominant cellular pattern (osteoblastic, chondroblastic, or fibroblastic) observed histologically. Variants of high-grade intramedullary osteosarcoma include telangiectatic (a lytic form) and small-cell osteosarcoma. A low-grade intramedullary variant of osteosarcoma is much less frequently observed.

Osteosarcomas that arise on the surface of the bone may exhibit both low- and high-grade characteristics. These osteosarcoma variants include conventional low-grade parosteal osteosarcoma, periosteal osteosarcoma, high-grade surface osteosarcoma, and dedifferentiated parosteal osteosarcoma.[5]

Localized pain and swelling are the hallmark clinical features of osteosarcoma. The pain is initially insidious in onset and intermittent in nature. It later becomes progressively more severe and unremitting over a period of weeks to months. Localized swelling and a firm, nonmobile soft-tissue mass with or without associated warmth and erythema may be present. A joint effusion may be observed. Range of motion of the adjacent joint may be limited and painful. Movement or weight-bearing of the involved extremity may exacerbate local symptoms. Often the pain is worse at night. Patients with osteosarcoma arising in the lower extremities may present with a painful limp. The neurovascular examination of the affected extremity is usually normal. Regional lymph nodes are involved rarely. A pathologic fracture may develop, although a history of pain prior to the fracture usually can be elicited from the patient.

Constitutional symptoms are rare. Blood studies reveal an increased alkaline phosphatase in approximately 50% of patients.

The diagnosis of conventional osteosarcoma or one of its variants must be made by clinical and radiographic evaluation (Fig. 23–2) and con-

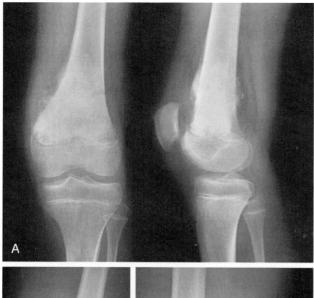
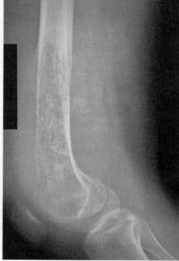
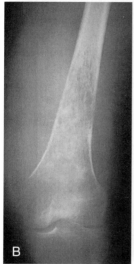

Figure 23–2 • Varied pattern of bone destruction secondary to osteosarcoma. *A*, AP and lateral views of the knee reveal a bone-forming lesion of the distal femur characterized by intramedullary osteoblastic changes, interrupted periosteal reaction, and ossification within the associated soft-tissue mass consistent with an osteoblastic osteosarcoma. *B*, AP and lateral views reveal lytic destruction of the distal femur with cortical erosion and soft-tissue mass consistent with the telangiectatic variant of osteosarcoma.

firmed by histopathologic analysis of biopsy-obtained tissue. Osteosarcoma is an inhomogeneous disease defined as a malignant spindle-cell proliferation that produces osteoid or immature bone. It can exhibit a varied radiographic pattern characterized by poorly marginated bone destruction and bony sclerosis, lysis, or a mixture of both, associated usually with an interrupted periosteal reaction and soft-tissue mass. Local staging using both CT and MRI delineates the extent of these changes. Conventional radiographs and CT of the chest are performed to detect pulmonary metastases (the site of approximately 85% of metastases). Radionuclide studies are useful to screen the skeleton for osseous metastases (the second most common type of metastases).

All current treatment protocols for newly diagnosed high-grade osteosarcomas include chemotherapy utilizing varying combinations of doxorubicin, cisplatin, high-dose methotrexate, and ifosfamide administered preoperatively. Surgical excision is performed by either amputation or a limb-sparing surgical procedure. Local tumor control can be accomplished successfully in more than 90% of patients. The specific methods of limb salvage that are applicable for all high-grade and some low-grade and benign tumors are discussed in this chapter.

Following surgery, an assessment of the tumor response, as measured by the degree of necrosis to preoperatively administered chemotherapy, is made on the resected specimen. The percentage of necrosis determines the postoperative chemo-therapy regimen. The response of the tumor to chemotherapy is considered favorable if there is greater than 90% necrosis and unfavorable if there is less than 90% necrosis. This histologically measured response to chemotherapy is the most powerful prognostic variable for patient survival.

Limb-salvage procedures have not adversely affected patient survival if performed appropriately. Current 5-year survival rates for patients with localized disease have increased from historical levels (without chemotherapy) of 15–20% to 60–75% (with chemotherapy).[6, 7] Patients with metastatic disease at presentation (10% to 20% of patients) have a poor prognosis, with an 11% 5-year survival.[8] Approximately 30% to 40% of patients who subsequently develop pulmonary metastases can be salvaged with re-induction chemotherapy and surgery.

Ewing's Sarcoma

Ewing's sarcoma is the second most common primary malignant tumor in children, accounting for approximately 1% of all cancers in patients under 15 years of age. This sarcoma can occur at any age, but the peak incidence is observed during the second decade of life. It is uncommon in children younger than 5 years of age and in patients older than 30. Males are more frequently involved than females (1.6:1). Ewing's sarcoma is rare (less than 2% incidence) in American or African blacks. Any bone can be involved, but more than half of all tumors develop in the pelvic girdle and lower extremity. The femur is the most common site of long-bone involvement. Classically, Ewing's sarcoma is described as a diaphyseal lesion, but it may arise in any region within the involved bone.

The most common presenting symptom, occurring in approximately 90% of patients, is pain. The pain may be of several months' duration and is commonly associated with localized soft-tissue swelling. Occasionally, constitutional symptoms may be observed, including low-grade fever, malaise, and weight loss. Pathologic fracture at the site of the tumor in long bones occurs approximately in 5% to 10% of patients.

Radiographically, Ewing's sarcomas exhibit a permeative destructive pattern with poor margination. Bony sclerosis may be the dominant pattern of bone involvement, but more frequently a mixed pattern of lysis and sclerosis is observed. A variety of periosteal reactions are observed. The lamellated reaction described as an "onion skin" appearance is common but not pathognomonic for Ewing's sarcoma. A soft-tissue mass is often present and usually large. The imaging study of choice to delineate the local extent of intra- and extraosseous involvement is the MRI. Staging studies for distant disease include a chest radiograph, CT scan of the chest, and bone marrow aspiration and biopsy.

Laboratory values that may be elevated include LDH and alkaline phosphatase. Leukocytosis, anemia, and an elevated sedimentation rate may be noted.

Ewing's sarcoma is an anaplastic, small-, round-cell tumor of unknown histogenesis. Histologically it is characterized by a monotonous sheet of densely packed, uniform, small round cells with abundant cytoplasm and no matrix production. Typically, the tumor cells demonstrate positivity for periodic acid–Schiff (PAS) stain, denoting the presence of glycogen. Ewing's sarcoma has shown reactivity to the monoclonal antibody HBA71 (MIC2), which recognizes a cell-surface glycoprotein p30/32mic2. These analyses help distinguish this tumor from other small-, round-cell tumors of childhood such as lymphoma of bone, embryonal rhabdomyosarcoma, metastatic neuroblastoma, and small-cell osteosarcoma.

The treatment of Ewing's sarcoma includes multiagent induction chemotherapy followed by local therapy by surgical excision, radiotherapy, or both. Chemotherapy regimens include a variable combination of known active agents including vincristine, cyclophosphamide, doxorubicin, ifosfamide, actinomycin-D, and etoposide. The response to chemotherapy is a critical factor to the overall outcome of the patients with Ewing's sarcoma and to the feasibility of safely performing a limb-sparing tumor excision (Fig. 23–3).

The role of surgery for localized Ewing's sarcoma has expanded and is currently recommended for all resectable lesions. Radiotherapy has been a mainstay of local treatment for this radiosensitive tumor, but local control has been inconsistently achieved. Late morbidity associated with irradiation, including limb-length inequality secondary to growth arrest, pathologic

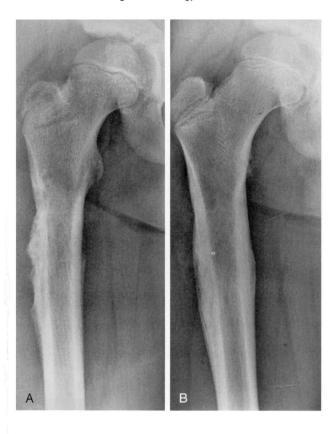

Figure 23–3 • Ewing's sarcoma of the proximal femur diagnosed in an 8-year-old girl with a 1-month history of thigh pain. *A*, Radiographic appearance prior to multiagent chemotherapy. *B*, Radiographic appearance following induction chemotherapy with vincristine, doxorubicin, and cyclophosphamide. Tumor necrosis was estimated to be 90% based on histologic examination of the resected specimen.

fracture through irradiated bone, soft-tissue fibrosis, joint ankylosis, and radiation-induced sarcoma, remains a concern. Currently, the principal application of irradiation is as a primary therapy for patients with unresectable tumors and as a postoperative therapy if the surgical resection margin is unsatisfactory.

No prospective randomized studies have been performed to define the relative role of each of these treatment modalities, but several retrospective studies suggest improved local tumor control and patient survival rates when surgery is satisfactorily performed.[9–14]

Prognostic factors for Ewing's sarcoma include tumor size (volume), anatomical site (peripheral versus central), the presence or absence of metastases at initial presentation, and the response to chemotherapy. Patient 5-year survival has improved with multimodality therapy from less than 20% (without chemotherapy) to approximately 70% (with chemotherapy) in patients with localized nonpelvic Ewing's sarcoma.[10] For patients with localized pelvic disease, 5-year survival has increased to approximately 50%.[11, 14, 15]

SURGICAL TREATMENT OF PRIMARY BONE MALIGNANCIES

Tumor Resection

The Musculoskeletal Tumor Society recommends a wide local excision either by amputation or limb-salvage procedure for high-grade osteosarcoma and Ewing's sarcoma. A wide excision removes the primary tumor en bloc, along with its reactive zone and a cuff of normal tissue in all planes (Figs. 23–4 and 23–5). Preoperative preparation is essential for successful tumor extirpation. A thorough assessment of the bone and soft-tissue extent of the primary disease is necessary before and after induction chemotherapy to assess the response of the tumor and extent of residual tumor. Plain radiographs, CT scan, and MRI of the affected extremity provide critical information necessary to plan the surgical procedure. Planning for the skeletal reconstruction and soft-tissue coverage procedures for patients deemed candidates for limb salvage must begin far in advance to permit adequate time to manufacture the prostheses or procure the bone-

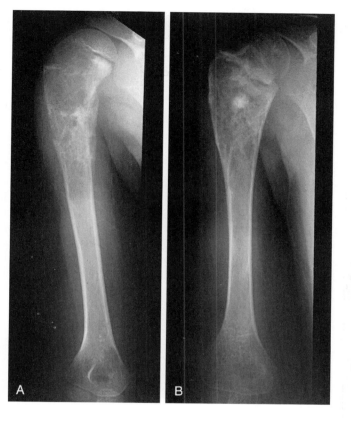

Figure 23–4 • Osteosarcoma diagnosed by needle biopsy in a 5 1/2-year-old male with a 2-month history of pain in the right shoulder. *A*, Radiographic appearance of the tumor associated with a pathologic fracture arising in the proximal humerus at the time of presentation. *B*, Radiographic appearance following preoperative chemotherapy with doxorubicin and cisplatin and ifosfamide demonstrates a healed fracture with reconstitution of the cortex. Tumor necrosis was estimated to be 92% based on histologic examination of the resected specimen.

graft materials for reconstruction. Consultation with a microvascular surgeon should be made if a rotation flap or free tissue transfer is considered likely for soft-tissue coverage.

The extent of the skeletal resection for both long-bone and pelvic tumors determines the functional deficit and influences the type of reconstruction offered to the patient. Preservation of bone stock, joint surfaces, and ligamentous structures of the joint results in a significant improvement in limb function, with a prospect of maintaining near normal function long term. Tumors associated with soft-tissue extension have been treated historically by extra-articular joint resection and sacrifice of the surrounding muscle because of concerns about soft-tissue invasion, intra-articular contamination, and tracking of tumor along ligamentous and capsular structures. But for selected tumors with minimal soft-tissue extension, or for tumors that have responded favorably to preoperative chemotherapy, the resection can be performed safely through the joint with maximal preservation of adjacent muscle.

Motor function can be optimized without compromising local tumor control. The preservation of these structures provides more favorable soft-tissue coverage of the reconstruction, decreases the risk of infection, increases joint stability, improves function, and produces a more cosmetic result.

With careful preoperative planning, the medical condition of the patient can be optimized in preparation for surgery to minimize intraoperative and postoperative risks. If management is properly coordinated, the interruption of chemotherapy will be brief and reinitiation can commence within 2–3 weeks postoperatively.

Amputation

All patients with extremity sarcomas are candidates for amputation. The level of amputation depends on the site and proximal extent of the tumor as determined on the preoperative radiographic imaging studies. Massive tumor size, tumor progression despite chemotherapy, patho-

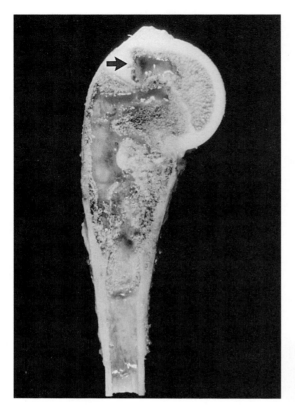

Figure 23–5 • Gross cut specimen of the widely excised osteosarcoma of the proximal humerus in a 6-year-old male. The en bloc excision included a margin of normal bone and cuff of normal soft tissue (stripped from specimen) about the tumor. Note the extension of the tumor across the growth plate into the epiphysis of the proximal humerus (*arrow*).

logic fracture with massive hemorrhage, unre-constructable limb following local resection, selected extremely young patients and major neurovascular involvement are absolute indications (Fig. 23–6).

Amputation continues to be a primary mode of achieving local tumor control in skeletally immature patients who have substantial skeletal growth remaining. A low-morbidity procedure with predictable wound-healing results, amputation is effective in local tumor control. Long-term problems include (1) phantom-limb pain, (2) stump pain, (3) stump-bone overgrowth, and (4) stump-prosthesis interface problems. Patients who undergo amputation generally adjust well to the absence of the limb and function well without favoring the affected extremity.[16] The level of function depends principally on the level of amputation.

Rotationplasty

Rotationplasty (intercalary amputation) is a common technique following resection of tumors arising in the distal femur or proximal tibia.[17, 18] The objective of this procedure is to lower the level of amputation, thereby improving function. Rotationplasty involves an intercalary resection of all structures within the region surrounding the tumor-bearing portion of the extremity, preserving only the neurovascular structures. The retained normal segment of the lower leg is rotated 180 degrees and reattached to the proximal bone remnant. The intact ankle joint serves as the knee joint, thereby creating a functional below-the-knee amputation. The patient must wear a modified external limb prosthesis (Fig. 23–7). The energy consumed with walking is less than that for above-knee amputees; however, the cosmetic result is undesirable for many patients.

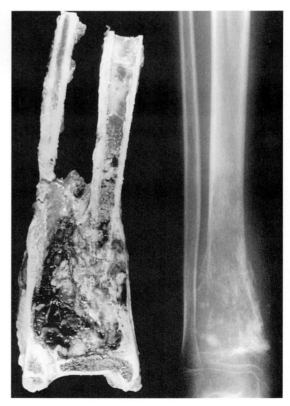

Figure 23–6 • Tumor in 10-year-old male with a 1-month history of pain in the ankle after injury. Despite multiagent chemotherapy, progression of the tumor was observed clinically and radiographically. The patient was treated by below-knee amputation. Tumor necrosis was estimated to be 34%.

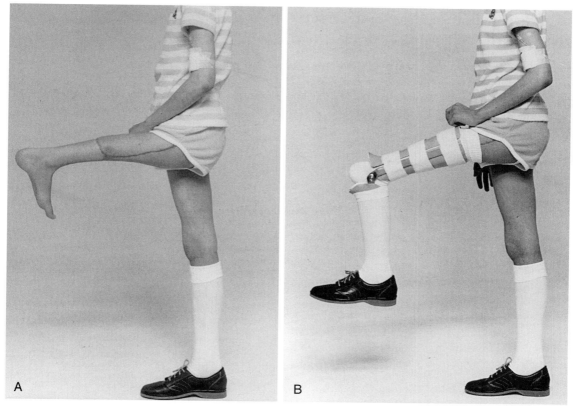

Figure 23–7 • Van Nes rotationplasty. *A*, Without modified below-knee-amputation prosthesis; *B*, with modified below-knee-amputation prosthesis.

Winkelmann has applied variations of this technique in which joints are transposed one level proximally to reconstruction following proximal femoral resection.[19] The overall complication rate of this procedure is low, but care must be taken in determining the proper level at which to place the ankle relative to the contralateral knee. The major objection to this procedure is cosmetic; many patients and their parents are initially shocked by the appearance of a shortened extremity with the "foot on backwards." In this regard, preoperative counseling for the patient and family is necessary. Videotapes showing the appearance of the operated limb with and without the prosthesis are helpful.

Rotationplasty is an excellent method for restoring function in children younger than 8 years. The procedure also offers a reconstruction with excellent durable function and a low risk of complications to the older patient who is able to accept the appearance of the extremity.

Limb Salvage

Techniques of skeletal reconstruction following segmental bone resection with and without sacrifice of the adjacent joint have proved successful in adults but are problematic when applied to growing children. The immature skeleton rapidly expands longitudinally, leading to the problem of limb-length inequality. The skeleton also expands circumferentially, causing early loosening of implants fitted to the intramedullary canal. Engineering limitations exist for the very young patient, particularly in reconstruction of the lower extremity. Children and adolescents frequently place great demands on implants, and as the proportion of osteosarcoma and Ewing's sarcoma survivors increases with effective chemotherapy, the life expectancy of the reconstructed limb is likely to be many times shorter than the life expectancy of the patient. The functional and psychological outcomes expected with amputation remain the standard against which any form of limb reconstruction must be measured.

Limb-salvage procedures have supplanted amputation as the principle surgical method of eradicating local disease in adults with primary sarcomas of the bone, regardless of histology or grade. As mentioned, the application of these techniques to the pediatric population continues to expand. In general, successful limb-salvage surgical management of the patient with a high-grade bone sarcoma is predicated on (1) complete extirpation of tumor, (2) effective skeletal reconstruction, and (3) adequate soft-tissue coverage. The reconstruction methods selected must be based on specific anatomical and oncologic factors, patient expectations, and anticipated functional demands. Experience with the limb-salvage approach over the past 20 years has resulted in improved function and cosmesis without compromising the overriding objective of satisfactory tumor extirpation.[20]

Preoperative planning for the operative procedure must begin far in advance to permit adequate time to procure the implant for reconstruction. Planning should be coordinated with (1) chemotherapy schedules, (2) anticipated recovery from bone marrow suppression, and (3) the time necessary to complete the manufacture of a prosthesis or to allow procurement of the desired reconstructive materials. Plain radiographs with a magnification marker or ruler must be obtained to provide accurate measurements of the dimensions of the bone segment and joint that must be resected in order to customize the reconstruction to the patient's anatomy.

Limb-sparing resections of the tumor-bearing bone fall into one of three types based on the anatomical site and extent of the involved bone to be excised: (1) tumor-bearing bone and adjacent joint, (2) tumor-bearing bone only, and (3) whole bone and adjacent joints. Since most bone sarcomas arise in the metaphysis of the long bone near the joint, the majority of the procedures that are performed for these tumors involve resection of both the segment of tumor-bearing bone and the adjacent joint (osteoarticular resection). Most of these resections are performed through the adjacent joint (intra-articular). When the tumor extends along the joint capsule or ligamentous structures or invades the joint, the entire joint (extra-articular) should be resected to avoid violating areas involved with tumor.

Less frequently encountered is the clinical situation in which a sarcoma arises within the diaphysis or shaft region of the long bone. Fewer than 10% of osteosarcomas arise within and remain confined to the diaphyseal portion of the long bones. Ewing's sarcoma more commonly arises in the shaft of the bone far enough from the adjacent joint that successful local tumor control can be achieved without sacrificing the adjacent joint. The tumor-bearing segment of bone alone is resected (intercalary resection).

Extensive tumor involvement in a long bone may require a whole-bone resection involving both the proximal and distal joints.

Pelvic resections represent a special challenge. A tumor arising in the pelvis can involve a segment of nonarticular bone, the acetabulum, or both. The extent of the skeletal resection determines the functional deficit and influences the decision regarding the type of reconstruction, if any, to be offered to the patient to optimize function.

Tumors arising within the sacrum and the vertebrae are rare and, because of the unique anatomical considerations, are seldom amenable to wide local excision.

Skeletal Reconstruction

Reconstruction alternatives have expanded as a result of advances in biomechanical engineering, prosthetic design and metallurgy, allograft biology, and microvascular techniques. These advances in bioengineering and the refinements in surgical techniques have increased the number of patients eligible for limb-salvage surgery. The reconstructive method chosen should be individualized. Numerous factors influence the type of reconstruction selected and the probability of successfully maintaining long-term function. Some of these factors are anatomical location, the integrity of surrounding structures, the extent of the resection, the risk and nature of potential early and late complications associated with a given type of reconstruction, and the patient's age, expectations, and anticipated functional demands. Current techniques for reconstructing and salvaging a functional extremity include prosthetic arthroplasty, osteoarticular allografts, and allograft/prosthesis composites for preservation of a mobile joint, as well as large-segment allografts and vascularized and nonvascularized segmental autografts for replacement of intercalary segments of bone and for arthrodesis across joints to establish a durable, nonmobile extremity. Method-specific complications affect both short- and long-term outcome. Regardless of the method of reconstruction, the principal perioperative concern is to prevent infection that could jeopardize the patient's limb and life. Reconstruction durability is the primary issue limiting long-term maintenance of meaningful function.

Prosthetic Arthroplasty

Prosthetic arthroplasty is the most frequent method of reconstruction following osteoarticular resection. This procedure is used primarily about the knee, hip, and shoulder when a mobile joint is desired. Anatomical and prosthetic design limitations restrict prosthetic replacement of the wrist (distal radius) or ankle (distal tibia) joints.

The current generation of implants are custom-designed and can be manufactured within 2–3 weeks. To further minimize delay and to provide intraoperative flexibility, oncologic prosthesis systems with modular components have been developed that can be utilized to fit a particular anatomical size and length of resected bone segment.

All prostheses for the knee are constrained (hinged) because of the obligatory resection of the ligamentous structures that support the joint. Prosthetic arthroplasties of the shoulders and hip are usually not constrained and require replacement only of the involved side of the joint in the majority of cases.

Fixation of the prosthesis into the host bone is usually accomplished with polymethylmethacrylate cement. The experience with alternative methods of fixation including cement-free fixation by bone ingrowth into the prosthesis stem has been encouraging, but this issue remains investigational.

The advantages of the prosthetic arthroplasty are (1) immediate joint stability without prolonged extremity immobilization and (2) early restoration of function and ambulation with low early morbidity. The reported low perioperative infection rate is low; for this reason, most primary reconstructions are performed using a prosthetic arthroplasty for the primary reconstruction

of osteoarticular defects in patients who require adjuvant chemotherapy.

Any mechanical device has inherent limitations in durability. The primary shortcoming of this type of reconstruction is loosening of the prosthesis at the bone-cement interface as a result of repetitive mechanical stresses and loads experienced during the activities of daily living.[21] All implants will need to be replaced at some point in the long-term survivor's lifetime. Most implants are revised long after active treatment for the primary disease has been completed; therefore, greater flexibility is afforded the orthopedic oncologist in planning for prosthesis salvage on an elective basis.

For patients with remaining skeletal growth who have had one or more growth plates resected along with the tumor specimen, the growth potential lost by the resection must be calculated and future limb growth predicted as a part of preoperative planning.[22] In the upper extremity, limb-length inequality is less a functional problem than a cosmetic one. In the lower extremity, a projected limb-length inequality of more than 2 cm must be addressed to avoid gait abnormalities and the development of leg and back pain.

Two different strategies are possible, each applied alone or in combination. If minimal limb-length discrepancies are anticipated, the limb may be lengthened by implanting a standard nonexpandable prosthesis that is longer than the resected bone segment, or an epiphysiodesis of the corresponding growth plate of the unaffected extremity can be performed. Or both procedures can be done. Epiphysiodesis (surgical closure of the growth plate) can overcome a substantial anticipated limb-length discrepancy but may leave certain patients unacceptably short in stature. The advent of the expandable prosthesis and modular prosthesis systems offers an alternative for this patient population.[23–25]

The goal of the expandable prosthetic reconstruction is to maintain a mobile joint and accommodate for the loss of the growth center of the bone. The expandable prosthesis has an intrinsic mechanism that allows it to be surgically modified periodically to achieve lengthening (Figs. 23–8 and 23–9). Length can be achieved by open, arthroscopic, or closed methods (knee manipulation, internal magnet, and external electromagnetic field).

All patients receiving an expandable prosthesis

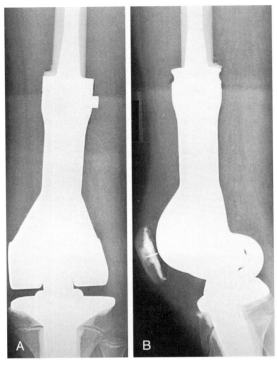

Figure 23–8 • A custom-made expandable knee prosthesis was used to reconstruct the segmental bone defect and adjacent knee joint. *A*, AP radiograph; *B*, lateral radiograph.

will require numerous operative procedures during the period of active skeletal growth. A limb cannot be lengthened more than about 2 cm at a time without risking major neurovascular complications. Yet multiple operative exposures of the implant increase the risk of infection. This need for multiple surgical procedures during the period of the patient's skeletal growth should be taken into account. At skeletal maturity, the expandable prosthesis can be exchanged for a nonexpandable prosthetic arthroplasty or can be converted to an arthrodesis if a more durable reconstruction is desired.

Mechanical failure of the expansion mechanism has been the principle limiting factor to the success of this method of reconstruction. In addition, although longitudinal bone growth is accommodated for by these implants, appositional growth is not. Loosening of both cemented and uncemented implants at the point of fixation to bone must be anticipated for long-term survivors. Modifications in the design of newer-generation prostheses may reduce the incidence of

prosthesis failure. Long-term follow-up is thus far lacking.

An alternative approach to the expandable prosthesis is a prosthesis system of modular intercalary components that can be exchanged to achieve incremental length at the time of reoperation. This system avoids the risks associated with the failure of the expansion mechanism in customized, expandable prostheses.

Clearly, not all children are candidates for this method of reconstruction even if wide surgical margins can be achieved without amputation. Anatomical limitations and constraints of prosthetic design and mechanics exist, particularly for very young patients. Patients who have undergone this type of reconstruction for the distal

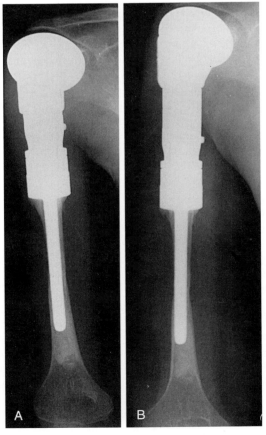

Figure 23–9 • Plain radiographs of an expandable prosthesis implanted following resection of an osteosarcoma of the proximal humerus in a 6-year-old male. *A*, Prior to insertion of expanded intercalary segment to maintain limb length equality; *B*, following insertion of segment.

femur expend less energy during gait but in general are more sedentary and protective of the affected extremity than patients who have undergone amputation, rotationplasty, or arthrodesis.[16, 26]

Massive Allografts

Allografts may be used as a primary reconstruction to replace the involved side of a joint (osteoarticular) or to bridge a defect in the diaphysis of a long bone with preservation of the adjacent joints (intercalary) or for arthrodesis (fusion) of a joint.[27, 28] Allografts offer several potential advantages over prosthetic arthroplasty as a reconstruction alternative. Foremost, the allograft is a biologic reconstruction that restores bone stock and the adjacent joint surface. Moreover, it can provide a site of attachment for host soft tissues and thus optimize active movement of the affected joint. Allografts avoid the principal limitations of prosthetic devices; that is, loosening and mechanical failure.

Two types of allografts are commonly used for skeletal reconstruction: large-segment osteoarticular allografts and intercalary allografts. Both are readily available from regional bone banks. Current cryopreservation techniques can maintain viable, articular cartilage, thus affording the potential for a long-term biologic reconstruction. Such reconstruction is particularly desirable for the area about the knee, where the majority of prosthetic failures occur. Therefore, osteoarticular allografts are applied most frequently for reconstruction about the knee.

Several significant disadvantages exist for large-segment allografts, however. The grafts must be fixed to the host bone and must heal to achieve the desired outcome. Prolonged limb immobilization, bracing or casting, and protected weight-bearing may be required for many months. Moreover, a high complication rate is associated with this method of reconstruction. Nonunions, fractures, and early infections are observed consistently in 15% to 20% of cases.[28] The risk of disease transmission following transplantation of allogeneic tissue remains an inherent disadvantage, too. Late complications include degenerative arthritis and joint instability.

The role of osteoarticular allografts as a method of primary reconstruction in patients with high-grade sarcomas remains controversial. The high rate of infection is problematic, particularly for patients who must undergo postoperative chemotherapy. Infection may place both limb and life in jeopardy for these patients. Yet, osteoarticular allografts offer the only chance at a truly biologic reconstruction of a joint surface in cases requiring resection of the epiphysis of a long bone. Therefore, they should be presented as a reconstruction option to appropriately selected patients. Patients considering such a reconstruction should be informed that there is a high rate of early complications (infection, nonunion, and fracture) and that the initial period of activity restriction is longer than that required for other forms of reconstruction. The use of osteoarticular allografts should be reserved for patients with less than 4 cm of remaining growth because these grafts are unable to remodel their transverse dimensions. The resultant size mismatch at the joint surface would eventually result in premature degradation of the joint surface.

No reconstruction that aims to preserve joint function will provide a lifelong solution in young patients who are long-term survivors of their disease. Although a nonmobile joint may be less desirable than a mobile joint to the majority of patients, in selected cases it may provide the best mode of reconstruction. It is the one method by which durable function can be achieved.[29]

Joint fusion is accomplished using either a large segment of allograft, autograft (i.e., fibula) or a combination of both. Plate fixation or intramedullary nail stabilization can support the construct until healing at the host-graft junction has been achieved. Once the grafted bone has been incorporated by the host, the reconstruction should last the patient's lifetime. This method of reconstruction is the treatment of choice for the wrist (distal radius) and ankle (distal tibia) joints and commonly is used for the shoulder (proximal humerus) and knee (distal femur or proximal tibia). Arthrodesis of the hip (proximal femur) is usually reserved for the young patient and is difficult to achieve. Arthrodesis utilizing allograft, autograft, or a combination of the two, has been successful in limb salvage following joint resection in growing patients. Poor results in children have resulted from the development of limb-length inequality. The technique of limb lengthening by distraction using external fixators and Ilizarov limb-lengthening methods may prevent these poor results secondary to limb-length discrepancy.

The most common method of reconstructing a

segmental bone defect is allograft reconstruction (Fig. 23–10). Nonvascularized or vascularized fibula autografts may serve as alternatives or augmentations to allograft reconstruction. In the non-weight-bearing upper extremity, fibular autografts are the most frequent choice for reconstructing segmental defects. Vascularized fibula grafts are particularly useful in patients with compromised host tissue beds (as in previously irradiated Ewing's sarcoma) and result in rapid healing. As this type of resection and reconstruction spares the patient's native joint, excellent long-term function can be anticipated.

The reported experience with intercalary allografts has been favorable, with better than 80% good or excellent outcomes in one large series.[30] Other researchers have advocated vascularized fibular autografts for the reconstruction of diaphyseal defects or a combination of intercalary allografts and vascularized fibular grafts. Extremely long intercalary allografts may not be suitable for the lower extremities of very young children with substantial growth potential, because the ability to lengthen such grafts, even after successful incorporation, has not been demonstrated.

Alloprosthesis

The alloprosthesis method of reconstruction combines the advantages of both allograft and prosthetic arthroplasty. The prosthesis is cemented into the allograft, which in turn must be fixed to the host bone to achieve incorporation. The allograft restores bone stock removed at the time of surgical resection, provides an attachment point for host soft tissues, and reduces the stresses on the prosthesis. The prosthesis provides a predictably stable joint articulation.

The experience with this approach has not been extensive.[31, 32] As a primary mode of reconstruction, alloprosthesis composites pose risks similar to those of osteoarticular allografts and prosthetic arthroplasty. The alloprosthesis is best suited to the proximal femur and proximal humerus when a mobile joint is the objective of reconstruction. It is the reconstruction method of choice at the University of Texas M.D. Anderson Cancer Center to salvage failed prosthetic arthroplasties.

Extensive intraosseous involvement may preclude adequate fixation of either a prosthesis or an allograft to a remnant of uninvolved host

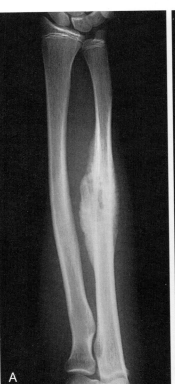
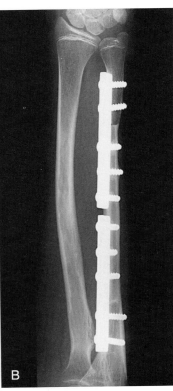

Figure 23–10 • Osteosarcoma diagnosed in a 12-year-old male with a 2-month history of pain in the forearm. *A*, Plain radiographs revealed an osteoblastic lesion of the midshaft of the ulna. The diagnosis was established as dedifferentiated parosteal osteosarcoma by needle biopsy. *B*, Resection and intercalary fibular allograft reconstruction with plate fixation was performed. The patient had full range of motion in the wrist and elbow 7 years following surgery.

bone. Replacement of the entire bone is a viable alternative to limb disarticulation. Two options are available for reconstruction: whole-bone (including adjacent proximal and distal joints); customized, expandable prosthetic arthroplasty, and whole-bone allograft–expandable prosthesis composite reconstruction. Too few of these types of reconstructions have been performed to comment on the incidence of complications or functional outcome anticipated.

PELVIS

Pelvic resections and reconstructions are the most challenging clinical issues in limb-salvage surgery. The surgical principles for resection of tumors arising within the bones of the pelvis are similar to those for resection of the long bones of the extremity. If a wide surgical margin can be achieved with limb preservation, an internal hemipelvectomy is a viable alternative to hindquarter amputation. Two aspects of this surgery remain unresolved. The first is the choice of reconstruction to be used for a given type of resection in order to provide optimal functional results. The second is the high incidence of complications resulting from the complex nature of the surgical procedure.

The choice of reconstruction method depends upon the extent of the resection. The pelvis may be left without reconstruction if a tumor is confined to the pubis, ischium, or iliac wing and the hip joint is preserved. Resection of the hip joint without reconstruction results in a flail and unstable hip, associated with significant limb shortening and weakness despite prolonged rehabilitation. Restoration of the disrupted pelvic ring or reconstruction of the hip joint may yield better short-term function than no reconstruction. But too few cases have been reported of any one reconstruction method to demonstrate superiority of one method over another, and scant long-term follow-up exists.

The reconstructive options for the pelvis vary depending upon the region resected and the age of patient. Methods to reconstruct the pelvis following tumor resection of the periacetabular region include large-segment allograft pelvis/hip prosthesis composite implant, pelvifemoral arthrodesis, or prosthetic spacer reconstruction (saddle prosthesis). The method of reconstruction must be based upon the clinical situation and the functional demands of the patient.

Regardless of the mode of reconstruction, judicious patient selection and careful preoperative counseling are important in view of the high complication rate (greater than 50%) reported in the literature associated with the various available reconstruction options.[33] Deep infection is the most commonly observed complication of pelvic reconstructions and can be devastating to the patient. If complications are avoided, lower extremity function and ambulation may be facilitated, at least in the short term.

SOFT-TISSUE MANAGEMENT

Adequate soft-tissue coverage is critical to the success of any limb-salvage procedure. Multiple intraoperative factors contribute to compromised wound healing. Microsurgical techniques represent a significant advance in limb-sparing surgery. Compromised wound healing and flap necrosis is a disastrous consequence of the surgical elevation of extensive soft-tissue flaps and resection of large segments of bone and surrounding soft tissues. The insertion of a massive prosthesis or allograft and the long duration of the surgical procedures coupled with the deleterious effects of chemotherapy on soft-tissue and bone healing render the surgical wound vulnerable to vascular compromise, necrosis, and deep infection. The development of these complications during the period of bone marrow suppression associated with adjuvant chemotherapy can place the patient's limb and life at risk and can lead ultimately to amputation.

Transposition muscle flaps and free tissue transfers have been extremely useful in overcoming tissue defects and in providing a healthy well-vascularized envelope of soft tissue to protect the reconstruction. The liberal application of these methods has significantly reduced the incidence of infections associated with limb-sparing procedures and of the potentially limb-threatening consequences of poorly placed or performed surgical biopsies.[34] Moreover, this technology has expanded the options afforded the orthopedic oncologist in addressing tumors that arise in compromised host tissue beds (for example, previously irradiated localized Ewing's sarcoma or radiation-induced sarcomas) and in anatomical regions for which host soft tissues may be inadequate for successful salvage (for example, tibial lesions). The utility of muscle flaps has been demonstrated in salvaging reconstructions associated with wound-related complications that might otherwise prompt amputation.[35]

Metastatic Disease

Metastatic bone disease can be a devastating consequence of advanced cancer that can threaten the structural integrity of the skeletal system. Incapacitating bone pain may persist despite local and systemic therapies secondary to significant bone destruction, joint instability, mechanical insufficiency, and fracture. Tumors that develop in children and metastasize to bone include neuroblastoma, Wilms' tumor, rhabdomyosarcoma, and lymphoma.

The primary treatment for advanced cancer involving bone is systemic therapy with radiation to the local site of metastases for pain palliation and fracture prophylaxis. Surgery is indicated to achieve these objectives when nonsurgical therapies fail. Surgical intervention can be an effective therapy to palliate pain, reduce patient anxiety, improve patient mobility and function, facilitate nursing care, prevent fracture, and control local tumor. Fracture treatment includes various techniques to provide stabilization of the long bones, including internal fixation, prosthetic joint replacement, and resection with segmental joint replacement. Spinal cord compression and vertebral fractures can result from vertebral metastases. Spinal cord decompression with vertebrectomy and spinal instrumentation and fusion can be performed for patients with spinal instability or progressive neurologic compromise.

Summary

Effective chemotherapy regimens have dramatically changed the surgical management of primary sarcomas of bone. Limb-salvage surgical procedures are possible in an ever increasing number of patients without a significantly increased risk of local tumor relapse. Advances in technology and surgical techniques have expanded the options available for skeletal reconstruction. End-result analyses have helped refine the application of this technology to maximize function. Novel approaches are focused on the preservation of the native joint and skeletal growth of the affected bone in selected pediatric patients.

Techniques to safely perform transphyseal resections in an attempt to preserve the growth plate as well as the integrity of the adjacent joint are currently being investigated. The application of bone-transport approaches such as the Ilizarov procedure may prove effective in overcoming a major limitation to limb salvage in patients with appreciable limb growth remaining. Further advances will be necessary to maintain function in the long-term cancer survivors of this young patient population.

MANAGEMENT CONSIDERATIONS FOR BENIGN TUMORS

Benign tumors of bone are more common than malignant tumors. Benign tumors may arise from any cellular constituent in bone, including osteogenic (osteoid osteoma, osteoblastoma), chondrogenic (chondroblastoma), and histiocytic and fibrohistiocytic (nonossifying fibroma, fibrous cortical defect, Langerhans-cell histiocytosis) elements. Other lesions with uncertain etiologies (aneurysmal bone cyst, unicameral bone cyst) also manifest principally in the immature patient.

The treatment recommendations for benign bone tumors have been developed in accordance with the biology of the specific tumor. The spectrum of behavior exhibited by benign lesions extends from relative quiescence to destructive aggressiveness. Treatment must be further individualized for each patient based on the patient's age, the site and extent of tumor involvement, and the proximity of tumor to important adjacent bone, growth plate, and joint structures. In general, the objectives of treatment of benign bone neoplasms are (1) local tumor control, (2) preservation of bone stock, growth plates, and adjacent joints; and (3) maintenance of normal extremity function. The surgical margin necessary for successful control of benign bone lesions varies, usually dictated by the biology of the tumor and its site and local extent. Intralesional excision by curettage provides local tumor control in the overwhelming majority of patients. Reconstruction alternatives of the resultant osseous defect include autogenous bone graft, allograft preparations, bone cement (polymethylmethacrylate), and bone graft substitutes.[36, 37]

The surgical staging system adopted by the

Musculoskeletal Tumor Society for benign tumors defines three stages[4]:

Stage 1 benign tumors are latent lesions that demonstrate limited local growth and have no metastatic potential. They commonly are asymptomatic and therefore are often discovered incidentally. These lesions may be treated by observation alone or by intralesional excision with curettage. Local recurrences are negligible.

Stage 2 benign tumors are actively growing lesions that almost never metastasize. They usually cause symptoms that prompt medical evaluation and are not infrequently associated with pathologic fracture. These lesions are usually treated by intralesional excision by curettage; however, because of their propensity to locally recur, physical or chemical adjuvants such as polymethylmethacrylate, liquid nitrogen (cryosurgery), or phenol may be used to extend the surgical margin.

Stage 3 benign tumors are aggressive lesions that often destroy the adjacent osseous tissue and extend into the surrounding soft tissues. Distant metastases can develop. The most reliable means of achieving a wide surgical margin is by en bloc excision. Unfortunately, en bloc excision may necessitate sacrifice of significant bone stock or resection of an adjacent joint. To avoid such disability, surgical margins can be extended by means of an effective adjuvant therapy following an intralesional excision as for a Stage 2 lesion. In this case, the potential for recurrence is greater than with a primary wide en bloc excision.

Osteoid Osteoma/Osteoblastoma

Osteoid osteoma and osteoblastoma are benign bone-forming lesions. Osteoid osteoma is characterized by a nidus (usually less than 1 cm) surrounded by a distinctive zone of reactive bone formation. These lesions constitute approximately 12% of all benign bone tumors.[38] They are characteristically found in children, adolescents, and young adults; Approximately 90% of such patients are under 30 years of age. Osteoid osteomas are more common in males than females (2:1) in reported series.

The characteristic symptom associated with osteoid osteoma is pain, usually persistent, dull, aching, intense, and often worse at night. Swelling and tenderness over the affected site are also commonly observed. Typically, symptoms respond dramatically to oral salicylates or other nonsteroidal anti-inflammatory agents, although that response is not universal.

Osteoid osteomas can occur in any bone and are most common in the long bones of the lower extremity; approximately one half of all cases occur in the femur and tibia. The majority of the femoral lesions occur in the region of the hip. Up to one fifth of all osteoid osteomas occur in the spine, with a noted predilection for the posterior elements. When affecting the spine, these lesions may be presented as a painful scoliosis.

The typical radiographic picture is that of a central, well-demarcated oval or round lucent nidus (less than 1 cm) surrounded by a variable amount of dense, sclerotic reactive bone. Osteoid osteomas usually arise in the cortex of the diaphysis of long bones but also can occur in the medullary or subperiosteal regions of the affected bone. When an exuberant osteoblastic reactive response is present, particularly in cortical lesions, a CT scan is often useful in localizing the nidus (Fig. 23–11). The role for MRI has not been established.

Currently, surgical excision of the nidus is necessary for a successful result. Removal of the surrounding sclerotic bone is unnecessary. Intraoperative localization of the nidus may be difficult, and therefore preoperatively administered tetracycline may be given.[39] Intraoperative localization is then performed by using a hand-held ultraviolet lamp and confirming complete excision of the nidus by the loss of fluorescence following removal of the lesion. In most instances, a thorough curettage of the nidus and perilesional bone will result in a cure.[40] The need for prophylactic internal fixation or bone graft is usually unnecessary unless the location of the bone and extent of material excised place the bone at risk for fracture.

Conservative management with salicylates, or, preferably, long-acting nonsteroidal anti-inflammatory agents may be effective. Evidence supporting the use of continuous administration (average duration 33 months) of a nonsteroidal anti-inflammatory agent to relieve the pain associated with osteoid osteoma and thus obviate surgical intervention has been reported.[41]

Osteoblastomas, although histologically similar to osteoid osteomas, are progressively growing

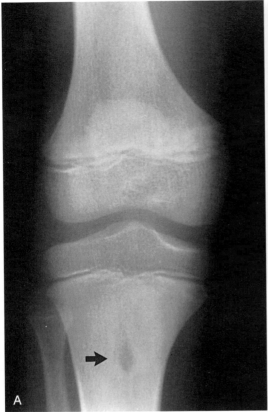

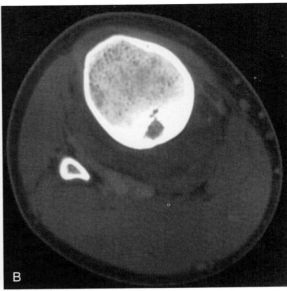

Figure 23–11 • Osteoid osteoma diagnosed in 9-year-old male with throbbing knee pain exacerbated at night. *A*, Plain radiographs revealed a radiolucency surrounded by bony sclerosis in the proximal tibia *(arrow)*. *B*, The diagnosis of osteoid osteoma was supported by the findings on CT scan.

lesions of a large size (greater than 2 cm). Osteoblastomas are less common than osteoid osteomas, accounting for approximately 3% of benign bone tumors.[38] The patient age and sex distributions are similar to that for osteoid osteoma.

Typically, patients present with insidious, dull pain that is usually less severe than that observed with osteoid osteoma. The clinical course for these patients is commonly prolonged. Nocturnal pain is not a characteristic feature of osteoblastoma. Symptomatic relief with salicylates is inconsistent. Spinal involvement may produce radicular symptoms in as many as one half of patients and may result in objective neurologic deficits in as many as 30%.[42] Painful scoliosis may be the presenting complaint in up to 75%.[42, 43]

The most common site for osteoblastoma is the axial skeleton (approximately one third of cases). Other frequent sites include the long bones of the appendicular skeleton and small bones of the hands and feet. The preferential sites of involvement of the spine are the posterior elements, both thoracic and lumbar segments equally. Involvement of the vertebral body is usually secondary to extension from the posterior elements. When associated with scoliosis, osteoblastomas are usually located at or near the apex of the concavity of the curve.

The radiographic features of osteoblastomas are not distinctive and vary with location. In long bones, osteoblastomas are usually observed in the metaphysis or diaphysis. The lesions are characteristically eccentric, well-circumscribed, lytic (greater than 2 cm), and expansile, with an intact thin shell of bone and no associated soft-tissue mass. The surrounding osteoblastic reaction is irregular and, although often scant, may be quite extensive. Spinal lesions are primarily lytic and may expand past the affected bone segment, encroaching on the spinal canal or extending into the adjacent paravertebral tissues (Fig. 23–12).

For osteoblastomas of small to moderate size, surgical treatment is similar to that for osteoid osteoma, consisting of thorough curettage with or without autogenous bone grafting. Even if removal of the tumor by curettage is incomplete,

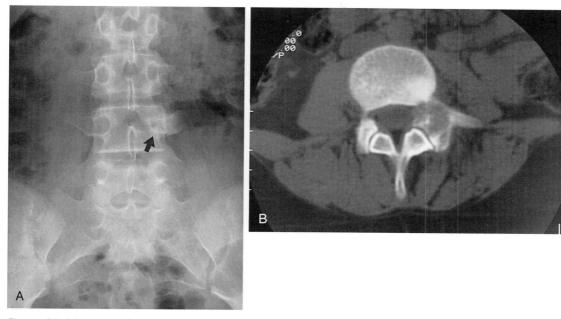

Figure 23–12 • Osteoblastoma diagnosed in a 15-year-old female with a history of several years of low back pain. *A,* Imaging studies revealed a blastic lesion in the left pedicle of the L4 vertebra *(arrow)*. *B,* CT scan delineated the extent of the mixed blastic and lytic lesion characteristic of an osteoblastoma.

the residual tumor may remain dormant and asymptomatic for many years. The recurrence rate for osteoblastoma varies up to 15% to 20% in reported series.[44]

A limited number of osteoblastic lesions that are atypical of the conventional osteoblastoma and fail to satisfy the criteria of osteosarcoma have been recognized. These aggressive osteoblastomas are so named because of their unusual clinical behavior and aggressive radiographic appearance.[45, 46] Atypical aggressive osteoblastomas may represent an intermediate lesion between typical benign osteoblastoma and osteosarcoma. These atypical lesions are more likely to recur following intralesional excision by curettage, and some of the more aggressive ones may metastasize.[47]

In light of these issues, many of which require further clarification, complete excision of all osteoblastomas should be considered when possible. Many investigators recommend marginal excision when feasible. Physical adjuvants, such as cryosurgery, can extend the surgical margins without unnecessarily compromising the integrity of the affected bone. Radiation therapy is rarely indicated for patients with benign osteoblastomas and is usually limited to those with unresectable or multiply-recurrent tumors.

Osteochondroma

Solitary osteochondroma is the most common primary benign lesion of bone, representing approximately 50% of all benign neoplasms (Fig. 23–13).[38] It is characterized as a cartilage-capped protuberance that arises adjacent to an epiphyseal plate and can develop in any bone performed in cartilage. This lesion is typically discovered in skeletally immature patients, particularly during the time of a growth spurt. Like the epiphyseal cartilage, the cartilaginous component of the osteochondroma undergoes endochondral ossification and can enlarge during skeletal growth. The growth of an osteochondroma ceases at maturity. The majority of lesions are asymptomatic. Symptoms may occur from nerve compression or mechanical irritation of adjacent soft-tissue structures.

Lesions in the distal femur and proximal tibia together account for approximately 50% of the osteochondromas observed. The proximal humerus, proximal femur, distal radius, distal tibia, and fibula are other common sites. Lesions of the spine are uncommon and involve the secondary centers of ossification. Osteochondromas are rare in the bones of the hand and feet.

The diagnosis of an osteochondroma can be

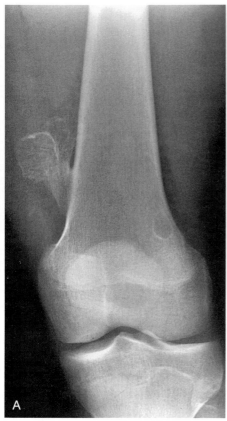

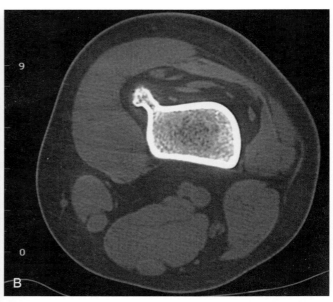

Figure 23–13 • Osteochondroma diagnosed in a 15-year-old male who presented with persistent discomfort in the medial distal thigh after athletic activities. *A*, Plain radiographs revealed a bony excrescence arising from the medial aspect of the distal femur. *B*, CT scan confirmed the presence of bony continuity of the exophytic lesion with the medullary canal of the distal femur consistent with the diagnosis of an osteochondroma.

made radiographically by the appearance of a bony excrescence (pedunculated or sessile) arising in the metaphysis of the affected bone and projecting away from the joint. The cortex of the affected bone is continuous with the cortical margin of the osteochondroma. The underlying trabecular pattern blends together with the intramedullary host bone. Occasionally the lesion is densely calcified centrally. The calcifications obscure these characteristics on plain radiographs. In these cases, a CT scan is recommended to confirm the suspected diagnosis.

The mere presence of an asymptomatic osteochondroma is not an indication for surgical intervention. Symptomatic or large, disfiguring lesions are best treated by surgical excision. The lesion is removed at its base at the level of the normal cortical bone. Care is taken to excise all of the cartilage cap and periosteum along with the lesion to prevent recurrence. As the stalk provides minimal mechanical strength to the bone, protective weight-bearing is necessary for only a limited period.

Growth of an osteochondroma after skeletal maturity should arouse suspicion of malignant transformation. This rare complication has been estimated to occur in less than 1% of cases. Radiographically, an irregular, thickened (greater than 1 cm) cartilaginous cap, the appearance of a soft tissue mass, or irregular blotchy calcifications within the cap should raise suspicion of a chondrosarcoma and prompt surgical excision.

Hereditary multiple exostoses are an autosomal dominant disorder with a prevalence of at least 1 in 50,000.[48] The majority of these patients have osseous deformities. Incidence of malignant transformation of a benign osteochondroma in these patients has been estimated at approximately 1%.

Chondroblastoma

Chondroblastoma is an uncommon entity that accounts for less than 1% of all primary bone tumors.[38] The peak incidence is in adolescence.

Males are affected more often (2:1) than females.

Symptoms are nonspecific. Localized pain and occasionally swelling may be observed in the region of the tumor and adjacent joint. Limitation in joint range of motion is commonly observed, along with muscular atrophy.

Chondroblastomas may occur in any bone of the axial or appendicular skeleton. Lesions in the femur, humerus, tibia, tarsal bones, and pelvis collectively account for approximately 75% of all cases. These lesions occur in the epiphysis or apophysis of skeletally immature, long tubular bones, occasionally extending into the adjacent metaphysis. Typically they are central, radiolucent, and round, with a smooth sclerotic rim. Occasionally punctate calcifications may be observed (Fig. 23–14).

Chondroblastomas are usually treated by intralesional excision with thorough curettage and bone grafting. Incidence of local recurrence after treatment is reported as 10% to 20%.[49] A few cases of patients developing pulmonary metastases have been reported.

Nonossifying Fibroma

Nonossifying fibromas are believed to represent one entity in a spectrum of benign fibrous lesions of bone ranging from the fibrous cortical defect to the benign fibrous histiocytoma. Nonossifying fibromas represent approximately 5% of benign bone tumors.[38] These lesions are rarely symptomatic and are usually discovered incidentally when radiographs are taken for unrelated reasons. They most often occur in children in the second decade of life. Males predominate in a ratio of 2:1 over females in most series. Most nonossifying fibromas occur in the long bones of the lower extremity, particularly the femur and tibia.

Nonossifying fibromas are usually eccentrically located in the metaphysis of long bones with the widest diameter oriented along the long axis of the affected bone. These fibromas are loculated, with a thin, well-defined sclerotic border. The cortex may be thinned or expanded, but remains intact. The diagnosis is made in the overwhelming majority of cases without biopsy, based only upon the typical radiographic presentation.

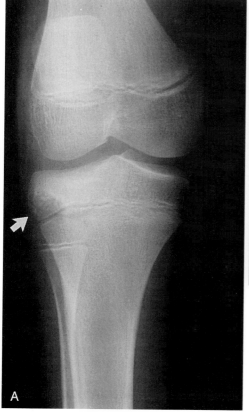

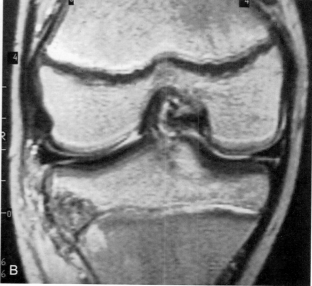

Figure 23–14 • Chondroblastoma diagnosed in a 13-year-old male with a 4-month history of knee pain with tenderness and soft-tissue swelling over the lateral aspect of the knee. *A,* Plain radiographs revealed a radiolucency along the lateral aspect of the proximal tibial epiphysis *(arrow). B,* The extent of the lesion was delineated by MR imaging. The diagnosis of chondroblastoma prompted curettage and particulate allograft bone reconstruction.

Observation alone usually is warranted if the lesion is found incidentally. Spontaneous healing of nonossifying fibromas may be anticipated with skeletal maturation. If the lesion is painful, has an unusual radiographic appearance, or involves an unusual location, a biopsy is recommended to confirm the diagnosis. Curettage and bone grafting are recommended if the lesion places the involved bone at risk for fracture. Internal fixation is generally not needed.

If pathologic fracture occurs, external immobilization of the bone is performed to allow healing to occur (Fig. 23–15). In some cases, the reparative process of fracture healing stimulates ossification of the nonossifying fibroma, making surgical intervention unnecessary.

Fibrous Dysplasia

Fibrous dysplasia is a benign developmental anomaly resulting in defective endochondral bone maturation. This disorder begins when a person is skeletally immature, but the age at onset of symptoms varies widely. In general, fibrous dysplasia clinically manifests in late childhood or adolescence with either a solitary, monostotic lesion or less frequently with polyostotic lesions. The skeletal lesions of fibrous dysplasia are not true neoplasms.

The clinical spectrum of fibrous dysplasia varies from asymptomatic monostotic lesions to painful solitary lesions to extensive skeletal deformities associated with polyostotic involvement. The polyostotic form can be associated with café-au-lait skin lesions and endocrinopathies (McCune-Albright syndrome). The monostotic form does not progress into the polyostotic form.

The majority of patients present with pain, but many remain asymptomatic into adulthood.[50] Swelling and localized tenderness of the affected region of the extremity may be observed. Often the disorder becomes clinically apparent after minor trauma precipitates a pathologic fracture.

Fibrous dysplasia usually occurs in the long bones of the lower extremity, typically in the proximal femur. The development of malignant change in fibrous dysplasia is rare, estimated to occur in less than 1% of both monostotic and polyostotic forms.[51]

The skeletal lesions present a variety of radiographic features. In the long bones, fibrous dysplasia appears in the metaphysis or diaphysis of the affected bone, characterized by a well-defined central or eccentric lesion. Radiographically, the lesion may vary from being completely radiolucent to having a more radiopaque, homogeneously "groundglass" appearance, depending upon the amount of bone within the lesion. Cystic and cartilaginous changes may be present. Endosteal scalloping and thinning of the cortex may be seen. The cortex may also be consider-

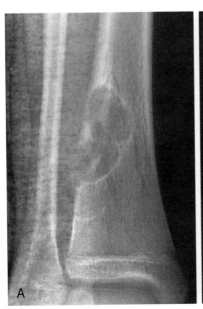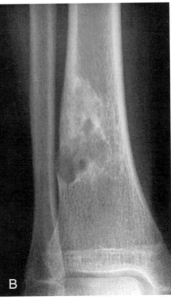

Figure 23–15 • Pathologic fracture in a 12-year-old female who sustained a twisting injury to the right ankle. *A*, AP radiograph of the distal tibia revealed a fracture through a geographic, lytic, eccentric metaphyseal lesion, the distal tibia characterized by well-defined sclerotic borders consistent with a nonossifying fibroma. *B*, AP radiograph shows healing of the fracture and lesion after cast immobilization.

ably thickened in some instances despite cortical erosions. Diffuse expansion of the bone contour can also be observed.

These bony changes often lead to structural weakness of the affected bone, resulting in fractures and secondary deformities. The femoral neck is particularly susceptible if involved. In the polyostotic form of the disease, multiple fatigue fractures may give rise to the "shepherd's crook" deformity associated with limb shortening, limp, and disabling pain.

Most lesions are asymptomatic and require no intervention. Treatment is indicated for established and impending fractures, persistent pain, or progressive deformity. Curettage, bone grafting, and stabilization, either with bracing or internal fixation, are required until osseous remodeling has been completed. Resorption of the bone graft and replacement with dysplastic immature bone are common. Progression of the disease may occur, leading to repeat fracture and failure of internal fixation. In this event, multiple surgical procedures are necessary. Autogenous cortical grafts and allografts have been shown to resorb more slowly than autogenous cancellous graft.[52, 53] Intramedullary devices are preferred for mechanical stabilization of the affected bone.

Solitary Bone Cyst

Solitary or unicameral bone cysts are benign, non-neoplastic, fluid-containing, unilocular lesions that occur mostly in children; 80% to 90% of all such lesions are found in patients younger than age 20. Solitary bone cysts are at least twice as frequent in males as in females.

Incidental trauma usually directs attention to the affected extremity. Pathologic fracture usually prompts medical attention. Healing of the fracture seldom stimulates healing of the underlying cyst.[54] The proximal femur and humerus are the sites of involvement in the overwhelming majority of cases (Fig. 23–16).

A unicameral bone cyst is characteristically centrally located within the medullary region of the metaphysis of long bones. The cyst is lytic and elongated in appearance, its length always greater than its width. The inner surface of the cyst cavity has sharply delimited margins. The overlying cortex is expanded and markedly thinned but is always intact. A sclerotic margin is apparent. Commonly, a free fragment of cortical

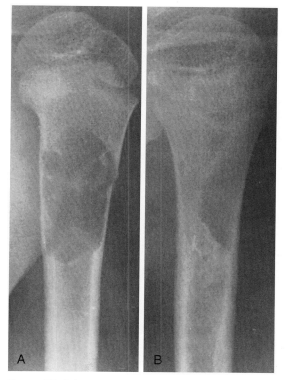

Figure 23–16 • Pathologic fracture of the left proximal humerus in a 6-year-old male after a fall. *A,* The radiographic appearance of the lesion was consistent with a unicameral bone cyst. The fracture was allowed to heal, after which time 125 mg of methyprednisolone was injected directly into the cyst. *B,* Complete healing of the cyst was noted after one injection.

bone will break off and settle to the dependent portion of the cyst—the so-called "fallen fragment sign."

At the time of presentation, a cyst may be abutting the epiphyseal plate. With skeletal maturity, the distance between the cyst and the physis may increase as a result of longitudinal growth of the affected bone.

Some believe that the lesion may be self-limited and spontaneously heal, thus accounting for the low incidence of unicameral bone cysts in adults. Limited intervention resulting in the least morbidity is therefore favored to affect a cure. Various methods of treatment have been advocated for unicameral bone cysts. The most commonly recommended treatment is intralesional methylprednisolone injection (80–200 mg, depending upon the size of the cyst) (Fig. 23–17). Although the etiology of these cysts is unknown,

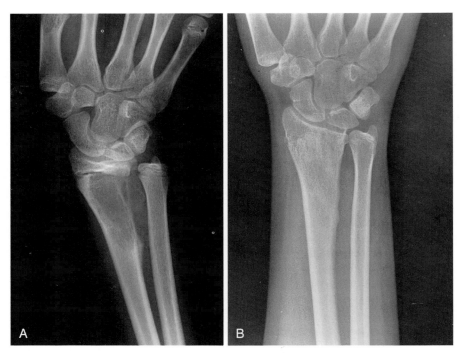

Figure 23–17 • Bone cyst in 13-year-old female with a history of several months of pain and swelling in the right wrist. *A,* Plain radiograph revealed a lytic lesion in the distal radius metaphysis that extended to the growth plate. Needle biopsy suggested the diagnosis of an aneurysmal bone cyst. The lesion was curetted and reconstructed with particulate allograft bone. *B,* The bone graft consolidated without evidence of local recurrence 2 years postoperatively.

elevated prostaglandin levels in the cyst may in part explain the relative effectiveness of corticosteroid injections.

Multiple steroid injections may be necessary to stimulate complete cyst healing. Injections are repeated as necessary every 6 weeks or less frequently until healing occurs. Follow-up must be continued after healing begins, as incomplete healing and recurrence may occur. One can expect approximately 50% to 70% of the cysts to heal completely, with at least partial healing of the remaining lesions.[54]

Cysts associated with pathologic fractures are immobilized and treated in a similar manner. One exception to this is a pathologic fracture of the proximal femur, which is commonly treated by curettage and autologous bone graft with cast immobilization or internal fixation (in an adolescent).

A similar technique with the injection of autologous bone marrow, the implantation of bone graft substitutes, or both, instead of injecting methylprednisolone has been reported. The early results of this method appear to be as effective

as or superior to corticosteroid injections. The recurrence rate appears to be related to age as much to the method of treatment.

Aneurysmal Bone Cyst

Aneurysmal bone cyst is a hemorrhagic, cystic lesion of bone that can arise de novo or secondarily with another benign primary lesion such as chondroblastoma, osteoblastoma, giant-cell tumor, chondromyxoid fibroma, or fibrous dysplasia.[55] These lesions have an equal sex distribution and occur most frequently in patients less than 20 years of age (80%).

Clinically, patients present with mild to moderate pain and associated swelling of varying duration. The long bones and posterior elements of the spine represent the most common sites of involvement. Spinal cord or nerve root compression may cause neurologic deficits.

Aneurysmal bone cyst appears as a purely lytic lesion radiographically. In long bones, it occurs eccentrically in the metaphysis with extension into the epiphysis when the physis is closed. The lesion is well-demarcated but usually lacks a well-defined sclerotic rim. It consistently expands and balloons the adjacent cortex, resulting in a soap-bubble appearance. In the spine, an aneurysmal bone cyst can extend into the vertebral body along the pedicle, expanding its contours and compressing the dural sac and spinal cord.

The treatment of aneurysmal bone cyst is intralesional excision with thorough curettage and bone grafting. A recurrence rate of up to 20% has been reported following treatment.[56, 57] The addition of cryosurgery can further decrease the local recurrence rate.[58]

Expendable bones can be resected. For unresectable lesions, radiotherapy with or without partial curettage can affect a cure in approximately 80% of patients.[56] The finite risk of the development of radiation-induced sarcoma in the involved field should caution one against injudicious use of this treatment. Transcatheter arterial embolization also has proved effective therapy for surgically inaccessible anatomical locations.[59]

Langerhans-Cell Histiocytosis (Eosinophilic Granuloma of Bone)

Localized Langerhans-cell histiocytosis (LCH) of bone is a rare, benign tumor-like condition that is characterized by a clonal proliferation of Langerhans-type histiocytes.[60] Patients usually present in the first decade of life with pain, tenderness, and swelling of the affected area. A male to female ratio of 2:1 has been noted in patients with primary bone presentation. The lesions are characteristically found in the skull, ribs, spine, pelvis, and the metaphyseal-diaphyseal regions of long bones, especially the femur and humerus. Lesions in the spine often cause vertebral collapse (vertebra plana) but infrequently cause neurologic deficits. Unifocal bone presentation is twice as common as multifocal bone involvement.

Although the pathogenesis remains undefined, the clinical course for most patients is generally benign. The clinical course can be highly variable, with lesions exhibiting healing (partial or complete) or recurrence after treatment and progression or spontaneous remission without treatment.[61]

The typical radiographic appearance of early localized LCH involving the long bones is characterized by lytic, well-defined, "punched out" lesions in the medullary region of the diaphysis or metaphysis. Less than half of the lesions will demonstrate marginal reactive sclerosis.

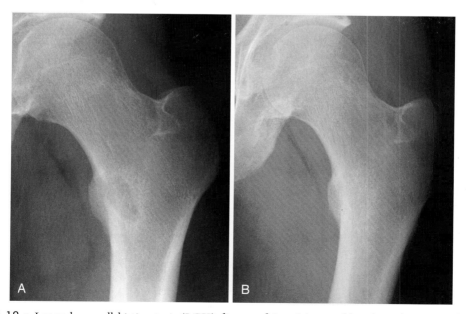

Figure 23–18 • Langerhans-cell histiocytosis (LCH) diagnosed in a 14-year-old male with a 4-month history of left hip pain. *A,* Plain radiographs demonstrated a lytic lesion for which the diagnosis of osteomyelitis and LCH were considered. A fine needle aspiration yielded cells consistent with LCH. The lesion was injected with 125 mg of methylprednisolone at the time the diagnosis was established. *B,* The patient's symptoms resolved within 1 week, and the bone lesion healed over the ensuing 2 months.

On occasion the lesions may be poorly demarcated with indistinct margins. Bone destruction may be irregular and patchy. Scalloping of the endosteum and thinning of the adjacent cortex may be noted. A smooth, uninterrupted periosteal reaction is characteristic, but the reaction may be highly variable. The pattern of reaction can be lamellated, suggesting a more aggressive lesion such as osteomyelitis or Ewing's sarcoma. Bone expansion occurs in patients with disease of long standing.

Various treatment options are available for long-bone lesions, including observation alone, curettage, and low-dose radiation therapy or intralesional injection of corticosteroids (Fig. 23–18).[52, 63] As some lesions appear to resolve spontaneously, relief of pain with minimal morbidity is the treatment goal. Vertebrae that collapse may partially reconstitute in height with healing regardless of the treatment given. For lesions treated by curettage, bone graft is not routinely performed unless the bone involved is structurally compromised. Low-dose radiation (300–600 cGy) has been advocated for inaccessible lesions.

The multifocal form may develop extraosseous manifestations such as diabetes insipidus, hepatosplenomegaly, and adenopathy. This form is best treated with low-dose chemotherapy including methotrexate, prednisone, and vinblastine, which have been found effective.[61]

Summary

Local tumor control is usually accomplished with preservation of the integrity of the affected bone, and therefore long-term function is preserved in the majority of patients. Minimally invasive techniques for the diagnosis and treatment of selected tumors continue to reduce perioperative morbidity. Ongoing investigation of effective synthetic bone-graft substitutes will expand the options for skeletal reconstruction and address a major obstacle to limb-defect reconstruction in children.

References

1. Mankin HJ, Lange TA, Spanier SS: The hazards of biopsy in patients with malignant primary bone and soft-tissue tumors. *J Bone Joint Surg Am* 64:1121–1127, 1982.

2. Mankin HJ, Mankin CJ, Simon MA: The hazards of the biopsy, revisited. *J Bone Joint Surg Am* 78:656–663, 1996.

3. Ayala AG, Ro JY, Fanning CV, et al: Core needle biopsy and fine-needle aspiration in the diagnosis of bone and soft-tissue lesions. *Hematol Oncol Clin North Am* 9(3):633–651, 1995.

4. Enneking WF, Spanier SS, Goodman MA: A system for the surgical staging of musculoskeletal sarcoma. *Clin Orthop* 153:106–120, 1980.

5. Raymond AK: Surface osteosarcoma. *Clin Orthop* 270:140–148, 1991.

6. Hudson M, Jaffe MR, Jaffe N, et al: Pediatric osteosarcoma: Therapeutic strategies, results, and prognostic factors derived from a 10-year experience. *J Clin Oncol* 8:1988–1997, 1990.

7. Meyers PA, Heller G, Healey J, et al: Chemotherapy for nonmetastatic osteogenic sarcoma: The Memorial Sloan-Kettering experience. *J Clin Oncol* 10:5–15, 1992.

8. Meyers PA, Heller G, Healey J, et al: Osteogenic sarcoma with clinically detectable metastasis at initial presentation. *J Clin Oncol* 11:449–453, 1993.

9. Bacci G, Toni A, Avella M, et al: Long-term results in 144 localized Ewing's sarcoma patients treated with combined therapy. *Cancer* 63:1477–1486, 1989.

10. Burgert EO Jr, Nesbit EM, Garnsey LA, et al: Multimodality therapy for the management of nonpelvic localized Ewing's sarcoma of bone: Intergroup study IESS-II. *J Clin Oncol* 8:1517–1524, 1990

11. Evans RG, Nesbit ME, Gehan EA, et al: Multimodal therapy for the management of localized Ewing's sarcoma of pelvic and sacral bones: A report from the second intergroup study. *J Clin Oncol* 9:1173–1180, 1991.

12. Yang R-S, Eckardt JJ, Eilber FR, et al: Surgical indications for Ewing's sarcoma of the pelvis. *Cancer* 76:1388–1397, 1995.

13. Toni A, Neff JR, Sudanese A, et al: The role of surgical therapy in patients with nonmetastatic Ewing's sarcoma of the limbs. *Clin Orthop* 286:225–240, 1993.

14. Frassica FJ, Frassica DA, Pritchard DJ, et al: Ewing's sarcoma of the pelvis. *J Bone Joint Surg Am* 75:1457–1465, 1993.

15. Scully SP, Temple HT, Keefe RJ, et al: The role of surgical resection in pelvic Ewing's sarcoma. *J Clin Oncol* 13:2336–2341, 1995

16. Harris IE, Leff AR, Gitelis S, et al: Function after amputation, arthrodesis, or arthroplasty for tumors about the knee. *J Bone Joint Surg Am* 72:1477–1485, 1990.

17. Cammisa FP Jr, Glasser DB, Otis JC, et al: The Van Nes tibia rotationplasty: A functionally viable reconstructive procedure in children who have a tumor of the distal end of the femur. *J Bone Joint Surg Am* 72:1541–1547, 1990.

18. Gottsauner-Wolf F, Kotz R, Knahr K, et al: Rotationplasty for limb salvage in the treatment

of malignant tumors at the knee. *J Bone Joint Surg Am* 73:1365–1375, 1991.

19. Winkelmann W: Hip rotationplasty for malignant tumors of the proximal part of the femur. *J Bone Joint Surg Am* 68:362–369, 1986.

20. Simon MA, Aschliman MA, Thomas N, et al: Limb-salvage treatment versus amputation for osteosarcoma of the distal end of the femur. *J Bone Joint Surg Am* 68:1331–1337, 1986.

21. Horowitz SM, Glasser DB, Lane JM, et al: Prosthetic and extremity survivorship after limb salvage for sarcoma. *Clin Orthop* 293:280–286, 1993.

22. Anderson M, Green WT, Messner MB: Growth and predictions of growth in the lower extremity. *J Bone Joint Surg Am* 45:1–14, 1963.

23. Eckardt JJ, Safran MR, Eilber FR, et al: Expandable endoprosthetic reconstruction of the skeletally immature after malignant bone tumor resection. *Clin Orthop* 297:188–202, 1993.

24. Finn HA, Simon MA: Limb-salvage surgery in the treatment of osteosarcoma in skeletally immature individuals. *Clin Orthop* 262:108–118, 1991.

25. Kenan S, Bloom N, Lewis MM: Limb-sparing surgery in skeletally immature patients with osteosarcoma: The use of an expandable prosthesis. *Clin Orthop* 270:223–230, 1991.

26. Otis JC, Lane JM, Kroll MA: Energy cost during gait in osteosarcoma patients after resection and knee replacements and after above-the knee amputation. *J Bone Joint Surg Am* 67:606–611, 1985.

27. Alma BA, DeBari A, Krajbich JI: Massive allografts in the treatment of osteosarcoma and Ewing's sarcoma in children and adolescents. *J Bone Joint Surg Am* 77:54–64, 1995.

28. Gebhardt MC, Flugstad DI, Springfield DS, et al: The use of bone allografts for limb salvage in high-grade extremity osteosarcoma. *Clin Orthop* 270:181–196, 1991.

29. Weiner SD, Scarborough M, Vander Griend RA: Resection arthrodesis of the knee with an intercalary allograft. *J Bone Joint Surg Am* 78:185–192, 1996.

30. Ortiz-Cruz E, Gebhardt MC, Jennings LC, et al: The results of transplantation of intercalary allografts after resection of tumors. *J Bone Joint Surg Am* 79:97–106, 1997.

31. Jofe MH, Gebhardt MC, Tomford WW, et al: Osteoarticular allografts and allografts plus prosthesis in the management of malignant tumors of the proximal femur. *J Bone Joint Surg Am* 70:507–516, 1988.

32. Gitelis S, Piasecki P: Allograft prosthetic arthroplasty for osteosarcoma and other aggressive bone tumors. *Clin Orthop* 270: 197–201, 1991.

33. Campanacci M, Capanna R: Pelvic resections: The Rizzoli Institute Experience. *Orthop Clin North Am* 22:65–86, 1991.

34. Horowitz SM, Lane JM, Healey JH: Soft-tissue management with prosthetic replacement for sarcomas around the knee. *Clin Orthop* 275: 226–231, 1992.

35. Eckhardt JJ, Lesavoy MA, Dubrow TJ, et al: Exposed endoprosthesis: Management protocol using muscle and myocutaneous flap coverage. *Clin Orthop* 251:220–229, 1990.

36. Nicholas RW, Lange TA: Granular tricalcium phosphate grafting of cavitary lesions in human bone. *Clin Orthop* 306:197–203, 1994.

37. Uchida A, Araki N, Shinto Y, et al: The use of calcium hydroxyapatite ceramic in bone tumor surgery. *J Bone Joint Surg Br* 74:298–302, 1990.

38. Unni KK: *Dahlin's Bone Tumors: General Aspects and Data on 11,087 Cases,* 5th ed. Philadelphia: Lippincott-Raven, 1996.

39. Ayala AG, Murray JA, Erling MA, et al: Osteoid-osteoma: Intraoperative tetracycline-fluorescence demonstration of the nidus. *J Bone Joint Surg Am* 68:747–751, 1986.

40. Frassica FJ, Waltrip RL, Sponseller PD, et al: Clinicopathologic features and treatment of osteoid osteoma and osteoblastoma in children and adolescents. *Orthop Clin North Am* 27(3):559–574, 1996.

41. Kneisl JS, Simon MA: Medical management compared with operative treatment for osteoid osteoma. *J Bone Joint Surg Am* 74:179–185, 1992.

42. Nemoto O, Moser RP, VanDam BE, et al: Osteoblastoma of the spine: A review of 75 cases. *Spine* 15:1273–1280, 1990.

43. Pettine KA, Klassen RA: Osteoid-osteoma and osteoblastoma of the spine. *J Bone Joint Surg Am* 68:354–361, 1986.

44. Lucas DR, Unni KK, McLeod RA, et al: Osteoblastoma: Clinicopathologic study of 306 cases. *Hum Pathol* 25:117–134, 1994.

45. Schajowicz F, Lemos C: Malignant osteoblastoma. *J Bone Joint Surg Br* 58: 202–211, 1979.

46. Dorfman HD, Weiss SW: Borderline osteoblastic tumors: Problems in the differential diagnosis of aggressive osteoblastoma and low-grade osteosarcoma. *Semin Diagn Pathol* 1:215–234, 1984.

47. Kenan S, Floman Y, Robin GC, et al: Aggressive osteoblastoma. A case report and review of the literature. *Clin Orthop* 195:294–298, 1986.

48. Schmale GA, Conrad EU, Raskind WH: The natural history of hereditary multiple exostoses. *J Bone Joint Surg Am* 76:986–992, 1994.

49. Springfield DS, Capanna R, Gherlinzoni F, et al: Chondroblastoma. A review of seventy cases. *J Bone Joint Surg Am* 67:748–755, 1985.

50. Harris WH, Dudley HR, Barry RJ: The natural history of fibrous dysplasia. *J Bone Joint Surg Am* 44:207–233, 1962.

51. Yabut Jr SM, Kenan S, Sissons HA, et al: Malignant transformation of fibrous dysplasia: A case report and review of the literature. *Clin Orthop* 228:281–289, 1988.

52. Enneking WF, Gearen PF: Fibrous dysplasia of the femoral neck: Treatment by cortical bone-grafting. *J Bone Joint Surg Am* 68:1415–1422, 1986.

53. Stephenson RB, London MD, Hankin FM, et al: Fibrous dysplasia: An analysis of options for treatment. *J Bone Joint Surg Am* 69:400–409, 1987.

54. Capanna R, Campanacci DA, Manfrini M: Unicameral and aneurysmal bone cysts. *Orthop Clin North Am* 27(3):605–614, 1996.

55. Martinez V, Sissons HA: Aneurysmal bone cyst: A review of 123 cases including primary lesions and those secondary to other bone pathology. *Cancer* 61:2291–2304, 1988.

56. Campanacci M, Capanna R, Picci P: Unicameral and aneurysmal bone cysts. *Clin Orthop* 204:25–36, 1986.

57. Vergel De Dios AM, Bond JR, Shives TC, et al: Aneurysmal bone cyst: A clinicopathologic study of 238 cases. *Cancer* 69:2921–2931, 1992.

58. Marcove RC, Sheth DS, Takemoto S, Healey JH: The treatment of aneurysmal bone cyst. *Clin Orthop* 311:157–163, 1995.

59. Chuang VP, Soo CS, Wallace S, et al: Arterial occlusion management of giant cell tumor and aneurysmal bone cyst. *Am J Roentgenol* 136:1127–1130, 1981.

60. Willman CL, Busque L, Griffith BB, et al: Langerhans-cell histiocytosis (histiocytosis X): A clonal proliferative disease. N Engl J Med 331:154–160, 1994.

61. Sessa S, Sommelet D, Lascombes P, Prevot J: Treatment of Langerhans-cell histiocytosis in children: Experience at the Children's Hospital of Nancy. *J Bone Joint Surg Am* 76:1513–1525, 1994.

62. Capanna R, Springfield DS, Ruggieri P, et al: Direct cortisone injection in eosinophilic granuloma of bone: A preliminary report on 11 patients. *J Pediatr Orthop* 5:339–342, 1985.

63. Shabb N, Fanning C, Carrasco CH, et al: Diagnosis of eosinophilic granuloma of bone by fine-needle aspiration with concurrent institution of therapy: A cytologic, histologic, clinical, and radiologic study of 27 cases. *Diagn Cytopathol* 9:3–12, 1993.

Nutritional Support

• *Walter Jakob Chwals, M.D.*

Malignancy visits three great dangers upon the child whom it attacks. The first is the danger of the tumor itself; the growth of the primary lesion into the healthy tissue of the organ system in which it arises; the progressive infiltration into the adjacent tissues as it expands despite the host's attempts to contain it, and the inexorable march throughout the body as it metastasizes, eventually destroying the organism upon which it feeds. The second danger stems from tumor-induced metastatic changes in the host that exhaust endogenous substrate stores and compromise organ function, gradually eroding the host's ability to defend itself against the neoplasm. The third danger is from the oncologic therapy itself, frequently harsh in nature and directed indiscriminately against malignant and nonmalignant tissue alike.

Often initiated in an already severely compromised host, oncology therapy can make the sick child even sicker. Because malignancy necessitates aggressive treatment, the oncologist must understand the metabolic alterations associated with a malignant tumor, the implications of the underlying host malnutrition that frequently ensues, and the metabolic consequences of acute injury states induced by oncologic treatment. The value of nutritional resuscitation in this setting is to provide exogenous substrate so that the child can recover or maintain adequate metabolic and immunologic function during the peritherapeutic period, thus withstanding the injury associated with the therapy and improving chances of survival.

CANCER CACHEXIA

Cancer cachexia is a complex and multifactorial phenomenon. Its components include weight loss, anorexia, organ dysfunction, and tissue wasting associated with significant alterations in protein, carbohydrate, and lipid metabolism. This condition appears to involve factors related to the tumor itself as well as factors stemming directly from the host response to stimuli induced by the tumor. Furthermore, interventions such as chemotherapy, radiation therapy, and surgery tend to worsen existing cachexia in the absence of exogenous nutritional support.

Anorexia

Anorexia is a principal feature of cancer cachexia. Hypophagia in patients with neoplastic disease exists despite the hypermetabolism (increased substrate demands) imposed by the tumor burden.[1, 2] In animal studies, hypermetabolism induced by cold exposure or exercise is compensated by increased food intake, but this normal adaptive response to increased energy expenditure is absent in tumor-bearing hosts. Several mechanisms have been proposed to account for this abnormality. One is related to the effect of tumor-stimulated neurotransmitters, such as serotonin, which depress the feeding control center located in the hypothalamus.[2] Another involves altered taste perception[3] and learned food aversions[4] associated with unpleasant symptoms from the tumor and various therapeutic interventions. Still other factors are psychological ones such as anxiety or depression.[5] Parental depression, restricted hospital menus, and the sometimes unpleasant environment of the hospital may affect a child's appetite negatively. Food aversions that develop in association with painful and physiologically upsetting complications of chemotherapy, radiation therapy, and surgery may persist in children even long after these sequelae have resolved. An example of this persistence is the anticipatory nausea frequently observed in adolescents and teenagers following chemotherapy.

Gastrointestinal Disorders

Stomatitis, resulting from mucosal injury following the administration of a number of chemotherapeutic modalities, is often associated with substantial pain that prevents adequate oral nutrient intake. Radiation therapy for malignancies of the head and neck can have a similar effect.

Nausea and gastrointestinal dysfunction are common clinical findings following surgery, chemotherapy, immunotherapy, and radiation therapy. Children, especially adolescents and teenagers, may also experience anticipatory nausea, which is a learned physiological phenomenon associated with previous discomfort.

Both chemotherapy and radiotherapy may be associated with injury to the intestinal mucosa causing malabsorption. But malnutrition itself is also known to cause malabsorption.[6] Certain tumors that invest the gut wall, such as Burkitt's lymphoma, can result in malabsorption as well.

Diarrhea commonly results from malabsorption due to any cause. Tumor products, such as the vasoactive peptides associated with neuroblastoma, can also produce diarrhea,[7] as can antibiotics that alter gut flora.

Another cause of hypophagia is mechanical obstruction or pain from tumors compressing or blocking the gastrointestinal tract. Radiotherapy to the gut can result in obstructive adhesions or luminal stricture. Chemotherapeutic agents such as vinblastine and vincristine can induce functional obstruction (ileus), as can narcotic analgesia.

The presence of any of these gastrointestinal disorders can further contribute to cachexia by decreasing or preventing enteral nutritional intake.

Corticosteroids

Corticosteroids can exacerbate cachexia owing to their counter-regulatory effects on protein metabolism (see the section on Metabolic Assessment). They promote endogenous muscle protein catabolism, which can result in decreased muscle strength and activity. Corticosteroids also contribute to muscle wasting by inhibiting the uptake of exogenous amino acids into muscle.

Immunosuppression

A number of studies have documented immunosuppression in association with malignancy.[8–11] Certainly, many chemotherapeutic agents can cause immunosuppression, but in one study of 81 newly diagnosed, untreated pediatric cancer patients, lymphocytes were significantly reduced in 49% of those with solid tumors, and mitogen reactivity of peripheral blood lymphocytes was significantly reduced in all those with malignant tumors (versus benign) disease.[11] The fact that immunologic status may also be influenced by nutritional status is suggested by some studies. These demonstrate that increased total body weight loss in pre-treatment, cancer-bearing adult patients was associated with anergy. This is in contrast to patients who had not experienced substantial changes in body weight and were immunocompetent.[9] The fact that this anergy can be reversed by adequate exogenous nutritional support (discussed next) suggests that malnutrition is a contributing cause.

Tumor-Associated Humoral Alterations

A variety of experimental models has been used to investigate the concept that tumors produce substances that directly affect the host organism. Toxohormone-L, a lipid-mobilizing substance isolated from tumor extracts, suppressed food and water intake by rats when injected into their lateral ventricles.[12] In addition, lipolytic factor produced by an experimental adenocarcinoma caused weight loss in mice despite no reduction in food intake.[13] The presence of another circulating metabolic mediator, thought to be released by tumor cells, has been suggested in a parabiotic experiment in which decreased food intake and weight loss was observed in the non-tumor-bearing partners of rats with sarcomas.[14] Other studies show that the serum of tumor-bearing patients induces anorexia and weight loss when infused into healthy rats.[15] The secretion of tumor-specific factors such as serotonin (carcinoid) and bombesin (small-cell lung carcinoma) are both known to suppress appetite.

Host-Associated Humoral Alterations

Although cachexia is a relatively common event in patients with cancer, the great majority of tumors studied have not as yet been found to produce humoral agents such as those discussed in the previous section. Instead, a wide variety of tumors that are clinically important in humans are thought to stimulate the production of powerful metabolic mediators by the host organism in response to the neoplastic insult. Prominent among these tumor-induced host mediators are the pro-inflammatory cytokines, including tumor

necrosis factor (TNF), interleukin-1 (IL-1), interleukin-6 (IL-6), and interferon-γ (IFN-γ) (see section on Metabolic Assessment).[16] These cytokines are secreted by macrophages and lymphocytes and are thought to represent a host defensive reaction to tumor cell invasion.

The administration of TNF to healthy adult human volunteers induces changes characteristic of cancer cachexia, including increased energy expenditure (hypermetabolism), increased acute-phase protein synthesis, lipolysis, muscle proteolysis, and anorexia.[17, 18] The severity of these alterations is dose-dependent.[19, 20] In animal models, continued exposure to TNF appears to impart resistance to the cachectic effects of this cytokine,[20] although the therapeutic use of TNF in this capacity in tumor-bearing patients has not reproduced these results.[19] Although serum concentrations of TNF have been inconsistently elevated in various studies of cancer patients, increased peripheral blood mononuclear cell production of both TNF and IL-6 have been found to be consistently elevated in conjunction with increased serum acute-phase protein concentrations and increased energy expenditure in pancreatic cancer. These findings suggest that local cytokine elaboration may cause substantial systemic metabolic changes.[21] The phenomenon leading to such metabolic changes may account for the failure to consistently detect systemic cytokine elevations in patients with cancer.

The effects of IL-1 are similar to those of TNF. In animal models, IL-1 administration has resulted in hypermetabolic response and anorexia.[22] The use of monoclonal antibodies directed against IL-1 receptors has been shown to improve food intake and reverse cachexia in anorexic, tumor-bearing animals.[23]

As with TNF and IL-1, increased IL-6 levels have been observed in tumor-bearing animal models.[20, 24] In contrast to TNF and IL-1, serum levels of IL-6 appear to be more consistently elevated in cancer patients.[21] Increased IL-6 serum concentrations have also been observed following TNF administration, reinforcing the concept of multiple cytokine activity to effect metabolic alterations.[19]

The principal features of cancer cachexia (e.g., weight loss associated with anorexia) have been demonstrated in animals receiving IFN-γ.[20, 24] In addition, IFN-γ appears to potentiate TNF activity.[19]

Tumor-Associated Metabolic Alterations

The normal response of the body to anorexia (starvation) is to conserve energy (decrease energy expenditure) and protein reserves (decrease proteolysis and gluconeogenesis) at the expense of endogenous carbohydrate and fat stores (increase glycogenolysis and lipolysis). But the tumor-induced host elaboration of cytokines results in a cascade of metabolic events that are characteristic of the acute metabolic stress response (see section on Metabolic Assessment). In addition to glycogenolysis and lipolysis, this response includes a marked increase in energy expenditure (hypermetabolism), proteolysis, and gluconeogenesis (protein hypercatabolism). In contrast to simple starvation, this response is paradoxical in that the depletion of endogenous energy and substrate stores is accelerated with decreased exogenous fuel substrate provision. In effect, cancer cachexia appears to result from a maladaption of the host to starvation.

Energy expenditure has generally been found to be elevated in cancer patients, but results are variable and inconsistent.[25–30] Although some of these differences have been attributed to the type of tumor, this criterion has failed to predict the degree of hypermetabolism. Instead studies suggest that the host metabolic response to the tumor insult is likely multifactorial and is related not only to the tumor type but also to the associated degree of malnutrition, the immunologic status of the patient, the tumor stage, the presence and effect of antitumor therapy, and the preexistence of associated underlying disease processes (e.g., diabetes and cirrhosis). Thus, patient heterogeneity may contribute to substantial interpatient variability in the metabolic response to tumor burden. Yet, in a report of a relatively homogeneous group of patients with metastatic pancreatic cancer, a 30% increase in energy expenditure was observed in patients who demonstrated an acute-phase protein response.[21] These data are important because they show that patients who are able to mount an acute metabolic stress response in association with the tumor burden also generate significant and associated hypermetabolism.

Protein metabolism is altered in cancer patients. The major factors contributing to these alterations are (1) the metabolic demands imposed by the tumor itself and (2) the host cytokine response elicited by the tumor. Characteristic changes include increased whole-body protein turnover, increased muscle catabolism, and increased hepatic and tumor protein synthesis despite associated anorexia and weight loss. Whole-body protein turnover has been shown to increase by 35% in malnourished patients with cancer, in contrast to malnourished control patients with benign disease or suffering the effects of simple starvation.[31]

Skeletal muscle protein wasting, resulting from increased muscle protein catabolism in association with decreased muscle protein synthesis, has been demonstrated in patients with malignancy versus age-matched, non-tumor-bearing controls.[32] Hepatic protein synthesis has been shown to increase by 60% in cancer patients with cachexia as compared with cancer patients who have not lost weight.[33] In this study, all patients were observed to have high tumor protein synthetic rates, independent of weight loss, and these rates increased in patients with tumor metastases relative to the primary lesion. Taken together, these studies suggest the possibility of futile cycling of protein during malignancy with increased hepatic and tumor-related protein synthesis at the expense of the muscle protein stores. The whole-body protein turnover rate increases acutely as a result of substantially greater protein catabolism versus protein synthesis in cachectic patients.[33] Furthermore, the hepatic conversion of amino acids (derived from muscle protein catabolism) to form glucose (gluconeogenesis) may be substantially increased to provide this tumor-preferred fuel substrate to malignant tissue.[34, 34a] These data support the concept that the tumor burden acts as a nitrogen trap and thus contributes significantly to cachexia.

The alterations in carbohydrate metabolism associated with malignancy are characterized by decreased glucose tolerance, increased glucose uptake, and increased lactate production. Insulin resistance (see section on Hormonal Alteration) has been suggested as the cause of glucose intolerance in a number of studies.[35–37] In one large study, glucose intolerance was observed in 37% of patients with cancer.[36] In another study, using a euglycemic clamp technique, significant glucose intolerance in cancer patients was reversed by graded increases in exogenous insulin infusion.[35] In some cases, insulin resistance has been reported to resolve following complete tumor resection.[37] In patients with cancer, hepatic glucose production is increased substantially, likely because of cytokine-induced gluconeogenesis.

Serum concentrations of gluconeogenic precursors such as alanine, lactate, and gycerol are elevated as a result of the catabolism of endogenous protein, carbohydrate, and fat stores. This accelerated hepatic metabolism of glucose may be due to increased tumor-related utilization of this substrate as a preferential fuel source. Increased tumor-dependent glucose uptake and utilization have been observed in both human and animal tumor models.[34, 38, 39] Increased tumor carbohydrate utilization is also associated with increased lactate production resulting from the anaerobic metabolism of glucose.[38] Lactate is metabolized through the Cori cycle to regenerate glucose, and this process has been associated with a 10% increase in energy expenditure in cancer patients.[40]

Alterations in lipid metabolism include increased lipolysis and fatty acid oxidation. Increased rates of glycerol and fatty acid turnover, which cannot be reversed by exogenous glucose, have been demonstrated in weight-losing versus weight-stable cancer patients.[41] Furthermore, increased fatty acid oxidation has been observed in patients with metastatic disease compared with normal controls.[42] Cancer patients who lose weight also have higher fatty acid oxidation rates than those who do not.[43]

In summary, cancer cachexia appears to result primarily from the increased metabolic demands imposed by the tumor burden itself, coupled with the acute stress response that malignancy elicits in the host. Generally, as the tumor burden increases, especially with metastases, the catabolism of endogenous substrate reserves becomes more profound, resulting in increasing weight loss and compromise of organ function. Malnutrition further reduces endogenous reserves, thus decreasing the host's ability to compensate for increased metabolic demands, putting the patient at higher risk of cachexia.

SIGNIFICANCE OF MALNUTRITION

The presence of malnutrition in pediatric patients with malignancy ranges widely from 6% to 50% depending on the type, stage, and location of the tumor.[44–47] Malnutrition is usually more severe in patients with more aggressive tumors in the later stages of malignancy. Therefore, as in the adult cancer population, malnutrition can be a helpful prognostic indicator of the degree of malignant disease in children.[44, 46] The more intensive treatment regimens necessitated by advanced malignancy and by relapse following initial therapy frequently exacerbate malnutrition for reasons previously discussed. In a retrospective study of 455 children with a variety of malignancies,[44] patients whose weight-to-height ratios prior to initiation of treatment were less than or equal to 80% of age-adjusted standards had significantly decreased survival following treatment (Fig. 24–1). This was especially evident in children with localized disease, in whom there was a 30% difference in survival, favoring the well-nourished group at 36 months following therapy (Fig. 24–2). Compromised nutritional status before initiation of therapy was also significantly associated with relapse following therapy in the solid-tumor subgroup of patients. These findings have also been observed in a second, smaller study of children with late-stage neuroblastoma.[48] Some evidence exists that malnutrition is associated with a higher risk of infectious complications. Higher infection rates have been documented in malnourished children in contrast to well-nourished children with metastatic bone disease.[49] The risk of opportunistic infection also appears to be increased in malnourished children with cancer.[50]

NUTRITIONAL ASSESSMENT

An accurate and detailed patient history is the crucial first step in the nutritional assessment of the pediatric cancer patient. In addition to data relative to the tumor itself, a complete dietary history should be obtained, including the nature and duration of any symptoms or signs related to compromised dietary intake. Primary among these is any history of recent weight loss or retardation of growth (in infancy through adolescence). The presence and duration of nausea, vomiting, food aversion, anorexia, early satiety, fatigue, weakness, diarrhea, abdominal pain, fever, and frequency of infections are all important potential indicators of malnutrition with potential for outcome significance.[44]

Anthropometric measurements should always include accurate weight and height data, which

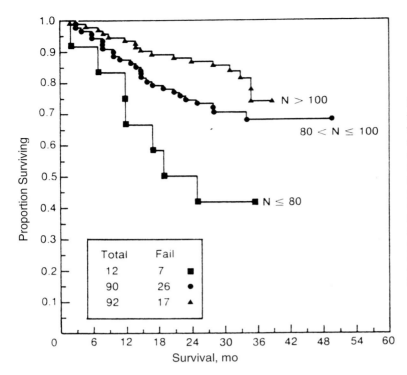

Figure 24–1 • Survival by nutritional status for eligible children with malignant disease who were not previously treated. N = ratio of weight and height at time of first referral compared with age-adjusted standard (expressed as percent of standard). (From Donaldson SS, Wesley MN, DeWys W, Suskind RM, Jaffe N, van Eys J: A study of the nutritional status of pediatric cancer patients. *Am J Dis Child* 135:1107–1112, 1981, with permission. Copyright 1981, American Medical Association.)

Figure 24–2 • Survival by nutritional status and stage of disease for eligible children with lymphoma who were not previously treated. N = ratio of weight and height at time of first referral compared with age-adjusted standard (expressed as percent of standard). (From Donaldson SS, Wesley MN, DeWys W, Suskind RM, Jaffe N, van Eys J: A study of the nutritional status of pediatric cancer patients. *Am J Dis Child* 135:1107–1112, 1981, with permission. Copyright 1981, American Medical Association.)

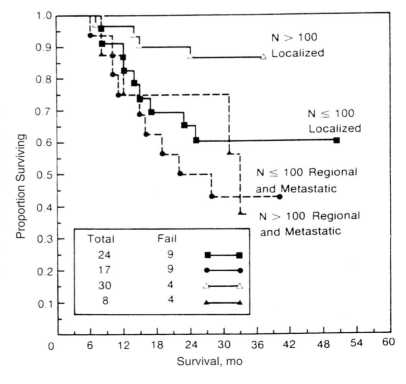

should be recorded on a growth chart appropriate for age. In infants, a head circumference measurement should also be obtained. Comparison with previous growth chart recordings should be carried out to establish growth velocity. Of these various measurements, weight for height, or weight/height percentile, is the best indicator of nutritional status (better than weight for age).[51] Weight/height percentile can be calculated from published National Center for Health Statistics data.[52]

Arm circumference and triceps skinfold measurements can be used to calculate muscle and fat compartments but are very operator-dependent and can provide misleading data if carried out incorrectly. It is important to measure with nonstretchable tape and to employ the same anatomical landmarks in measuring.[53] For instance, mid–upper *arm circumference* (AC) should be measured exactly halfway between the acromion and the olecranon. *Triceps skinfold thickness* (TSF) should be measured at this same point with skinfold calipers.[54] *Arm muscle circumference* (AMC), which is representative of the muscle compartment, can then be calculated as follows:

$$AMC = AC - TSF$$

TSF assesses the thickness of the subcutaneous adipose layer. In contrast to adults, fat stores in children are almost exclusively confined to the subcutaneous fat compartment. This compartment constitutes the major body energy reserve and diminishes as a function of malnutrition severity.

In children with cancer, a significant correlation exists between weight/height percentile and both TSF and AMC.[55] Caveats, in addition to operator-associated variability, including compartment-fluid shifts induced during acute metabolic stress states (caused for instance by inflammation, infection, surgery, intensive chemotherapy, and so on) and malignancy-related fluid accumulations (ascites). All can lead to gross inaccuracies in the interpretation of anthropometric data.

Biochemical assessment includes evaluation of visceral proteins. Although serious hypoalbuminemia (≤3.0 g/dl) is not observed in the majority of nonstressed malnourished pediatric cancer patients, it is sometimes present and has been associated with compromise of muscle function.[44] Shorter half-life visceral proteins such as prealbumin and transferrin also accurately reflect protein compartment losses resulting from malnutrition-related catabolism (see section on Visceral Protein Status).

Two nonspecific markers of protein nutrition that may reflect immunologic competence can be assessed clinically by calculating total lymphocyte counts and delayed cutaneous hypersensitivity. Data suggesting that *total lymphocyte count* (TLC) is a marker of malnutrition stem from studies that have documented malnutrition-related pediatric thymic atrophy[56] and reduced TLC (<2500/mm³) in about 20% of malnourished children (versus no reduction below this number in well-nourished children).[57] Low TLC (<1500/mm³ versus >2000 mms³ for nutritionally repleted patients) has also been documented in hospitalized adult patients[58] but does not correlate well with outcome parameters such as mortality and morbidity.[59] Reasons for lack of correlation may be related to the wide range of normal TLC (1000–4000/mm³) and the fact that TLC does not reflect helper-to-suppressor T-cell ratios.

Calculations of TLC may be performed by multiplying the total white blood cell count by the percent lymphocytes. This value remains questionable, though, as a marker of protein malnutrition and immunocompromise in the metabolically nonstressed child *prior* to oncologic therapy, particularly chemotherapy. During acute metabolic stress and oncologic therapy, TLC is valueless as a measure of malnutrition, but increasing counts following therapy may be related to accelerated bone marrow recovery made possible by nutritional support.[60]

Delayed cutaneous hypersensitivity (DCH) is a measure of impaired antibody reactivity to a series of skin-test antigens.[61] The synthesis of antibodies may be impaired as a result of malnutrition (and resulting decreased protein synthesis).[62] In addition to T-cell dysfunction, DCH is one possible contributing factor to the anergy-related immunocompromise observed during cancer cachexia.

Anergy established on the basis of DCH has been associated with a reduced lymphocyte proliferative response in malnourished children.[57] In a large population of adult surgical patients (with and without cancer), anergy has been associated with a significantly increased incidence of sepsis and mortality as compared with immunocompetent patients.[63] These immunologic assessment modalities assume previous exposure of the child to the antigens tested and are valueless during periods of acute metabolic stress and following chemotherapy.

METABOLIC ASSESSMENT

Acute Metabolic Stress: Overview

In response to a variety of local or systemic injury stimuli (such as tissue injury, sepsis, acute inflammatory conditions), a series of metabolic changes that characterize the acute stress state occur (Fig. 24–3). Among the early features of injury response are the release of cytokines followed rapidly by important alterations in the hormonal environment: increased counter-regulatory hormone levels associated with insulin and growth hormone resistance. As a result, a sequence of metabolic events is initiated that includes the catabolism of endogenous stores of protein, carbohydrate, and fat to provide essential substrate intermediates (primarily amino acids) and energy necessary to fuel the ongoing response process. Amino acids from catabolized proteins flow to the liver, where they provide substrate for the synthesis of acute-phase proteins and glucose (gluconeogenesis). The acute metabolic stress response represents a hypermetabolic, hypercatabolic state[64] that results in the loss of endogenous tissue[65] and can lead to poor clinical outcome in the absence of appropriate exogenous support.[66] As the acute response resolves, adaptive anabolic metabolism ensues to restore catabolic losses.[67] In children this phase is characterized by the resumption of somatic growth. The goal of metabolic and nutritional resuscitation in the critically ill child is to provide the proper balance of exogenous substrates, thereby minimizing the loss of lean body mass so as to preserve vital organ function as well as to maintain or restore immunocompetence and to promote the earlier and more complete evolution to growth recovery.

Cytokines

Cytokines are secreted by a number of cells—including macrophages, monocytes, lymphocytes,

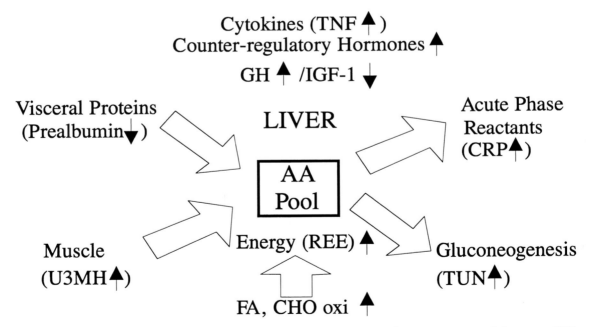

Figure 24–3 • Metabolic response to acute injury. TNF = tumor necrosis factor; GH = growth hormone; IGF-1 = insulin-like growth factor 1; AA = amino acid; CRP = C-reactive protein; TUN = total urinary nitrogen; FA, CHO oxi = fatty acid and carbohydrate oxidation; U3MH = urinary 3-methylhistidine; REE = resting energy expenditure. (From Chwals, WJ: Infant and pediatric nutrition. In Zaloga, GP (ed): *Nutrition and Critical Care*, 1st ed. Chicago: Mosby-Year Book, Inc., 1994, p. 737, with permission.)

and vascular smooth muscle—in response to a variety of metabolic stress stimuli. They have important regulatory functions in mediating the metabolic and immune responses to injury. Although these peptides are secreted in small amounts and have relatively short serum half-lives, they appear to individually or synergistically mediate a cascade of events with widespread metabolic and immunologic effects.[68, 69] Cytokines have been shown to play an important role in the host response mechanism to a variety of inflammatory, neoplastic, and acute injury states.[68, 69] Cytokines bond to specific membrane receptors on the cell wall of target organs and thus induce intracellular metabolic events that alter gene expression and proliferation, which are important for immunocompetence and wound healing. One of the most significant consequences of cytokine release, in terms of the acute metabolic stress response, is related to the potent cytokine stimulus of counter-regulatory hormone release.

In addition to these endocrine effects, cytokines act in a paracrine fashion to facilitate direct cell-to-cell communications. Although the actions of many cytokines result from the elaboration and secretion of the metabolic regulators (such as counter-regulatory hormones) that they induce, these peptides also have direct effects on nutrient substrate metabolism. The features of cytokine activity that are related to cancer cachexia have been discussed previously (see section on Host-Associated Humoral Alterations). Further general injury–response characteristics are discussed next to provide a more comprehensive understanding of the acute metabolic stress response that usually accompanies periods of intense oncologic therapy.

Among many other effects, TNF induces neutrophil release from bone marrow (leukocytosis), activates neutrophils and monocytes to promote microbial killing, stimulates T and B lymphocytes, regulates neutrophil degranulation and superoxide production, causes increased endothelial permeability, and causes release of IL-1, IL-6, and *prostaglandin E_2* (PGE$_2$) in vitro and in vivo.[70, 71] These actions underscore TNF function in maintaining immunocompetence and in limiting the spread of infection. TNF appears to promote muscle catabolism[72] and decrease muscle amino acid uptake while increasing hepatic uptake of amino acids. TNF stimulates glucose transport by the de novo synthesis of glucose transporters that are inserted into the plasma membrane.[73] Hepatic gluconeogenesis from alanine is stimulated by IL-1.[74] Protein metabolism is also directly altered by TNF, which has been demonstrated to stimulate specific hepatic amino acid transport systems.[75] Elevations of TNF are associated as well with increases in the serum concentrations of acute-phase proteins[76] and adrenocorticotropic hormone (ACTH) levels. Systemic manifestations associated with TNF such as fever and tachycardia are blocked by ibuprofen,[77] suggesting that these responses involve cyclooxygenase-mediated intermediates of arachidonic acid such as PGE$_2$.

The systemic and metabolic effects of IL-1 are generally similar to those of TNF.[68] They include fever, neutrophilia, anorexia, lethargy, increased synthesis of hepatic acute-phase proteins, decreased synthesis of hepatic visceral proteins, increased ACTH secretion, increased IL-6 concentrations, hypozincemia, and hypoferremia. At higher levels, IL-1 induces hypotension and leukopenia. In addition, IL-1 stimulates fibroblast proliferation and collagen production,[68] both of which influence wound healing. Studies also show an early decrease in serum *insulin-like growth factor 1* (IGF-1) levels following administration of IL-1,[78] an effect that may contribute substantially to pediatric growth retardation during acute metabolic stress. Like TNF, IL-1 can activate both T and B lymphocytes.[68] In addition, IL-1 may be instrumental in stimulating T-helper cells to produce interleukin-2 (IL-2).[79]

IL-6 plays a dominant role in inflammation. Its principal effect appears to be the stimulation of hepatic synthesis of acute-phase proteins.[80] Following acute injury, serum IL-6 concentrations increase prior to, and correlate well with, subsequent elevations in serum CRP concentrations in patients with normal liver function.[81] High IL-6 levels are also associated with elevated IgM and IgG serum concentrations and thrombocytosis,[80] indicating strong bone marrow stimulation. IL-6 can act in concert with IL-2 or IFN-γ to stimulate myeloid cell growth and T-cell differentiation.[82]

IL-2 and IFN-γ have important immunomodulatory functions and are elevated in response to antigen-antibody interactions. The most dominant effect of IL-2 is its tumoricidal activity, but it also induces elevation of counter-regulatory hormones and is associated with systemic symptoms such as malaise, fever, and tachycardia.[83] IL-2 may also stimulate the release of IFN-γ.[84]

Hormonal Alterations and the Catabolic Response

Insulin is a potent anabolic hormone responsible for (1) glycogen synthesis and the storage of carbohydrate, (2) lipogenesis and the storage of fat, and (3) new protein synthesis. Insulin and IGF-1 are essential hormones for somatic growth in infants and children. Acute metabolic stress is characterized by substantial increases in serum concentrations of catecholamines, glucagon, and cortisol, referred to as counter-regulatory hormones because they counteract, or oppose, the anabolic effects of insulin, thus leading to insulin resistance. Serum concentrations of these metabolic stress-related hormones increase as a result of cytokine release.[77]

Glucagon induces glycolysis and gluconeogenesis. These effects counteract the synthetic effects of insulin. Increased glycolysis, which results in increased serum lactate and alanine levels, thus providing the substrate necessary for the endogenous regeneration of glucose (Cori cycle and alanine cycle), is a major contributor to altered carbohydrate metabolism during acute metabolic stress.[85]

Cortisol induces muscle proteolysis and promotes gluconeogenesis. Glucocorticoids cause the muscle proteolysis associated with cytokine release[86] and have been shown to be predictors of protein breakdown and hypermetabolism in acutely stressed adults.[87] The major amino acid sources for gluconeogenesis are alanine[88] and glutamine[89] from skeletal muscle and gut. Hepatic uptake of these amino acids is accelerated during acute metabolic stress. Like glucagon, cortisol also causes insulin resistance. Although insulin levels may be elevated during acute metabolic stress, its anabolic effects are inhibited.

Catecholamines cause hyperglycemia by promoting hepatic glycogenolysis, by causing conversion of skeletal muscle glycogen to lactate, which is then transported to the liver for conversion to glucose (Cori cycle), and by suppression of the pancreatic secretion of insulin. Catecholamines also induce lipolysis, which results in the mobilization of *free fatty acids* (FFAs). Moreover, catecholamines, in addition to glucagon and cortisol,

induce hypermetabolism, which results in an increase in the basal metabolic rate.

In health, the major actions of *growth hormone* (GH) are to decrease protein catabolism and promote protein synthesis, to promote fat mobilization and the conversion of FFAs to acetyl coenzyme A, and to decrease glucose oxidation while increasing glycogen deposition. The anabolic effects of GH, particularly as they are related to protein metabolism, are mediated principally by IFG-1.[90] During acute metabolic stress, IGF-1 levels fall and IGF-1 inhibitory binding protein concentrations rise (anabolic GH resistance). In this state, the substrate-mobilizing effects of GH prevail, resulting in increased lipolysis and FFA oxidation.[91]

Visceral Protein Status

The liver normally synthesizes a number of proteins that constitute labile pools within the serum compartment. Among others, these proteins include albumin, transferrin, prealbumin, and retinol-binding protein. These proteins, sometimes referred to as "reserve proteins," constitute labile protein stores. They account for early nitrogen losses resulting from catabolism induced by injury (or starvation). As compared with albumin (t½ = 20 days), both prealbumin (t½ = 2 days) and retinol-binding protein (t½ = 10 hours) have shorter serum half-lives and constitute smaller protein pools. Visceral proteins with shorter half-lives correlate better than albumin with other variables of malnutrition.[92]

Although serum albumin and prealbumin concentrations both decrease precipitously in response to surgical trauma, prealbumin concentrations appear to be more significantly depressed.[93] Prealbumin is of greater clinical utility than albumin as a marker of nutritional repletion following acute injury.[92] Studies in children and teenagers undergoing bone marrow transplantations as treatment for a variety of malignancies have also demonstrated that prealbumin is a better marker of nutritional repletion than albumin or transferrin (Fig. 24–4).[94, 95]

Total Urinary Nitrogen

Protein and fat catabolism during acute metabolic stress results in increased urinary nitrogen

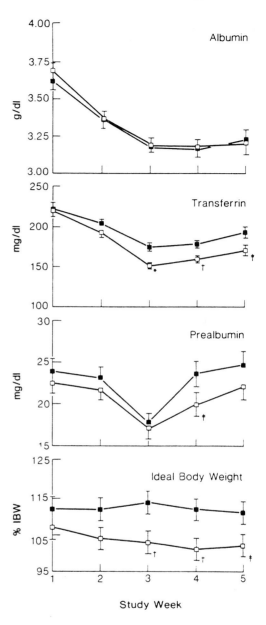

Figure 24–4 • Parameters indicating nutritional status in total parenteral nutrition prophylaxis patients (-■-) compared with those in control patients (-□-). Mean albumin levels were similar in both groups, with significant decreases seen in the week before transplantation (study week 1) and the first week following transplantation. Mean transferrin levels dropped below normal in both groups, with the control group mean being significantly lower than the TPN group mean during the second through the fourth week after transplant. Mean prealbumin decreased in both groups also, with slower recovery in the control group, giving a significantly lower mean prealbumin during the third week after transplant. Mean ideal body weight was not significantly different at baseline (study week 1) but was higher in the TPN prophylaxis group. The TPN prophylaxis patients maintained their body weight during the study period, and the control patients showed a significant decrement by the second week (study week 3) post-transplant. (From Weisdorf SA, Lysne J, Wind D, et al: Positive effect of prophylactic total parenteral nutrition on long-term outcome of bone marrow transplantation. *Transplantation* 43:833–838, 1987, with permission.)

losses. Protein catabolism increases the size of the pool of hepatic free amino acids. The liver deaminates a substantial portion of these amino acids to synthesize glucose (gluconeogenesis), resulting in increased nitrogen that is excreted in the urine as urea.[96] Fat catabolism (lipolysis) yields increased FFAs, which, when oxidized, result in ketone body formation. These ketoacids are buffered by ammonia and excreted in the urine.[97]

Because urea nitrogen losses correlate poorly with ammonia nitrogen losses in the urine during injury states, it is preferable to measure 24-hour *total urinary nitrogen* (TUN).[98] Serial urinary nitrogen measurements reflect the degree and duration of catabolism resulting from various categories of injury and correlate grossly with hypermetabolism (increased stress-related energy expenditure).[64] Therefore, this technique can be employed to monitor the acute metabolic stress response and may be valuable in determining injury severity.[99] Small (0.2–0.5 g N_2) but signifi-

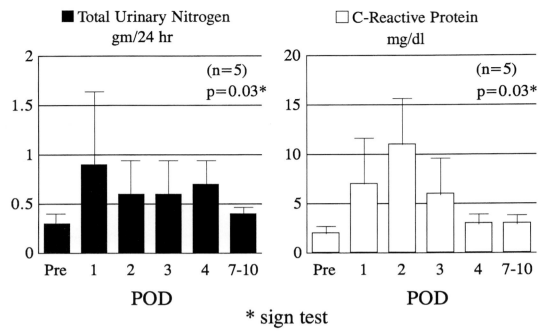

Figure 24–5 • Infant metabolic response to surgical stress. Pre = values obtained within 24 hours before surgery; POD = postoperative day. (From Chwals, WJ: Infant and pediatric nutrition. In Zaloga, GP (ed): *Nutrition and Critical Care*, 1st ed. Chicago: Mosby-Year Book, Inc., 1994, p. 737, with permission.)

cant increments in TUN during the first 2–4 days following major surgery in infants return to normal levels by postoperative days 7 through 10 (Fig. 24–5). Similar changes have been noted by other investigators[100] and may reflect nutritional repletion as the acute stress response resolves.[101]

Acute-Phase Response

One of the key features of the acute metabolic stress response is an increase in the hepatic synthesis of certain specialized proteins. These acute-phase proteins, so called because they were found in serum obtained from patients acutely ill with infectious disease, are now known to appear in response to a variety of stimuli such as tissue injury, inflammation, bacterial infection, antigen-antibody interaction, and endotoxin challenge.[102] The acute-phase response is mediated by cytokines, principally IL-6,[81] that selectively redirect hepatic protein synthesis such that the synthesis of acute-phase proteins is increased while the synthesis of visceral proteins is retarded. The reprioritization of hepatic protein synthesis in response to injury has been elegantly demonstrated in a guinea-pig burn model[103] that indicates the process is cytokine-induced.[81]

These proteins appear to carry out a number of important immunologic and repair functions during the acute stress period.[102] *C-reactive protein* (CRP) is an acute-phase protein that, among its several known biologic functions, is capable of activating the complement pathway in the absence of immunoglobulin. In the presence of activated complement, it can also induce monocyte phagocytosis of bacteria and enhance *natural killer* (NK) cell activity.

After injury, there is a latent period of 6 to 16 hours followed by increased serum levels that generally peak at 24 to 48 hours. Because serum half-life is 4 to 6 hours, decreases in the hepatic synthesis of CRP (as the acute metabolic stress response resolves) are promptly reflected in decreased serum levels of this acute-phase protein. In children, marked increases in serum CRP concentrations have been observed following a variety of metabolic stress stimuli,[104, 105] even in immunosuppressed hosts.[106] The perioperative acute-phase response in healthy infants is characterized by significant increases in serum CRP concentrations on postoperative day 1 (relative to preoperative values), which return toward normal values by postoperative day 4. These changes in serum acute-phase protein levels appear to coincide with urinary nitrogen excretion, demonstrating two important aspects of altered protein metabolism during acute metabolic stress (see Fig. 24–5). A serum CRP concentration of less than 2.0 mg/dl is usually associated with resolution of the acute metabolic stress response and resumption of the growth potential in children.[107]

Indirect Calorimetry

Energy expenditure is a characteristic feature of metabolism that can be measured according to the amount of heat released. This measurement is based upon the principle of *direct calorimetry*,[96] in which energy release is quantified by the amount of heat required to raise the temperature of 1 ml of water by 1°C from 15 to 16°C (1 calorie). The methodology of direct calorimetry involves confining the subject in a closed calorimeter for extended time periods, making it impractical for clinical use. In contrast, *indirect calorimetry* can be carried out at the patient's bedside. Indirect calorimetry involves the measurement of the differences in O_2 and CO_2 concentrations between a known volume (minute ventilation) of inspired and expired gas. In this way, oxygen consumption ($\dot{V}O_2$) and carbon dioxide production ($\dot{V}CO_2$) can be calculated. These calculations[108] are carried out based upon known and constant relationships between $\dot{V}O_2$, $\dot{V}CO_2$, and heat produced (energy expenditure) for many metabolic processes. The metabolic processes include, among others, (1) oxidation of various carbohydrates, fats, and proteins and (2) lipogenesis. *Respiratory quotient* (RQ), which may be expressed as $\dot{V}CO_2/\dot{V}O_2$, is also specific and constant for each of these processes; for instance, the total oxidation of carbohydrate (RQ = 1.0) or fat (RQ = 0.7). For lipogenesis (the synthesis of fat from carbohydrate), RQ equals 2.75.[109]

The value of indirect calorimetry in the intensive care setting lies in the fact that estimations of energy expenditure based on other clinical criteria are notoriously inaccurate.[110] Actual *measured energy expenditure* (MEE) is frequently much less than predicted values based upon clinical grounds.[111, 112] Whereas average MEE values in large patient series tend to differentiate various degrees of injury,[64] individual patients may respond to similar injury states with widely diverse MEE values.[113] A study of 20 critically ill children demonstrated a 3.5-fold difference in MEE (adjusted for age and weight) between lowest and highest interpatient values.[114]

MEE has been shown to correlate well with weight gain following nutritional repletion of malnourished children.[115] In the critical care setting, indirect calorimetry may be helpful in accurately determining caloric needs during acute metabolic stress to avoid overfeeding (discussed shortly) and promote optimal growth recovery.

Accurate MEE can be obtained in mechanically ventilated children with noncuffed endotracheal tubes if no audible air leak is present.[116] Adequate MEE usually requires 20 to 30 minutes and correlates well with 24-hour MEE values in acutely stressed adult and pediatric population.[117, 118]

OVERFEEDING

Overfeeding occurs when the administration of calories or specific substrate exceeds the requirements to maintain metabolic homeostasis. These requirements are substantially altered during periods of injury-induced acute metabolic stress such as those caused by intensive oncologic therapy. Excess nutritional delivery during this period can further increase the metabolic demands of an acute injury and place an added burden on the lungs and liver. The result is to not only increase pulmonary and hepatic pathophysiology but also to increase the risk of mortality.[119] It is important, therefore, to ensure that caloric intake not exceed demand.

Precise caloric delivery is best determined during acute injury states by measuring energy expenditure. Owing to substantial interpatient variability, estimates of energy needs on the basis of disease categories, subject age, or body composition can be misleading and usually result in overfeeding. Overfeeding cannot reverse tissue catabolism until the acute metabolic stress response has resolved. In acutely stressed children, MEE constitutes the total energy requirement, and caloric delivery in excess of this amount should be avoided until metabolic stress parameters indicate resolution of the acute injury state.[119]

GENERAL NUTRITIONAL GUIDELINE FOR NONSTRESSED CHILDREN

Nutritional needs can be divided into the general categories of energy, protein, and nonprotein substrate delivery. Amounts differ in children

Table 24–1 • Age-Adjusted Energy Requirements

	Energy Delivery°	
Age (yr)	kcal/kg/day	kcal/day
0–1	120–90	500–1000
1–7	90–75	1000–1500
7–12	75–60	1500–2000
12–18	60–30	2000
>18	30–25	2000+

°The left-sided values in each column indicate requirements at the lowest age of the interval (e.g., 120 kcal/kg/day or 500 kcal/day at the age of 0 years).

Adapted from Wretlind A: Complete intravenous nutrition. Theoretical and experimental background. *Nutr Metab* 14(suppl.):1–57, 1972.

as compared with adults, primarily because of increased requirements for growth and activity in children. During early infancy, visceral organ growth is rapid and extensive relative to muscle and fat growth.

Energy can be partitioned into maintenance metabolic needs (basal metabolic rate, activity, and heat loss to the environment) and growth. Energy requirements are age-related and are three to four times higher for infants than for adults (Table 24–1). During acute metabolic stress states in patients, if indirect calorimetry is unavailable, care should be taken to prevent calorie intake from exceeding basal metabolic rate. The basal metabolic rate is approximately 50 to 55 kcal/kg/day in infancy and gradually declines to about 20 to 25 kcal/kg/day during adolescence.[120]

Protein requirements correlate with basal metabolic rate (as assessed by resting energy expenditure) and decrease with age.[121] Protein caloric delivery is therefore relatively constant and should constitute approximately 7% to 10% of the total caloric intake. In hospitalized patients, protein repletion should provide 2.0 to 2.5 g/kg/day to infants up to 2 years of age, 1.5 to 2.0 g/kg/day to children 2 to 10 years of age, and 1.0 to 1.5 g/kg/day to children older than 10 years of age. Approximately 35% of the daily caloric requirement should be provided as fat.

Recommended dietary allowances (RDAs) for vitamins, minerals, and trace elements have been suggested for healthy infants and children.[122] Children with malignancy should be screened for zinc and iron deficiency, both of which may result from malnutrition. Furthermore, existing zinc

and iron deficiencies may be exacerbated during acute metabolic stress due to IL-1 activity (see section on Metabolic Assessment). The importance of these noncaloric nutrients is that they support immunocompetence (cell-mediated immunity).[123, 124] Tumor-associated immunocompromise can be impaired by uncorrected deficiencies in these nutrient pools.

INDICATIONS FOR SUPPLEMENTAL NUTRITION

Criteria for identifying children with malignancy who are malnourished differ somewhat in various published reports.[125–127] Generally, the following surveillance criteria can be used to identify children with malignancy who are malnourished or likely to require supplemental nutritional support:

1. Interval or total weight loss of greater than 5% relative to pre-illness body weight.
2. Weight-to-height ratio less than or equal to 90% or weight/height percentile less than or equal to the 10th percentile.
3. Serum albumin less than or equal to 3.2 g/dl (in the absence of recent acute metabolic stress within the past 14 days).
4. Adipose energy reserves as determined by TSF less than or equal to the 5th percentile for age and gender.
5. A decrease in the current percentile for weight (or height) of at least two percentile channels (for instance, pre-illness weight of the 75th to 90th percentile might decrease to the 25th to 50th percentile for age and gender).
6. Voluntary food intake less than 70% of estimated requirements for 5 days for well-nourished patients.
7. Anticipated gut dysfunction for more than 5 days for well-nourished patients.
8. High-nutritional-risk patients based upon tumor type and oncology treatment regimens required (Table 24–2).
9. Bone marrow transplantation as a treatment for any tumor type.
10. DCH-established anergy in any child older than 2 years[128] prior to treatment.

EFFICACY OF NUTRITIONAL SUPPLEMENTATION

The value of nutritional support in published reports involving both adults and children is of-

Table 24–2 · Types of Neoplastic Diseases with High and Low Risk as Well as Examples of Oncologic Treatments That Contribute to PEM

Tumor Type	Examples of Portions of Oncologic Regimens That Contribute to PEM†
High Nutritional Risk	
Advanced diseases during initial intense treatment:	
Stages 3 and 4 Wilms' tumor and unfavorable-histology Wilms' tumor	National Wilms' Tumor Study 3: Operative removal of tumor at diagnosis, actinomycin D ± Adriamycin (doxorubicin), maximal age-adjusted abdominal irradiation.
Stages 3 and 4 neuroblastoma	(1) Cyclophosphamide and DTIC every 3 weeks: abdominal irradiation within first 10 weeks—Stage 3 only.
	(2) Melphalan weeks 1 and 4, cyclophosphamide and DTIC week 7; resection and abdominal irradiation may occur during 1st and 19th weeks.
Pelvic rhabdomyosarcoma or Ewing's sarcoma	Actinomycin D, Adriamycin (doxorubicin), cyclophosphamide every 3 to 4 weeks, pelvic irradiation.
Some non-Hodgkin's lymphoma°	Irradiation to the esophagus, pharynx, or large abdominal fields.
Acute nonlymphocytic leukemia	Daunamycin, high-dose or continuous intravenous cytosine arabinoside every 14 days.
Some poor-prognosis acute lymphocytic leukemias	(1) Daunamycin, cytosine arabinoside, cyclophosphamide, L-asparaginase, irradiation to bulk disease.
	(2) Daunamycin, L-asparaginase.
Multiple-relapse leukemia	Daunamycin, cytosine arabinoside, VM26, L-asparaginase.
Medulloblastoma	Operative resection, cranial and spinal irradiation.
Low Nutritional Risk	
Good-prognosis acute lymphocytic leukemia	
Nonmetastatic solid tumors	
Advanced diseases in remission during maintenance treatment	

°Tumor extent significantly impairs gastrointestinal function.

† Bone marrow transplantation for any reason constitutes high nutritional risk.

Adapted from Rickard KA, Grosfeld JL, Coates TD, Weetman R, Baehner RL: Advances in nutrition care of children with neoplastic diseases: A review of treatment, research, and application. *J Am Diet Assoc* 86:1666–1676, 1986, with permission.

ten difficult to clearly establish owing to heterogeneous outcome-related factors. These include the type and stage of the tumor, variations in antitumor therapy, presence or absence of complications such as infection, immunologic status of the patient, inconsistencies in the type and adequacy of nutritional support in various subgroups, and interpatient response variability compounded by generally small patient numbers in the subgroups analyzed in various trials. Given these drawbacks, certain reasonable conclusions can still be drawn from the existing data.

It is useful to group children with malignancy into two categories (well-nourished and malnour-ished) based on the surveillance parameters (discussed previously) obtained prior to initial therapy. Furthermore, patients may be considered at high or low risk of malnutrition developing or being exacerbated on the basis of tumor type and stage as well as planned therapeutic regimen (see Table 24–2).

Although few studies evaluate aggressive enteral feeding (using a nasogastric or nasoduodenal feeding tube) in tumor-bearing children, it is evident that in some well-nourished children in the low-risk category, adequate nutriture can be maintained with tube-delivered enteral nutrition.[129] Platelet counts should be above 75,000/

μl to decrease the risk of gastrointestinal bleeding. If oral nutrition is provided, strict attention is necessary to ensure that daily protein and caloric intake reach at least 90% of RDA values. When patients are malnourished at the time of initial evaluation or are in the high-risk malignancy group (requiring intensive therapeutic intervention), oral intake alone is generally inadequate to maintain acceptable nutriture during the toxic treatment period.[45, 130] High-risk children with advanced solid tumors or relapsed leukemia and lymphoma who underwent intensive combined therapy were observed to lose an average of 16% body weight during the first month of treatment while receiving an oral diet that averaged 48% of the RDA despite comprehensive dietary encouragement.[131] Patients with Wilms' tumors lost an average of 22% body weight during this period. This trend of weight loss was also observed in orally fed patients undergoing aggressive therapy for advanced-stage neuroblastoma.

In contrast, in a study of adult patients with unresectable gastrointestinal malignancies, standard oral diet supplemented with an oral elemental formula improved skin test reactivity.[132] Furthermore, in adult patients with head and neck cancers receiving intensive enteral nutrition via a nasogastric tube—while undergoing an 8-week regimen of radiotherapy—experienced reduced weight loss and normal serum albumin concentrations at the end of therapy.[133] An orally fed control group did not. Such studies suggest the potential utility of enteral tube nutritional delivery in pediatric cancer patients with adequate gut function. If the gastrointestinal tract is patent but functionally compromised, an elemental formula may be tolerated. New formulations are very palatable, and if the patient is nevertheless unable to ingest them, they can be delivered by nasogastric or nasoduodenal feeding tubes. The caloric requirement does not all need to be delivered enterally; a small fraction of the total caloric requirement is adequate to protect against enterocyte atrophy and to maintain the gut mucosa barrier.

Because of complications associated with the parenteral route (as explained later), careful vigilance and considered daily evaluation of the patient's clinical gastrointestinal status along with the route of delivery should be carried out. This avoids the use of parenteral nutrition for the sake of convenience alone. Enteral delivery of partially predigested formulations containing short-chain polypeptides, modified lipid substrates, and simple sugars should be advanced to increased delivery rates (while weaning the patient from TPN) and then switched to nonelemental, complete enteral preparations as early as possible. Provided that protein-calorie intake is adequate (at least 90% RDA), oral feedings have also been shown to maintain acceptable nutritional status in pediatric patients with Stages 3 and 4 neuroblastoma after the conclusion of intensive chemotherapy.[130]

The body of pediatric studies pertaining to children with cancer supports the use of parenteral nutrition for those who are malnourished at the time of initial presentation or who are in the high-nutritional-risk group (see Table 24–2) based upon diagnosis and treatment.

The general areas in which nutritional support in the form of TPN has been shown to be of benefit are in (1) reversing malnutrition, (2) improving immunologic status, (3) improving muscle function and promoting a sense of well-being, (4) decreasing oncologic therapy–associated complications, and (5) improving survival rates.

Reversing Malnutrition. As a practical definition, return to pre-illness anthropometric values (including interim calculations for anticipated growth) constitutes reversal of malignancy-associated malnutrition. This reversal includes a return of serum albumin concentrations to greater than 3.2 g/dl (assuming the absence of an acute metabolic stress insult within 2 weeks prior to measurement).

In contrast to an exclusively oral diet, parenteral nutrition that delivers at least 90% of RDA energy and approximately 2.5–3.0 g protein/kg/D has been shown to reverse preexisting malnutrition in children with late-stage malignancies and recurrent leukemia or lymphoma who required aggressive, toxic antitumor therapy.[131] In this study, improved nutritional status was established by normalization of weight/height percentile, TSF thickness, albumin, and transferrin serum concentrations, all of which occurred with 28 days of TPN in contrast to an oral ad libitum diet, which delivered less than 50% RDA calories. But premature cessation of TPN (at 9 to 14 days) prior to the completion of toxic oncologic therapy failed to resolve malnutrition.

Other studies in well-nourished children also demonstrate improved maintenance of body weight, fat, and muscle reserves in patients administered TPN compared with control patients receiving an oral ad libitum diet during periods of extensive abdominal irradiation[125] and intense chemotherapy.[60, 130]

Improvement of Immunologic Status. The TPN-associated reversal of anergy has been documented in children malnourished prior to treatment while they were receiving chemotherapy.[131] This finding has been confirmed in other studies involving both pediatric and adult cancer patients.[134–136] Furthermore, an improved response to chemotherapy has been obtained in cancer patients who had positive skin test reactivity.[137] Adult cancer patients who become anergic during therapy have been found to have a 100% mortality compared with 11% mortality in immunocompetent patients.[135] The putative relationship between correction of malnutrition and maintenance of immunocompetence is further supported by a study documenting rates of infection significantly lower in well-nourished children compared with malnourished children with metastatic bone disease who were receiving TPN.[49]

Improvement in Muscle Function. Performance status (as an index of muscle function) was evaluated in well-nourished and malnourished children with malignancies requiring abdominal/pelvic radiotherapy, sometimes with adjuvant chemotherapy.[125] All (100%) children in both well-nourished (10 of 10 patients) and malnourished (4 of 4 patients) subgroups were able to maintain or improve performance status while receiving TPN. Of well-nourished children receiving oral ad libitum nutrition, 65% (8 of 12 patients) were able to maintain or improve muscle performance.

Decreased Therapy-Related Complication Rates. A number of studies have documented fewer drug treatment delays caused by marrow suppression and fewer drug dose reductions (improved drug tolerance) in patients who maintained good nutritional status while receiving TPN.[48, 49, 130, 137] However, other studies, involving extensive abdominal radiotherapy, have failed to show fewer treatment-related complications.[125, 137] In fact, the last two studies of parenteral versus enteral nutritional delivery have not

shown any advantage of TPN-induced bowel rest in patients receiving combination abdominal irradiation and chemotherapy.[125, 137]

In a small, randomized, prospective study, children receiving intensive induction chemotherapy for treatment of nonlymphocytic leukemia who were administered TPN (approximately 60 kcal/kg/D; 2 g protein/kg/D) experienced accelerated bone marrow recovery (significantly higher total white blood cell, absolute granulocyte, and platelet counts) as compared with the control group (oral intake approximately 40 kcal/kg/D; 1 g protein/kg/D).[60] Evaluation of an older patient group (teenagers and young adults) with advanced-stage sarcomas receiving aggressive combined therapy failed to demonstrate significant improvement of myelosuppression with TPN.[138] These patients, however, all likely experienced protracted periods of acute metabolic stress (as suggested by fevers greater than 38.5°C), which may have impeded nutrition-related bone marrow recovery.

In adult patients who underwent surgery for esophageal cancer, preoperative TPN has been shown to decrease postoperative complications related to healing.[139] This is especially true if severe malnutrition exists prior to planned surgical intervention.[140]

Improved Clinical Outcome. Earlier studies of children with malignancy failed to demonstrate improved remission and survival rates following adequate nutritional support during antitumor therapy. But a study of patients undergoing bone marrow transplantation (including children older than 1 year of age, teenagers, and young adults) who received TPN from 1 week prior to transplantation through the fourth week following marrow transplant demonstrated a significantly improved 2-year survival rate (50% for TPN versus 35% for control) and a significantly decreased percentage of relapse (35% for TPN versus 60% for control at 2 years).[95] Moreover, malnourished adult patients who underwent surgery for gastrointestinal carcinomas and had nutritional repletion from TPN during the postoperative period also had an improved survival rate in contrast to patients who did not have TPN.[141]

METHODS OF NUTRITIONAL SUPPORT
Enteral Delivery

A large body of literature now exists to establish the substantial advantages of enteral as compared with parenteral nutritional delivery. The advantages include better maintenance of the structural and function integrity of the gastrointestinal tract, decreased risk of bacterial translocation, greater ease and safety of administration, more efficient physiologic utilization of nutrient substrates, decreased hepatobiliary complications, improved outcome, and improved cost effectiveness.[142] As previously discussed, patients who are incapable of adequate oral intake can usually be fed via a small, flexible nasogastric or nasoduodenal feeding tube. Patients in whom placement of this type of tube is difficult (e.g., those with head and neck malignancies) can receive supplement enterally via a gastrostomy or jejunostomy tube.[143]

Although enteral feeding is generally safer than parenteral feeding, complications can occur from improper administration, poor gastric emptying, feeding-tube migration, bacterial contamination of the formula, underlying illness, or reactions to medications.[144] The most frequent serious complication associated with nasogastric or gastrostomy tube feeding is the pulmonary aspiration of formula. This risk of pulmonary aspiration can be reduced by (1) elevating the upper torso to a 30° angle or by keeping the younger child in a prone position and (2) advancing the nasogastric tube to a transpyloric position, preferably beyond the ligament of Treitz.

Inadequate absorption can result in diarrhea or poor growth. Measuring the biochemical products of malabsorption is more useful than measuring the volume of diarrhea to evaluate feeding intolerance.[145] Carbohydrate malabsorption can be documented by a fecal pH of less than 5.5 and the presence of more than 0.25 g/dl of reducing substances in the stool. Fat malabsorption is assessed by the fat content of a 72-hour stool collection. After 6 months of age, healthy children should absorb 90% of ingested fat.

Parenteral Delivery

Parenteral nutrition is necessary in patients who are unable to tolerate adequate enteral nutritional delivery for an extended time period (conventionally 5 days or more) owing to prolonged gastrointestinal dysfunction. In addition, parenteral nutrition is frequently given to supplement protein-calorie needs in critically ill patients who can tolerate only limited enteral nutritional delivery. As highly concentrated (more than 12.5 g/dl) carbohydrate solutions quickly induce thrombophlebitis in peripheral veins, these solutions must be administered through a central venous catheter. The catheter tip is usually advanced to the junction of the superior vena cava with the right atrium to facilitate rapid dilution of the infused hyperosmolar solution with blood in a large, high-flow chamber. The development of small-caliber, soft, polyurethane catheters has reduced complications associated with erosion of the catheter tip through the vessel wall. The addition of heparin (1 U/ml) to the solution may reduce the risk of central vein thrombosis.

Peripheral-vein parenteral nutrition (PPN) may be given for periods of 1 to 2 weeks, either as the sole source of nutritional support or as a supplement to enteral nutritional delivery.[146] To reduce the risk of thrombophlebitis, solution osmolality should not exceed 600 mOsm/L, and dextrose concentrations should not exceed 12.5 g/dl. Glycerol, an alternative carbohydrate energy source to dextrose, offers the advantage of lower osmolality and thus can be delivered in higher concentrations. The addition of heparin (1 U/ml) and hydrocortisone (1 mg/dl) to the solution further reduces the risk of thrombophlebitis. The addition of lipid emulsions, either in combination with protein and carbohydrate (3-in-1 compounded solutions) or piggybacked into polyurethane catheters with protein-carbohydrate solutions, decreases the irritative effects of hypertonic carbohydrate infusion.

These modifications enable the safe nutrient delivery of up to 85 kcal/kg/D (approximately 850 mOsm). PPN avoids the complication of central vein thrombosis as well as the technical and mechanical complications (such as pneumothorax and catheter tip–induced central vein and right atrial erosion or perforation) associated with the placement of central catheters. The short-term use of femoral venous catheters has proved a safe alternative for PPN delivery, associated, in one study, with a low catheter-related sepsis rate of 1.9%.[147]

In children requiring long-term TPN during bone marrow transplantation, cyclic delivery has been shown to be safe and effective.[94] The cyclic administration of carbohydrate mimics, to some extent, the intermittent nature of oral feeding. When TPN is cycled, serum glucose and insulin concentrations fall, lipid oxidation increases, and lipid storage decreases. All of these factors have potential benefit in reducing liver dysfunction, a complication frequently observed in children receiving long-term TPN.[119] Furthermore, the TPN infusion-free period allows for easier administration of chemotherapy, blood products, and so forth.

During the period of toxicity associated with intense oncologic therapy, when the child is generally dependent on the parenteral administration of nutrients for adequate caloric delivery, some nutritional supplementation, even a small amount, can frequently be given enterally.[119] This amount may be as little as 5 ml/h of a predigested, partially elemental formula delivered via an enteral feeding tube or orally, in sips. The putative advantage of this nutritional strategy is to support the gut mucosal barrier (see later discussion) and potentially decrease the risk of infectious complications related to the translocation of intestinal flora. In a randomized study of children with advanced-stage neuroblastoma or Wilms' tumor, patients were able to tolerate 25% of their RDA caloric requirement in oral formulations to supplement nutritional delivery by peripheral parenteral infusion. Thus, malnutrition was effectively resolved.[46]

The complications associated with parenteral feeding, some of which are discussed here, may be categorized as mechanical/technical (related to catheter, pump, or placement), metabolic (related to fluids, electrolytes, or organ functions), nutritional (related to excessive or inadequate nutrient delivery), and infectious. In one study, the overall infection rate associated with TPN administration was 5%, with considerable variability according to site of placement and lumen number.[148] In particular reference to intravenous catheter-related infection rates in children with malignancy, earlier studies suggested no difference between the oncologic and nononcologic subgroups in those receiving TPN.[149] Others suggested an increased risk of infection associated with tumor-related immunosuppression but not with TPN.[150] Later evaluations of pediatric cancer patients have demonstrated a significantly increased risk of infection associated with TPN. In a study of patients (children and teenagers) receiving bone marrow transplantation, there was a 50% increase in bacteremia in the group randomized to receive TPN when compared with the control group.[95] In another retrospective

study, this time of 310 pediatric cancer patients with indwelling central venous catheters, there was a 2.4-fold increase in the risk of infection, primarily with gram-positive organisms, associated with the infusion of TPN.[151] The risk of many or all of these complications is substantially reduced if a complete nutritional support team, including well-trained physicians, nurses, dieticians, and pharmacists, takes part in nutritional delivery.

Enteral Versus Parenteral Delivery

Advantages associated with enteral versus parenteral feeding administration in a variety of animal models include improved gut mass and function, decreased translocation, decreased infectious complications, and improved survival rates.

Enteral nutritional delivery is critical in preventing bacterial translocation.[152] Parenteral nutrition (without glutamine supplementation) is associated with mucosal atrophy. In contrast, enteral formulations stimulate trophic gut hormone secretion and nourish the mucosa. Enterally fed, stressed humans have been found to have fewer postoperative septic-related complications when compared with those parenterally fed.[153] In guinea pigs, early versus late enteral feeding has been shown to reduce the hypermetabolic response to burn injury and promote gut mucosal growth.[154] This effect on energy expenditure is possibly due to decreased translocation resulting in a decreased metabolic stress response. In rats, immediate postoperative enteral feeding is associated with improved wound strength and less weight loss when compared with late feeding.[155]

In addition, enteral feeding, even in small amounts, appears to protect the liver against TPN-related complications.[156] A prospective study of severely injured adult trauma patients has demonstrated increased constitutive and decreased acute-phase protein levels following enteral versus parenteral nutrient delivery, suggesting early resolution of the acute metabolic stress response if the gut is supported.[157] In all of these studies, better maintenance of intestinal barrier function with early enteral nutrition is the most probable reason for improved outcome.

In humans, the evaluation of TPN versus enteral nutritional delivery in acutely stressed high-risk patients (including children) has now been evaluated in a substantial number of randomized, prospective trials. Recent meta-analysis of eight of these trials (involving high-risk surgical patients) shows a significant reduction in septic complications (18% versus 35%) in the enterally fed patient group.[158] Moreover, a study of 39 patients with greater than 50% total body surface area burns demonstrated significantly increased mortality in the group randomized to receive TPN supplementation of enteral calories versus enteral calories alone (63% versus 26%).[159] In a single-center study[160] of 98 adult trauma patients (abdominal trauma score ≥15) prospectively randomized to receive either enteral or parenteral nutrition, the infection rate was significantly lower in the enteral versus the parenteral group, as determined by fewer cases of pneumonia (11.8% versus 31%) and fewer intra-abdominal abscesses (1.9% versus 13.3%). These data support the preferential use of enteral nutritional delivery to the degree clinically feasible.

SPECIALIZED NUTRITIONAL STRATEGIES

Short-chain Polypeptides Versus Free Amino Acids

Considerable debate has focused on whether short-chain polypeptide (2–5 carbon length) formulations are absorbed by intestinal mucosa better than formulations consisting primarily of free amino acids. In unstressed animals, short-chain polypeptide as compared with amino acid diets are associated with decreased translocation,[161] improved bowel growth,[162] trophic gut hormone secretion,[163] and somatic growth and IGF-1 production.[162] Short-chain polypeptide diets also improve early somatic growth recovery[164] and survival rates[165–168] when compared with amino acid diets in metabolically stressed animals. Furthermore, short-chain polypeptide diets are superior to amino acid diets in decreasing diarrhea, improving visceral protein synthesis, and decreasing hospital stay in trauma patients.[169] These data suggest that short-chain polypeptide diets are better than amino acid diets in supporting bowel function during acute injury states.

Glutamine

Glutamine is the most abundant amino acid in plasma and skeletal muscle, but serum levels of glutamine fall precipitously following acute metabolic stress, primarily because of increased uptake and metabolism by the gut.[170] Glutamine is a major energy source for intestinal mucosa[171] and may stimulate increased protein synthesis in enterocytes during acute injury states such as sepsis.[172] Glutamine is also deaminated by the gut to form alanine, which then flows via the splanchnic circulation to the liver. During acute stress, this gut-to-liver pathway provides a major contribution to the hepatic amino acid pool.[173] Provision of standard parenteral nutrition is associated with atrophy of the intestinal mucosa.[174] In contrast, glutamine-enriched parenteral nutrition has been shown to increase gut mucosal weight and DNA content,[175] stimulate villous growth,[176] and improve gut glutamine utilization. Moreover, glutamine-supplemented TPN decreases bacterial translocation as compared with standard TPN.[177] Parenteral glutamine supplementation may have the additional benefit of protecting the liver against TPN-induced hepatic steatosis.[176] The safety of parenterally administered glutamine has been demonstrated in humans.[178]

During acute metabolic stress, gut glutamine uptake is enhanced. Improved survival rates have been achieved in septic rats with glutamine-enriched TPN.[179] This effect may be due to enhancement of the immunologic rather than the physical gut-barrier function. In addition to its role as a primary fuel source for enterocytes and colonocytes, glutamine is an important fuel source for lymphocytes and macrophages. Whereas it is considered nonessential to health, glutamine appears to become essential during acute metabolic states when its uptake by ingesting and by immunologically active cells exceeds its synthesis and release from skeletal muscle.

Marked glutamine deficiency has been documented in cancer patients.[180] In a study of cancer patients undergoing bone marrow transplantation, administration of TPN supplemented with glutamine versus standard TPN resulted in improved nitrogen balance, fewer infections, and shorter hospital stay.[178]

Modified Lipid Substrates

Medium-chain triglyceride (MCT) preparations contain saturated fatty acids with 6 to 12 carbon-chain lengths. MCTs are directly absorbed into the circulatory system from the gut and do not require bile. They are rapidly cleared from the bloodstream, exhibit rapid mitochondrial uptake, and do not require carnitine for metabolism. In contrast to *long-chain triglycerides* (LCTS),[181] MCTs do not appear to impair reticuloendothelial system clearance of bacteria.[182, 183] MCTs are incorporated in several enteral formulations and can improve fat absorption from dysfunctional bowel. Studies have also demonstrated potentially beneficial effects of short-chain fatty acids (butyrate) in promoting intestinal growth delivered both enterally[184] and parenterally.[185]

NUTRITIONAL IMMUNOMODULATION

Data have suggested that several dietary components can exert a variety of effects on the immune system. Because increased metabolic stress severity is associated with substantially increased immunocompromise, the potential ability to enhance immunologic function by dietary alterations offers the possibility of improving clinical outcome following injury. Research interest has focused on three major substrate subgroups: omega-3 fatty acids, nucleotides, and arginine.

Omega-3 Polyunsaturated Fatty Acids (ω-3 PUFA)

In addition to providing an important substrate for energy, essential fatty acids, fat-soluble vitamins, and cell membranes, lipid metabolism may also modulate immune function via arachidonic acid synthetic pathways.[79] Increased intake of *linoleic acid* (ω-6 PUFA), an important precursor of arachidonic acid, has been shown to inhibit immune function by impeding neutrophil chemotaxis, phagocytosis, and bacteriocidal activity, thereby reducing macrophage phagocytosis and lymphocyte proliferation.[186] The metabolism of linoleic acid via the cyclooxygenase pathway yields mono and dienoic prostaglandins (such as PGE_2), known to have widespread macrophage and lymphocyte immunosuppressant effects at high serum concentrations ($>10-^8M$) associated with severe metabolic stress conditions, such as sepsis and burn trauma.[186]

In contrast, diets high in ω-3 PUFA (fish oil) result in comparatively less arachidonic acid production and yield the less potent trienoic prostaglandins. Consequently, PGE_2 production and immunosuppression are reduced. Diets rich in ω-3 versus ω-6 PUFA have been shown to improve immunologic function in burned animals.[187, 188] They have also been associated with improved survival rates in acutely stressed human[189] and animal[190] study populations.

In a study of postsurgical cancer patients, early postoperative feeding with an enteral diet containing a fish oil/medium-chain, triglyceride-structured lipid resulted in a 50% decline in gastrointestinal complications and infections compared with an isonitrogenous, isocaloric diet without ω-3 PUFA.[191]

Nucleotides

In vitro investigations have suggested that the metabolism of stimulated lymphocytes is nucleotide dependent.[192] Enhanced immunologic function has been demonstrated in animal studies by increased allograft rejection,[193] greater resistance to bacterial challenge,[194] and improved delayed hypersensitivity[195] associated with nucleotide-supplemented versus nucleotide-free diets. Immunosuppression resulting from the absence of dietary nucleotides appears to be due primarily to increased helper T-cell suppression and decreased IL-2 production. These findings seem to be uracil-dependent.[195]

Arginine

The immune effects of in vitro arginine are to enhance lymphocyte activation—that is, improve mitogenesis and increase synthesis of nucleic acids and protein.[196] Arginine administration increases T-cell immunity and is associated with increased thymic mass and cellularity. Arginine may become an essential amino acid during acute metabolic stress states as a result of insufficient endogenous production and increased demands. Animal studies demonstrate improved survival rates with arginine-supplemented diets following burn injury and peritonitis,[197, 198] presumably by improving T-lymphocyte-dependent immunocompetence. This concept is supported by studies with postoperative human subjects showing an increase in mitogenic response of circulating lymphocytes with arginine supplementation.[196, 199] Arginine-enriched diets have also been associated with improved wound healing,[200] and they may inhibit the growth and development of malignant tumors because of enhanced immune function.[196]

Arginine is a precursor of nitric oxide synthesis. Arginine-induced augmentation of macrophage and NK-cell activity may be due, in part, to enhanced nitric oxide production. Of special potential importance from a pediatric surgical prospective, arginine induces increased pituitary growth hormone secretion,[201] and it may be necessary for optimal growth in healthy human children.[196]

NUTRITION AND TUMOR GROWTH

The fact that in a number of animal models tumor growth rates have correlated positively with nutritional status[202] and exogenous nutritional delivery[203] has prompted concern. The results, however, of providing intravenous nutrition to malnourished, tumor-bearing rats have been to restore body weight and immunocompetence without adversely stimulating tumor growth out of proportion to the growth of the host.[8] Furthermore, clinical studies of children with malignancy receiving exogenous nutritional support have failed to demonstrate increased tumor growth or decreased survival rates despite improved host nutritional status.[204]

References

1. Morrison SD, Moley JF, Norton JA: Contribution of inert mass to experimental cancer cachexia in rats. *J Natl Cancer Inst* 73:991–998, 1984.
2. Norton JA, Peacock JL, Morrison SD: Cancer cachexia. *CRC Crit Rev Oncol Hematol* 7:289–327, 1987.
3. DeWys WD, Walters K: Abnormalities of taste sensation in cancer patients. *Cancer* 36:1888–1896, 1975.
4. Bernstein IL, Sigmundi RA: Tumor anorexia: A learned food aversion. *Science* 209:416–418, 1980.
5. Daly JM, Hoffman K, Lieberman M, et al: Nutritional support in the cancer patient. *JPEN* 14(suppl.):244S–248S, 1990.
6. Alleyve GAO, Hay RW, Picou DI: *Protein Energy Malnutrition.* London: Edward Arnold Publishers, Ltd. 1977.
7. Mitchell CH, Sinatra FR, Chrast FW: Intractable watery diarrhea, ganglioneuroblastoma and vasoactive intestinal peptide. *J Pediatr* 89:593–595, 1976.
8. Daly JM, Copeland EM, Dudrick SJ: Effects of intravenous nutrition on tumor growth and host immunocompetence in malnourished animals. *Surgery* 84:655–658, 1978.
9. Daly JM, Dudrick SJ, Copeland EM: Evaluation of nutritional indices as prognostic indicators in the cancer patient. *Cancer* 43:925–931, 1979.
10. Donaldson SS, Lenon RA: Impact of chemotherapy and radiation therapy. *Cancer* 43:2036–2052, 1979.
11. Ramirez I, van Eys J, Carr D, et al: Immunologic evaluation in the nutritional assessment of children with cancer. *Am J Clin Nutr* 41:1314–1321, 1985.
12. Masuno H, Yamasaki N, Okuda H: Purification and characterization of a lipolytic factor (toxohormone-L) from cell free fluid of ascites sarcoma 180. *Cancer Res* 41:284–288, 1981.
13. Beck SA, Tisdale MJ: Production of lipolytic and proteolytic factors by a murine tumor-producing cachexia in the host. *Cancer Res* 47:5919–5923, 1987.
14. Norton JA, Moley JF, Green MV, Carson RE, Morrison SD: Parabiotic transfer of cancer anorexia/cachexia in male rats. *Cancer Res* 45:5547–5552, 1985.
15. Illig KA, Maronian N, Peacock JL: Cancer cachexia is transmissible in plasma. *J Surg Res* 52:353–358, 1992.
16. Fong Y, Moldawer LL, Shires T, Lowry SF: The biologic characteristics of cytokines and their implication in surgical injury. *Surgery* 170:363–378, 1990.
17. Selby P, Hobbs S, Viner C, et al: Tumor necrosis factor in man: Clinical and biological observations. *Br J Cancer* 56:803–808, 1987.
18. Starnes HF, Warren SR, Jeevanandam M, et al: Tumour necrosis factor and the acute metabolic response to tissue injury in man. *J Clin Invest* 82:1321–1325, 1988.
19. Langstein HN, Norton JA: Mechanisms of cancer cachexia. *Hematol Oncol Clin North Am* 5:103–123, 1991.
20. McNamara JJ, Alexander HR, Norton JA: Cytokines and their role in the pathophysiology of cancer cachexia. *JPEN* 16(suppl.):50S–55S, 1992.
21. Falconer JS, Fearon KCH, Plester CE, Ross JA, Carter DC: Cytokines, the acute-phase response, and resting energy expenditure in cachectic patients with pancreatic cancer. *Ann Surg* 219:325–331, 1994.
22. Moldawer LL, Georgieff M, Lundholm K: Interleukin-1, tumor necrosis factor-α (cachectin) and the pathogenesis of cancer cachexia. *Clin Physiol* 7:263–274, 1987.
23. Gelin J, Moldawer LL, Lonnroth C, Sherry B, Chizzonite R, Lundholm K: Role of endogenous tumor necrosis factor α and interleukin-1 for experimental tumor growth and the development of cancer cachexia. *Cancer Res* 51:415–421, 1991.
24. Moldawer LL, Rogy MA, Lowry SF: The role

of cytokines in cancer cachexia. *JPEN* 16(suppl.)43S–49S, 1992.

25. Dempsey DT, Feurer ID, Knox LS, et al: Energy expenditure in malnourished gastrointestinal cancer patients. *Cancer* 53:1265–1273, 1984.

26. Fredrix EWHM, Soeters PB, Wouters EFM, et al: Effect of different tumour types on resting energy expenditure. *Cancer Res* 51:6138–6141, 1991.

27. Fredrix EWHM, Wouters EFM, Soeters PB, et al: Resting energy expenditure in patients with non-small cell lung cancer. *Cancer* 68:1612–1621, 1991.

28. Hansell DT, Davies JWL, Burns HJG: The relationship between resting energy expenditure and weight loss in benign and malignant disease. *Ann Surg* 203:240–245, 1986.

29. Hyltander A, Christer D, Korner U, Sandstrom R, Lundholm K: Elevated energy expenditure in patients with solid tumours. *Eur J Cancer* 27:9–15, 1991.

30. Warnald I, Lundholm K, Schersten T: Energy balance and body composition in cancer patients. *Cancer Res* 38:1801–1807, 1978.

31. Jeevanandam M, Legaspi A, Lowry SF, Horowitz GD, Brennan MF: Effect of total parenteral nutrition on whole-body protein kinetics in cachectic patients with benign or malignant disease. *JPEN* 12:229–236, 1988.

32. Lundholm K, Edstrom S, Ekman L, Karlberg I, Bylund A, Schersten T: A comparative study of the influence of malignant tumor on host metabolism in mice and man: Evaluation of an experimental model. *Cancer* 42:453–461, 1978.

33. Shaw JHF, Humberstone DM, Douglas RG, Koea J: Leucine kinetics in patients with benign disease, non-weight-losing cancer, and cancer cachexia: Studies at the whole-body and tissue level and the response to nutritional support. *Surgery* 109:37–50, 1991.

34. Albert JD, Legaspi A, Horowitz GD, Tracey KJ, Brennan MF, Lowry SF: Peripheral tissue metabolism in man with varied disease states and similar weight loss. *J Surg Res* 40:374–381, 1986.

34a. Humberstone DA, Shaw JHF: Metabolism in hematologic malignancy. *Cancer* 62:1619–1624, 1989.

35. Cersosimo E, Pisters PWT, Pesola G, et al: The effect of graded doses of insulin on peripheral glucose uptake and lactate release in cancer cachexia. *Surgery* 109:459–467, 1991.

36. Glicksman AS, Rawson RW: Diabetes and altered carbohydrate metabolism in patients with cancer. *Cancer* 9:1127–1134, 1956.

37. Yoshikawa T, Noguchi Y, Matsumoto A: Effects of tumor removal and body weight loss on insulin resistance in patients with cancer. *Surgery* 116:62–66, 1994.

38. Kallinowski F, Schlenger KH, Runkel S, et al: Blood flow, metabolism, cellular

39. microenvironment and growth rate of human xenografts. *Cancer Res* 49:3759–3764, 1989.

39. Nolop KB, Rhodes CG, Brudin LH, et al: Glucose utilization in vivo by human pulmonary neoplasms. *Cancer* 60:2682–2689, 1987.

40. Young VR: Energy metabolism and requirements in cancer patients. *Cancer Res* 37:2336–2347, 1977.

41. Shaw JHF, Wolfe RR: Fatty acid and glycerol kinetics in septic patients and in patients with gastrointestinal cancer: The response to glucose infusion and parenteral feeding. *Ann Surg* 205:368–376, 1987.

42. Arbeit JM, Lees DE, Corsey R, Brennan MF: Resting energy expenditure in controls and cancer patients with localized and diffuse disease. *Ann Surg* 199:292–298, 1984.

43. Hansell DT, Davies JWL, Burns HJG, Shenkin A: The oxidation of body fuel stores in cancer patients. *Ann Surg* 204:637–642, 1986.

44. Donaldson SS, Wesley MN, DeWys W, Suskind RM, Jaffe N, van Eys J: A study of the nutritional status of pediatric cancer patients. *Am J Dis Child* 135:1107–1112, 1981.

45. Rickard KA, Baehner RL, Coates TD, Weetman RM, Provisor AJ, Grosfeld JL: Supportive nutritional intervention in pediatric cancer. *Cancer Res* 42(suppl.):766S–773S, 1982.

46. Rickard KA, Foland BB, Detamore CM, et al: Effectiveness of central parenteral nutrition versus peripheral parenteral nutrition plus enteral nutrition in reversing protein-energy malnutrition in children with advanced neuroblastoma and Wilms' tumor: A prospective randomized study. *Am J Clin Nutr* 38:445–456, 1983.

47. Van Eys J: Malnutrition in children with cancer. Incidence and consequence. *Cancer* 43:2030–2039, 1979.

48. Rickard KA, Detamore CM, Coates TD, et al: Effect of nutrition staging on treatment delays and outcome in stage IV neuroblastoma. *Cancer* 52:587–598, 1983.

49. Van Eys J, Copeland EM, Cangir A, et al: A clinical trial of hyperalimentation in children with metastatic malignancies. *Med Pediatr Oncol* 8:63–73, 1980.

50. Hughes WT, Price RA, Sisko F, et al: Protein-calorie malnutrition: A host determinant for *Pneumocystis carinii* infection. *Am J Dis Child* 128:44–52, 1974.

51. Trowbridge FL: Clinical and biochemical characteristics associated with anthropometric nutritional categories. *Am J Clin Nutr* 32:758–766, 1979.

52. Rao KV, Singh D: An evaluation of the relationship between nutritional status and anthropometric measurements. *Am J Clin Nutr* 23:83–93, 1970.

53. Grant A: *Nutritional Assessment Guideline*. Cutter Laboratories 1979, pp. 11–22.

54. Hamil PVV, Drizd TA, Johnson C, Reed RB,

Roche AF, Moore WM: Physical growth: National Center for Health Statistics percentiles. *Am J Clin Nutr* 32:607–629, 1979.

55. Carter P, Carr D, Van Eys J, Coody D: Nutritional parameters in children with cancer. *J Am Diet Assoc* 82:616–622, 1983.

56. Smythe PM, Brereton-Stiles GG, Grace JH, et al: Thymolymphatic deficiency and depression of cell-mediated immunity in protein-calorie malnutrition. *Lancet* 28:939–944, 1971.

57. Chandra RK: Immunocompetence in undernutrition. *J Pediatr* 81:1194–1200, 1972.

58. Bistrian BR, Blackburn GL, Scrimshaw N, Flatt JP: Cellular immunity in semistarved states in hospitalized adults. *Am J Clin Nutr* 28:1148–1155, 1975.

59. Mullen JL, Buzby GP, Matthews DC, Smale BF, Rosato EF: Reduction of operative morbidity and mortality by combined preoperative and postoperative nutritional support. *Ann Surg* 192:604–613, 1980.

60. Hays DM, Merritt RJ, White L, et al: Effect of total parenteral nutrition on marrow recovery during induction therapy for acute nonlymphocytic leukemia in childhood. *Med Pediatr Oncol* 11:134–140, 1983.

61. Neumann CG, Lawlor GJ, Stiehm ER, et al: Immunological responses in malnourished children. *Am J Clin Nutr* 28:89–104, 1975.

62. Law DK, Dudrick SJ, Abdou NI: The effect of dietary protein depletion on immunocompetence. *Ann Surg* 179:168–173, 1974.

63. Pietsch JB, Meakins JL, McLean LD: The delayed hypersensitivity response: Application to clinical surgery. *Surgery* 82:349–355, 1977.

64. Long CL, Schaffel N, Geiger JW, Schiller WR, Blakemore WS: Metabolic response to injury and illness: Estimation of energy and protein needs from indirect calorimetry and nitrogen balance. *JPEN* 3:452–456, 1979.

65. Kinney JM, Elwyn DH: Protein metabolism in the traumatized patient. *Acta Chir Scand* 522(suppl.):45–56, 1984.

66. Cerra RB: Hypermetabolism, organ failure, and metabolic support. *Surgery* 101:1–14, 1987.

67. Moore FD: Bodily changes in surgical convalescence.I. The normal sequence: Observations and interpretations. *Ann Surg* 137:289–315, 1953.

68. Dinarello CA: Interleukin-1 and interleukin-1 antagonism. *Blood* 77:1627–1652, 1991.

69. Rock CS, Lowry SF: Tumor necrosis factor-α. *J Surg Res* 51:434–445, 1991.

70. Ertel W, Morrison MH, Ayala A, Chaudry IH: Mechanisms responsible for the increase of interleukin-6 synthesis. *Surg Forum* 43:88–90, 1992.

71. Warner SJC, Libby P. Human vascular smooth muscle cells: Target for and source of tumor necrosis factor. *J Immunol* 142:100–109, 1989.

72. Flores EA, Bistrian BR, Pomposelli JJ, et al: Infusion of tumor necrosis factor/cachectin promotes muscle catabolism. A synergistic effect with interleukin-1. *J Clin Invest* 83:1614–1622, 1989.

73. Lee MD, Zentella A, Pekala PH, et al: Effect of endotoxin-induced monokines on glucose metabolism in the muscle cell line L6. *Proc Natl Acad Sci USA* 84:2590–2594, 1987.

74. Roh MS, Moldawer LL, Ekman LG, et al: Stimulatory effect of interleukin-1 upon hepatic metabolism. *Metabolism* 35:419–425, 1986.

75. Pacitti AJ, Inoue Y, Souba WW: Tumor necrosis factor stimulates Na+-dependent amino acid uptake in plasma membrane vesicles. *J Clin Invest* 91:474–483, 1993.

76. Warren RS, Starnes HF, Jr., Gabrilove JL, et al: The acute metabolic effects of tumor necrosis factor administration in humans. *Arch Surg* 122:1396–1400, 1987.

77. Michie HR, Spriggs DR, Manogue KR, et al: Tumor necrosis factor and endotoxin induce similar metabolic responses in human beings. *Surgery* 104:280–286, 1988.

78. Lazarus DD, Lowry SF, Moldawer LL: Cytokines acutely decrease circulating insulin-like growth factor-1 (IGF-1) and IGF binding protein-3 (IGFBP-3). *Surg Forum* 43:92–94, 1992.

79. Kinsella JE, Lokesh B, Broughton S, et al: Dietary polyunsaturated fatty acids and eicosanoids: Potential effects on the modulation of inflammatory and immune cells: An overview. *Nutrition* 6:25–44, 1990.

80. Nijsten MWN, Hack CE, Helle M, et al. Interleukin-6 and its relation to the humoral immune response and clinical parameters in burned patients. *Surgery* 109:761–767, 1991.

81. Ohzato H, Yoshizaki K, Nishimoto N, et al: Interleukin-6 as a new indicator of inflammatory status: Detection of serum levels of interleukin-6 and C-reactive protein after surgery. *Surgery* 111:201–209, 1992.

82. Koj A: The role of interleukin-6 as the hepatocyte-stimulating factor in the network of inflammatory cytokines. *Ann NY Acad Sci* 557:1–8, 1989.

83. Michie HR, Eberlein TJ, Spriggs DR, et al: Interleukin-2 initiates metabolic responses associated with critical illness in humans. *Ann Surg* 208:493–503, 1988.

84. Levi R, Krell RD: Biology of leukotrienes. *Ann NY Acad Sci* 524:91, 1988.

85. Wolfe RR, Jahoor F, Herndon DN, Miyoshi H: Isotopic evaluation of the metabolism of pyruvate and related substrates in normal adult volunteers and severely burned children: Effect of dichloroacetate and glucose infusion. *Surgery* 110:54–67, 1991.

86. Zamir O, Hasselgren PO, O'Brien WO, et al: Muscle protein breakdown during endotoxemia in rats and after treatment with interleukin-1 receptor antagonist (IL-1ra). *Ann Surg* 216:381–387, 1992.

87. Arnold J, Campbell IT, Samuels TA, et al: Increased whole body protein breakdown predominates over increased whole-body protein synthesis in multiple organ failure. *Clin Sci* 84:655–661, 1993.

88. Consoli A, Nurjhan N, Reilly JJ, et al: Contribution of liver and skeletal muscle to alanine and lactate metabolism in humans. *Am J Physiol* 259:E677–E684, 1990.

89. Smith RJ, Wilmore DW. Glutamine nutrition and requirements. *JPEN* 14(suppl.);94S–99S, 1990.

90. Chwals WJ, Bistrian BR: Role of exogenous growth hormone and insulin-like growth factor I in malnutrition and acute metabolic stress: A hypothesis. *Crit Care Med* 19:1317–1322, 1991.

91. Anand KJS, Brown MJ, Bloom SR, et al: Studies on the hormonal regulation of fuel metabolism in the human newborn infant undergoing anesthesia and surgery. *Hormone Res* 22:115–128, 1985.

92. Chwals WJ, Fernandez ME, Charles BJ, et al: Serum visceral protein levels reflect protein-calorie repletion in neonates recovering from major surgery. *J Pediatr Surg* 27:317–321, 1992.

93. Fletcher JP, Little JM, Guest PK: A comparison of serum transferrin and serum prealbumin as nutritional parameters. *JPEN* 11:144–147, 1987.

94. Reed MD, Lazarus HM, Herzig RH, et al: Cyclic Parenteral Nutrition During Bone Marrow Transplantation in Children. *Cancer* 51:1563–1570, 1983.

95. Weisdorf SA, Lysne J, Wind D, et al: Positive effect of prophylactic total parenteral nutrition on long-term outcome of bone marrow transplantation. *Transplantation* 43:833–838, 1987.

96. Wilmore DW. *The Metabolic Management of the Critically Ill.* New York: Plenum Press, 1977.

97. Felig P, Marliss EB, Cahill GF, Jr: Metabolic response to human growth hormone during prolonged starvation. *J Clin Invest* 50:411–421, 1971.

98. Loder PB, Kee AJ, Horsburgh R, et al: Validity of urinary urea nitrogen as a measure of total urinary nitrogen in adult patients requiring parenteral nutrition. *Crit Care Med* 17:309–312, 1989.

99. Bistrian BR: A simple technique to estimate severity of stress. *Surg Gynecol Obstet* 148:675–678, 1979.

100. Rickham PP: *The Metabolic Response to Neonatal Surgery.* Cambridge, MA: Harvard University Press, 1957, pp. 7–93.

101. Helms RA, Mowatt-Larssen CA, Boehm KA, et al: Urinary nitrogen constituents in the postsurgical preterm neonate receiving parenteral nutrition. *JPEN* 17:68–72, 1993.

102. Pepys MB, Baltz ML: Acute phase proteins with special reference to C-reactive protein and related proteins (Pentaxins) and serum amyloid A protein. *Adv Immuno* 34:141–212, 1983.

103. Dickson PW, Bannister D, Schreiber G: Minor burns lead to major changes in synthesis rates of plasma proteins in the liver. *J Trauma* 27:283–286, 1987.

104. Nudelman R, Kagan BM: C-reactive protein in pediatrics. *Adv Pediatr* 30:517–547, 1983.

105. Peltola H, Ahlqvist J, Rapola J, et al: C-reactive protein compared with white blood cell count and erythrocyte sedimentation rate in the diagnosis of acute appendicitis in children. *Acta Chir Scand* 152:55–58, 1986.

106. Gonn M, Slordahl SH, Skrede S, et al: C-reactive protein as an indicator of infection in the immunosuppressed child. *Eur J Pediatr* 145:18–21, 1986.

107. Letton RW, Chwals WJ, Jamie A, Charles B: Early postoperative alterations in infant energy utilization increases the risk of overfeeding. *J Pediatr Surg* 30:988–993, 1995.

108. Weir JB: New methods for calculating metabolic rate with special reference to protein metabolism. *J Physiol* 109:1–9, 1949.

109. McGilvery RW: *Biochemistry: A Functional Approach.* Philadelphia: W.B. Saunders Co., 1979, p. 532.

110. Cortes V, Nelson LD: Errors in estimating energy expenditure in critically ill surgical patients. *Arch Surg* 124:287–290, 1989.

111. Baker JP, Detsky AS, Stewart S: Randomized trial of total parenteral nutrition in critically ill patients: Metabolic effects of varying glucose-lipid ratios as an energy source. *Gastroenterology* 87:53–59, 1984.

112. Fredrix EW, Soeters PB, Von Meyenfeldt MF, Saris WHM: Resting energy expenditure in cancer patients before and after gastrointestinal surgery. *JPEN* 15:604–607, 1991.

113. Swinamer DL, Phang PT, Jones RL, et al: Twenty-four hour energy expenditure in critically ill patients. *Crit Care Med* 15:637–643, 1987.

114. Chwals WJ, Lally KP, Woolley MM, et al: Measured energy expenditure in critically ill infants and young children. *J Surg Res* 44:467–472, 1988.

115. Salas JS, Dozio E, Goulet OJ, et al: Energy expenditure and substrate utilization in the course of renutrition of malnourished children. *JPEN* 15:288–293, 1991.

116. Chwals WJ, Lally KP, Woolley MM: Indirect calorimetry in mechanically ventilated infants and children: Measurement accuracy with absence of audible airleak. *Crit Care Med* 20 (6):768–770, 1992.

117. Pierro A, Carnielle V, Filler RM, et al: Partition of energy metabolism in the surgical newborn. *J Pediatr Surg* 26:581–586, 1991.

118. Powell K, Albernaz L, Skipper E, et al: Does measurement of 20-minute energy expenditure represent the 24-hour energy expenditure in the critically ill? *JPEN* 15:37S, 1991.

119. Chwals WJ. Overfeeding the critically ill child: fact or fantasy? *New Horizons* 2:147–155, 1994.

120. Talbot FB: Basal metabolism standards for children. *Am J Dis Child* 55:455–459, 1938.

121. Young VR, Steffee WP, Pencharz PB, et al: Total human body protein synthesis in relation to protein requirements at various ages. *Nature* 253:192–194, 1975.

122. Committee on Dietary Allowances Food and Nutrition Board: Recommended dietary allowances. Washington, D.C. National Academy of Sciences/National Research Council, 1980.

123. Good RA, West A, Fernandes G: Nutritional modulation of immune responses. *Fed Proc* 39:3098–3104, 1980.

124. Strauss RG: Iron deficiency, infections, and immune function: a reassessment. *Am J Clin Nutr* 31:660–666, 1978.

125. Donaldson SS, Wesley MN, Ghavimi F, Shils ME, Suskind RM, DeWys WD: A prospective randomized clinical trial of total parenteral nutrition in children with cancer. *Med Pediatr Oncol* 10:129–139, 1982.

126. Mauer AM, Burgess JB, Donaldson SS, et al: Special nutritional needs of children with malignancies: A review. *JPEN* 14:315–324, 1990.

127. Rickard KA, Grosfeld JL, Coates TD, Weetman R, Baehner RL: Advances in nutrition care of children with neoplastic diseases: A review of treatment, research, and application. *J Am Diet Assoc* 86:1666–1676, 1986.

128. Stiehm ER, Winter HS, Bryson YJ: Cellular (T cell) immunity in the human newborn. *Pediatrics* 64:814, 1979.

129. Lingard CD, Rickard KA, Jaeger BL: Planning and implementing a nutrition program for children with cancer. *TICN* 2:71–86, 1986.

130. Rickard KA, Loghmani ES, Grosfeld JL, et al: Short- and long-term effectiveness of enteral and parenteral nutrition in reversing or preventing protein-energy malnutrition in advanced neuroblastoma. A prospective randomized study. *Cancer* 56:2881–2897, 1985.

131. Rickard KA, Grosfeld JL, Kirksey A, Ballantine TV, Baehner RL: Reversal of protein-energy malnutrition in children during treatment of advanced neoplastic disease. *Ann Surg* 190:771–781, 1979.

132. Douglass Jr., Milliron S, Nava H, et al: Elemental diet as an adjuvant for patients with locally advanced gastrointestinal cancer receiving radiation therapy: A prospectively randomized study. *JPEN* 2:682–686, 1978.

133. Daly JM, Hearne B, Dunaj J, et al: Nutritional rehabilitation in patients with advanced head and neck cancer receiving radiation therapy. *Am J Surg* 148:514–520, 1984.

134. Copeland EM, Daly JM, Dudrick SJ, et al: Nutrition, cancer, and intravenous hyperalimentation. *Cancer* 43:2108, 1979.

135. Harvey KB, Bothe A, Blackburn GL: Nutritional assessment and patient outcome during oncological therapy. *Cancer* 43:2065, 1979.

136. Teitell-Cohen B, Herson J, van Eys J: Recall antigen response in pediatric cancer patients receiving parenteral hyperalimentation. *JPEN* 4:9–11, 1980.

137. DeWys WD: Anorexia as a general effect of cancer. *Cancer* 43:2013, 1979.

137a. Ghavimi R, Shils ME, Scott BF, et al: Comparison of morbidity in children requiring abdominal radiation and chemotherapy, with and without total parenteral nutrition. *J Pediatr* 101:530–537, 1982.

138. Shamberger RC, Pizzo PA, Goodgame JTJ, et al: The effect of total parenteral nutrition on chemotherapy-induced myelosuppression. A randomized study. *Am J Med* 74:40–48, 1983.

139. Daly JM, Massar E, Giacco G, et al: Parenteral nutrition in esophageal cancer patients. *Ann Surg* 196:203–208, 1982.

140. Buzby GP, Blauin G, Colling CL, et al (Veterans Affairs Total Parenteral Nutrition Cooperative Study Group): Perioperative total parenteral nutrition in surgical patients. *N Engl J Med* 325:525–532, 1991.

141. Muller JM, Brenner U, Dienst C, Pichlamaier H: Preoperative parenteral feeding in patients with gastrointestinal carcinoma. *Lancet* 1:68–71, 1982..

142. Chellis MJ, Price MB, Dean JM: Cost effectiveness of early enteral feeding in critically ill children. *Crit Care Med* 22:A156, 1994.

143. Andrassy RJ, Mahour GH, Harrison MR, et al: The role and safety of early postoperative feeding in the pediatric surgical patient. *J Pediatr Surg* 14:381–385, 1979.

144. Brown RO, Carlson SD, Cowan GSM, et al: Enteral nutritional support management in a university teaching hospital: Team versus non-team. *JPEN* 11:52–56, 1987.

145. Roberts P, Meredith JW, Black K, Zaloga G. Diarrhea does not alter impaired small bowel absorption following trauma. *JPEN* 17:34S, 1993.

146. Payne-James JJ, Khawaja HT. First choice for total parenteral nutrition: The peripheral route. *JPEN* 17:468–478, 1993.

147. Friedman B, Kanter G, Titus D: Femoral venous catheters: A safe alternative for delivering parenteral alimentation. *Nutr Clin Pract* 9:69–72, 1994.

148. Kemp L, Burge J, Choban P, Harden J, Mirtallo J, Flancbaum L: The effect of catheter type and site on infection rates in total parenteral nutrition patients. *JPEN* 18:71–74, 1994.

149. Merritt RJ, Ennis CE, Andrassy RJ, et al: Use of Hickman right atrial catheter in pediatric oncology patients. *JPEN* 5:83–85, 1981.

150. van Eys J, Wesley MN, Changir A, et al: Safety of intravenous hyperalimentation in children with malignancies: A cooperative group trial. *JPEN* 6:291, 1982.

151. Christensen ML, Hancock M, Gattuso J, et al: Parenteral nutrition associated with increased

infection rate in children with cancer. *Cancer* 72:2732–2738, 1993.

152. Alverdy JC, Aoys E, Moss GS: Total parenteral nutrition promotes bacterial translocation from the gut. *Surgery* 104:185–190, 1988.

153. Moore F, Feliciano D, Andrassy R, et al: Enteral feeding reduces postoperative septic complications. *JPEN* 15(suppl.):22, 1991.

154. Mochizuki H, Trocki O, Dominioni L, et al: Mechanism of prevention of postburn hypermetabolism and catabolism by early enteral feeding. *Ann Surg* 200:297–310, 1984.

155. Bortenschlager L, Zaloga G, Black KW, et al: Immediate postoperative enteral feeding decreases weight loss and improves wound healing following abdominal surgery in rats. *Crit Care Med* 20:115–118, 1992.

156. Zamir O, Nussbaum MS, Bhadra S, Subbiah MTR, Rafferty JF, Fischer JE: Effect of enteral feeding on hepatic steatosis induced by total parenteral nutrition. *JPEN* 18:20–25, 1994.

157. Herndon DN, Barrow RE, Kunkel KR, et al: Effects of recombinant human growth hormone on donor-site healing in severely burned children. *Ann Surg* 12:424–431, 1990.

158. Moore FA, Feliciano DV, Andrassy RJ, et al: Early enteral feeding, compared with parenteral, reduces postoperative septic complications. The results of a meta-analysis. *Ann Surg* 216:172–183, 1992.

159. Herndon DN, Barrow RE, Stein M, et al: Increased mortality with intravenous supplemental feeding in severely burned patients. *J Burn Care Rehabil* 10:309–313, 1989.

160. Kudsk KA, Groce MA, Favian TC, et al: Enteral *versus* parenteral feeding. *Ann Surg* 215(5):503–513, 1992.

161. Shou J, Ruelaz EA, Redmond HP, et al: Dietary protein prevents bacterial translocation from the gut [# 75]. *JPEN* 15(suppl.):29S(abstract), 1991.

162. Zaloga GP, Ward KA, Prielipp RC: Effect of enteral diet on whole body and gut growth in unstressed rats. *JPEN* 15:42–47, 1991.

163. Rerat A, Nunes CS, Mendy F, et al: Amino acid absorption and production of pancreatic hormones in non-anesthetized pigs after duodenal infusions of a milk enzymatic hydrolysate or of free amino acids. *Br J Nutr* 60:121–130, 1988.

164. Imondi AR, Stradley RP: Utilization of enzymatically hydrolyzed soybean protein and crystalline amino acid diets by rats with exocrine pancreatic insufficiency. *J Clin Invest* 104:793–801, 1974.

165. McAnena OH, Harvey IP, Bonau RA, et al: Alteration of methotrexate toxicity in rats by manipulation of dietary components. *Gastroenterology* 92:354–360, 1987.

166. Stanford JR, King D, Carey L, et al: The adverse effects of elemental diets on tolerance for 5-FU toxicity in the rat. *J Surg Oncol* 9:493–501, 1977.

167. Trocki O, Mochizuki H, Dominioni L, et al: Intact protein versus free amino acids in the nutritional support of thermally injured animals. *JPEN* 10:139–145, 1986.

168. Zaloga GP, Knowles R, Ward K, et al: Total parenteral nutrition (TPN) increases mortality following hemorrhage. *Crit Care Med* 19:54–59, 1991.

169. Meredith JW, Dietsheim JA, Zaloga GP: Visceral protein levels in trauma patients are greater with peptide diet than intact protein diet. *J Trauma* 30:825–829, 1990.

170. Souba WW, Smith RJ, Wilmore DW: Glutamine metabolism by the intestinal tract. *JPEN* 9:608–617, 1985.

171. Windmueller HG: Glutamine utilization by the small intestine. *Adv Enzymol* 53:201–237, 1982.

172. Higashiguchi T, Frederick JA, Zamir O, et al: Effect of glutamine on protein synthesis in isolated enterocytes from septic rats. *Surg Forum* 43:26–28, 1992.

173. Souba WW, Herskowitz K, Austgen RT, et al: Glutamine nutrition: Theoretical considerations and therapeutic impact. *JPEN* 14(suppl.):237S–243S, 1990.

174. O'Dwyer ST, Smith RJ, Hwang TL, et al: Maintenance of small bowel mucosa with glutamine-enriched parenteral nutrition. *JPEN* 13:579–585, 1989.

175. Hwang TL, O'Dwyer ST, Smith RJ, et al: Preservation of small bowel mucosa using glutamine-enriched parenteral nutrition. *Surg Forum* 38:56, 1987.

176. Grant J: Use of L-glutamine in total parenteral nutrition. *J Surg Res* 44:506–513, 1988.

177. Burke D, Alverdy JC, Aoys E, et al: Glutamine-supplemented TPN improves gut immune function. *Arch Surg* 124:1396–1399, 1989.

178. Ziegler TR, Young LS, Benfell K, et al: Clinical and metabolic efficacy of glutamine-supplemented parenteral nutrition after bone marrow transplantation: A randomized, double-blind controlled study. *Ann Intern Med* 116:821–828, 1992.

179. Inoue Y, Grant JP, Snyder PJ: Effect of glutamine-supplemented intravenous nutrition on survival after *Escherichia coli*–induced peritonitis. *JPEN* 17(suppl.):41–46, 1993.

180. Souba WW: Glutamine and cancer. *Ann Surg* 218:715–728, 1993.

181. Katz S, Plaisier BR, Folkening WJ, et al: Intralipid adversely affects reticuloendothelial bacterial clearance. *J Pediatr Surg* 26(8):921–924, 1991.

182. Hamawy KJ, Moldawer LL, Georgieff M, et al: Effect of lipid emulsions on the reticuloendothelial system function in the injured animal. *JPEN* 9:559–565, 1985.

183. Sobrado J, Moldawer LL, Pomposelli JJ, et al: Lipid emulsions and reticuloendothelial system function in healthy and burned guinea pigs. *Am J Clin Nutr* 42:855–863, 1985.

184. Kripke SA, Fox AD, Berman JM, et al: Stimulation of intestinal growth with intracolonic infusion of short-chain fatty acids. *JPEN* 3:109–116, 1989.

185. Koruda MJ, Rolandelli RH, Zimmaro DM, et al: Parenteral nutrition supplemented with short-chain fatty acids: Effect on the small bowel mucosa in normal rats. *Am J Clin Nutr* 51:685–689, 1989.

186. Kinsella JE, Lokesh B: Dietary lipids, eicosanoids, and the immune system. *Crit Care Med* 18(suppl.):S94–S113, 1990.

187. Alexander JW, Saito H, Trocki O, et al: The importance of lipid type in the diet after burn injury. *Ann Surg* 204:1–8, 1986.

188. Mochizuki H, Trocki O, Dominioni L, et al: Optimal lipid content for enteral diets following thermal injury. *JPEN* 8:638–646, 1984.

189. Alexander JW, Gottschlich MD: Nutritional immunomodulation in burn patients. *Crit Care Med* 18(suppl.):S149–S153, 1990.

190. Peck MD, Ogel CK, Alexander JW: Composition of fat in enteral diets can influence outcome in experimental peritonitis. *Ann Surg* 214:74–82, 1991.

191. Kenler AS, Swails WS, Driscoll DF, et al: Early enteral feeding in postsurgical cancer patients: Fish oil structured lipid-based polymeric formula versus a standard polymeric formula. *Ann Surg* 223:316–333, 1996.

192. Rudolph FB, Kulkarni AD, Fanslow WC, et al: Role of RNA as a dietary source of pyrimidines and purines in immune function. *Nutrition* 6:45–52, 1990.

193. Van Buren CT, Kulkarni AD, Schandle VP, et al: The influence of dietary nucleotides on cell-mediated immunity. *Transplantation* 36:350–352, 1983.

194. Kulkarni AD, Fanslow WC, Rudolph FB, et al: Modulation of delayed hypersensitivity in mice by dietary nucleotide restriction. *Transplantation* 44:847–849, 1988.

195. Kulkarni AD, Fanslow WC, Rudolph FB, et al: Effect of dietary nucleotides on response to bacterial infections. *JPEN* 10:169–171, 1986.

196. Barbul A: Arginine and immune function. *Nutrition* 6:53–62, 1990.

197. Madden HP, Breslin RJ, Wasserkrug HL, et al: Stimulation of T-cell immunity enhances survival in peritonitis. *J Surg Res* 44:658–663, 1988.

198. Saito H, Trocki O, Wang S, et al: Metabolic and immune effects of dietary arginine supplementation after burn. *Arch Surg* 122:784–789, 1987.

199. Daly JM, Reynolds JV, Thom A, et al: Immune and metabolic effects of arginine in the surgical patient. *Ann Surg* 208:512–523, 1988.

200. Nirgiotis JG, Hennessee PJ, Andrassy RJ: The effects of an arginine-free enteral diet on wound healing and immune function in the postsurgical rat. *J Pediatr Surg* 26:936–941, 1991.

201. Merimee TJ, Rabinowitz D, Riggs L: Plasma growth hormone after arginine infusion: Clinical experiences. *N Engl J Med* 276:434–439, 1967.

202. Lowry SF, Goodgame JT, Norton JA, et al: Effect of chronic protein malnutrition on host tumor composition and growth. *J Surg Res* 26:79, 1979.

203. Daly JM, Copeland EM, Dudrick SJ, et al: Nutritional repletion of malnourished tumor-bearing and nontumor-bearing rats: Effects of body weight, liver, muscle, and tumor. *J Surg Res* 28:507, 1980.

204. Van Eys J: Nutrition and cancer: Physiological interrelationships. *Annu Rev Nutr* 5:435–461, 1985.

Abdominal Complications

• *Cynthia A. Corpron, M.D.* • *Richard J. Andrassy, M.D.*

Surgeons involved in the care of children with cancer may be called upon to evaluate and treat complications of therapy. Diagnosis of abdominal processes may be much more difficult in these patients. Symptoms and physical findings may be altered by severe neutropenia and by the effects of steroids, narcotics, and antiemetics used to treat tumor symptoms. In patients with severe neutropenia, the inflammatory response may be blunted by lack of neutrophils. Infectious processes such as perforation that are likely to be contained in patients with normal immune function are likely instead to become generalized in patients with severe neutropenia. Hemorrhage may result from tumor, mucosal ulceration, thrombocytopenia, or coagulation defects.

GASTRIC AND DUODENAL ULCERS

Children receiving high-dose corticosteroids or nonsteroidal anti-inflammatory drugs, and children with increased intracranial pressure, are at increased risk for gastric and duodenal ulcers (such as stress ulcers and Cushing's ulcers).[1] These ulcers may be presented with pain or hemorrhage. Prophylactic treatment with a histamine blocker (e.g., cimetidine or ranitidine) should be considered for children at risk because of high-dose steroids or nonsteroidal anti-inflammatory drugs.[1] Treatment of bleeding ulcers should include lavage with endoscopy and correction of coagulation abnormalities and thrombocytopenia. Uncontrollable bleeding may require either endoscopic or surgical treatment.

PANCREATITIS

The differential diagnosis of nausea and abdominal pain in the pediatric cancer patient should include pancreatitis. Children being treated with steroids or L-asparaginase are at higher risk of developing pancreatitis.[2] Diagnosis may be made by serum and urine amylase and lipase levels. Ultrasound or CT imaging of the pancreas can serve as a baseline evaluation.

Patients with a confirmed diagnosis of pancreatitis should be treated with bowel rest and fluid resuscitation. Secondary infection and pancreatic abscess may be treated conservatively with antibiotics or may require open debridement and drainage. If pancreatitis progresses to a pseudocyst, 6 to 8 weeks of medical management may facilitate internal or CT-guided percutaneous drainage.[3]

CHOLECYSTITIS AND BILIARY OBSTRUCTION

Acalculous cholecystitis may occur in children who are severely ill, septic, or dehydrated. Symptoms include leukocytosis, fever, right upper quadrant pain, and frequently a right upper quadrant mass. Diagnosis may be confirmed by ultrasound or nonvisualization on nuclear medicine scans. Treatment should include broad-spectrum antibiotics to counter gram-positive, gram-negative, and anaerobic bacteria and fungi in the neutropenic patient. Failure of medical management may require percutaneous or operative cholecystotomy or cholecystectomy.

BOWEL OBSTRUCTION

The differential diagnosis of small bowel obstruction includes obstipation from *Vinca* alkaloids or narcotics, postoperative adhesions or strictures, post-radiation strictures, and intussusception. Children who have undergone resection of a retroperitoneal tumor are at especially high risk for postoperative small bowel obstruction. Ritchey and coworkers[4] reviewed bowel obstructions occurring after resection of Wilms' tumor. The etiology of the obstruction was bowel adhesions in 104 cases, intussusception in 17, internal hernia in 2, and uncertain in the remaining 8 children.[4]

HEMORRHAGIC CYSTITIS

Cyclophosphamide and ifosfamide are the most common causes of hemorrhagic cystitis. An acrolein dye that is a by-product of cyclophospha-

mide metabolism causes edema, ulceration, and fibrosis of the bladder mucosa and submucosa. Although the incidence of hemorrhagic cystitis may be decreased by vigorous hydration, acidification of the urine, and administration of sodium-2-mercaptoethanesulfonate (mesna), hemorrhagic cystitis should be included in the differential diagnosis of dysuria and hematuria. Treatment consists of hydration, correction of coagulation abnormalities and thrombocytopenia, transfusion as needed, and removal of clots by bladder irrigations or cystoscopy.[5] Continued hemorrhage may require cystoscopic electrocoagulation or instillation of formalin or alum into the bladder. Alum is preferred for patients with uterovesical reflux because of the effects of formalin on the ureters and kidneys. Uncontrollable bleeding may require emergency cystectomy.

ACUTE ABDOMINAL PAIN

Children with cancer are at normal risk of causes of acute abdominal pain such as appendicitis, gastroenteritis, and Meckel's diverticulum, but these children are at greater risk of some other causes of acute abdominal pain. For example, those who have received a bone marrow transplant and are suffering from severe graft-versus-host disease may present with crampy abdominal pain, nausea, diarrhea, and thickened bowel wall on imaging studies. Pediatric cancer patients with severe neutropenia are at risk for neutropenic enterocolitis (sometimes referred to as typhlitis), which is a necrotizing enterocolitis limited to the cecum and right colon. Series have reported symptoms of an acute abdominal pain requiring surgery in 5% to 30% of patients being treated for hematologic malignancies. Incidence may vary with intensity of therapy.[6-8] Shamberger and coworkers[9] found that one third of patients with acute myelogenous leukemia had documented enterocolitis during induction therapy.

Diagnosis of neutropenic colitis in the neutropenic patient can be made on the basis of symptoms of fever, nausea, right lower quadrant or diffuse abdominal pain, and sometimes an associated right lower quadrant mass. Radiographic studies, including plain films, ultrasound, and CT scan, may show diffuse thickening of the cecal wall and pneumatosis intestinalis.

Treatment of neutropenic colitis is controversial and has not been well studied in a prospective, randomized fashion. Shamberger and associates[9] suggest four criteria for surgical intervention in neutropenic enterocolitis: (1) evidence of intra-abdominal perforation, (2) development of symptoms of an intra-abdominal process that would require operation in non-neutropenic patients, (3) clinical deterioration requiring treatment with large volumes of fluid or vasopressors, and (4) persistent gastrointestinal hemorrhage despite correction of thrombocytopenia and clotting abnormalities. Under these criteria, 80% of patients can be treated medically using broad-spectrum antibiotics to combat gram-negative and anaerobic bacteria and achieve hydration and intravenous hyperalimentation. Sauter and coworkers[10] reported results of peritoneal lavage in ruling out perforation in patients with neutropenic enterocolitis.

Treatment of bowel malignancies, especially non-Hodgkin's lymphoma, may result in bowel perforation when tumor response to therapy is rapid. These patients should be treated in a similar manner to other patients with perforation—that is, by diversion, resection, and primary repair as dictated by the clinical situation.

Neutropenic patients treated with antibiotics are also at risk for antibiotic-related pseudomembranous colitis. *Clostridium difficile* is isolated in the majority of cases. Symptoms are related to toxin production by the bacteria and include fever, watery diarrhea, and abdominal pain.[11] Patients should be evaluated by stool cultures and assays for *Clostridium difficile* toxin. Treatment of documented cases requires either oral vancomycin or metronidazole. *Clostridum difficile* may be transmitted as a nosocomial infection, and patients with documented *Clostridium difficile* enterocolitis should be placed on enteric isolation.

RADIATION ENTERITIS

The most common abdominal complication of irradiation seen in pediatric patients is radiation enteritis.[12] Radiation enteritis has an acute phase associated with abdominal pain and ileus. A chronic phase may be associated with low-grade intestinal obstruction and malabsorption. Operative resection of involved areas is usually delayed until therapy is completed and the patient has returned to a normal hematologic and nutritional status. Acute obstruction may require diversion.

Hirschl and associates[13] have described use of a "sling" to move the small bowel out of the radiation field; similar techniques may have application in patients undergoing wide-field abdominal radiation.

References

1. Ross AJ III, Siegel KR, Bell W, et al: Massive gastrointestinal hemorrhage in children with posterior fossa tumors. *J Pediatr Surg* 22:633–636, 1987.
2. Eden OB, Shaw MP, Lilleyman JS, et al: Non-randomized study comparing toxicity of *Escherichia coli* and *Erwinia* asparaginase in children with leukemia. *Med Pediatr Oncol* 18:497–502, 1990.
3. Caniano DA, Browne AF, Boles ET: Pancreatic pseudocyst complicating treatment of acute lymphoblastic leukemia. *J Pediatr Surg* 20:452–455, 1985.
4. Ritchey ML, Kelalis PP, Etzioni R, et al: Small bowel obstruction after nephrectomy for Wilms' tumor. A report of the National Wilms' Tumor Study-3. *Ann Surg* 218:654–659, 1993.
5. Shepherd JD, Pringle LE, Barnett MJ, et al: Mesna versus hyperhydration for prevention of cyclophosphamide-induced hemorrhagic cystitis in bone marrow transplantation. *J Clin Oncol* 9:2016–2020, 1991.
6. Wagner M, Rosenberg H, Fernbach D, et al: Typhlitis: A complication of leukemia in childhood. *Am J Roentgenol* 109:341–350, 1970.
7. Exelby PR, Ghandchi A, Lansigan N, et al: Management of the acute abdomen in children with leukemia. *Cancer* 35:826–829, 1975.
8. O'Brien S, Kantarjian HM, Anaissie E, et al: Successful medical management of neutropenic enterocolitis in adults with acute leukemia. *SMJ* 80:1233–1235, 1987.
9. Shamberger RC, Weinstein HJ, Delorey MJ, et al: The medical and surgical management of typhlitis in children with acute nonlymphocytic (myelogenous) leukemia. *Cancer* 57:603–609, 1986.
10. Sauter ER, Vauthey JN, Bolton JS, et al: Selective management of patients with neutropenic enterocolitis using peritoneal lavage. *J Surg Oncol* 45:63–67, 1990.
11. Bartlett JG, Chang TW, Gurwith M, et al: Antibiotic-associated pseudomembranous colitis due to toxin-producing *Clostridia*. *N Engl J Med* 298:531–534, 1978.
12. Donaldson SS, Jundt S, Ricour C, et al: Radiation enteritis in children. *Cancer* 35:1167–1178, 1975.
13. Meric F, Hirschl RB, Mahboubi S, et al: Prevention of radiation enteritis in children using a pelvic mesh sling. *J Pediatr Surg* 29:917–921, 1994.

Index

Note: Page numbers in *italics* refer to illustrations; page numbers followed by t refer to tables.

ISBN 0-7216-6378-8

90038

9 780721 663784